ROUTLEDGE HANDBOOK OF YOUTH SPORT

The *Routledge Handbook of Youth Sport* is a comprehensive survey of the latest research into young people's involvement in sport. Drawing on a wide diversity of disciplines, including sociology, psychology, policy studies, physical education and physiology, the book examines the importance of sport during a key transitional period in the life-course, from the later teenage years into the early twenties, and therefore helps us develop a better understanding of the social construction of young people's lives.

The book covers youth sport in all its forms, from competitive game-contests and conventional sport to recreational activities, exercise and lifestyle sport; and at all levels, from elite competition to leisure-time activities and school physical education. It explores youth sport across the world, in developing and developed countries, and touches on some of the most significant themes and issues in contemporary sport studies, including physical activity and health, lifelong participation, talent identification and development, and safeguarding and abuse.

No other book brings together in one place such a breadth and depth of material on youth sport or the extent of the engagement of young people in physical activity. The *Routledge Handbook of Youth Sport* is therefore important reading for all advanced students, researchers, practitioners and policy-makers with an interest in youth sport, youth culture, sport studies or physical education.

Ken Green is Professor of Sociology of Physical Education and Youth Sport and Head of Sport and Exercise Sciences at the University of Chester, UK, as well as Visiting Professor at Hedmark University College, Norway, and the University of Wolverhampton, UK. He is Editor-in-Chief of the *European Physical Education Review* and his books include *Understanding Physical Education* (2008) and *Key Themes in Youth Sport* (2010). His main research interests revolve around physical education and youth sport.

Andy Smith is Professor of Sport and Physical Activity at Edge Hill University, UK, where he is also Associate Head of the Department of Sport and Physical Activity. His research interests and publications focus on sport, physical activity and health and on youth, sport policy and development. He is co-author of *Sport Policy and Development* (with Daniel Bloyce, 2010), *An Introduction to Drugs in Sport* (with Ivan Waddington, 2009) and *Disability, Sport and Society* (with Nigel Thomas, 2009), and co-editor of *Doing Real World Research in Sports Studies* (with Ivan Waddington, 2014). Andy is also former co-editor of the *International Journal of Sport Policy and Politics*, which he launched with Barrie Houlihan and Daniel Bloyce in 2009, and an Editorial Board member of *Leisure Studies* and the *European Physical Education Review*.

ROUTLEDGE HANDBOOK OF YOUTH SPORT

Edited by Ken Green and Andy Smith

Routledge
Taylor & Francis Group

LONDON AND NEW YORK

First published in paperback 2018

First published 2016
by Routledge
2 Park Square, Milton Park, Abingdon, Oxon OX14 4RN

and by Routledge
711 Third Avenue, New York, NY 10017

Routledge is an imprint of the Taylor and Francis Group, an informa business

British Library Cataloguing-in-Publication Data
A catalogue record for this book is available from the British Library

Library of Congress Cataloguing in Publication Data
Routledge handbook of youth sport/edited by Ken Green and Andy Smith.
pages cm
Includes bibliographical references and index.
1. Sports for children—Great Britain. 2. Exercise for children—Great Britain.
I. Green, Ken (Professor of applied sociology of sport) II. Smith, Andy, 1979–
GV709.2.R66 2016
796.083—dc23
2015025496

ISBN: 978-0-415-84003-3 (hbk)
ISBN: 978-0-8153-5739-1 (pbk)
ISBN: 978-0-203-79500-2 (ebk)

Typeset in Bembo and Minion Pro
by Florence Production Ltd, Stoodleigh, Devon, UK

This Handbook is dedicated to Ken Roberts:
mentor, inspiration and friend.

CONTENTS

CONTRIBUTORS

Nida Ahmed is an independent scholar and graduate of Georgetown University. Her research focuses on sports for development, Muslim women in sports, cross-cultural understanding, and social and political uses of new media with sports movement. She has developed, managed and implemented educational and sports exchange programmes for the US Department of State and US embassies abroad. The following are publications she has co-authored: *Youth, Action Sports and Political Agency in the Middle East: Lessons from a Grassroots Parkour Group in Gaza* (2013), and *Transnational Families in Armenia and Information Communication Technology Use* (2013).

Laura Azzarito is an Associate Professor of Physical Culture and Education at Teachers College, Columbia University, New York, USA. Her research examines the links among young people's construction of the body, identity and inequality issues from a pedagogical and sociocultural perspective. Her current research aims to understand the ways in which the intersectionality of gender/sex, race/ethnicity, and social class impacts on young people's embodiment in urban, multicultural school contexts. Laura has published widely in refereed international journals and book chapters in PE and sport pedagogy, sociology of sport, qualitative methods, visual studies and curriculum studies. Her most recent book is *Pedagogies, Physical Culture and Visual Methods* (2013). She has presented her research findings at the conventional venues of state, national and international conferences, and also at alternative sites like schools, museums and community art centres that engage research participants and the general public. Laura is currently serving as an Associate Editor of *Journal of Teaching in Physical Education*.

Roald Bahr is Professor of Sports Medicine in the Department of Sports Medicine at the Norwegian School of Sport Sciences and Chair of the Oslo Sports Trauma Research Center. He also holds a clinical appointment in the Medical Department at the National Olympic Training Center, where he has been the Chief Medical Officer and Chair of the Health Department since 2011. Professor Bahr also joined Aspetar as the Head of the Aspetar Sports Injury and Illness Prevention Programme in October 2012. He is authorized as a Sports Medicine Physician by the Norwegian Society of Sports Medicine and is a fellow of the American College of Sports Medicine. He serves as Team Physician for the beach volleyball national teams. He is past chair of the National Council on Physical Activity, past president of the Norwegian Society of Sports

Medicine and current member of the Sports Medicine Council of the Norwegian Olympic Committee and Confederation of Sports. Roald is the President of the FIVB Medical Commission and a member of the IOC Medical Commission – Medical and Scientific Group. His main research area is sports injury prevention, and he has published more than two hundred original research articles, review papers and book chapters, in addition to ten books. Roald is the main editor of the widely acclaimed textbook *IOC Manual of Sports Injuries* and the new *Handbook of Sports Injury Prevention*, both published in several languages. In October 2008 at Buckingham Palace, Roald was presented with the Prince Philip Medal for his outstanding and original contribution to the advancement of medical knowledge in Sports and Exercise Medicine by His Royal Highness The Prince Philip, The Duke of Edinburgh. He is also a former national team volleyball player and coach.

Julie Borgers is a PhD student within the Policy in Sports and Physical Activity Research Group in the Department of Kinesiology at the University of Leuven, Belgium. She graduated as a Master of Science in Kinesiology and Physical Education at the University of Leuven in 2011. Her doctoral research focuses on the social-organizational aspects of sports participation. For her current research activities, Julie is affiliated to the Flemish Policy Research Centre on Sports (supported by the Flemish government).

Camilla Brockett is a Senior Research Fellow and Senior Sport Consultant at the Institute of Sport, Exercise and Active Living (ISEAL), Victoria University (VU), where she manages projects and partnerships with key university partners. Her research career began in sports science, specifically muscle physiology, but she soon transitioned into high-performance sport management focusing on benchmarking elite sport systems and programmes during her nine years at the Australian Institute of Sport (AIS). More recently, Camilla has led a VU–AIS collaboration to identify sport policy factors that impact on Australia's sporting success as part of an international comparative study known as SPLISS, and she is currently engaged with the SPLISS consortium to extend this research by examining national paralympic-sports systems. Camilla has consulted to various national and international sporting organizations and is currently delivering sport development initiatives and high-performance sport consultancy to state governing bodies and the national government of India.

Johannes Brug is Dean and member of the executive board at the VU University Medical Centre in Amsterdam, the Netherlands. He is Professor of Epidemiology and an Honorary Professor at the School of Nutrition and Exercise Sciences of Deakin University, Melbourne, Australia. Johannes's main research interests are in behaviour epidemiology, with a special interest in behavioural nutrition and physical activity. The scope of his research covers studies on the determinants of nutrition and physical activity behaviours, small-scale experimentation with innovative ICT-supported health education interventions, and larger-scale field experiments in which the efficacy and external validity of health-promoting interventions are tested. He has co-authored more than 400 international scientific publications and is the first editor of the Dutch handbook on health education and behaviour change.

Shushu Chen joined Edge Hill University, UK, in 2014 as Lecturer in Sport Development and Management having obtained her PhD from Loughborough University. She has a particular interest in sport policy analysis and programme evaluation, and has published in these areas. Shushu is a visiting researcher at the Centre for Olympic Studies and Research at Loughborough University.

Jay Coakley is a Professor Emeritus of Sociology at the University of Colorado in Colorado Springs, USA. His research over the past forty-five years has investigated the relationship between sports, culture and society. Jay was the founding editor of the *Sociology of Sport Journal*, and his book, *Sports in Society: Issues and Controversies*, is now in its 11th edition (2015). It has been adapted multiple times for students in Canada, Europe, Australia and Southern Africa, and it has been translated into Chinese, Japanese and Korean. Most recently, he has done research on the relationship between sport, development, and national identity and the legacies of mega-sport events. Jay is an internationally respected scholar, author and journal editor and has received many teaching, service and professional awards. Additionally, he continues to work with a number of advisory and policy making groups related to sports with the goal of making sport participation a source of enjoyment and development for people of all ages.

Fred Coalter is Professor of Sports Policy at Leeds Metropolitan University, UK, and was previously a Professor of Sports Policy at the University of Stirling. His research interests relate to sport's claimed contributions to various aspects of social policy. His published work includes *Sport-in-Development: A Monitoring and Evaluation Manual* (2006), *A Wider Social Role for Sport: Who's Keeping the Score?* (Routledge, 2007), *Sport-for-Development Impact Study Comic Relief* (2010) and *Sport-for-Development: What Game are we Playing?* (Routledge, 2013). He has undertaken extensive monitoring and evaluation work with youth organizations in the UK, Kenya, Uganda, Tanzania, South Africa, Zimbabwe, Zambia, Mumbai and Kolkata. Fred is a member of the Scientific Advisory Board of the Swiss Academy Development and a Board member of the Nairobi-based Mathare Youth Sport Association's Leadership Academy.

Steve Cobley is a Senior Lecturer in Motor Control and Skill Acquisition and Sport and Exercise Psychology within the Faculty of Health Sciences at the University of Sydney, Australia. His research interests examine developmental factors that constrain learning, development and performance. Steve's research and applied work has led to the evaluation, modification and writing of athlete and coaching programmes and policy for both sport governing bodies and associated organizations; this work has also included general consultancy for individual athletes and organizations. He recently co-edited *Talent Identification and Development: International Perspectives* (Routledge, 2012).

Sean Cumming is a Senior Lecturer in Sport and Exercise Sciences in the Department for Health at the University of Bath, UK. Adopting a bio-cultural perspective, his research explores how the processes of growth and maturation contribute towards adolescent health and development in the contexts of sport and exercise. He also works in consultancy and research roles with a number of leading sports organizations and professional clubs, including the Premier League, the English Football Association, the Lawn Tennis Association and Bath Rugby.

Manuel Coelho-e-Silva is Professor in the Faculty of Sport Science and Physical Education, University of Coimbra, Portugal. He organized and chaired the 2013 Pediatric Work Physiology Meeting and edited the proceedings, *Children and Exercise XXVIII* (Routledge). Manuel is member of a very active network that emerged in the late 1990s under the enthusiastic coordination of Robert Malina at the Institute for the Study of Youth Sports, Michigan State University, USA.

Jean Côté is Professor and Director in the School of Kinesiology and Health Studies at Queen's University in Kingston, Canada. His research interests are in the areas of youth sport, coaching, sport expertise and positive youth development. Jean is regularly invited to present his work to both sport governing organizations and academic conferences throughout the world. In 2009, he was the recipient of the fourth EW Barker Professorship from the Physical Education and Sport Science department at the National Institute of Education in Singapore. He received the Queen's University Award for Excellence in Graduate Supervision for 2013. In collaboration with Dr Ronnie Lidor, Jean has recently completed the first comprehensive book on talent development in children's sport, published in 2013 by Fitness Information Technology.

Veerle De Bosscher is Professor in the Department of Sports Policy and Management (Faculty of Physical Education) in the Vrije Universiteit Brussel (VUB), Belgium, and visiting professor at Utrecht University, the Netherlands. Her research expertise is in the area of elite sport, sport development, sport policy and management, effectiveness, benchmarking and competitiveness. Veerle has published in diverse refereed journals, written book chapters and edited and authored several English and Dutch books (e.g. the *Global Sporting Arms Race*; *Managing High Performance Sport*). She is leading a worldwide international network on research in high performance sport, called SPLISS (Sports Policy factors Leading to International Sporting Success), which was also the subject of her PhD in 2007. Veerle is co-editor of the *International Journal of Sport Policy and Politics* (*IJSPP*), board member of the *European Sport Management Quarterly* (*ESMQ*), the European Association of Sport Management (EASM) and the Steering Committee of elite sport in Belgium (Flanders). She has also counselled the elite sport development of several organizations and countries over the years.

Ulf Ekelund is Professor in Physical Activity and Health at the Department of Sport Medicine, Norwegian School of Sport Sciences, Oslo, Norway. He is also a senior investigator scientist at the MRC Epidemiology Unit, University of Cambridge, UK. Ulf's main research interests are related to measurement and population levels of physical activity; the role of physical activity in the prevention of non-communicable diseases, especially metabolic diseases; and to understand the biological basis for physical activity and sedentary behaviour during a life. Ulf has published more than original peer-review articles including publications in *The Lancet*, *JAMA*, *PLOS Medicine* and *Nature Genetics*. His current H-index is sixty. He serves as an associate editor for *Medicine and Science in Sport* and *Exercise and the Journal of Physical Activity and Health*. Ulf is a fellow of the American College of Sports Medicine and received the British Nutrition Silver Medal for excellence in Science in 2013.

Karl Erickson is an Assistant Professor in the Institute for the Study of Youth Sports, in the Department of Kinesiology at Michigan State University, USA. In the broadest sense, Karl's research interests explore the facilitation of positive youth development via participation in sport and physical activity settings. Karl's research focuses on athlete development and coaching in youth sport, and is primarily concerned with understanding youth sport as a context for personal development. Prior to joining MSU, Karl completed his undergraduate and graduate work at Queen's University, Canada, and a postdoctoral fellowship at Tufts University, USA.

William Falcão is a PhD candidate in Sport Psychology in the Department of Kinesiology and Physical Education at McGill University, in Montreal, Canada. His research focuses on teaching coaches how to promote youths' psychosocial development through sport, utilizing a coach training protocol that fosters athletes' personal development, health, and well-being. William is also the mental performance consultant for the McGill men's and women's soccer teams, as well as a consultant for a non-profit youth sport organization in Montreal.

Guy Faulkner is a Professor in the School of Kinesiology at the University of British Columbia, and is a Canadian Institutes of Health Research-Public Health Agency of Canada (CIHR-PHAC) Chair in Applied Public Health. He is also a research scientist with the Centre for Addiction and Mental Health (CAMH) and a Research Affiliate of the Alberta Centre for Active Living. He serves on the ParticipACTION research advisory committee (2010–present) and is a member of the Research Work Group for the Active Healthy Kids Canada Report Card on Physical Activity for Children and Youth. Broadly, his research has focused on two interrelated themes: the effectiveness of physical activity promotion interventions, and physical activity and mental health. He is the founding editor of the Elsevier journal *Mental Health and Physical Activity*.

Scott Fleming is Professor of Sport and Leisure Studies and is the Director of Research and Graduate Studies at Cardiff Metropolitan University, Wales, as well as Honorary Professor at Plymouth University, UK, and Honorary Research Fellow at Zhejiang University, China. Scott trained as a physical education teacher and has published widely around the themes of race relations and youth sport, and continues to publish research broadly linked to sport and leisure cultures and research ethics, methodology and methods. Scott was Chair of the Leisure Studies Association, UK, between 2004 and 2009, and is Managing Co-Editor of the *Leisure Studies* journal.

Jessica Fraser-Thomas is an Associate Professor in the School of Kinesiology and Health Science at York University in Toronto, Canada. Her research focuses on child and youth development through sport, with a particular interest in positive youth development, psychosocial influences (i.e. coaches, family, peers) and withdrawal. Currently she is working on projects exploring children's earliest introductions to organized sport, characteristics of sport programmes that facilitate optimal youth development, and how youth sport models may inform Masters athletes' development; all projects are supported by the Social Sciences and Humanities Research Council of Canada (SSHRC) and Sport Canada's Sport Participation Research Initiative (SPRI). Jessica has (co-) authored more than thirty book chapters and articles in peer-reviewed international journals, recently co-editing *Health and Elite Sport: Is High Performance Sport a Healthy Pursuit?* (2015). She is a recipient of the Canadian Society for Psychomotor Learning and Sport Psychology Young Scientist Award (2007) and the Province of Ontario Volunteer Service Award (2012).

Laura Gale is a Lecturer in Sports Coaching at the University of Hull, UK. Her research principally focuses on the everyday working lives of community sports coaches and the personal, emotional and socio-political complexities of practice.

Michael Gard is Associate Professor of Health, Sport and Physical Education at the University of Queensland. He teaches, researches and writes about how the human body is and has been used, experienced, educated and governed. Among a range of publications he has authored several books, including *The Obesity Epidemic: Science, Morality and Ideology* (with Jan Wright) and *Men Who Dance: Aesthetics, Athletics and the Art of Masculinity*.

Paul Gilchrist is Senior Lecturer in Human Geography in the School of Environment and Technology at the University of Brighton. His research focuses on the geographies of sport, leisure and popular culture. He has published on a range of themes, including leisure theory and the social regulation of public space, countercultural and lifestyle sport, histories of mountaineering, and the politics of countryside recreation. He is co-editor of *The Politics of Sport: Community, Mobility, Identity* (2011) and *Coastal Cultures: Liminality and Leisure* (2014). Paul's current research, funded by the Arts and Humanities Research Council, investigates the ways in which people connect through food and farming, and the cultural heritage of minor waterways and canals. He is founding convenor of the Political Studies Association's Sport and Politics study group and is a member of the Executive Committee of the Leisure Studies Association.

Donna Goodwin is a professor and Associate Dean, Graduate Programs in the Faculty of Physical Education and Recreation, University of Alberta, Canada. Her research focuses on bringing to light literal, metaphorical and political voices of people with impairments as they negotiate social and cultural impediments to self-determined health and wellness through physical activity. Donna was the Executive Director of the Steadward Centre for Personal and Physical Achievement (2006–2011) at the University of Alberta. The Centre provides exercise and physical activity programming for adults, youth and children with impairments. She is also interested in the process of transition from rehabilitation settings to community programmes and the hidden labour involved for those transitioning and their families. Donna has been a visiting professor in China, Hong Kong, Ireland, Japan, Korea and Norway.

Ken Green is Professor of Sociology of Physical Education and Youth Sport and Head of Sport and Exercise Sciences at the University of Chester, UK, as well as Visiting Professor at Hedmark University College, Norway, and the University of Wolverhampton, UK. He is Editor-in-Chief of the *European Physical Education Review* and his books include *Understanding Physical Education* (2008) and *Key Themes in Youth Sport* (2010). His main research interests revolve around physical education and youth sport.

Laurent Grélot is Professor of Physiology at the Faculty of Sport Sciences of the Aix-Marseille University, France. He obtained his PhD in Neurosciences in Marseille in 1989 and began his career investigating the neurophysiology and neuropharmacology of breathing, coughing and vomiting in animal models. He then shifted to sport sciences focusing his research on the physiological and behavioural determining factors in sport performance. He served two terms as chairman of the Physiological Research Department of the Faculty of Sport Sciences, and then was elected Dean of the Faculty. Laurent is author or co-author of about eighty-five peer-reviewed articles and twenty book chapters.

Mike Hartill is a Senior Lecturer in the Sociology of Sport at Edge Hill University, UK. His main interests are childhood, masculinity and sexual violence in sport. His research publications have focused on the abuse of children in sport settings, with a particular focus on the sexual exploitation of young male athletes. He has also conducted some of the first research into child protection in sport policy, examining how it is implemented and received within the sports community. He has recently participated in two European projects on the prevention of sexual violence in sport and coordinates the Sport Respects Your Rights campaign against sexual violence in sport in the UK. He collaborates with many sport and victim-support organizations across the UK and Europe and continues to conduct narrative research with survivors of childhood sexual abuse in sport.

David Haycock is an independent researcher in the sociology of youth sport and leisure. He has worked as a lecturer on a number of taught undergraduate and postgraduate programmes focused on physical education, sport development and management and the sociology of sport at Edge Hill University, UK. He has also published a range of peer-reviewed articles in the sociology of physical education, sport, leisure and youth that appear in journals including *Leisure Studies; Sport, Education and Society*; and the *British Journal of Sociology of Education*. David was awarded his PhD entitled University Students' Sport Participation: The Significance of Sport and Leisure Careers from the University of Chester in 2015.

Maria Hildebrand is a PhD student at the Department of Sport Medicine, Norwegian School of Sport Sciences, Oslo, Norway, and will be finishing her studies in autumn 2016. Her research predominantly focuses on objective assessment of physical activity and sedentary time in children and adults, and understanding determinants for physical activity and sedentary time in young people. Maria has a BSc in Physiotherapy from Oslo and Akershus University College of Applied Sciences and an MSc in Sports Physiotherapy from the Norwegian School of Sport Sciences, where she also graduated top. She has published original peer-review articles in *The American Journal of Clinical Nutrition* and *Medicine and Science in Sport and Exercise*, and served as reviewer for *Medicine and Science in Sport and Exercise*.

Nicholas L. Holt is a Professor in the Faculty of Physical Education and Recreation at the University of Alberta, Canada, where he is the director of the Child and Adolescent Sport and Activity Laboratory. His research focuses on psychosocial aspects of participation in sport and physical activity among children, adolescents and their families. His research has received consistent funding from major Canadian funding agencies, including the Social Sciences and Humanities Research Council of Canada and Canadian Institute of Health Research. He has published over 120 peer-reviewed articles and book chapters on topics such as youth sport, active free play and paediatric weight management. His books include *Positive Youth Development Through Sport* (2008), *Lifelong Engagement in Sport and Physical Activity* (2011) and *Parenting in Youth Sport* (2014). He has served as the President of the Canadian Society for Psychomotor Learning and Sport Psychology and as Associate Editor of *The Sport Psychologist*.

Ben Ives is a PhD student and Graduate Teaching Assistant in the Department of Sport, Health and Exercise Science at the University of Hull, UK. His research principally focuses on the socio-political and emotional complexities of community sports coaching.

Evan James is a fourth year medical student at the University of Minnesota, USA, Medical School. He has published more than twenty-five peer-reviewed papers in orthopaedic sports medicine. His work has been presented at national and international meetings including ESSKA, ISAKOS, EFORT, AOSSM, AOFAS and AANA. His research interests include clinical outcomes, biomechanics and musculoskeletal imaging of the knee and foot and ankle, which he focused on under the mentorship of Robert F. LaPrade during a year-long research fellowship at the Steadman Philippon Research Institute. Evan is a graduate of the University of Notre Dame, USA, and is a recipient of Notre Dame's Braco Award for Excellence in Cell Biology Research.

Melanie Lang is a sociologist and former international youth athlete and journalist who now works as a Senior Lecturer in Child Protection in Sport at Edge Hill University. Her work centres on the policy and practice of safeguarding, child protection and children's rights in sport and features regularly in the national media. Melanie has been involved in the EU-funded project *Safer, Better, Stronger! The Prevention of Sexual Harassment and Abuse in Sport* and is co-editor of the books *Bullying and the Abuse of Power: From the Playground to International Relations* (2010) and *Safeguarding, Child Protection and Abuse in Sport: International Perspectives in Research, Policy and Practice* (2015, Routledge). She sits on the NSPCC Child Protection in Sport Unit Research Evidence and Advisory Group, the editorial board of the *Irish Journal of Sociology* and on the editorial advisory board of the British Sociological Association's Network publication.

Robert F. LaPrade MD, PhD is a complex-knee surgeon at the Steadman Clinic and the Chief Medical Officer for the Steadman Philippon Research Institute. He has published more than 225 peer-reviewed publications and is most well known for his comprehensive research on the posterolateral knee, posterior cruciate ligament, medial collateral ligament and meniscal roots. His research group has received the OREF Clinical Research Award, the Excellence in Research Award (twice) from AOSSM, the Nicola Young Investigator and Smith and Nephew Ligament Awards from ESSKA, and the Trillat and Achilles Awards from ISAKOS. Robert is on the Editorial Boards of the *American Journal of Sports Medicine (AJSM)* and *Knee Surgery Sports Traumatology, Arthroscopy (KSSTA)*. He has been very active on committees within AOSSM, ESSKA and ISAKOS. LaPrade is also an adjunct professor at the University of Minnesota and affiliate faculty at Colorado State University.

Håkan Larsson is Professor of Physical Education and Sport Pedagogy at the Swedish School of Sport and Health Sciences in Stockholm. Since 2006, he has led a research group for physical education and sport pedagogy that dates back to the mid-1980s. At present, the group includes seven senior researchers and nine PhD students who are researching educational issues in physical education (as a school subject), child and youth sport, and recreational sport among adults. Professor Larsson is currently doing research within two major research strands: gender and heteronormativity in both club sports and physical education in schools, and teaching and learning in physical education. During the last decade, the work of Professor Larsson and colleagues has been influential in developing policy regarding school physical education as well as gender equality and children's and adolescents' rights in sports.

Fabrice Lorenté is a Lecturer at the University of Perpignan Via Domitia, France, where he teaches epidemiology and psychosociology. Fabrice obtained a PhD in Sport Sciences at the University of Aix-Marseilles in 2003 with a dissertation on use of substances and sports participation among youth. Since 2012, he has been the President of the University of Perpignan Via Domitia.

Doune Macdonald is a Professor of Health and Physical Education, Pro-Vice-Chancellor (Teaching and Learning) and Director of the Institute of Teaching and Learning Innovation at the University of Queensland, Australia. From 2011 she undertook the role of Lead Writer for the Australian Curriculum: Health and Physical Education. She serves on a number of committees and boards including the International Association for Physical Education in Higher Education, Sport, Education and Society, and Physical Education and Sport Pedagogy. Doune is currently the principle investigator on two Australian Research Council grants looking at the health work undertaken by generalist and specialist teachers and an international study investigating the global patterns of outsourcing the health and physical education curriculum.

Her publication record of nine books and some 150 book chapters and refereed journal articles includes writing on curriculum, policy and inclusion in physical activity and sport.

Robert Malina is Professor Emeritus in the Department of Kinesiology and Health Education, University of Texas at Austin, USA, and Research Professor in the Department of Kinesiology, Tarleton State University, Stephenville, Texas, USA. His primary area of interest is the biological growth and maturation of children and adolescents with a focus on motor development and performance, youth sports and young athletes and the potential influence(s) of physical activity and training for sport. A related area of interest is the growth, nutritional status, performance and physical activity of school-age children in Oaxaca, southern Mexico. The research in Mexico began in 1968 and continues to the present day.

Clifford Mallett is an Associate Professor of Sport Psychology and Coaching, and Director of the Australian Centre for Sport, Physical and Health Education Research in the School of Human Movement Studies at The University of Queensland. Cliff is Associate Editor for the *International Sports Coaching Journal* and previously the *International Journal of Sport and Exercise Psychology* and serves on the Editorial Board for *International Journal of Sport Science and Coaching*. He is Co-Chair (Research) for the International Council for Coaching Excellence (ICCE). Cliff has published over ninety peer-reviewed papers and book chapters on sport and coach motivation, motivational climate, mental toughness, coach learning and development.

Nanna L. Meyer is an Associate Professor in the Department of Health Sciences at the University of Colorado (UCCS). Nanna's background is in nutrition for exercise and sport. Nanna developed the UCCS Sport Nutrition Graduate Program. She has been a research working-group member of the International Olympic Committee Medical Commission related to winter sport nutrition, body composition, health and performance, and relative energy deficiency in sport. Nanna is the past president of the international organization of Professionals in Nutrition for Exercise and Sport (PINES) and has been in Olympic sport nutrition for nearly 20 years.

Aaron L. Miller is an independent scholar specializing in the study of education, sports, culture, power and violence. He was most recently Assistant Professor and Hakubi Scholar at Kyoto University, Japan, and Visiting Scholar at Stanford University's Center on Adolescence. His first book, *Discourses of Discipline: An Anthropology of Corporal Punishment in Japan's Schools and Sports*, was published by the Institute for East Asian Studies at the University of California, Berkeley, USA, in 2013. He is currently writing a new book tentatively entitled, *The Idea of Education in Modern Sports*, which traces the historical roots of sports education from Victorian England to Japan and the United States and explores its significance today.

Atsushi Nakazawa is Associate Professor in the Graduate School of Social Sciences, Hitotsubashi University, Tokyo, Japan. His research explores the social and historical relationships between education and sport, especially focusing on school sport in secondary education in Japan, the United States and the UK. Atsushi has published widely in his native Japanese, and he has also recently contributed to the English language edited volume, *Safeguarding, Child Protection and Abuse in Sport: International Perspectives in Research, Policy and Practice* (Routledge, 2014).

Kacey Neely is a doctoral student in the Faculty of Physical Education and Recreation at the University of Alberta, Canada, and a research assistant in the Child and Adolescent Sport and

Activity Laboratory. She is interested in psychosocial aspects of youth sport, particularly positive youth development through sport. Her dissertation research focuses on deselection in competitive youth sport. She has received funding for her doctoral research through the Social Sciences and Humanities Research Council of Canada and Sport Canada.

Lee Nelson is a Senior Lecturer in the Department of Sport and Physical Activity at Edge Hill University, UK. His research interests include micro-politics, emotions and pedagogy in coaching and coach education contexts.

Mai Chin A Paw is University Research Chair Professor at VU University Medical Center in Amsterdam, the Netherlands. She takes a translational approach from science to society by combining scientific expertise in human movement science and epidemiology resulting in innovative studies in real-world situations. Her research focuses on determinants and health consequences of physical activity (PA) and sedentary behaviour (SB), with a strong interest in underlying mechanisms and innovations in risk-factor research. She is also acknowledged for her innovations in methodology, for example, mediation analyses, participatory action methods with children and novel analytical methods of accelerometer data providing detailed, unique information on SB and PA patterns. Mai's significant contributions to science and major societal issues were rewarded with an appointment as University Research Chair, a selective and privileged appointment as full professor (www.vu.nl/nl/onderzoek/onderzoekers/university-research-chair/mai/index.asp). She chairs the section Child Health and Care Research and theme group Youth and Lifestyle within VU University Medical Center. Mai is also director of the EMGO Institute for Health and Care Research (EMGO+) research programme Lifestyle, Overweight and Diabetes and vice-chair of the Academic Collaborative Center, Youth and Health, an important collaboration between VU University Medical Center and five Municipal Health Services in North-Holland aiming to improve evidence-based child health-care practice. She is associate editor of *The Journal of Science and Medicine in Sport* and member of the editorial board of the *International Journal of Behavioral Nutrition and Physical Activity*.

Patrick Peretti-Watel is Research Director in the French National Institute for Medical Research. He obtained his PhD in Sociology in Paris in 1999. His major research areas throughout his career have been the sociology of risk and the sociology of health. During the last decade, he coordinated a series of research projects dealing with licit and illicit drug uses as well as other risky behaviours, both among the general population and specific subpopulations, including young athletes, with a special focus on social inequality issues. Patrick is author or co-author of about 150 peer-reviewed articles and a dozen books.

Chris Platts was awarded a PhD in 2012 from the University of Chester for his study entitled Education and Welfare in Professional Football Academies and Centres of Excellence: A Sociological Study. The research, which was undertaken at twenty-one professional football clubs across England and Wales, explored the experiences of 303 players between the ages of sixteen and eighteen and is one of the largest academic studies of the lives of young players to have so far been published. For three years, Chris was the Editorial Assistant for the *International Journal of Sport Policy and Politics* and has published his work in various peer-reviewed academic journals. Since 2011, Chris has been a Senior Lecturer at Sheffield Hallam University, UK, and teaches on various aspects of Sport Development, Sport Coaching and Sport Business Management.

Paul Potrac is Professor of Sports Coaching at the Department of Sport and Physical Activity, Edge Hill University, UK, and an Honorary Professor at the University of Hull, UK. His research focuses on the micro-political and emotional features of practice in coaching and coach education. He has co-authored several books on sports coaching including *Sports Coaching Cultures: From Practice to Theory, Routledge Handbook of Sports Coaching, Research Methods in Sports Coaching, Understanding Sports Coaching: The social, cultural and pedagogical foundations of coaching practice* (third edn), and *A Sociology of Sports Coaching*. Paul is also an Associate Editor of the *Sports Coaching Review*.

Thomas Quarmby is a Senior Lecturer in Physical Education and Sport Pedagogy at Leeds Beckett University, UK. His research interests focus on the socio-cultural influences that constrain or facilitate young people's engagement with sport and physical activity, especially as they pertain to the family and different family structures. He is interested in exploring the role of sport and physical activity for underprivileged young people from low socioeconomic backgrounds and their in/exclusion from it. Thomas is currently engaged in research projects that explore looked-after children's engagement with sport and physical activity and the role it plays within their daily lives. He has published in peer reviewed journals and books in the area of sport sociology, physical education and health.

Karin Redelius is Associate Professor of Physical Education and Sport Pedagogy and pro vice-chancellor at The Swedish School of Sport and Health Sciences. She is also a Guest Professor at Linnaeus University in Sweden. From 2005 to 2011 she was a board member of the Swedish Sport Confederation and in that position responsible for the confederation's sport research. Her major research areas are children and youth sport and questions concerning children's rights in sport, as well as school physical education and questions concerning student learning in relation to assessment and grading. At present she is responsible for several large research projects on policy implementation and the consequences of early specialization in youth sport.

Alba Reguant Closa is a Registered Dietitian from the University of Navarra (Spain), with a Masters in Sports Performance from the Spanish Olympic Committee and the Autonomic University of Madrid. In 2011, she completed the International Olympic Committee Diploma in Sports Nutrition. As recipient of a Fullbright scholarship, Alba is currently finishing a Masters degree in sports nutrition at the University of Colorado, Colorado Springs, USA. Her research is focused on validating the Athlete's Plate educational tool. Previously, Alba has been the head dietician in the sports medicine clinic VitalSport, in Andorra, where she collaborated with different sport and health organizations, such as the Andorran Olympic Committee. Alba is interested in sports nutrition and performance, but also focuses her efforts on raising awareness regarding sustainability and food sovereignty.

Ken Roberts is Emeritus Professor of Sociology at the University of Liverpool and Visiting Professor at the University of Chester, UK. His major research areas throughout his career have been the sociology of leisure, and youth life stage transitions. After 1989, he coordinated a series of research projects in East-Central Europe and the former Soviet Union. His current research is UK based, and is into the development of educational and vocational aspirations during secondary education, the role of higher education in social mobility, and leisure and class re-formation in Britain. Professor Roberts' latest books are *Key Concepts in Sociology* (2009), *Youth in Transition: Eastern Europe and the West* (2009), *Class in Contemporary Britain* (2011) and *Sociology: An Introduction* (2012).

Bettina Rulofs is a Senior Lecturer at the German Sport University Cologne, Germany, in the Institute of Sociology and Gender Studies in Sport. Her main areas of research are social inequality, child protection, the prevention of violence and diversity management in sport. She has been a member of the National Working Group on Child Protection in Sport since 2010, and in 2011, she compiled a set of guidelines for child protection in sport for the organization German Sport Youth. Since 2012, Bettina has been a spokesperson for the sport sociology section within the German Association for Sport Sciences.

Lotte Salome is currently a Lecturer at the University of Amsterdam in the Netherlands, in the Department of Communication Science. She has a strong focus on Marketing Communication, specifically in the field of sports and health. In 2012, she obtained a PhD degree at the University Utrecht after finishing her dissertation about lifestyle sports, entitled *Indoorising the Outdoors: Lifestyle Sports Revisited*.

Michael Sam is a Senior Lecturer in the School of Physical Education, Sport and Exercise Sciences at the University of Otago, New Zealand. His research interests broadly encompass areas of policy, politics and governance as they relate to the public administration/management of sport. Michael has published widely in both sport and parent-discipline journals including the *International Review for the Sociology of Sport* and *Policy Sciences*. He has also co-edited two books: *Sport in the City: Cultural Connections* (2011) and *Sport Policy in Small States* (2015). He serves on the editorial board of the *International Journal of Sport Policy and Politics* and is an executive board member of the International Sociology of Sport Association (ISSA).

Jan Seghers received his PhD in Kinesiology in 2003 and currently holds the position of Associate Professor at the Physical Activity, Sports and Health Research Group within the Department of Kinesiology at the KU Leuven, Belgium. He is occupied with a research, educational and consultancy task within the scientific fields of sport and exercise pedagogy, physical-activity epidemiology and health promotion. His research activities are focused on the study of (psychological and environmental) determinants of physical activity and sedentary behaviour across the lifespan and the effectiveness of physical activity interventions in different populations. Jan has research collaborations with universities worldwide and is actively involved in the HEPA-Europe Network (Health Enhancing Physical Activity).

Jeroen Scheerder is Associate Professor in the Department of Kinesiology and Head of the Policy in Sports and Physical Activity Research Group at the University of Leuven, Belgium. His research focuses on policy-related and socio-economic aspects of sport and leisure-time physical activity. He has (co-)authored more than fifty articles in peer-reviewed international journals, and is editor/author of about twenty books on sport, participation and policy. He is (co-) supervisor of PhD projects in the fields of sport policy, sport sociology and sport marketing and is member of the editorial board of the *European Journal for Sport and Society*. Together with colleagues from the Mulier Institute (the Netherlands), he initiated the MEASURE project, which is a European research network on sport participation and sport policy. In 2014, he was appointed as the president of the European Association for Sociology of Sport (EASS). Jeroen Scheerder lectures in the fields of public sport policy and sport management and is a guest professor at the universities of Brussels, Cassino, Cologne, Jyväskylä, Kaunas and Porto. From 2005 to 2007, he was a visiting professor in sport sociology at the Faculty of Political and Social Sciences, Ghent University, Belgium.

Amika Singh is a senior researcher who conducts and supervises research in the Child Health and Care Research section at the VU University Medical Centre in Amsterdam, the Netherlands. Her research focuses on the development and evaluation of school-based interventions, aimed at improving physical activity and dietary behaviour. As scientific project manager, she coordinated the ENERGY-project, aimed at promoting healthy energy-balance related behaviours in children across Europe. In recent years, Amika has focused upon unravelling the relationship between physical activity and cognitive performance in children. Amika has co-authored more than fifty international scientific articles.

Andy Smith is Professor of Sport and Physical Activity at Edge Hill University, UK, where he is also Associate Head of the Department of Sport and Physical Activity. His research interests and publications focus on sport, physical activity and health, and on youth sport policy and development. He is co-author of *Sport Policy and Development* (with Daniel Bloyce, 2010), *An Introduction to Drugs in Sport* (with Ivan Waddington, 2009) and *Disability, Sport and Society* (with Nigel Thomas, 2009) and co-editor of *Doing Real World Research in Sports Studies* (with Ivan Waddington, 2014). Andy is also former co-editor of the *International Journal of Sport Policy and Politics*, which he launched with Barrie Houlihan and Daniel Bloyce in 2009, and an Editorial Board member of *Leisure Studies* and the *European Physical Education Review.*

Jorunn Sundgot-Borgen is Professor of Physical Activity and Health in the Department of Sports Medicine at the Norwegian School of Sport Sciences, Oslo, Norway. She received a Masters degree at Arizona State University in 1985 and her PhD at the Norwegian School of Sport Sciences in 1993. Jorunn has worked at the Norwegian Olympic Training Centre, leading the Nutrition Department. She has been Deputy Chairman and Acting Head of the National Council for Physical Activity, and is currently Vice-President of the Nordic Society for Eating Disorders. Jorunn's research areas include eating disorders, weight regulation, menstrual disorders and bone health.

Saskia te Velde is an Assistant Professor at the Department of Epidemiology and Biostatistics at the VU Medical Center, Amsterdam, the Netherlands, and Associate Professor at the Department of Public Health, Sport and Nutrition at the University of Agder, Kristiansand, Norway. Her research addresses health promotion and intervention development with a special focus on physical activity and dietary behaviours. She has special interest in social determinants of health behaviours and the evaluation of interventions, including mediation and moderation analyses. She has (co-)authored more than eighty articles in peer-reviewed international journals and lectures in the field of epidemiology and behaviour change. Saskia te Velde was actively involved in several European projects such as the Pro Children Project, ENERGY and ToyBox.

Katherine Tamminen is an Assistant Professor in the Faculty of Kinesiology and Physical Education at the University of Toronto, Canada. Her research examines youth sport experiences and adolescent athletes' coping in sport. She also conducts research on interpersonal emotion regulation and social processes related to coping and emotion in groups and teams, to understand how individuals' coping and emotions impact others. Her research is supported by the Social Sciences and Humanities Research Council of Canada and has been published in journals such as *Psychology of Sport and Exercise, Journal of Sports Sciences* and *Qualitative Research in Sport, Exercise, and Health.*

Holly Thorpe is Senior Lecturer in Te Oranga, School of Human Development and Movement Studies, at the University of Waikato, New Zealand. She is a sociologist of sport and physical culture with particular interests in youth culture, action sports, Sport for Development and Peace (SDP), girls' and women's health and well-being, social theory and qualitative methods. She has published more than forty academic journal articles and book chapters on these topics, and is co-editor of various special issues and books, including *The Berkshire Encyclopedia of Extreme Sport* and the five-part *Greenwood Guides to Extreme Sports* series. She is author of *Snowboarding Bodies in Theory and Practice* (2011) and *Transnational Mobilities in Action Sport Cultures* (2014), and is currently co-editing both the *Routledge Handbook of Physical Cultural Studies* and *Women in Action Sport Cultures: Politics, Identity, Experience and Pedagogies*. She has been the recipient of both a Leverhulme Fellowship and a Fulbright Visiting Scholar Award, and continues to serve on the editorial boards for the *International Review for the Sociology of Sport* and *Qualitative Research in Sport, Exercise and Health*.

Jennifer Turnnidge is a fourth year PhD student in the School of Kinesiology and Health Studies at Queen's University, Canada. She completed a Masters degree in Sport Psychology, a Bachelors degree in Science, and a Bachelors degree in Physical Health and Education at Queen's University. Her research interests are in transformational leadership and coaching, peer relationships and positive youth development in sport. More specifically, she is interested in how social interactions can promote positive development in youth, both in able-bodied and disability-sport environments.

Maarten van Bottenburg is Professor and Head of the Department of Sport Policy and Sport Management of Utrecht University School of Governance, the Netherlands. Maarten has focused on themes like the globalization and commercialization of sport, elite sport policy, sports participation trends, the societal meaning of sport, and sport management. Among many other books, he was author of *Global Games* (2001) and co-author of *Managing Social Issues. A Public Values Perspective* (2013) and *The Global Sporting Arms Race* (2008). He also published articles in journals such as the *American Behavioral Scientist, Leisure Studies, Journal of Sport Management, Sport Management Review, European Sport Management Quarterly* and the *International Review for the Sociology of Sport*.

Hanne Vandermeerschen is a sociologist and conducts research at the Policy in Sports and Physical Activity Research Group, University of Leuven (Belgium). Her research interests lie in the area of Sports for All (social stratification of sports participation, Sports for All policies) as well as poverty and social exclusion. The sports participation of underprivileged people and opportunities for social inclusion in and through sports are currently the main focus of her research. She is preparing a doctoral thesis on this topic.

Bart Vanreusel is Professor at the Department of Kinesiology at the University of Leuven (KU Leuven) in Belgium. As a member of the Policy in Sport and Physical Activity research group, his focus is on the sociology of sport and physical activity. He has published in international journals and has books on sport, culture, participation, socialization, policy, governance and development. He was chair of the Sport Council in Flanders, Belgium, and Advisory Board for Sport Policy. Bart cooperated with the University of the Western Cape, among others, in South African projects on sport and development. Recently, he contributed to the fiftieth anniversary issue of the *International Review for the Sociology of Sport*. Longitudinal socialization and physical activity, as presented in the anniversary issue, is an ongoing topic of his research, started and continued by former and upcoming generations of scholars in his research group.

Willem van Mechelen is Professor of Occupational and Sports Medicine at the VU University Medical Center in Amsterdam and Honorary Professor at both the University of Queensland and University of Cape Town. He has a unique combined background in physical education, human movement sciences, epidemiology, (occupational and sports) medicine and public health. After a career as classroom physical education teacher and occupational physician, he completed a PhD at the age of forty. In the last ten years, Willem has been a driving force in the development of lifestyle interventions for various subgroups of the general population (children, working-age people and elderly) in different settings (e.g. schools, the worksite and the community at large). Willem is member of many (inter-)national expert committees and professional boards. He is an often-asked speaker at international scientific meetings. He has received a number of prestigious international prizes and awards. He also has a prize named after him.

Charlotte van Tuyckom is research coordinator at Howest School of Applied Sciences, Department Sport and Movement Sciences, Bruges, Belgium. She lectures in the field of (local) sport and health policy, marketing, and sport and movement activities for socially vulnerable target groups. Charlotte holds a PhD in Health Sociology, a Masters degree in Sociology and in Quantitative Analysis. In the past, she was affiliated as assistant professor with Ghent University (Belgium), and as a research fellow with the Sporthochschule in Cologne, Germany, and the World Health Organization in Geneva, Switzerland. She is author of several books and international publications, mainly focusing on cross-national differences in sport and leisure-time physical activity among Europeans. Her current research is into (local) community aspects of sport and the use of apps and wearables.

Maïté Verloigne is a postdoctoral researcher at Ghent University in Belgium. She is part of the research group Physical Activity, Fitness and Health led by Professor Ilse De Bourdeaudhuij and Professor Greet Cardon. Her research focuses on the promotion of physical activity and the reduction of sedentary behaviour among youngsters. As part of her PhD, she was involved in the ENERGY-project that had the aim to develop an evidence-based intervention to prevent overweight and obesity in ten- to twelve-year-old children across Europe.

Matthew Vierimaa is a PhD candidate in sport psychology in the School of Kinesiology and Health Studies at Queen's University in Kingston, Ontario, Canada. His research broadly focuses on understanding how social relationships and contextual factors influence young athletes' performance, participation and personal development in sport. Funded by the Social Sciences and Humanities Research Council of Canada, his doctoral research explores youths' experiences and personal development in an exemplary community sport programme.

Kristin Walseth is an Associate Professor at Oslo and Akershus University College of Applied Sciences in Norway. She teaches sport sociology and coordinates the masters programme in PE and Education Science and is leader of the research group Body, Learning and Diversity. Her major research area has been the sociology of sport, particularly sport among Muslim youth. She has published articles on Islam, Muslim youth, identity work and integration. Her current research project is on sport, Islam and Muslim organizations in Norway.

Hans Westerbeek is Professor of Sport Business and the Dean of the College of Sport and Exercise Science, and of the Institute of Sport, Exercise and Active Living (ISEAL) at Victoria University, in Melbourne, Australia. He holds a visiting Chair position at the Free University of Brussels in Belgium and at the Real Madrid Graduate School in Madrid in Spain. He also sits on numerous academic advisory boards for institutions in several countries and until recently was a Board member of the Australian Football League (AFL) Europe, based in London. He has published twenty-three books and more than two hundred articles in sport management, sport business, sport marketing and sport policy, and his work has been translated into Chinese, Russian, Dutch, Arabic, Portuguese and Greek. He is an international consultant to more than fifty organisations including the FIFA, IMG London, Giro D'Italia, Royal Dutch Football Association, AFL, Cricket Australia, the Dutch Olympic Committee and to governments in India (current), New Zealand, United Arab Emirates, the Netherlands and Belgium to name a few. One of the major projects that he is involved in is SPLISS – sport policy factors leading to international sporting success – which involves comparing elite sport policy and sporting systems in fifteen different nations. He is also working with the Australian Institute of Sport and telecommunications giant Telstra, on a project that involves the creation of a digital interface between elite athletes and government in regard to supporting athletes during and after their active careers. He is frequently approached by international media and has delivered presentations and keynote addresses at over 120 conferences in more than twenty-five nations around the world.

Belinda Wheaton is an Associate Professor in Sport and Leisure Studies at the University of Waikato, New Zealand. Previously she was a reader in Sport and Leisure Cultures at the University of Brighton, UK. She is known internationally for her research on the politics of identity in lifestyle sport, which includes a monograph, *The Cultural Politics of Lifestyle Sports* (2013), and edited collections including *Understanding Lifestyle Sport* (2004), and *The Representation and Consumption of Lifestyle Sport* (2012). She is also co-editor of *Leisure and Environmental Politics* (2013). Current projects include the sportization of parkour, surfing, embodiment and ageing, and the racialization of surfing culture and space.

Lauren Wolman is a doctoral student at York University in the School of Kinesiology and Health Science, Toronto, Canada. Her research interests are within sport development, particularly around athlete recruitment and retention. Her Masters research explored the role of community sports clubs in supporting youth to continue participating in organized sports in adulthood, while her doctoral research is focused on optimizing contexts for sport participation among immigrant children and youth. For over twenty years, Lauren has been actively involved in girls' and women's rugby, as a coach and administrator in both Canada and the UK.

Jan Wright is a Professorial Fellow in the Faculty of Social Sciences at the University of Wollongong and Guest Professor at Deakin University, Australia. Her research draws on feminist poststructuralist theory to critically engage issues associated with embodiment, culture and health. Her most recent work has focused on the place and meaning of health and physical activity in children and young people's lives. She is co-editor of *Body Knowledge and Control* (Routledge, 2004), *Critical Inquiry and Problem Solving in Physical Education* (Routledge, 2004), *Biopolitics and the Obesity Epidemic* (Routledge, 2009) and *Young People, Physical Activity and the Everyday* (Routledge, 2010) and co-author with Michael Gard of *The Obesity Epidemic: Science, Ideology and Morality* (Routledge, 2005).

Chen XueDong is a Lecturer in Sport and Physical Education in the Civil Aviation University of China. He obtained his MA degree in Physical Education and Training from Nanjing Sport

Institute (China). His research and teaching broadly encompass physical education, sport pedagogy, football and badminton tactics, and sport development in general in higher education. He has published widely in the representative core journals of China.

Jiri Zuzanek is Emeritus Professor in the Faculty of Recreation and Leisure Studies at the University of Waterloo, Ontario, Canada. Prior to his appointment at Waterloo, Jiri taught sociology at universities in Czechoslovakia, Sweden and New York. His interests in the sociology of leisure, mass culture, fine-arts audiences and participants, and life quality among the elderly, are reflected in his four books and about seventy articles and chapters in edited works. His work has been supported by over thirty grants, mainly from Canadian government agencies involved in the arts, communications, commerce, fitness, international relations, social science research and statistics, and others. Jiri has been Associate Editor or reviewer for several sociology and leisure journals and has reviewed grant proposals for the Canada Council, the Social Science and Humanities Research Council, National Endowment for the Arts and other agencies. He has given invited papers throughout the United States and Canada and a dozen other countries.

ACKNOWLEDGEMENTS

First and foremost, we would like to thank all the contributors to the Handbook for giving so generously of their time and expertise. We are particularly pleased by the mix of established figures and the next generation of names represented in the Handbook.

We are indebted to Simon Whitmore and Will Bailey at Routledge for their unflinching good humour, support and forbearance.

We must also thank Ian 'Pritch' Pritchard at the University of Chester for keeping us attuned to the pitfalls of referencing!

Ken Green and Andy Smith

GENERAL INTRODUCTION

Ken Green and Andy Smith

The production of this *Routledge Handbook of Youth Sport* is indicative of the growing interest in youth sport across a range of fields (including physical education, public health, sports development and government policy) as well as a breadth of academic disciplines and sub-disciplines (ranging from sociology through psychology to physiology and sports medicine). It is also indicative of a critical mass of research and researchers generated within and by these fields and disciplines. Nowadays, very many academic and professional conferences have youth sport strands. This buoyancy is expressed in a raft of publications (in both journal and book forms) on youth sport. Many of the topics covered by these publications are mirrored in the content of the Handbook. In part, the growth of interest among academics is an expression of growing concern in various professional arenas with the participation of young people and youth in physical activity and exercise, particularly via sport. As the contributions in Section 1 make clear, it is also an expression of the prolonged and changing nature of youth as a transitional life-stage, the growth and diversity of leisure activities in which young people are now engaged, and the increasing social, cultural and economic significance of youth sport.

Although all the themes in the book are initially defined and interpreted, the two central terms – youth and sport – probably need some explanation at the outset. The age band thought to constitute youth (or terms often treated as *de facto* synonyms such as adolescence and teenager, despite their focus on the biological changes of puberty associated with growing up and/or the years thirteen to nineteen) varies over time as well as within and between societies: '[T]he chronological ages when youth begins and ends have varied greatly by time and place, and both the beginnings and ends are "fuzzy" in all modern societies' (Roberts, 2009: 12). It is unsurprising, therefore, that attempts to define youth can be problematic, not least because youth cannot be tied rigidly to 'specific age ranges, nor can its end point be linked to specific activities, such as taking up paid work or having sexual relations' (Furlong, 2013: 1). Instead, youth is perhaps most adequately recognized as a 'period of semi-dependence that falls between the full dependency that characterizes childhood and the independence of adulthood' (Furlong, 2013: 3).

Notwithstanding the difficulties involved, we have chosen to define youth as a life-stage that, in chronological terms, can be very broadly mapped onto the latter teenage years, with some leeway at the upper end to include the post-teen years up to young adulthood. Thus, youth is regarded as a period of transition ranging from roughly sixteen to twenty-five years. This allows for coverage of those youngsters whose leisure lives are quite precocious and those young adults whose lives continue to resemble closely that of teenagers. Maintaining fluid boundaries to the concept of youth enables the text to incorporate contributions germane to young people's past (in other words, their childhood) as well as their (adult) futures and the significance of both of these for their relationships with sport and other uses of leisure. In the process, it implicitly encourages a relational view of youth sport: recognizing the many and varied ways in which young people are interdependent with a wide variety of people and networks (including, for example, their parents and family, schools, peers and friends, the countries they inhabit and, within these, the various government and regional policies towards sport) whose actions constitute the kinds of sporting and cultural practices that are examined in this Handbook.

The second central term is sport and this too requires some initial consideration. As Coalter (2007: 7; original emphasis) observes, in a sense 'sport is a collective noun which hides more than it reveals'. Indeed, there are 'almost endless variations of sport processes, mechanisms, participants and experiences – individual, partner or team sports; motor or perceptually dominated sports; those which require physical or mental dexterity; tasks verses ego orientation and so on' (Coalter, 2007: 7). In this Handbook, sport will (unless indicated) be used in a general sense to incorporate not only competitive game-contests (that is to say, conventional sports such as football, hockey, basketball and badminton) but also less competitive, less organized, recreational versions of these sports as well as more recreationally oriented physical activities and exercise (swimming, aerobics, cycling, skateboarding, surfing, cheerleading, parkour and so forth), often referred to as lifestyle or lifetime sports and activities. On occasions, phrases such as 'sport and physical activities' or 'active recreation' will be used in order to highlight the significance of recreational or lifestyle activities to the point being made. Here again, these stipulated uses of the various terms will give way to the specific terms used in the research, which provides the evidence base for particular themes. Contributors have been encouraged to work with the editors' operational definitions of the two key terms, youth and sport. Cutting across these, however, has been the need to allow authors leeway to employ the terminology and language of their respective sub-disciplines and their own research, as well as the terms that accurately reflect the particular socio-cultural contexts under consideration. On occasions, the contributors have used terms such as 'adolescents', 'teenagers' and 'teens' as these have been deployed by the authors whose work they cite, while others have referred to periods of adolescence alongside discussions of the transitional life-stage that is typically used to refer to changes in the life course that occur within the broad age categories used to define youth in this Handbook.

The Handbook charts and examines some significant changes in not only the character of youth sport (the rise of so-called lifestyle sports, for example) but also the breadth and depth of research, which indicates the growing maturity of youth sport as a field in which inter-disciplinary enquiries are increasingly common. Although it is clear from some of the contributions that, in some countries and particular social contexts, youth sport is often regarded as being inseparable from phenomena such as school-based physical education, in many others it has emerged as a much broader social practice that is not necessarily defined narrowly by the kinds of sports and physical activities that are provided in schools. This is perhaps because we are witnessing an increasing disconnection between physical education (which is often linked synonymously with school sport) on the one hand, and youth sport on the other, where youth sport is linked to education but not necessarily defined by the activities and priorities of schools and other educational institutions. Yet, in some countries such as Britain, the rapid growth and cultural significance of what is referred to as youth sport has sometimes meant it is difficult to separate youth sport from physical education. Despite the conceptual differences thought to exist between the two, and the different ways in which they are enacted in practice, it is now just as common for the terms 'youth sport' and 'physical education' to be used interchangeably just as they are considered separately.

Regardless of the ways in which youth is conceptualized, and the blurring of boundaries between each of the contexts in which they engage in sport, physical activity and other uses of leisure, young people and many features of their lives not only remain of interest to politicians and the media, but are the subject of much academic discussion. Where this discussion has been most useful has been when researchers have been willing to subject to critical scrutiny many of the common-sense claims that underpin the assumptions that are frequently made about young people's lives, and to bring much needed clarity to the reality of youth as a life-stage. Discussions of young people's participation in sport and physical activity, for example, often generate more heat than light and as a consequence has limited our understanding of not only these dimensions of youth lifestyles, but also of related matters including young people's use of leisure and their health and well-being. This is perhaps most clearly expressed in the avalanche of publications, media reports and government policy that have in part provided the foundations upon which a supposed moral panic has emerged surrounding young people's participation in sport, physical activity and its consequences for their physical, mental and social health.

What is particularly striking about contemporary concerns regarding the state of youth lifestyles is their near universal acceptance across a range of societies in the Western world and beyond. In both more- and less-developed societies, there is a now a broad consensus that declining participation in sport and physical activity, alongside the growing prevalence of unhealthy diets, declining levels of daily energy expenditure, an increasing preference for engaging in sedentary leisure activities and the increasing incidence of mental illness are among the central causes of a health crisis identifiable in children and youth. Although frequently portrayed as a present-day problem of youth lifestyles, young people's engagement in sport, physical activity and other uses of leisure that have implications for their health and well-being have been sources of concern for over a century or more. Thus, while these features of young people's lives, to varying degrees, among the most prominent headline social problems (Cohen, 2002 [1972]) in the twenty-first century, the uncritical reporting of certain so-called facts amplify and exaggerate the supposed problems of contemporary youth lifestyles. Accordingly, among less critical observers, the one-sided presentation of young people as inactive, unhealthy and disinterested in sport because of the appeal of other uses of leisure is liable to perpetuate misleading emotional generalizations based on the lives of some young people, which are then assumed to accurately reflect the reality of all youth lifestyles.

It is hoped that the contributions to this Handbook serve as a useful corrective to these tendencies and, to that end, Section 1 contextualizes youth sport by exploring social change among youth as well as youth leisure as the context for youth sport, time use, and how these collectively help us to understand the interdependence between young people's sport and leisure careers. This is followed, in Section 2, by a snapshot of youth sport in countries and regions around the world which, as the various contributions make clear, reveals a complex and diverse, but in other ways similar, picture of youth sport participation. The insights provided in this section are then extended in Section 3 in which some of the major trends in youth sport are explored, including the growth of so-called lifestyle sports and the indoorization of, among other examples, outdoor and adventurous activities. The fourth section focuses upon the key dimension of socialization into sport and focuses on the roles played in this process by family and peers and how these contribute to the tendency for young people to remain locked in, or out, of sport. Subsequently, in Section 5, the effects of various social dynamics, such as social class, ethnicity, gender and sexuality, on youth sport participation are examined. In the next two sections, six and seven, two particular related issues come under scrutiny: first, the relationship between youth sport, health and physical activity and, second, elite youth sport, which examines issues of talent development, the 'logic' of youth sports work and child abuse. The Handbook is rounded off, in Section 8, with an overview of some key features of politics and policy in youth sport, with each contribution addressing some of the major themes that are examined in earlier chapters.

The authors and topics included in the Handbook are intended not merely to offer coverage of significant dimensions to the study of youth sport but also, wherever possible, to show the international breadth of interest and expertise in the field of youth sport. The selection of each has, of course, been entirely ours and we accept responsibility where and when this does not meet with approval!

References

Coalter, F. (2007). *A wider social role for sport: who's keeping the score?* London: Routledge.
Cohen, S. (2002 [1972]). *Folk devils and moral panics.* (30th anniversary edition). London: Routledge.
Furlong, A. (2013). *Youth studies: an introduction.* London: Routledge.
Roberts, K. (2009). *Youth in transition. Eastern Europe and the West.* Basingstoke: Palgrave Macmillan.

SECTION 1

Youth sport in context

1

INTRODUCTION

Ken Green

The four authors in Section 1 explore change and transformation in youths' lives and the implications for the context in which the remaining topics in the Handbook need to be understood. In Chapter 2, *Young people and social change*, Ken Roberts outlines the ways in which the youth life-stage has been reshaped in all Western countries, with most other countries increasingly resembling the West. There have been several key developments in the overall reshaping of youth, which Roberts identifies as extension, destandardisation and individualisation. In keeping with the notion of youth as a life stage (see the General introduction), youth has been extended, but with huge variations in how long it now lasts, depending on individual circumstances. In addition, some of the transitions experienced during youth (for example, from living with parents to living alone, and from being in education to gaining paid employment) have been destandardised in the sense that there is no longer a single, normal sequence followed by the vast majority of youth. These developments have led to the increased individualisation of youth biographies. Although youth has been reshaped, what Roberts refers to as 'the major landmarks' in the transition from youth to adulthood remain: completing full-time education, obtaining an adult job, marriage and parenthood. Indeed, as Roberts observes, the wider changes in the life stage of youth appear to have no direct implications for sports careers. These tend to have their own structure and momentum. While sports careers have always been individualised, the wider changes in the youth life stage have altered the context in which youth sports careers develop (or do not develop). The upshot is that although youth sports careers can endure relatively independently of wider changes to the life stage of youth, such changes require us to rethink how sport is presented and delivered to young people. The rest of this Handbook teases out some of the issues in need of reflection and, perhaps, action.

In Chapter 3, *Youth leisure as the context for youth sport*, Roberts follows up his outline of *Young people and social change* by asking the question: 'how does a wider leisure context add to our understanding of youth and sport?' In short, his response is two-fold: first, we come to recognise that 'most of the young people who do little if any sport, and those who take part less often as they grow older, are rarely becoming couch potatoes but rather, they are diverting their time, money and attention to other forms of leisure; second, we realise that youth is not the life stage when individuals are most likely to be drawn into sport and in which they remain for life'. Youth is the life stage when drop-out from sport peaks and the explanation, Roberts notes, lies in the greater appeal of other uses of leisure. Consequently, sport tends to be repositioned during youth as the age group divides into peer groups that align with different youth sub-cultures. As a useful lead into Jiri Zuzanek's chapter on time use among youth, Roberts shows how, against several measures, sport is not a major use of leisure among youth – especially when compared with such things as TV viewing and computer usage. At the same time, however, he notes how quantitative yardsticks overlook sport's cultural traction among adults and children as well as youth. Sport is rivalled for cultural pull, he adds, only by popular entertainment. However, sport has some major advantages: people think sport is a good thing – sport matters. Youth and sport appear a natural couplet, according to Roberts, not least because nearly all younger children have had sport built into their routines. Childhood is the life stage when there is mass recruitment into sport. So the vast majority of young people enter the post-child life stage with foundations in sport already laid. As explained elsewhere in the Handbook, these foundations are not all equally strong. Roberts goes on to introduce very many of the issues dealt with in the Handbook, including: the assumed relationship between sport and health, socialisation into sport, drop-off and drop-out from sport, the significance of parents and friends, levels of physical activity and participation, elite youth sport and the benefits of youth sport compared with other uses of leisure, to name but a few. In the process, he teases out what distinguishes the minority of young people who continue to play sport regularly into young adulthood.

Historic gains in free time have gone disproportionately to the young and the elderly. Childhood has grown as a result of children being required to remain longer in compulsory education and the life stage of youth has been prolonged by, among other things, more youngsters remaining in education until their early twenties. Simultaneously, the elderly have (until recently, at least) been retiring earlier and living longer. In *Youths' use of time from comparative, historical and developmental perspectives*, Jiri Zuzanek considers the impact of lifestyle changes that have accompanied technological advancements in the form of automobiles, TV, mobile phones and the internet, and their seeming impact upon physical activity and sedentary lifestyles. Like Roberts before him and Haycock and Smith subsequently, Zuzanek highlights the fact that sports involvement typically diminishes with age, beyond the early teenage years. A range of health-related issues have contributed to an intensification of research into youths' time use and, in particular, the place of sport and other active uses of leisure time. Thus, drawing upon time use surveys over a period of several decades, Zuzanek examines the place of sport and physically active leisure in the lives of youth and, more specifically, how much of it is allocated to physically active leisure and sports. He reveals how the decline in sports participation characteristic of the teenage years and beyond tends to be relatively modest in some countries while pretty steep in others. Among the many policy implications of youths' time use, Zuzanek picks out several that he considers 'particularly serious', including what he refers to as the dangers of sedentary lifestyles resulting, in part, from the growth of mass and electronic media and youths' 'excessive media exposure'. Zuzanek argues that greater attention needs to be paid not only to physically active leisure but to adolescents' overall patterns of (and balances between) daily life – especially sleep, eating habits, mass media consumption, extra-curricular activities and relationships with parents and peers. In this regard, Zuzanek argues that a balanced use of time rather than an exponential growth of selective activities is at the root of higher quality of youths' lives and their physical, emotional and intellectual well-being; hence, what Zuzanek perceives as the need to avoid focusing solely on expanding youths' participation in one particular group of activities, such as sport.

In *Youth, sport and leisure careers*, David Haycock and Andy Smith bring the section to a close by developing Roberts' observation that until their mid-twenties, the largest concentration of young people is in education, and higher education, like primary and secondary education, is an obvious location for youth sport. Drawing upon research conducted with university students, Haycock and Smith examine some of the benefits, as well as the difficulties, of injecting a longitudinal dimension into the study of young people's lives using panel research designs, and how these can be particularly beneficial for understanding the interrelationships between sport and leisure careers. Central to the explanation of youth sport and leisure careers, they argue, is the differential contribution made by the construction of young people's habituses and capitals, which help provide the foundations upon which participation and tastes for sport in later life are based. Following Roberts and others in this book, Haycock and Smith show that it is childhood, rather than youth, which is the most critical life stage in which the predispositions for subsequent sport participation are frequently laid. Accordingly, since the observed differences in sport participation first emerged during childhood, widened between the ages of twelve to thirteen, and remained relatively set from age sixteen onwards, the subsequent inequalities in sport participation among university students could not be attributed to a higher education effect, as previous research has suggested.

Taken together, the contributions to Section 1 can help us understand just why the growth of participation in post-compulsory education, in countries such as the UK, has not been followed by an increase in adult sports participation of the kind anticipated – given that young people staying on in education are likely to have their sporting predispositions reinforced and enhanced by the availability of opportunities, like-minded friends and peers, the availability of subsidised, close-to-hand facilities and so forth (Roberts, 2010). It seems that the expected effects of prolonged involvement in education on youth sport participation may only operate amid other favourable factors of the kind explored elsewhere in this Handbook.

Reference

Roberts, K. (2010). Personal communication. Wednesday, 1 December 2010.

2

YOUNG PEOPLE AND SOCIAL CHANGE

Ken Roberts

Introduction

This chapter reviews how the youth life stage has changed during the current era, which is variously described as post-industrial, post-modern, globalised, neo-liberal, an information age and post-welfare. The preceding industrial age is inevitably the benchmark against which subsequent changes are assessed. Hence the importance of stressing the brevity of the industrial era, which was when most modern sports were invented.

The chapter begins with a brief sketch of pre-modern youth, then proceeds to how youth was reconstructed, and became more structured, universal and less gendered during the industrial age. The main subsequent changes in the life stage – extension, destandardisation and individualisation – are then described. The concluding section explains that youth sport careers have their own structure and momentum that are unaffected by wider changes. Even so, these wider changes make the case for a rethink on how sport is presented and delivered to young people.

Pre-modern youth

It is impossible to generalise except to state that youth has not been a universal life stage. In some societies, in some social groups, children started to work in their homes and in the fields as soon as they were able to do so. Children were treated as mini adults and were expected to grow up quickly (Aries, 1973). Marriage could be at any age from puberty onwards. Pre-pubertal children could be betrothed (contracted to marry), and were sometimes actually married, though invariably with an assumption that these relationships would not be consummated before puberty.

When it was a distinguishable life stage, youth was often a mark of privilege for those who could be allowed to delay adulthood while they completed their education, trained for a profession or practised the arts of warfare. Sometimes the delay was enforced, usually when inheritance of a title or property was involved.

In pre-modern times, youth was always gendered. Often all the youths were males. Full adulthood for high status young men could be delayed until an aristocratic title was inherited and family property passed down to the rising generation. For such males, major landmarks in the transition through youth could be completion of formal education or an apprenticeship, or participation in a military campaign, but always marriage, which made it possible for men to father legitimate children. It was usually possible for the sisters of these young men to marry at any age after puberty whereupon they became adult women. Until they married or were betrothed, they were maidens, available for offers. However, practices changed in early modern Europe's aristocratic families when it became normal to delay girls coming out until the late-teenage years. In England, these debutantes were formally presented at the court of the monarch. This practice ended in 1958, but London society still organises a season of balls and other events that are attended by eligible daughters and possible suitors. Whereas a male could become accepted as an adult without marrying, this was usually impossible for a daughter unless she inherited family property (in the absence of a male heir). Once passed child-bearing age, single women became spinsters and could not expect this status to change.

Youth in the industrial age

When countries became industrial and urban, youth was always reconstructed. In this process youth always became a more firmly structured, and thereby a more distinct, life stage. Also, youth always became universal within the countries, meaning that it became a distinct life stage for all social groups, and it became less gendered than in the past.

The reconstruction was due mainly to the multiplication of laws specifying age-related rights, responsibilities and prohibitions (Wallace and Kovacheva, 1998). There were laws specifying the ages between which children and young people had to attend school, and the ages from which they could undertake paid employment, sometimes, at first, with restrictions on the hours that they could work and the kinds of work that they could do. There were laws stipulating the ages from which young people could purchase alcohol and tobacco, watch adult entertainment and engage in consensual sexual activity. Then there were the ages at which young people became eligible to vote and hold public office, which became relevant for all young people when the franchise was extended to all adults, male and female. There were also ages at which young people became eligible for full adult welfare entitlements – sickness and unemployment benefits, and housing assistance for example. There was never a single age at which all the new rights and responsibilities took effect. Thus, youth became the life stage during which new adult rights and responsibilities were gradually bestowed. That said, completing full-time education, obtaining an adult job, marriage and parenthood remained the really major landmarks. Once passed these, you were an adult. Youth became a life stage for males and females, and in this sense was less gendered than in the past. However, it remained normal for males and females to be educated differently and to be employed in gendered occupations, and for girls, marriage and parenthood were somewhat more significant landmarks than for men, though for the latter it usually meant becoming the main breadwinner while the woman's main role was henceforth domestic.

As youth became a distinct life stage, special youth services were introduced. There were youth courts and sentences deemed appropriate for young offenders who were usually kept out of adult prisons. Special services and new professions were created to provide young people with education and career advice, and assistance in finding suitable jobs. Apprenticeships were joined by additional juvenile jobs thus creating an intermediate stage for everyone between being a child and an adult employee. Additional youth services offered legal, health and housing advice. Special housing was allocated for young people, especially full-time students who needed to move away from their parents' homes. Civil society organisations – churches, trade unions and political parties – created youth sections. The same applied in sports clubs and associations. Dedicated youth agencies were created – scouts, guides, and youth clubs with various sponsors.

As countries became more prosperous, various commercial goods and services were targeted as a distinct youth market – fashion, music, films, holidays, motor bikes and scooters.

This is how a 'classical' youth life stage was constructed. It is inevitably the benchmark against which more recent changes are assessed. So it is useful to bear in mind that the classical youth life stage lasted for less than a century in most countries, and in much of the world, especially in the global south, the countries and their young people are currently skipping the industrial stage. Youth move from traditional lives in traditional villages into cities where a post-modern type of youthhood awaits them.

Ideas that survive into the present about the age group that can be described as youth were formed in the industrial period. The precise ages before and after which it is inappropriate to describe someone as a youth vary from country to country. In North America, youth are passing through the high school years (twelve to eighteen/nineteen). In England, it is the fourteen to twenty-one age group for whom local education authorities were made responsible for the provision of youth services in the 1918 Education Act. In Germany, youth included anyone still serving an apprenticeship or in higher education (which could be up to the mid-twenties). In communist Eastern Europe, the Komsomol (the communist party youth organisation) had members up to age twenty-eight after which they could progress to full party membership. The age limits varied from place-to-place, but in all industrial countries the word youth became associated with a specific age group.

The wider societies' thinking about this life stage was influenced profoundly by a theory of adolescence first formulated by the American psychologist, G. Stanley Hall (1904). He argued that adolescence began with puberty and lasted until the physiological changes that were set in motion were complete. He suggested that the intervening years were traumatic for young people and all those around them: a period of storm and stress that lasted until adolescents had come to terms with their new bodies and emotions. This theory of adolescence was woven into the Freudian psychology that was influential in the mid-twentieth century, and suggested that the life stage was complete when a young person had formed a stable adult identity (Erikson, 1968). Puberty was universal, and therefore adolescence was regarded as a universal life stage. The American social anthropologist Margaret Mead (1935, 1971) challenged this view, claiming that Pacific island teenagers passed through the life stage without any storm and stress. Subsequently, instead of trying to identify universal characteristics, sociologists have stressed the extent to which youth has always been socially constructed: that the ages when it begins and ends have varied by time and place, and often between social groups in the same places and at the same time. The very evident reconstruction of youth – as societies have become post-industrial – has led to sociology replacing psychology as the lead discipline in youth studies (Furlong and Cartmel, 2007).

Youth in the post-industrial age

During the last forty years, the youth life stage has been reshaped in all Western countries, and most other countries have increasingly resembled the West in the character of the life stage. Specifically, the life stage has been generally extended, but with huge variations in how long it now lasts. Second, the several youth life stage transitions have been destandardised, meaning that there is no longer a single, normal sequence. Third, these developments have led to the increased individualisation of youth biographies.

For present purposes, there is no need to debate the contributions of economic and occupational restructuring (the switch of employment from manufacturing to services, and from manual into non-manual occupations), the increased appetite of parents and young people for educational qualifications, the role of new information and communication technologies, the neo-liberal economic and social policies of governments, and the normalisation of the use of the contraceptive pill by single young women. The crucial point for present purposes is that the youth life stage has been reshaped.

Extended youth

The construction of youth in the industrial era involved the introduction of compulsory schooling, initially at elementary and lower secondary levels (up to age sixteen). Subsequently in post-industrial societies it has become more common, and it is now compulsory in many countries, for young people to complete upper secondary education (up to age eighteen or nineteen), and increasing numbers have been enrolling in tertiary education – a name that is replacing higher education as the systems transform from elite to mass. In some countries (Slovenia in Europe and South Korea in Asia, for example), around eighty per cent of young people now progress into tertiary education. Part of the explanation is that there are fewer low-level jobs for which no qualifications are required, and more jobs where entry requires advanced qualifications. However, educational expansion has outpaced occupational upgrading, and an outcome has been the devaluation of educational credentials. Upper secondary qualifications can now be demanded of applicants for jobs that sixteen-year-olds formerly entered. University qualifications are now necessary for entry to jobs for which upper secondary qualifications were once sufficient. Young people who complete university courses today find that their qualifications do not guarantee access to graduate jobs. All they have earned is admission to the pools that are allowed to compete for these occupations.

Another development that has extended education-to-work transitions has been the insertion of intermediate stages between initial employment and jobs from which it is possible to build an adult career. Entrants to the labour market, whatever their qualifications, now face layers of screens. These are composed of internships, training programmes, part-time and temporary jobs. All these are stages from which young people may (but will not necessarily) progress to permanent full-time employment that pays an adult salary. An outcome is that most young people today reach their mid-twenties or beyond before they establish themselves in what they can regard as career jobs.

Education-to-work transitions have lengthened for most young people, but not for everyone. There are still some sixteen-year-olds who obtain then manage to hold onto full-time employment. There are still university graduates who step straight from their courses into graduate career jobs. Overall, transitions into working life have been extended, and simultaneously these transitions have become more varied in length.

A related trend has been for young people to delay marriage and parenthood until their late-twenties or into their thirties. Intermediate stages have been inserted into family and housing life-stage transitions. In the working class communities in South Wales that Diana Leonard (1980) studied in the 1960s and early 1970s, it was not uncommon for a young couple to each leave their family homes, marry, start life in their own marital home, and sometimes lose their virginity all within a single day. Nowadays, such compressed transitions are extremely rare. Young people exit their parents' homes to live singly or in shared housing. They typically rent accommodation. Some start to do so when students then continue for many years after leaving education (Heath and Kenyon, 2001). The age when it is normal to first become a home-owner has shifted upwards into mid-thirties and even beyond (Claphamet al., 2010). Marriage is now usually preceded by cohabitation, which is usually preceded by several sexually active relationships.

However, we should note that some young people have prosperous and generous parents who can enable their children to become property owners while still students, and some young women start their careers as mothers while teenagers. It is remarkable that behaviour that was regarded as perfectly normal fifty years ago – young motherhood, and starting work in a job without formal training at age sixteen to eighteen – are now seen as problems and signs of disadvantage.

The upward extension of youth has not been compensated by a delay in the start of the life stage. If anything, youth is starting earlier than ever before as a result of the marketing of youth fashions and music to the pre-teens amid fears over the premature sexualisation of children. However, typical ages of puberty have remained stable in post-industrial countries where there was a decline in the mid-twentieth century, which was associated with rising standards of living and nutrition and improved medical services. Likewise, in these countries, typical ages of first full sexual experience have remained stable at fifteen to seventeen.

There are several unresolved issues. One is whether we should talk of an extended youth or sub-divide the life stage into youth and young adulthood or emerging adulthood as proposed by American sociologist Jim Arnett (2005). The problem with sub-division is where to draw the boundary. The end of the high school years may feel right in North America but less so in countries where twenty-somethings are comfortable with the youth label. Indeed, throughout the global south all those still waiting to advance into leadership roles in business and politics like to identify with the youth of their countries.

Another issue concerns the extent to which young people are choosing to delay taking on adult responsibilities as opposed to being held back by the absence of opportunities. Would twenty-somethings hop from one short-lived job to another, adding bytes to lengthening CVs, if the option of a steady career job was available?

A further issue concerns whether delayed transitions to full adulthood are resulting in young people's socio-psychological development being permanently arrested as argued by Canadian sociologist James Côté (2000). This has been a long-running issue in Southern European countries where it remained normal throughout the modern era (as it was before then) for young people to remain living with their parents until their late-twenties or into their early-thirties (Cavalli, 1997). The argument of Southern European critics, and Côté, is that young adults can become permanently reluctant and maybe incapable of taking-on responsibilities as heads of families, becoming parents, and needing to hold down career jobs. Will young adults who continue to rely on the bank of mum and dad throughout an extended life stage ever become reliable bankers for their own children?

A final issue is whether, for some young people, the extension of youth may prove never ending through the poverty of their employment opportunities rather than their own choices. Experience of prolonged unemployment when young increases the risks of long-term labour-market precarity (Ainley and Allen, 2010). These risks are known to be class-related.

Destandardisation

There are two ways in which youth life stage transitions have been destandardised. First, in the previous industrial era, there was a standard, proper order in which these transitions were made, and the vast majority of young people followed what was regarded as the correct sequence. You began by completing education, then establishing yourself in employment, following which you became financially independent and able, with a partner, to maintain an independent household whereupon you could marry and become a parent. Today it is so common as to be considered normal for young people to depart from this standard sequence. They may cohabit prior to completing full-time education. Couples are likely to become parents before they marry. In fact they may dispense with marriage entirely. Any order of life events has become socially acceptable.

Second, transitions were formerly treated as non-reversible, and were rarely reversed. When you left education, you had left for ever: school days were behind you. There was little chance that you would return to a classroom. When you married you expected the relationship to be for life. Today it has become more common and acceptable for young people to yo-yo or boomerang (Pais, 2003). They may return to full-time education after experiencing full-time employment. They may plan this sequence, using a period in work as a way of saving to part-fund their studies. Or the return to education may not have been envisaged, but made upon realising that their career opportunities would improve if they added to their qualifications. Young people today may leave, then subsequently return to live with their parents. This sequence may occur on leaving home to pursue full-time education in another city, then returning after graduating and being unable to obtain a job paying a salary that would enable them to live independently. Couples may cohabit, even marry, then separate and rejoin the singles while they are still twenty- or thirty-something.

There is no dispute that the youth life stage has been destandardised in these ways. The debates are about the significance of these trends. Is it really the case that anything goes, and that any order will do for young people today? Or are boomeranging or yo-yoing signs of disadvantage and failure rather than new, liberating options? For example, leaving education to seek employment then returning to school may be a response to bleak labour market prospects rather than a favoured route onwards in life (Furlong et al., 2005). Likewise boomeranging back to the parental home is more likely to be enforced than a step on a young adult's preferred life course. Young people who are able to do so appear to continue to drive their lives forward and do not boomerang. On the other hand, any former stigma associated with back-stepping appears to have dissipated.

Individualisation

According to German sociologist Ulrich Beck (1992), this trend began after the Second World War. Full employment and rising real incomes made households less dependent on extended families and neighbours. Meanwhile, secularisation was diminishing the size of and weakening religious congregations. Also, stronger welfare states were bestowing rights upon individuals: education, health care, sickness and unemployment benefits, access to social housing and so on. Beck claims that an outcome was not just to allow, but to require young people to take responsibility for their own educational and career choices, and thus for their future lives.

In the post-industrial age, as the youth life stage has been extended, individualisation is said to have accelerated. Every individual builds a unique biography of educational courses, modules, qualifications, experience in part-time and full-time jobs, peer relationships, housing and leisure. It no longer tells a prospective employer sufficient to know your family background, the place where you were brought up and the school that you attended. Everyone needs a personal CV. No two biographies are identical. These are sometimes described as choice biographies. Every person is deemed responsible for the previous steps that they have taken, and for planning their own futures. Each biography becomes a personal project.

This here-and-now can be contrasted with a past in which young people could see their future life courses laid out before them. Your parents would arrange, and maybe pay for your schooling, and could possibly ensure your progression into a specific business or profession. You would be expected to marry someone from the same neighbourhood, school or church.

By looking at a slightly older age group, individuals could see the futures that lay in store for them. Often young people attended the same elementary schools as others in their neighbourhoods, then entered employment in the same local mines or factories. They would marry one another, have children at around the same time, and continue to live and work in the districts where they were born. It was possible to break-out, to rebel, but this required there to be an expected future life plan that could be rejected. It was as if most young people from a given background boarded the same public transport vehicle when young, then journeyed through life together. Today, the metaphor is boarding private motor cars and plotting personal itineraries.

Beck and Beck-Gernsheim (2009) have drawn attention to the normality of geographical mobility among young people today. They move for education and employment as well as for leisure (as tourists), sometimes with a mixture of motives, and they do this within and between countries. Students in higher education find themselves in cosmopolitan settings in which students from numerous countries and with different nationalities and religions feel equally at home. Future life plans cease to be bounded by place of birth and nationality.

In practice, however, it is not always like this. There can be obstacles to individualisation. Migrants seeking jobs and housing may encounter hostility from locals. This increases their dependence on diasporic communities. Migrants tend to move along paths and to destinations where others from their home communities have already settled. Also, some of the trends that have fostered individualisation are now being reversed. The weakening and withdrawal of some state welfare rights makes young people more dependent on their families. That said, most parents do not try to reassert control but do their best to support children in the latter's own life projects. Needless to say, the support that young people can expect varies enormously by social class origins. The metaphorical private motor cars in which they embark on their life journeys have differently powered engines. Yet despite this, individualisation can still operate in so far as it is incumbent on young people themselves to use whatever kinds and levels of support that are available to them.

Implications for youth sport

The wider changes in the post-industrial youth life stage have no direct implications for sports careers; these have their own structure and momentum. Young people progress in sport as they grow physically and improve their skills. At any age from early-teens, depending on the sport, young people are able to compete in all-age events. There is no need to delay players in youth leagues because they are spending longer in education any more than prolonged education must lead to a postponement of sexual experience. There is no reason why sport careers should be destandardised to any greater extent than has always been the case. Back-stepping has always occurred when players have tried to advance too quickly or to levels beyond their ultimate capabilities. Sport careers have always been individualised. This applies even in team sports where players progress to teams, clubs and leagues that match their personal abilities. Players rise and sometimes fall-back to levels that match their individual talents.

The wider changes in the youth life stage alter the context in which youth sports careers develop (or do not develop). Provisions (facilities and facilitators) operate within a changing context. In the case of sport providers, this is an increasingly favourable context. Most modern sports were invented in the nineteenth century and the principal sites of invention were secondary schools and universities. The sports that were promoted were suited to these contexts: teams of male competitors who competed against each other, and by the end of their education (which would be late-teens or early-twenties) they would be able to play in all-age teams, clubs and leagues. Nothing has changed here except that much higher proportions of young people now benefit from upper-secondary and higher education. Until their mid-twenties, the largest concentration of young people is in education. This is an obvious location for youth sports except that students are thereby separated from other adult competitors, and young people who complete their education earlier are likely to be disadvantaged. The way to avoid separation from other adults was pioneered a century ago: college teams compete against all-age opponents. The disadvantages of early leavers from education are long-standing, but these young people are now a minority rather than the majority of the age group.

Beyond lower secondary education, players do not need special youth facilities and leaders. They are normal players who do not need anything age-specific. It is veterans (past their peak), family groups, and young teens and children who need age-specific provisions. Other young people today simply need facilities.

If the aim is life-long sports participation, then the youth problem is not recruitment but retention throughout what is now a prolonged life stage during which individuals and peer groups are seeking places to go and things to do. Facilities need to be attractive to the age group —as attractive as the leisure competition. Higher education has successful models. The problem, of course, is cost. Exercise can be free but sports that require halls, courts and pools or playing fields are an entirely different proposition.

References

Ainley, P. and Allen, M. (2010). *Lost Generation? New Strategies for Youth and Education*. London: Continuum.

Aries, P. (1973). *Centuries of Childhood*. Harmondsworth: Penguin.

Arnett, J. J. (2005). *Emerging Adulthood: The Winding Road from Late Teens Through the Twenties*. Oxford: Oxford University Press.

Beck, U. (1992). *Risk Society: Towards a New Modernity*. London: Sage.

Beck, U. and Beck-Gernsheim, E. (2009). Global generations and the trap of methodological nationalism for a cosmopolitan turn in the sociology of youth and generation, *European Sociological Review*, 25, 25–36.

Cavalli, A. (1997). The delayed entry to adulthood: is it good or bad for society?. In J. M. Pais, and L. Chisholm (eds) *Jouvens em Mundanca* (pp. 179–186). Lisbon: Instituto de Ciencias Socias, University of Lisbon.

Clapham, D., Buckley, K., Mackie, P., Orford, S. and Stafford, I. (2010). *Young People and Housing in 2020: Identifying Key Drivers for Change*. York: Joseph Rowntree Foundation, York.

Côté, J. (2000). *Arrested Adulthood: The Changing Nature of Maturity and Identity. What Does it Mean to Grow Up?* New York: New York University Press.

Erikson, E. H. (1968). *Identity, Youth and Crisis*. New York: Norton.

Furlong, A. and Cartmel, F. (2007). *Young People and Social Change*. Maidenhead: Open University Press. Second edition.

Furlong, A., Cartmel, F., Biggart, A., Sweeting, H. and West, P. (2005). Complex transitions: linearity and labour market integration in the West of Scotland. In C. Pole, J. Pilcher. and J. Williams (eds) *Young People in Transition: Becoming Citizens?* (pp. 12–30). Basingstoke: Palgrave Macmillan.

Hall, G.S. (1904). *Adolescence*. New York: Appleton.

Heath, S. and Kenyon, L. (2001). Single young professionals and shared household living, *Journal of Youth Studies*, 4, 83–100.

Leonard, D. (1980). *Sex and Generation*. London: Tavistock.

Mead, M. (1935). *Sex and Temperament in Three Primitive Societies*. London: Routledge.

Mead, M. (1971). *The Coming of Age in Samoa*. Harmondsworth: Penguin.

Pais, J. M. (2003). The multiple faces of the future in the labyrinth of life, *Journal of Youth Studies*, 6, 115–126.

Wallace, C. and Kovacheva, S. (1998). *Youth in Society: The Construction and Deconstruction of Youth in East and West Europe*. London: Macmillan.

3

YOUTH LEISURE AS THE CONTEXT FOR YOUTH SPORT

Ken Roberts

Introduction

How does a wider leisure context add to our understanding of youth and sport? It makes two important contributions. First, we realise that most of the young people who do little if any sport, and those who take part less often as they grow older, are rarely becoming couch potatoes. Rather, they are diverting their time, money and attention to other forms of leisure. Second, we realise that youth is not the life stage when individuals are most likely to be drawn into sport and in which they remain for life. This applies with visits to pubs and bars. Quite the reverse applies with sport. Youth is the life stage when drop-out from sport peaks and the explanation lies in the greater appeal of other uses of leisure.

This chapter proceeds by comparing sport with other uses of leisure. It then examines how sport is repositioned during youth when the age group divides into peer groups that align with different youth sub-cultures. The chapter then assesses the short- and longer-term benefits of remaining sports-active throughout youth against the appeal of alternative ways, and possibly more reliable ways, of using leisure to secure benefits of at least equal value. Finally, the chapter asks what distinguishes the minority of young people who continue to play sport regularly into young adulthood, and explains why, in the context of alternative uses of leisure, it proves difficult to enlarge the size of the sports-active group.

Sport and the rest of leisure

Uses of leisure can be ranked according to the amounts of time and money that they command, and the proportion of a population that is involved. These yardsticks place sport as a low to middle rank use of leisure. The amounts of time spent playing and watching sport are tiny compared with hours spent watching television. Spending on admissions, memberships, sports equipment and special clothing is vastly exceeded by spending on hospitality (which includes out-of-home eating and drinking) and tourism. The proportion of the population that takes part in sport is depressed because drop-out begins during youth then continues, whereas television, holidays and alcohol are popular in all age groups and among both women and men.

However, these quantitative yardsticks overlook sport's cultural traction: the number of non-participants who nevertheless follow a team, sport or competition, and feel elated or dejected depending on the result. People may follow their teams daily in newspapers and on websites, and track progress during and then the result following every game. Or they may do this just occasionally such as when a national side reaches the final stages of a world championship, or when a national competitor is a contender for an Olympic medal. The cultural appeal of sport is indicated by the number of back pages in newspapers, the television channels and programmes that are devoted to sport, and the regular sports slots in general news bulletins. The strength of sport's cultural traction is also indicated by it being the content that is most likely to sell subscriptions to television channels and pay-per-view programmes, the value of team and player endorsements in marketing non-sports goods and services, the widespread use of sports clothing and footwear as general leisure attire and sport's attraction as an object for gambling. Perhaps as significant as anything else, sport is a reliable topic for small talk. This matters: small talk is an essential lubricant in forming and maintaining social relationships, including friendships among young people. A point to note is that people can be attracted to and attached to sport, and can follow sport in all these ways without actually playing.

Sport is rivalled for cultural pull only by popular entertainment: films, music and television programmes about which 'everyone' can be assumed to possess some level of knowledge and interest. However, sport has some major advantages. First, popular entertainment is regarded as lightweight. Taking it seriously is a misuse of intelligence. This is due to comparisons with high culture where there are rules against which performances and compositions can be judged, and experts who interpret and apply the rules. Sport is more like high culture than popular entertainment in this respect. Sport can be taken seriously. There are experts who write and commentate authoritatively. Ordinary fans and players are allowed to take their sports seriously – to miss classes and to take time off work, to disrupt household routines and defer family obligations because they just have to be present at an event.

Second, sport has an immediacy that popular entertainment cannot rival. The value of watching an event live is far greater than a recording. It is impossible to derive the same intensity of enjoyment when watching an event over and over again once the outcome is known. Music is different. Also, sports events can never be repeated. Each is unique and can therefore be unmissable.

Third, everyone of consequence appears to agree that sport is a good thing. The numerous presumed benefits of sport are discussed later but they mean that there is no serious opposition to encouraging children and young people to play. The value of sport is endorsed by virtually all parents, teachers and other public authority figures. Politicians like to demonstrate that sport has their backing. Tony Blair, UK prime minister at the time, gave his government's backing for sport his personal endorsement: 'The government does not and should not run sport. Sport is for individuals, striving to succeed – either on their own, or in teams. However, these individuals, together or alone, need the help of others – to provide the facilities, the equipment, the opportunities' (Department for Culture, Media and Sport, 2001, p 2). Spending tax-payers' money on participant sport is less likely to encounter opposition than spending on almost anything else. Attending high profile sports events and behaving like other fans show that politicians have the common touch without making them look frivolous. Sport has always been part of school education, and it has been among the activities typically offered by youth organisations.

All this makes it unsurprising that school children play a lot of sport. In Britain most play several sports, on several occasions each week, in school and out of school (Department for Culture, Media and Sport, 2008; Sport England, 2003). Children are encouraged to take part by parents, teachers, youth leaders, politicians and, of course, by sportsmen and sportswomen, and by representatives of all the associations that run and promote all the different sports.

Youth careers in sport and leisure

If youth and sport appear a natural couplet, this is because nearly all younger children have had sport built into their routines. Childhood is the life stage when there is mass recruitment into sport. So the vast majority of young people enter the post-child life stage with foundations in sport already laid. As explained below, these foundations are not all equally strong.

Sport is widely believed to be especially beneficial for young people (the reasons are discussed below), and young people are more likely to play sports than any older age groups. Hence the common impression that young people are especially keen on sport. However, the peak age for sport participation in most countries is twelve to fourteen. Thereafter many young people maintain and some even increase their sport participation, but year-on-year the overall trend is for young people to do progressively less. Young people may spend more time playing, and play more sports than adults, but youth is the life stage when players are most likely to begin to reduce their activity or drop-out altogether. This is not necessarily because they become less interested in sport. As noted above, sport has an unrivalled ability to attract and retain followers. Nor is it because young people who play less than when they were younger become over-weight couch potatoes. Rather, it is because they acquire wider ranges of leisure options, and certain disadvantages of sport as a leisure activity begin to kick in as young people approach adulthood.

Children play at times, with friends, in places and at activities that are chosen and supervised by adults – parents, teachers and others to whom the care of dependents is entrusted. It is under these conditions that the young first play most of the sports that they will ever play, and most of them play more sports, and play more frequently, than they will at any later stage in their lives. Thus, as regards sport participation, the youth life stage begins at a high point. By age fourteen, thirteen, twelve or even earlier, young people begin escaping into their own worlds. Adults begin to lose control. Children begin to express independent desires. They begin choosing their own friends and meeting unsupervised, or subject to looser and less obtrusive adult supervision than formerly. They do this in school playgrounds, on the streets, in parks and in study/play/bedrooms (Hendry et al., 1993). Close friends are sometimes part of larger, looser reputational crowds, which may be part of wider, possibly international, youth sub-cultures (Thurlow, 2001). Cliques and peer groups form around tastes in music, styles of dress and preferred uses of free time. These divisions may or may not map onto broader gender, ethnic, religious and other divisions. By sixteen-plus, peer relationships tend to reflect divisions between educational tracks (academic and vocational, for example), and thereafter they tend to reflect the even clearer division between those continuing in education and those who have started or are trying to start full-time labour market careers.

Teenagers can usually name the main crowds in their own schools – those who are into particular kinds of music, the sports enthusiasts, technos who can do astonishing things with computers, and very likely geeks and others who excel academically and otherwise conform with adults' expectations (Currie et al., 2006; Wood, 2003). Reputations matter in these emotionally charged social networks (Carter et al., 2003). Style failure invites ridicule (Croghan et al., 2006). Amid these developments, relationships with sport change. Sport becomes central in some peer groups' lives and relatively marginal in others (Kreme et al., 1997). Young people do not want to be the same as everyone else. They need to be able to display difference vis-à-vis other cliques and crowds. They need to fit in while expressing individuality among their own close friends. Young people need to establish identities in this way. Becoming an adult means creating an identity that is not ascribed by family background, and the identities and reputations established within youth sub-cultures remain important for as long as adult destinations remain unknown, which is usually late-twenties (or even beyond) nowadays (Miles, 2000).

The new media have added new dimensions to peer-group life. Mobile phones enable friends and others to be in touch at any time, wherever they are. Peer relationships can multiply via interactive websites. Cyberspace can be an arena in which friendships are strengthened, and also a site for bullying. As they exit childhood, young people face the unavoidable challenge of establishing and defending reputations and identities in these hyper-charged twenty-four-hour milieu (Lehdonvirta and Rasenen, 2011; Mattar, 2003).

As they grow older, young people experience widening choices over friendships, things to do and places to go. When they are earning their own money they have greater access to commercial facilities – cinemas, music events, bars and cafes as well as sports clubs and stadiums. Sport faces more competition than among younger teenagers. Those who remain in sport tend to specialise in the sports that they most enjoy and at which they are most proficient (MacPhail and Kirk, 2006). Different sports compete for young people's loyalty, and all sports compete with other tastes and places that can act as sources of friends, identities and reputations. The choice is not between sport and idleness. Sport has to compete in a marketplace of leisure activities, styles and identities.

In this marketplace, sport has two serious handicaps that kick in as young people leave childhood behind. First, sports are competitive. It may be true that people with all levels of ability can enjoy and benefit from sport but playing is most rewarding for those who can win. Reputations among players depend on ability. Young people who are hopeless at sport are unlikely to use this as their preferred source of identity. Children who enjoyed playing sports at primary school often find, later on, that they are unwanted in sports clubs that are interested in recruiting and retaining only those players who will strengthen their teams (Clark, 2012). They may also find themselves marginalised in secondary school sport in which encouragement, resources and reputations follow sporting ability. In music-based sub-cultures it is unnecessary to be able to sing or play: knowledge is sufficient to earn status and respect. Sport is more demanding in this respect except that anyone can remain vaguely interested in sport, able to take part in the relevant small talk, without being a player. Young people will not risk basing reputations and identities on sport if they are regarded as hopeless performers, or if their appearances when taking part invite ridicule.

Sport's second handicap is that competitions are usually gender divided: males play with and against other males while females play with and against other females. This fits with young teenagers' normal modes of socialising, but these modes change as young people grow older. Physically energetic recreation can be non-competitive in which case the sexes can surf, swim and ski together. This will be one reason why the trend with age is out of competitive team sports and into lifestyle sports. These have additional advantages. They can be played individually or in a group of any size and sex and age composition. Lifestyle sports can be played flexibly, for short or longer periods and at times that suit the participants. This makes them compatible with the routines of today's teenagers and adults. Young people aged sixteen-plus typically balance the schedules of study, part-time or full-time jobs, family obligations and self-maintenance, which includes time to just relax, doing nothing in particular. Organised competitive sport is demanding, not in the total amount of time spent playing but in the need to be available regularly at set times for events and practice sessions. This means making sport a pivotal, fixed reference point in one's life. Lifestyle sports are more like other youth sub-cultural activities in their flexibility and are therefore more compatible with other demands on a player's time.

Also, and very importantly, adult venues where alcohol is served have one huge advantage for older young people – they are kid-free zones, and they differ from most sport facilities in this respect. Disengaging from sport can be part of a lifestyle strategy for growing up, looking and feeling like an adult.

Benefits of youth sport compared with other uses of leisure

Sport has a multitude of vocal supporters and hardly any visible opposition. Most sports are administered by voluntary associations that are passionate advocates for their games, and members who are even more passionate about their own teams and clubs. No other activity attracts as many volunteers (Gratton and Taylor, 2000). Mega events are overwhelmed by applicants seeking to work as unpaid helpers. The mass media promote sport daily. As we have seen, nearly all politicians, governments and oppositions want to position themselves on the side of sport. Most significant for our purposes, involving and retaining young people is usually seen as a way of capturing their lifelong enthusiasm. Sports can be advocated for sport's own sake. No further justification is absolutely necessary, but throughout the history of modern sports their promoters have alleged instrumental benefits. These have three common features. First, the claims of instrumental benefits are often implausible and usually unproven. Second, they present youth as the age group that has most to gain in both the short and longer runs. Third, they ignore the possibility that other uses of leisure may offer the same or equally attractive benefits.

Sport has always been recommended as a way of keeping young people out of trouble and saving those who are deemed at risk. Nowadays social mobility is a common slogan. We know that sport can work (Feinstein et al., 2006), but the crucial process appears to be to involve those individuals who are otherwise at risk in law abiding, higher-ranked or upwardly mobile social groups. Sport may or may not do this. Other leisure activities, especially those based on church or arts groups, are more reliable. Sports provisions that are swamped by at-risk cases absorb and may amplify their existing cultures (Nichols, 2004; Skogen and Wichstron, 1996). In any case, family origins and educational attainments are far better predictors of adult outcomes than whether young people play sport or practise any other kind of leisure. The link between sport participation and all manner of good outcomes in cross-sectional data sets is due mainly to the types of people who play rather than the effects of participation.

Sport's advocates claim that society will reap health and fitness benefits and savings in health-care costs. The problem here is that the physical health benefits depend on play being energetic, aerobic, of at least twenty minutes duration, at least three times per week, and this regime must be maintained for life in order to gain lifelong benefits (American College of Sports Medicine, 1990). Few people achieve this target. Currently less than one-fifth of England's adult population does so. Only a proportion of these will continue throughout adult life, and if they do so the risks of sports injuries are likely to eliminate the benefits (Roberts and Brodie, 1992). If today's young people's lifestyles are less healthy than was the case in the past (British Medical Association, 2003), this is not because they are playing less sport. Rather, sport is unable to compensate for the loss of activity since the time humans were hunters and gatherers, then engaged in agriculture and then in heavy extractive and manufacturing industries, before mechanical transport and domestic labour–saving technologies. The obesity crisis is due to diet (eating too much and eating unhealthy foods) and it is inconceivable that the population's excess body weight might be burnt off by playing sport. Less frequent and more moderate sport participation may deliver social and psychological health benefits, but the same applies to any form of leisure that is active (incompatible with an armchair) and social.

Encouraging more young people to play more sport may be advocated as a means of producing sport champions. There is no doubt that the public loves to cheer its champion athletes to victory.

One problem here is that mass participation is superfluous and, if elite success is the priority, a waste of resources. The best-known success strategy is to sift the child population for talent, then hothouse and continuously sift elite squads (Green and Oakley, 2001). Another problem is that there can be only one winner per event. The quest for success is zero-sum. In sport there have to be losers, though the continuous invention of new sports and events enables more countries, schools, colleges, cities and individual athletes to win at something.

Sport for sport's sake may sound naïve, but it is probably the strongest, least vulnerable argument for promoting this use of leisure. Sport for sport's sake simply means making the intrinsic satisfactions of playing and watching as widely available as possible even if there are no extrinsic benefits (gains in health and fitness, less crime, or more Olympic champions, for example). If this argument is used, youth may still appear to be the right age group to engage individuals in sport after which there will be good chances that they will remain in sport for life. How convincing is the relevant evidence?

Foundations for lifelong sport participation

It is certainly the case that lifelong players have usually built up, continued to practise and maintained frequent participation in a wide range of sports throughout the youth life stage. If these foundations are not built by this stage and sustained throughout youth, it is unlikely that individuals will play sport regularly into and then throughout adulthood (Roberts and Brodie, 1992). However, what this overlooks is that there is a heavy dropout rate from sport throughout the youth life stage. This is more typically a time for cutting down rather than building up sport repertoires. Also, the sport repertoires that lead to lifelong participation appear to have been built prior to youth – during childhood – in sports-active families.

Sports promoters need to confront some uncomfortable truths. There are always new initiatives for involving young people in sport, and they usually appear to work in so far as young people are attracted onto the schemes. Youth is the life stage when lifestyles are fluid: individuals are available for recruitment. Yet in Britain the rate of sport participation throughout the general population, including the youth age group, has remained unchanged since the late-1980s. What has happened to all the young players who took part in successive initiatives? Young people who remain in full-time post-compulsory education, especially higher education students, have above average chances of remaining sports-active into their late-teens and early-twenties. In Britain, the proportion of the age group entering higher education has doubled since the 1980s, but this has not fed through into higher rates of adult (or even youth) sports participation. The only plausible explanations of this evidence are that any additional recruits to and stayers-on in sport have dropped out soon afterwards and/or that the programmes targeted at youth have recruited those who would have played in any case, and that young people who would otherwise have remained sports–active have been over-represented among the additional higher education students. Attempts to boost lifelong sports participation by targeting young people do not work. They would stand a far better chance if they did not have to compete with alternative uses of leisure. Whether young people remain in sport in the face of the competition appears to depend on whether strong foundations have already been laid.

Childhood, not youth, is probably the really critical life stage for laying secure foundations for long-term careers in sport, and in many other forms of leisure also (Birchwood et al., 2008; Nagel, 2010; Quarmby and Dagkas, 2010). It is not self-evident that schools, youth or sports organisations can be substitutes for the power of family socialisation, which operates daily throughout childhood. If excess young people are drawn into sport, they may simply drop out at a later point during the transition to adulthood. If there is latent suppressed demand to play sport, then building facilities that enable this demand to become manifest may boost long-term levels of sport participation. This appears to have happened in the UK during the opening of new indoor sport and leisure centres between the 1960s and 1980s. However, if the demand is not there, further investment in facilities may simply provide better accommodation for existing players. This appears to have been the outcome of the flow of new funds into UK sport since the introduction of the National Lottery in 1994. As stated above, since the late-1980s, rates of sport participation in the UK have remained stable in all age groups despite the injection of new money, and throughout all the twists and turns in government sport policies. The relatively high levels of sport participation in Scandinavian countries such as Norway are inexplicable except, for example, in terms of Norwegians being born that way, meaning that the country has a long history of sport as a normal part of family life (Green et al., 2013).

Conclusions

Notwithstanding the above, it must be emphasised that most young people do play sport. The young players include those whose frequency of participation declines. How often young people play and whether sport is a central part of their leisure lives, appear to depend on sporting talent and predispositions. Their sporting lives are affected by, but they are not the cause of, young people splitting into different peer and lifestyle groups among which the hyper-active in sport become a distinct sub-culture. Whether others remain active, and if so how active, will depend partly on opportunities – the facilities that are available and accessible. Providers can facilitate, but they cannot boost participation above young people's predispositions, and they cannot hope to overwhelm all the leisure competition.

The continued appeal of sport among young people may be considered a triumph for the facilitators. There has been no decline despite all the competitor attractions that have been introduced since the mid-twentieth century. In Britain, youth (and adult) sport participation rates rose in the decades up to the 1980s. Since then the rates have settled on a plateau, but unlike cinema attendances, there has been no decline in the face of competition from television, coffee bars, pubs and latterly from all the new media.

The cultural traction of sport appears to have grown stronger from decade to decade. The globalisation of television has boosted sport's media audiences. Sports stars have become international celebrities. Children and young people are socialised as consumers of sport. As adults, they pay television channel subscriptions. They purchase sports clothing and footwear as everyday attire. Young people's interest in sport is retained and boosted with the result that the consumption of sport has become a normal part of media-led everyday youth and adult leisure and related small talk. This may not boost, but neither is it at the expense of, participation by those who are sufficiently predisposed, talented and facilitated.

References

American College of Sports Medicine (1990). The recommended quantity and quality of exercise for developing and maintaining cardiorespiratory and muscular fitness in healthy adults, *Medicine and Science in Sports and Exercise*, 22, 265–274.

Birchwood, D., Roberts, K. and Pollock, G. (2008). Explaining differences in sport participation rates among young adults: evidence from the South Caucasus, *European Physical Education Review*, 14, 283–300.

British Medical Association (2003). *Adolescent Health*. London: British Medical Association.

Carter, D. S. G., Bennetts, C. and Carter, S. M. (2003). "We're not sheep": illuminating the nature of the adolescent peer group in effecting lifestyle choice, *British Journal of Sociology of Education*, 24, 225–241.

Clark, S. (2012). Being "good at sport": talent, ability and young women's sporting participation, *Sociology*, 46, 1178–1193.

Croghan, R., Griffin, C., Hunter, J. and Phoenix, A. (2006). Style failure: consumption, identity and social exclusion, *Journal of Youth Studies*, 9, 463–478.

Currie, D. H., Kelly, D. M. and Pomerantz, S. (2006). "The Geeks shall inherit the earth": girls' agency, subjectivity and empowerment, *Journal of Youth Studies*, *9*, 419–436.

Department for Culture, Media and Sport (2001). *A Sporting Future for All*. London: Department for Culture, Media and Sport.

Department for Culture, Media and Sport (2008). *Taking Part: England's Survey of Culture, Leisure and Sport. Headline Findings from the Child Survey 2007*. London: Department for Culture, Media and Sport.

English Sports Council (1999). *The Development of Sporting Talent 1997*. London: English Sports Council.

Feinstein, L., Bynner, J. and Duckworth, K. (2006). Young people's leisure contexts and their relation to adult outcomes, *Journal of Youth Studies*, 9, 305–327.

Gratton, C. and Taylor, P. (2000). *The Economics of Sport and Recreation*. London: Spon.

Green, K., Thurston, M., Vaage, O. and Roberts, K. (2013). '[We're on the right track, baby] We were born this way'! Exploring sports participation in Norway', *Sport, Education and Society*, DOI: 10.1080/ 13573322.2013.769947

Green, M. and Oakley, B. (2001). Elite sports development systems and playing to win: uniformity and diversity in international approaches, *Leisure Studies*, 20, 247–267.

Kremer, J., Trew, K. and Ogle, S. (1997). *Young People's Involvement in Sport*. London: Routledge.

Hendry, L. B., Shucksmith, J. and Glendinning, A. (1993). *Young People's Leisure and Lifestyles*. London: Routledge.

Lehdonvirta, V. and Rasenen, P. (2011). How do young people identify with online and offline peer groups? A comparison between UK, Spain and Japan, *Journal of Youth Studies*, 14, 91–108.

MacPhail, A. and Kirk, D. (2006). Young people's socialisation into sport: experiencing the specialisation phase, *Leisure Studies*, 25, 57–74.

Mattar, Y. (2003). Virtual communities and hip-hop music consumers in Singapore: interplaying global, local and subcultural identities, *Leisure Studies*, 22, 283–300.

Miles, S. (2000). *Youth Lifestyles in a Changing World*. Buckingham: Open University Press.

Nagel, I. (2010). Cultural participation between the ages of 14 and 24: intergenerational transmission or cultural mobility? *European Sociological Review*, 26, 541–556.

Nichols, G. (2004). Crime and punishment and sports development, *Leisure Studies*, 23, 177–194.

Quarmby, T. and Dagkas, S. (2010). Children's engagement in leisure time physical activity: exploring family structure as a determinant, *Leisure Studies*, 29, 53–66.

Roberts, K. and Brodie, D. A. (1992). *Inner-City Sport: Who Plays and What are the Benefits?* Culemborg: Giordano Bruno.

Skogen, K. and Wichstrom, L. (1996). Delinquency in the wilderness: patterns of outdoor recreation activities and conduct problems in the general adolescent population, *Leisure Studies*, 15, 151–169.

Sport England (2003). *Young People and Sport in England: Trends in Participation 1994–2002*. London: Sport England.

Thurlow, C. (2001). The usual suspects? A comparative investigation of crowds and social-type labelling among young British teenagers, *Journal of Youth Studies*, 4, 319–334.

Wood, R.T. (2003). The straightedge youth sub-culture: observations on the complexity of sub-cultural identity, *Journal of Youth Studies*, 6, 33–52.

4

YOUTHS' USE OF TIME FROM COMPARATIVE, HISTORICAL AND DEVELOPMENTAL PERSPECTIVES

Jiri Zuzanek

Much of public attention to sports and physically active leisure is focused today on professional sports and is driven by commercial interests, in particular interests of mass media. Paradoxically this attention to professional sports is often accompanied by a rise of passive lifestyles among the population at large. Put simply, the interest in professional sports, which should ideally serve as a stimulus for participation in physically active pursuits, often produces growing numbers of couch potatoes. Lifestyle changes accompanying technological advancements of industrial and post-industrial societies, such as automobiles, TV, mobile phones and the internet have reduced the need and the realm for active physical activity and increased the risk of sedentary lifestyles. Under these circumstances, the question about youths' participation in sports and outdoor and physically active leisure assumes particular importance. As a life-cycle group, youth was always positioned ahead of other population groups in sports and outdoor activities. Sports involvement usually subsides with aging due to economic, employment and family constraints. The decline of involvement in physical activities is, however, particularly steep among individuals who missed the opportunity of such involvement when they were young.

Heightened concern with sedentary habits, obesity, risk behaviours and the emotional well-being of youth (King *et al.*, 1996; Millstein *et al.*, 1993; Ozer *et al.*, 2002), as well as growing awareness of the fact that early child and adolescent development play a critical role in determining a population's health and well-being during the adult stages of the life cycle (Dietz, 1998; Wabitsch, 2000), have contributed to intensified national and international research efforts directed at the understanding of the role of adolescents' time use and leisure as determinants of health and well-being.

The role of sports and physically active leisure in the lives of the youth will be examined in this chapter primarily through the lens of time use. It is contended that important determinants of adolescents' physical and mental health are embedded in young people's daily behaviour and their leisure choices and preferences. The analyses reported in this chapter will be preceded by a brief discussion of the research strategies used in the study of adolescent time use and well-being. I will then examine how adolescents spend their time and how much of it is allocated to physically active leisure and sports. Next I will discuss how adolescents' time use and involvement in physically active leisure changed over the past several decades. Analyses of time use trends will be followed by an examination of the well-being and health implications of participation in different types of activities. The concluding part of the chapter will focus on policy challenges posed by the observed time use trends.

Time use and well-being: research strategies and data sources

Findings reported in this chapter are based on data from three major sources. These sources are:

1. National time use surveys conducted from the 1980s to the early 2000s by statistical agencies in Australia, Belgium, Canada, Finland, France, Germany, the Netherlands, Norway, UK and the United States.

2. Information about time use and its developmental outcomes reported by authors from some of the observed countries.

3. The *Survey of Adolescents' Time Use and Well-Being* (OATUS/ESM) conducted in 2003 in the Canadian province of Ontario by the Research Group on Leisure and Cultural Development at the University of Waterloo.[1]

According to Robinson and Converse (1972), a 24-hour day can be visualised as the available input of lifestyle resources, with the output represented by the choice of activities and the time allocated to each of them. To Larson and Verma (1999), time can be conceptualised as a resource that is used for the development of a wide range of adolescent faculties, including 'social competencies and dispositions related to healthy emotional adjustment' (p. 702).

Compared to recall questions, which ask respondents to estimate the amount of time or frequency of participation in selected activities in the past year, month or week, time diaries focus on time use during the survey day or the day preceding it. By focusing on short time intervals (usually 10 minutes long) on the diary day and covering the whole range of human activities rather than a group of activities or a single activity (leisure, sports, etc.), time use surveys reduce recall errors and make the reporting of activities less susceptible to social desirability biases.

In the past, national time use surveys in many countries focused on the labour force population only and did not sample respondents under the age of 15. This situation has changed. In a number of countries, particularly in Europe, respondents aged 12 years and older are now included in the survey samples (Belgium, Finland, Germany, Netherlands, UK, Australia).

Comparative data on adolescents' time use were collected in 1992 and 1993 by the European Research Network. This study focused on similarities and differences in the time use of school-aged adolescents in thirteen European countries (Alsaker and Flammer, 1999). Interesting information about time use practices of adolescents in industrial and developing countries can be found in Larson and Verma (1999), and about the time use of U.S. youth in Hofferth and Sandberg (2001) and Juster, Ono and Stafford (2004).

Unlike time diary studies, which focus on quantitative dimensions of daily life (duration) and use attitudinal measures independent of their immediate behavioural context, Experience Sampling Surveys (ESM), initiated in the 1970s at the University of Chicago by Csikszentmihalyi and associates, focus on the daily behaviour as a structured sequence of qualitative experiences precisely anchored in time (Csikszentmihalyi and Larson, 1987). In the ESM surveys, respondents are typically signalled (beeped) eight times per day and asked – at the time of the beep – to complete short self-reports, in which they answer questions about what they were doing, where and who they were with, as well as report their experiential states (feeling happy, sad, lonely, pressed for time, etc.). By providing researchers with an opportunity to assess immediate and circumstantial meanings and motivations of human activity, ESM surveys offer a unique opportunity to examine the emotional and health effects of adolescents' time use in the course of daily life.

Most of the ESM data reported in this chapter are taken from the *2003 Ontario Survey of Adolescent Time Use and Emotional Well-being* (OATUS/ESM), which combined the time diary method with an ESM survey of adolescents' time use and experiential states. The time diary part of the survey was administered in eleven Ontario schools (grades seven to thirteen) and sampled 2,213 high-school students aged 12 to 19. The follow-up Experience Sampling Survey collected data from 219 students, who took part in the time diary survey. A total of 9,731 self-reports were collected from these students (Zuzanek, 2005). Information about adolescents' time use, experiential states and emotional well-being of U.S. teens can be found in Csikszentmihalyi and Larson (1984), Csikszentmihalyi and Schneider (2000) and Larson (2001).

Time use of youth at the beginning of the millennium

The study of youth's time use poses serious measurement problems. Teens' time use undergoes considerable changes with age and varies with gender. Time use of teens attending schools differs from the time use of youth seeking early employment. For the school population, we need to take into account differences between the use of time during the school year and the summer holidays, and within the school year between the time use on school days and days off. To assess adolescent time use and examine historical trends in its use, it was necessary to choose a comparable population universe, a task that is complicated by different sampling and methodological practices in countries collecting time use data.

Analyses reported in this chapter focus on the time use of school-attending adolescents aged 15–19. Time use patterns are reported for school days, weekend days and average days. The latter are calculated as a mean of five weekdays and two weekend days. This averaged hybrid does not resemble any distinct day, but by providing a single measure eases the interpretation of gender and age differences, as well as historical trends in adolescent time use.

Time use on school days

Of all teens' daily activities, night sleep takes most time. The length of teens' sleep on school days wavers around 8 hours. The longest sleep was reported by students of the Netherlands, Australia and France (8.7–8.8 hours). Norwegian, Canadian, German and U.S. students' sleep on school days was the shortest – fewer than 8 hours (Table 4.1).

The second largest group of teens' daily activities is school attendance. Cross-national comparisons show that at the end of the 1990s and in the early 2000s, students in most industrial countries spent 5–6 hours on schooldays attending classes and 1–1.5 hours of homework.

There is considerable difference in the length of school-related time between the surveyed countries. Belgian students spent 8.8 hours in school-related activities on school days (including travelling to school). The comparable figures were 8.5 for Canada, 7.8–8 hours in the UK, United States, Australia and France, and 7.2–7.5 hours for students from Germany, Finland, Norway and the Netherlands. Doing homework on school days occupied as little as 45 minutes in Finland and as much as 1.7 hours in Belgium, with students from other countries reporting around 1 hour of homework per day (Table 4.1).

Table 4.1 Adolescent time use on school days: A cross-national comparison*

	Australia (1997)	Belgium (1999)	Canada (1998)	Finland (1999/00)	France (1998)	Germany (2001/02)	Netherlands (2000)	Norway (2000)	UK (2000)	USA (2003)
N=	862	291	230	267	606	582	99	175	403	512
School-related time	8:01	8:46	8:31	7:11	8:01	7:23	7:34	7:19	7:46	7:53
Attending classes	5:31	6:02	6:07	5:35		5:11	4:53	5:29	5:41	6:31
Homework	1:25	1:42	1:34	0:45		1:08	1:30	0:56	0:58	0:56
Paid and domestic work	1:07	0:57	1:15	1:05	0:41	1:06	1:28	1:18:	1:04	1:07
Personal needs	10:16	9:54	9:09	9:45	11:31	9:45	10:38	9:24	10:02	9:41
Sleep	8:48	8:16	7:52	8:09	8:51	7:57	8:43	7:44	8:34	7:59
Eating	0:44	0:53	0:32	0:50	1:54	0:57	0:57	0:47	0:38	0:47
Personal care	0:44	0:44	0:45	0:46	0:46	0:51	0:50	0:52	0:49	0:55
Voluntary and religious activities	0:02	0:04	0:04	0:07	0:01	0:10	0:05	0:03	0:03	0:12
Free time	4:29	4:18	5:02	5:53	3:46	5:36	4:22	6:06	5:06	4:57
Watching TV and video	1:44	1:34	1:48	1:45	1:35	1:42	1:17	1:48	2:06	1:38
Social leisure	1:17	0:57	1:41	0:59	0:43	1:29	1:24	1:51	1:28	0:52
Physically active leisure	0:39	0:33	0:43	0:58	0:18	0:33	0:28	0:30	0:21	042
Reading	0:08	0:15	0:09	0:25	0:12	0:17	0:14	0:12	0:06	0:06
Movies, sports, culture	0:05	0:03	0:06	0:03	0:12	0:17	0:04	0:22	0:07	0:16
Computer & video games	0:09	0:14	0:05	0:21	0:14.	0:29	0:28	0:18	0:12	0:18
Internet & surfing the web	0:03	0:07	0:05	0:15	.	0:15	.	0:15	0:12	0:19
Other free and unspecified time	0:24	0:31.	0:26	1:00	0:33	0:31	0:27	0:45	0:36	0:35
Daily total	24:00	24:00	24:00	24:00	24:00	24:00	24:00	24:00	24:00	24:00

* Time use of 15- to 19-year-old teens, who reported 60 or more minutes of class time on the diary day. Differences in coding of travel time required adjustment of time allocated to leisure activities in Australia and the Netherlands. Eating did not include dining out in restaurants attributed to social leisure.

Personal hygiene and eating accounted for approximately three quarters of an hour each on school days. There was little time left for paid work, household help, volunteering and religion.

The third largest segment of the school day was allocated by teens to free-time activities. German, Finnish, and Norwegian students reported having access to 5.5–6 hours of free time on school days, the U.S., Canadian, and UK students to about 5 hours, and French students to fewer than 4 hours. The low figure of free time reported by the French students may be accounted for by cultural differences as well as differences in coding. The scarcity of free time was compensated by French teens with much longer sleep and eating time than in other countries. This trend was observed already in the 1992–1993 European Research Network study (Alsaker and Flammer, 1999).

Watching TV and socialising with friends occupied on school days about half of teens' free time. Participation in physically active pursuits and sports took only 20–30 minutes per day, with the exception of Finland, where it amounted to almost an entire hour.

Time use on weekends

Teens' weekend time use, as expected, differed from the time use on school days. Teens' involvement in paid labour, domestic work and shopping increased to 1.5–3 hours per day. Paid work on weekends was almost entirely absent among school-attending teens in Belgium, France, Germany and Finland, but in Norway and the Netherlands it averaged 1.5–2 hours. Higher amounts of paid labour were also reported by students in Australia, Canada and the US (Table 4.2).

The big difference between the time use on school days and weekend is apparent in the length of sleep. Teens in most countries compensated for a shorter sleep on school days by close to 10 hours of sleep on weekends (Paakkonen, 2005). Teens' free time on weekends almost doubled its amount on school days. In most countries, teens reported having on weekends access to approximately 8 hours of free time, with German students reporting as many as 9 hours and French teens as little as 7.3 hours.

The proportionate allocation of free time on weekends did not differ significantly from its distribution on school days. Watching TV and socialising with friends occupied over half of teens' weekend free time. The greatest amounts of TV viewing were reported in Finland, the U.S., UK and Australia (2.8–3 hours). Socialising with friends in most countries amounted to between 1.5 and 2 hours, with as little as 1.2 hours reported in the United States and over 3 hours in Norway, the Netherlands and Canada. Reading occupied less than 20 minutes in most countries on weekend days, with the US and UK teens reporting the lowest amounts – less than 10 minutes per day (Table 4.2).

Growing amounts of teens' free time began to be spent at the end of the 1990s on playing computer and video games and surfing the web. The size and the rising role of these two activities in the lives of the teens will be commented upon in the next section dealing with the historical trends in adolescent time use.

Physically active leisure and sports occupied on weekend days less than 1 hour of teens' time. Finnish and Canadian adolescents were physically most active, reporting 1.2–1.4 hours of sports and outdoors per day.

Gender differences in adolescent time use

Gender differences are remarkably similar across most of the surveyed countries. Boys spent somewhat more time than girls in classes, while girls spent more time doing homework. In

Table 4.2 Adolescent time use on weekend days: A cross-national comparison*

	Australia (1997)	Belgium (1999)	Canada (1998)	Finland (1999/00)	France (1998)	Germany (2001/02)	Netherlands (2000)	Norway (2000)	UK (2000)	USA (2003)
N=	367	359	128	328	340	242	99	47	162	688
School-related time	0:41	1:48	1:16	0:47	1:33	0:56	0:56	0:42	1:13	0:48
Paid work	2:12	0:05	1:21	0:19	0:04	0:14	1:55	1:27	1:18	0:58
Domestic work & shopping	1:42	1:31	1:14	1:28	1:32	1:16	1:00	1:10	1:26	1:35
Personal needs	11:38	12:11	11:15	12:12	13:30	12:12	12:05	11:43	12:02	12:15
Sleep	10:00	10:09	9:46	10:30	10:22	10:11	9:53	9:44	10:21	10:28
Eating	0:49	1:11	0:43	0:55	2:19	1:07	1:06	0:46	0:49	1:00
Personal care	0:49	0:48	0:46	0:46	0:49	0:54	1:00	0:51	0:52	0:47
Voluntary organizations	0:03	0:15	0:09	0:12	0:02	0:11	0:11	0:00	0:04	0:11
Religious activities	0:06	0:02	0:14	0:05	0:01	0:04	0:09	0:02	0:06	0:24
Free time	7:38	8:01	8:30	8:55	7:18	9:07	7:46	8:54	7:52	7:37
Watching TV and video	2:44	2:25	2:30	2:59	2:19	2:34	1:43	1:57	2:45	2:46
Listening to radio & music	0:07	0:15	0:08	0:31	.	0:21	0:14	0:08	0:18	0:11
Social leisure	1:48	2:15	3:07	1:40	1:38	2:14	3:07	3:22	2:41	1:13
Physically active leisure	1:04	0:55	1:27	1:12	0:58	0:41	0:48	0:54	0:40	0:58
Reading	0:17	0:23	0:12	0:27	0:19	0:24	0:17	0:14	0:09	0:08
Movies, sports, culture	0:19	0:32	0:30	0:18	0:29	0:41	0:17	0:48	0:20	0:32
Hobbies	0:09	0:12	0:03	0:11		0:15	0:10	0:07	0:07	
Rest & relaxation	0:23	0:17	0:02	0:15	0:06	0:09	0:16	0:20	0:14	0:13
Computer & video games	0:20	0:26	0:16	0:34	0:43	0:53	0:49	0:10	0:17	0:34
Internet, surfing the web	0:02	0:07	0:09	0:11		0:24		0:15	0:20	0:22
Other free or unspecified time	0:25	0:17.	0:02	0:26	.0:47	O:10	0:05	0:05	0:21.	0:54
Daily total	24:00	24:00	24:00	24:00	24:00	24:00	24:00	24:00	24:00	24:00

* Time use of 15- to 19-year-old teens attending school on weekend days. For coding of eating and adjustments of travel time, see footnote to Table 1.4.1.

most countries, boys spent more time working for pay, while girls spent, on average, 60–70 per cent more time in domestic activities. Girls also spent 1.5–2 times more time than boys on personal care (Zuzanek, 2005).

In all surveyed countries, boys reported having almost an hour more of free time than girls. The gap between boys' and girls' access to free time was the biggest in France and the Netherlands (20 per cent) and the smallest in the UK (9 per cent). Boys spent more time than girls watching television, engaging in sports and outdoor activities, playing computer and video games. Girls read more than boys and spent more time on hobbies (Blanke and Cornelißen, 2005; Glorieux *et al.*, 2005; Short, 2005; Soupourmas, 2005). The gender gap in sporting participation and computer use was rather large at the end of the 1990, but may have narrowed lately. In 2003, Ontario girls reported 34 minutes of surfing the internet, compared to boys' 37 minutes, that is, only 3 minutes less (Kleiber and Powell, 2003; Zuzanek, 2013).

Age differences in adolescents' time use

There is a strong cross-national similarity in how adolescents' age affects their allocation of time to most activities. Older adolescents spend more time doing homework and less time attending classes. In countries where adolescents work for pay, their workloads peak in the final years of school. At the ages of 12–14, students in Canada, the UK and the Netherlands reported virtually no involvement in paid work, while in the final years of schooling their weekly workloads amounted to 8, 9 and 15 hours respectively (Zuzanek, 2005).

In contrast to paid and domestic work, older adolescents report fewer hours of sleep and free time than their younger counterparts. In Canada, the night sleep of adolescents aged 18–19 was, on average, 1 hour shorter than among the 12–14-year-olds, and their free time 51 minutes shorter than of the 15–17-year-olds.

Playing computer and video games and participation in physically active leisure are probably most affected by age. Computer and video games are particularly popular among the 12–14-year-old boys. The interest in these activities subsides among older teens.

The decline of sports and outdoor participation among older adolescents is relatively modest in some countries, yet alarmingly steep in others. In Finland, the 17–19-year-olds reported only 12 per cent less time of physical activities than the 12–14-year-olds (Paakkonen, 2004), but in Canada the 18–19-years old Ontario teens reported in 2003 on school days only 24 minutes of physically active leisure, compared to 45 minutes of the 12–14-year-olds.

Time use in other countries

Larson and Verma (1999) compared time use of adolescents in developed industrial societies of Western Europe and North America with the time use of teens in developing countries and industrially advanced countries of Eastern Asia (Japan, Korea). They concluded that, in contrast to Western countries, teens in non–industrial populations allocate much more time to household labour. Time use of teens in Japan and Korea differed substantially from the time use of teens in the United States and Europe. In East Asia, schoolwork accounted for a third to a half of adolescents' waking hours, and much less time than in North America was spent on leisure activities. According to Larson and Verma (2004), European teens spend more time than their North American counterparts on homework but work less for pay. Time use by European youth thus represents, in the opinion of Larson and Verma, 'a middle course between the pattern for East Asian and North American adolescents' (p. 725).

Historical trends in adolescent time use

Cross-national analyses allow us to compare not only adolescents' current time use but also its changes over the past 15–20 years. Has adolescent time use in different countries evolved in a similar way? Can some conclusions be drawn from the past and present trends about the future directions of adolescent time use? These are some of the questions asked by parents, policy makers and the public at large. Analyses of time use trends in different countries require considerable caution, however, since one inevitably faces the difficult task of distinguishing between universal and country-specific trends, as well as counter-trends or quasi-trends resulting from measurement differences.

It seems that by the end of the 1990s and at the beginning of the 2000s, teens in most countries spent less time in class and doing homework than they did a decade earlier. In Canada, 15–19-year-old students' weekly school load was almost 4 hours shorter in 2010 than it was in 1992. In France, the school load shortened between 1986 and 1998 also by over 4 hours. In Finland, the decline from 1988–2000 was over 2 hours. Time spent by U.S. adolescents in school-related activities has also declined between 1981 and 2002 (Juster *et al.*, 2004). Germany appears to be an exception to this trend. German students reported almost 2 hours more of school-related time in 2001 than in 1991.

In some countries, reduced school loads were accompanied by greater participation in part-time paid work. There are social and economic reasons for increased levels of adolescents' labour participation. Paid work provides teenagers with discretionary money and contributes to their greater independence from parents. For the employers, students represent a relatively cheap source of flexible labour. Students' involvement in paid work increased in the 1990s in Norway and the Netherlands, but its levels often depend on the state of the economy. The low levels of students' job involvement in Finland, France and Germany are probably embedded in social policies, employment standards as well as historical and cultural traditions of these countries.

Adolescents' contribution to housework did not change much during the past two decades. If there were changes, they usually meant slightly less rather than more time spent in domestic work. Domestic work was cut short by 20 minutes in Germany, by around 15 minutes in Norway and the Netherlands and by 10 minutes in France.

The amount of time allocated by adolescents to eating declined virtually in all countries. Much of this drop was due to the diminished amount of eating at home. In 2005 and 2010, Canadian teens spent approximately 15 minutes less time per day eating meals at home than they did in the early 1990s. Norwegian and Dutch adolescents cut their meals at home during the 1990s by 5–7 minutes.

In some countries, adolescents shortened their night sleep. Norwegian and German students reported 10 minutes less of sleep in 2001 than they did at the beginning of the 1990s. In the United States, the shortening of sleep affected in particular the 12–14-year-old age group (Juster *et al.*, 2004). There is some evidence that this trend can be attributed to the late watching of TV and surfing the web.

In most surveyed countries, adolescents have, in the 1990s, retained or made small gains of free time. This applies to France, Finland and Australia. A question that has been often asked with regard to free time trends concerns the repertoire of adolescents' leisure choices. Has it changed over the years and, if so, how did it change in the surveyed countries? Most countries have seen over the past two decades of the twentieth century increases in adolescent television and video viewing. In Norway, watching television and videos increased between 1980 and 2000 by 40 minutes per day (Vaage, 2004). Increases in adolescents' television viewing in France, Finland, and Germany ranged from 14–17 minutes per day. In Canada, levels of television and video viewing peaked in the mid-1980s, but remained stable or declined slightly thereafter. A similar trend seems to have taken place in the Netherlands and, lately, in the United States (see Huysmans *et al.*, 2005; Juster *et al.*, 2004).

The late 1990s saw a dramatic rise of computer use among adolescents. Younger teenagers were attracted by computer and video games, while teenagers aged 15 and over spent growing amounts of time surfing the internet and participating in on-line chat groups. Time use surveys conducted in the late 1990s did not capture this phenomenon fully. General Social Survey data show that internet surfing among Canadian school-attending teens increased from 3 minutes in 1992 to 37 minutes in 2010. Playing computer and video games increased during this same period five-fold – from 6 minutes in 1992 to 32 minutes in 2010. Part of the time for computer games and internet may have been gained at the expense of television viewing (Table 4.3).

Other trends that are common to most surveyed countries include falling levels of social leisure and reading. In the late 1990s, adolescents in most countries reported less socialisation with friends and the family than they did in the 1980s. In countries where participation in social leisure has declined (Finland, Australia, U.S., Norway, Netherlands), this may have happened due to the re-channelling of free time from social activities to computer use or television viewing, or due to added hours of paid work.

The amount of reading reported in the late 1990s and at the beginning of the new millennium has also fallen compared to the levels reported in the 1980s. Norwegian adolescents reported only 15 minutes of reading in 2000, compared to 36 minutes in 1980 (Vaage, 2004). Dutch students' reading fell during the same period from 34–15 minutes per day, and Finnish students' from 46–26 minutes (Paakkonen, 2005). Canadian students' reading declined between 1981 and 2005 by 15 minutes. Ontario (2003) and U.S. (2003) data suggest, however, that this trend may have slowed down lately, perhaps due to the success of Harry Potter and electronic books.

Another trend that has serious life style and health implications is falling levels of participation in physically active leisure. Adolescents' participation in sports and outdoor activities declined in Germany, Norway, Australia, and the United States, and remained at approximately the same levels as in the late 1980s in France, Finland, and the Netherlands. In Germany, adolescents aged 15–19 spent 38 minutes per day in sports and outdoor activities in 2001, compared to 57 minutes in 1990. In Norway, teens' participation in physically active leisure fell between 1990 and 2000 by three quarters of an hour per week, and in Australia between 1992 and 1997 by approximately 20 minutes per week. In 1992, Canadian teens reported 65 minutes of physically active leisure per day, but by 2005 and 2010 this figure fell to 48 minutes.

Another concern brought to light by the time use surveys is growing amount of time spent by adolescents alone. In 1986, 15–19-year-old Canadian adolescents attending school spent 3.3 hours per day alone. In 2005, this figure has risen to 5 hours. This trend is associated, in part, with teens' rising use of mass and electronic media. According to the 2005 GSS time use survey, teens spent daily, past 6:00 pm, on average, 2.5 hours watching TV, surfing the web or playing computer and video games. Over 70 per cent of time was spent surfing the web or playing computer and video games, and almost 50 per cent of time spent watching TV were spent alone (Zuzanek, 2013).

Teens' time use, physical health and emotional well-being

According to Larson (2001), assessment of time spent in different activities provides a useful starting point for evaluating a population's set of developmental experiences (p. 160).

Table 4.3 Historical trends in teens' time use

	Canada 1992	Canada 2005	Canada 2010	Finland 1988	Finland 1999/00	Germany 1991	Germany 2001	Norway 1990	Norway 2000	France 1986	France 1998
N=	340	583	363	717	658	962	1024	238	160	559	1198
School-related time	5:32	5:22	5:04	4:41	4:23	4:32	4:48	5:15	5:31	5:01	4:23
Attending classes	3:12	3:17	3:08	3:24	3:10		3:11	3:45	3:52	4:25	3:56
Homework	1:14	1:05	1:04	0:50	0:43		0:51	0:53	0:59		
Travel to / from school	0:34	0:29	0:26	0:27	0:30	0:32	0:41	0:35	0:40	0:37	0:27
Paid work incl. travel	0:46	1:00	0:45	0:17	0:13	0:20	0:18	0:24	0:43	0:16	0:11
Domestic work incl. travel	0:51	0:51	0:50	1:11	1:20	1:29	1:08	1:25	1:10	1:19	1:09
Personal needs	10:15	10:23	10:34	10:47	10:43	10:38	10:33	10:07	9:56	11:07	11:26
Sleep	8:31	9:03	9:07	9:05	9:04	8:57	8:45	8:24	8:15	9:21	9:36
Eating	0:47	0:29	0:32	0:53	0:52	0:59	0:57	0:56	0:52	1:48	2:03
Personal care	0:51	0:42	0:48	0:48	0:47	0:42	0:51	0:47	0:50	0:58	0:47
Voluntary organizations	0:08	0:03	0:04	0:06	0:07	0:08	0:02	0:05	0:02	0:02	0:01
Religious activities	0:04	0:04	0:06	0:02	0:03			0:01	0:01	0:01	0:01
Free time	6:22	6:16	6:37	6:57	7:11	6:54	7:11	6:35	6:38	5:14	5:49
Watching TV and video	2:10	1:34	1:41	1:57	2:14	1:46	2:02	1:19	1:43	1:51	2:05
Social leisure	1:47	1:55	1:41	1:41	1:18	2:03	2:02	2:52	2:30	0:52	1:15
Physically active leisure	1:05	0:49	0:48	0:59	1:00	0:57	0:38	0:50	0:43	0:41	0:43
Reading	0:15	0:10	0:10	0:46	0:26	0:16	0:30	0:28	0:14	0:21	0:17
Movies, sports, culture	0:10	0:12	0:18	0:10	0:08	0:31	0:24	0:18	0:27	0:22	0:20
Hobbies	0:11	0:05	0:09	0:13	0:10	0:20	0:12	0:13	0:08		
Listening to radio, CD	0:11	0:04	0:02	0:27	0:22	0:16	0:13	0:16	0:08		
Rest and relaxation	0:03	0:10	0:28	0:06	0:13	0:11	0:08	0:06	0:11	0:05	0:07
Computer and video games	0:07	0:23	0:32		0:27		0:37		0:18		
Surfing the web, comp. use	0;04	0:38	0:37	0:08	0:13		0:20		0:16	1:00	
Other free & unspecified time				0:30	0:40	0:38	0:05	0:03			
Daily total	24:00	24:00	24:00	24:00	24:00	24:00	24:00	24:00	24:00	24:00	24:00

In the 1990s, a shift in reference group orientation from the parents to peers and growing amounts of time spent by adolescents in the presence of mass and electronic media signaled worrisome trends (Gecas and Seff, 1990). Adolescents' use of time became an issue of national concern. Emotional and academic implications of changing adolescents' time use practices became a focus of intense inquiry. After-school hours were identified as the time of risk (Larson, 2001). Research reports abounded with negative observations.

Adolescents' TV viewing unlike that of their parents' was diagnosed as a solo rather than a social activity (Saxbe *et al.*, 2011, p. 181). Time spent watching TV was held responsible for a decline of socialising with family and friends (Bickham and Rich, 2006). Watching TV more than 3–4 hours per day was associated with teens' lower grade averages (Larson, 2001). Frequent internet use was suspected of enforcing social isolation (Kraut *et al.*, 1998). Prolonged involvement with friends in unstructured activities correlated with greater risks of problem behaviours (Bartko and Eccles, 2003; Osgood *et al.*, 1996). Too little time allocated to homework jeopardised academic standing of North American students compared to students from other countries (Larson and Verma, 1999).

Developmental benefits and potential liabilities of time use varied, according to researchers, across uses and users, but in the end adolescents often chose entertaining rather than challenging activities, which put them at the risk of social and psychological disadvantage (Larson, 2001, p. 163).

Most problems with regard to the well-being effects of adolescent time use stem from the fact that some activities enjoyed by the teens are developmentally unchallenging and at times physically and emotionally problematic. Time use and ESM findings show that homework contributed to teens' better performance in school, but it correlated negatively with teens' emotional well-being. The conflict between the academic and emotional implications of teens' time use is also apparent with regard to free time. Leisure activities top the list of adolescents' favourite pursuits but greater access to free time is, according to ESM findings, associated with lower rather than higher grade averages.

According to Larson (2001), time spent by teens in structured voluntary activities, such as arts, sports, and organizations, fosters 'initiative, identity, and other positive developmental outcomes' (p. 160). Unstructured leisure, on the other hand, is often a waste of time in developmental terms.

Academic and emotional correlates of many leisure activities are bi-directional. Of four large groups of free time activities – watching TV, surfing the web, socialising with friends and participating in sports – only the last one was associated with positive emotional and academic outcomes. Socialising with friends and watching television correlated positively or neutrally with teens' emotional well-being, but were accompanied by lower grade averages in school. Surfing the web, while popular among adolescents, correlated negatively with both teens' academic performance and emotional well-being (Table 4.4).

In the 1980s and 1990s, relationships between time use and emotional well-being became a focus of numerous studies using ESM (Csikszentmihalyi and Larson, 1984, Csikszentmihalyi and Mai Ha-Wong, 1991; Csikszentmihalyi and Schneider, 2000; Larson and Richards, 1994). These studies documented that instantaneous valuations of daily activities sometimes conflicted with well-being effects of prolonged participation in the same activities. At the instantaneous beep level, watching TV and videos was assessed by the teens positively, but frequent watching of TV and videos was associated with lower affect scores. In short, generalised or momentary assessments of daily activities do not take into account that repeated exposure to the same activity can alter its initial emotional assessment. Observations that emotional outcomes of prolonged involvement in different activities may reverse their instantaneous ratings posed before researchers the problem of time balance.

Table 4.4 Well-being correlates of teens' time use (Pearson "r")

	2005 GSS – all days			2003 OATUS – school days			2003 ESM self-reports – weekly summation			
	Health (1–5)	Life satisfaction (1–10)	Feeling happy (1–4)	Grade average	Physically fit (1–5)	SWB	Grade average	Affect (1–7)	Anxiety (1–7)	Feeling challenged (0–9)
Homework	ns	-.07	-.07	.23	ns	-.08	.32	-.04	.18	.18
Watching TV and video	-.05	-.03	-.10	-.18	ns	ns	-.06	-.04	-.09	-.13
Socialising with friends	.06	.07	.09	-.17	ns	ns	ns	.10	ns	-.07
Physically active leisure	.14	.10	.13	.07	.21	.07	ns	.10	-.14	.28
Computer & video games	-.04	-.02	-.04	-.11	-.10	ns	ns	ns	-.06	.09
Internet / surfing the web	-.05	-.06	-.06	.08	ns	ns	-.29	-.21	.20	-.05

Time use of 15 to 19 years old teens attending school. In the 2003 OATUS, SWB was defined as a composite of feeling happy, sociable and not depressed (Alpha=.75) In 2003, ESM affect was defined as a composite of feeling happy, good and cheerful (Alpha=.83) and anxiety as feeling worried, upset and tense (Alpha=.84).

Policy implication of teens' time use trends

It is impossible in a short report to outline all policy implications of teens' time use. What follows are, therefore, five policy challenges that appear particularly serious in view of the observed time use trends.

The high cost of sleep deficit

Health research suggests that adolescents need 8–9 hours of sleep to perform well at school and in life generally (Caerscadon, 1990). Yet in a number of countries (Finland, Norway), students slept less than 8 hours on school days and in some countries, the amounts of teens' sleep declined over the past decade. ESM findings suggest that 27 per cent of Ontario students slept fewer than 7 hours on school days and 14 per cent went to bed after midnight.

The length of sleep – particularly on school days – negatively affects adolescents' emotional well-being and health. Students, who slept fewer than 7 hours on school days reported higher levels of perceived time pressure and stress and lower levels of self-assessed health than students who slept longer hours. Going early to bed, on the other hand, was associated with less time pressure, less fatigue on the way to school and fewer emotional problems (Zuzanek, 2005).

Doing things together as a family

The importance of doing things together as a family in the lives of teens is best illustrated by the consistency of findings about positive emotional outcomes of family dinners. Joint suppers and meals synchronise family life and provide an opportunity for informal face-to-face communication. Keeping this tradition alive in a rapidly desynchronising world serves as an instrument of social cohesion and contributes to teens' emotional well-being. Correlation between eating together with parents and teens' emotional well-being in the 2003 home-based ESM questionnaire was 0.33. It is symptomatic that taking personal interaction out of the family meals nullifies their positive impact. Having TV turned on during the family supper reversed positive relationship between having a meal and emotional well-being of the teens to -.09 (Feldman *et al.*, 2007; Offer, 2013; Zuzanek, 2013). In this regard, there is a difference between being together and doing things together. The feeling of togetherness requires that the 'minds meet' and that 'closeness is shared' (Larson and Richards, 1994, p. 8). Regular family suppers, joint involvement in sporting and outdoor activities, and attendance of cultural events in the company of parents contribute to teens' sense of feeling good and happy. Joining parents for shopping or watching TV has, on the other hand, little or no effect on teens' subjective well-being (Zuzanek, 2013).

Mass and electronic media: dangers of sedentary lifestyles

Rising rates of overweight and obesity among adolescents in Canada, the United States and throughout the industrialized world represent a major health and policy challenge. Adolescents' excessive media exposure and the expansion of sedentary lifestyles raised risks of obesity (The Henry J. Kaiser Family Foundation, 2004; Tjepkema and Shields, 2005). OATUS time diary data show that *obese* teens spent on school days 35 per cent more time watching TV and almost double the time playing computer and video games than *normal weight* teens (Hilbrecht and Zuzanek, 2005). It should not be surprising, therefore, that along with nutrition, sedentary lifestyles and mass media are most frequently named as contributing factors to obesity (Schneider, 2000).

Adolescents' sports and well-being: men's sana in corpore sano

Teens' participation and interest in sporting activities is positively associated with teens' well-being and health. Physically active leisure is associated with greater time use satisfaction, fewer emotional problems and a happier outlook of life. OATUS data testify to the fact that, of all leisure pursuits, sporting activities generate most positive emotional outcomes. A comparison of the emotional texture of participation in sporting activities with that of watching TV suggests that both activities are perceived by teens as interesting and enjoyable, but watching TV was seen as unchallenging and unimportant while the opposite was true of sports and outdoor activities (Table 4.4).

Of time use balance

Analyses of time diaries and ESM self-reports show that relationships between teens' time use and subjective well-being are often curvilinear rather than linear and the emotional outcomes of involvement in these activities depend on the amount of time allocated to them. Conflicting conclusions with regard to the well-being effects of different activities are caused, among others, by ignoring their duration. Put simply, the emotional connotations of the same activities, such as watching TV or socialising with friends, could change from positive to negative if pursued excessively rather than moderately.

OATUS teens, who reported having more than 10 hours of free time on Sundays (upper 25 per cent of the sample) or little or no free time at all felt less happy than teens, whose free time amounted to 6–10 hours (middle 50 per cent of the sample). A similar observation applies to socialising with friends. Teens, who reported socialising in excess of 2 hours on school days or in excess of 5 hours on Sundays, and teens, who reported none or minimal socialising felt less happy than teens reporting moderate levels of socialising. There is also some evidence that too much sporting may negatively affect teens' academic performance (Zuzanek, 2009).

Findings reported in this chapter demonstrate that concerns with adolescents' health and well-being require greater attention to be paid not only to physically active leisure but to adolescents' overall patterns of daily life, including sleep, eating habits, mass media consumption, extra-curricular activities as well as relationships with parents and peers. Not just expanding participation in one particular group of activities, but rather a balanced use of time is at the core of adolescents' physical, emotional and intellectual well-being. A balanced use of time rather than an exponential growth of selective activities is at the root of higher quality of teens' life (Zuzanek, 2009). The everlasting dilemma of the ant and the grasshopper, or the emotionally pleasing as opposed to physically and intellectually challenging use of time, is not so much a dilemma about the choice of activities as it is about the proportionate distribution of time allocated to these activities.

Note

1 The 2003 OATUS/ESM survey was directed by Jiri Zuzanek (principal investigator) and Roger Mannell, and supported by grants from the Social Sciences and Humanities Research Council of Canada and Canadian Institute for Health Information (CIHI). The author would like to thank all participants of the Comparative study of adolescent time use, funded by CIHI and associated with the International Association for Time Use Research (IATUR) for collecting and standardising the data that were used in this chapter. These thanks are extended to Karen Blanke, Andries van den Broek, Alain Chenu, Waltraub Cornelißen, Ignace Glorieux, Frank Huysmans, Margo Hilbrecht, Laurent Lesnard, Roger Mannell, Hannu Paakkonen, Sandra Short, Faye Soupourmas, Odd Vaage, Jessie Vandeweyer, Margaret Vernon and Elke Zeijl.

References

Alsaker, F.D. and Flammer, A. (eds) (1999). *The Adolescent Experience: European and American Adolescents in the 1990s*. Hillsdale, NJ: Lawrence Erlbaum Associates.

Bartko, W.T. and Eccles, J.S. (2003) Adolesecent participation in structured and unstructured activities: A person-oriented analysis. *Journal of Youth and Adolescence, 32(4)*, 233–241.

Bickham, D. and Rich, M. (2006) Is television viewing associated with social isolation? Roles of exposure time, viewing context, and violent content. *Archives of Paediatric and Adolescent Medicine, 160*, 387–392.

Blanke, K. and Cornelißen, W. (2005) German adolescents' time use from 1991 to 2001: Is gender symmetry in sight? *Loisir et Société/Society and Leisure, 28(2)*, 511–530.

Caerscadon, M.A. (1990). Patterns of sleep and sleepiness in adolescents. *Pediatrician, 17*, 5–12.

Csikszentmihalyi, M. and Larson, R. (1984). *Being Adolescent*. New York: Basic Books.

Csikszentmihalyi, M. and Larson, R. (1987). Validity and reliability of the Experience Sampling Method. *Journal of Nervous and Mental Disease, 175(9)*, 526–37.

Csikszentmihalyi, M. and Mai Ha-Wong, M. (1991) The situational and personal correlates of happiness: A cross national comparison; in Strack, F., Argyle, M. and Schwarz, N. (eds) *Subjective Well-being: An Interdisciplinary Perspective*. Oxford: Pergamon Press. 193–212.

Csikszentmihalyi, M, and Schneider, B. (2000). *Becoming Adult. How Teenagers Prepare for the World of Work*. New York: Basic Books.

Dietz, W.H. (1998). Health consequences of obesity in youth: Childhood predictors of adult disease. *Pediatrics, 101(3)*, 518–525.

Feldman, S., Eisenberg, M., Neumark-Steiner, D. and Sory, M. (2007) Association between watching TV during family meals and dietary intake among adolescents. *Journal of Nutrition Education and Behaviour, 29(5)*, 257–263.

Gecas, V. and Seff, M.A. (1990) Families and adolescents: Review of the 1980s. *Journal of Marriage and the Family, 34*, 627–634.

Glorieux, I., Stevens, F. and Vandeweyer, J. (2005). Time use and well-being of Belgian adolescents: Research findings and time use evidence. *Loisir et Société/Society and Leisure 28(2)*, 481–510.

Hilbrecht, M. and Zuzanek, J.(2005). Adolescent time use, eating habits, and obesity. *Loisir et Société/Society and Leisure, 28(2)*, 611–631.

Hofferth, S. and Sandberg, J. (2001). How American children spend their time. *Journal of Marriage and Family, 63(2)*, 295–308.

Huysmans, F., Zeijl, E. and van den Broek, A. (2005). Adolescents' leisure and well-being in the Netherlands: Trends and correlates. *Loisir et Société/Society and Leisure 28(2)*, 531–548.

Juster, F.T., Ono, H. and Stafford, F.P. (2004). *Changing Times of American Youth*. Ann Arbor: Institute for Social Research.

King, A., Wold, B., Tudor-Smith, C. and Harel, Y. (1996). *The Health of Youth: A Cross-national Survey*. Copenhagen: WHO.

Kleiber, D.A. and Powell, G.M. (2005). Historical change in leisure activities during after-school hours; in J.L. Mahoney, R.W. Larson, and J.S. Eccles (eds). *Organized Activities as Contexts of Development* (pp. 23–43). Mahwah, N.J.: Lawrence Erlbaum Associates.

Kraut, R., Patterson, M., Lundmark, V., Kiesler, S. Mukhopadhyay, T. and Sherlis, W. (1998) Internet paradox. A social technology that reduces social involvement and psychological well-being. *American Psychologist 53(9)*, 1017–1031.

Larson, R. (2001). How US children and adolescents spend time: What it does (and doesn't) tell us about their development. *American Journal of Community Psychology, 29(4)*, 565–597.

Larson, R. and Richards, M. (1994). *Divergent Realities: The Emotional Lives of Mothers, Fathers, and Adolescents*. New York: Basic Books.

Larson, R. and Verma, S. (1999) How children and adolescents spend time across the world: Work, play, and developmental opportunities. *Psychological Bulletin, 125(6)*, 701–736.

Millstein, S.G., Petersen, A.C. and Nightingale, E.O. (eds). (1993). *Promoting the Health of Adolescents. New Directions for the Twenty-first Century*. New York: Oxford University Press.

Offer, S. (2013). Assessing the relationship between family mealtime communication and adolescent emotional well-being using the experience sampling method, *Journal of Adolescence 36*, 577–585.

Osgood, D.W., Wilson, J.K., O'Malley, P.M., Bachman, J.G. and Johnston, L.D. (1996). Routine activities and individual deviant behaviour. *American Sociological Review, 61*, 635–655.

Ozer, E.M., Macdonald, T. and Irwin, C.E. (2002). Adolescent health care in the United States: Implications and projections for the new millennium; in J.T. Mortimer and R. Larson (eds). *The Changing Adolescent Experience*. Cambridge: Cambridge University Press.

Paakkonen, H. (2004) Teens' time use trends in Finland (working tables sent to me by H. Paakkonen (Statistics Finland) as part of the comparative study of adolescent time use).

Paakkonen, H. (2005) What do schoolchildren in Finland do with their time? *Loisir et Société/Society and Leisure, 28(2)*, 425–442.

Robinson, J. and Converse, P. (1972). Social change as reflected in the use of time; in A. Campbell, and P. Converse (eds) *The Human Meaning of Social Change*. New York: Russell Sage Foundation, 17–86.

Saxbe D., Graesh, A. and Alvik, M. (2011). Television as a social or solo activity: Understanding families' everyday television viewing patterns. *Communication Research Reports, 28(2)*, 180–189.

Schneider, D. (2000). International trends in adolescent nutrition. *Social Science and Medicine, 51(6)*, 955–967.

Short, S. (2005). Adolescents' health and well-being in the United Kingdom. *Loisir et Société/Society and Leisure 28(2)*, 591–610.

Soupourmas, F. (2005). Work, rest and leisure – trends in late adolescent time use in Australia in the 1990s. *Loisir et Société/Society and Leisure 28(2)*, 571–590.

The Henry J. Kaiser Family Foundation (2004). *The Role of Media in Childhood Obesity – Issue Brief* (Report No 7030). Menlo Park: CA.

Tjepkema, M. and Shields, M. (2005). *Measured Obesity: Overweight Canadian Children and Adolescents* (Report No 82–620-MWE2005001). Ottawa: Statistics Canada.

Vaage, O.F. (2004) Adolescent time use trends in Norway (working tables sent to me as part of the comparative study of adolescent time use).

Vaage, O.F. (2005). Adolescent time use trends in Norway. *Loisir et Société/Society and Leisure 28 (2)*, 443–460.

Wabitsch, M. (2000). Overweight and obesity in European children: definition and diagnostic procedures, risk factors and consequences for later health outcome. *European Journal of Pediatrics, September; 159 Suppl. 1*, 8–13.

Zuzanek, J. (2005). Adolescent time use and well-being from a comparative perspective. *Loisir et Société/Society and Leisure 28(2)*, 379–421.

Zuzanek, J. (2009). Time use imbalances: Developmental and emotional costs; in K. Matuska and C. Christiansen, *Life Balance: Biological, Psychological and Sociological Perspectives on Lifestyle and Health*. Bethesda: AOTA Press. 207–222.

Zuzanek, J. (2013). Do parents matter? Teens' time use, academic performance and well-being. Paper presented at the Workshop on children's time diaries, London, UK (10–11 June, 2013).

5

YOUTH, SPORT AND LEISURE CAREERS

David Haycock and Andy Smith

Introduction

In very many countries, there has been a longstanding interest among academics, policy makers, politicians, the media and other interested parties in the lives of young people. This is not surprising for, as Furlong (2013: 5) has noted, 'there is always a high level of interest in young people when they are perceived to be a problem' whether as a consequence of their threat to social order (e.g. through urban disorders), their engagement in so-called risk activities (e.g. via the use of legal and illegal drugs) and their contribution to social integration and economic competitiveness and efficiency (e.g. in terms of rates of unemployment and labour market supply and demand). To this might be added young people's participation in sport and other uses of leisure, both of which are often bound-up in discussions about the *state* of youth and their lifestyles (most notably in relation to health and well-being). In addition, there is an almost irresistible tendency to regard young people and their lifestyles as both a cause of, and a solution to, declines in regular sport participation and engagement in leisure pursuits that are considered unhealthy to individuals, their communities and the wider society.

The focus of this chapter, however, is young people's participation in sport and leisure and their careers in these domains. More particularly, we will examine some of the benefits, and some of the challenges, of studying young people's lives biographically and longitudinally and how such an approach has a number of advantages for researchers interested in making sense of youth, sport and leisure careers. In doing so, we shall argue that because 'there has long been a tendency to study (interrelated) aspects of people's lives – and, for that matter, people themselves in isolation' (Green 2014a: 160), a vital pre-requisite of any analysis of young people's lives involves locating these within the complex interdependencies to which they belonged in the past, and continue to form in the present. While such an approach might seem axiomatic to sociologists of sport and leisure, 'most of the literature on young people and physical activity ignores the complexity and diversity of young people's lives' (Wright and MacDonald 2010: 1). In other words, many studies fail frequently to take into account how young people's choices and participation in activities such as sport and leisure 'are made in the context of their personal biographies and the political, economic, cultural and geographical contexts of their everyday lives' (Wright and MacDonald 2010: 2). In this chapter, we shall argue that two dimensions of youth biographies – habitus formation and capital development – are among the key processes that need to be better understood if we are to make more adequate sociological sense of the reality of young people's sporting and leisure lives, and the contexts in which their lives are enacted.

Longitudinal studies of (young) people's lives

In many countries, there are several large-scale longitudinal studies that seek to explain the ways in which people's lives change across the life course, including changes that occur in their personal biographies and in the structure of the societies of which they are a part. In Britain, the British Household Panel Survey, which began in 1991, is among the most well-known investigations and was conducted annually before being replaced in 2010 by *Understanding Society*, a *UK Household Longitudinal Study* that reports annual data on the social and economic circumstances, attitudes, health and behaviours of representative samples of individuals drawn from across the UK (Institute for Social and Economic Research [IESR] 2015). For adults aged sixteen and above, these survey data include participation in various leisure activities, current and future labour market aspirations, experiences of education, family and other social relationships, and health-related lifestyle behaviours (e.g. diet, drinking, smoking, and mental well-being) (IESR 2015). Modified versions of the survey are also undertaken with ten- to fifteen-year-olds that permit detailed analysis of various uses of leisure including media use, sport participation and other markers of well-being (including mental health) (e.g. Booker *et al.* 2015).

Other longitudinal studies include the 1970 British Cohort Study (BCS70), which follows the lives of just under 17,200 people born in England, Scotland and Wales in a single week of 1970. Currently managed by the Centre for Longitudinal Studies (CLS) at the Institute of Education in London, the BCS70 provides important insights on how participants' lives have changed, including in relation to their health, physical, educational and social development, as well as their socio-economic circumstances (CLS 2015a). The CLS also retains responsibility for Next Steps (formerly known as the Longitudinal Study of Young People in England [LSYPE]), which began in 2004 when approximately 16,000 cohort members were 13–14-years old. As with the BCS70, Next Steps provides information on, and investigates the relationships between, several inter-related features of young people's lives such as their education and employment, their economic circumstances and family life, their physical and emotional heath and wellbeing, and their social participation and attitudes (e.g. CLS 2015b; Department for Education, 2011). In this regard, Next Steps is similar to the multi-disciplinary Millennium Cohort Study, which follows the lives of approximately 19,000 children born in the UK in 2000–01, and explores the influence of family contexts on a whole range of outcomes throughout childhood, into adolescence and subsequently through adulthood. These include: parenting styles and behaviour; child behaviour and cognitive development; child and parental health; parents' employment and education; income and poverty; and social capital and ethnicity (CLS 2015c).

These kinds of panel studies yield significant insights into how people's lives unfold from childhood to youth and into adulthood, can help identify change at the individual and aggregate levels, and the data generated by such studies are publically available via the UK Data Archive for further investigation. In this regard, longitudinal investigations such as the UK Household Longitudinal Study, BCS70 and Next Steps (as well as their international equivalents) are particularly useful for researchers interested in understanding the interdependence between various features of people's lives as they get older, though they remain a much under utilized resource in sociological studies of youth sport and other leisure activities. This may in part be a reflection of researchers' preferences for other approaches and methods, but it is also the case that undertaking detailed panel studies are typically expensive, generate often largely quantitative data the full implications of which can take a long time to be published, and such studies are frequently beset by a range of methodological difficulties (like all methods) including participant attrition. In the next section, we consider another approach – known as the retrospective method – to the study of youth sport and leisure careers, which, while suffering serious recall problems, can 'yield fast results which appear realistic, particularly for structured, time-bounded leisure activities . . . and can plot both individual and aggregate changes' (Roberts *et al.*, 2009: 265) in the activities being studied, including sport participation. Another advantage of this approach, Roberts *et al.* (2009: 265–66) argue, is that it 'avoids biases due to sample attrition (which plague panel studies), and it also avoids the complications that historical change can inject into cross-sectional snapshots covering successive age groups'.

Studying youth leisure careers biographically and longitudinally

Although there are important exceptions (e.g. Aldridge *et al.*, 2011; Hendry *et al.*, 1993; Hendry *et al.*, 2002; MacDonald and Shildrick, 2007), the value of injecting a longitudinal, biographical dimension into studies of young people's leisure has often been overlooked (Roberts *et al.* 2009). Researchers have instead most often been concerned with generating cross-sectional data that permit the comparison of 'participation rates in different leisure activities, purchasing patterns and sub-cultural affiliations (if any) in different socio-demographic groups' (Roberts *et al.*, 2009: 262). Where a longitudinal, biographical dimension has been deployed in investigations of young people's leisure careers, this has typically been in relation to single leisure activities such as drug use (e.g. Aldridge *et al.*, 2011; MacDonald and Shildrick, 2007; Parker *et al.*, 1998; Parker *et al.*, 2002). The findings of studies that have examined drug use as an aspect of youth leisure careers have concluded that drug-using biographies need to be understood in terms of the 'processual, longer-term, complex and multi-dimensional nature of young people's transitions to adulthood' (MacDonald and Shildrick, 2007: 342). This is because, for many young people, the use of illicit drugs has been shown to be an experimental and fleeting activity that does not always become a part of their adult lives despite earlier experience of drugs, while for others drug use may become a more or less established feature of their repertoire of adult leisure activities and is most often related to earlier life circumstances (e.g. Aldridge *et al.*, 2011; MacDonald and Shildrick, 2007; Parker *et al.*, 1998; Parker *et al.*, 2002).

In their study of working-class youth in Teesside, north-east England, MacDonald and Shildrick (2007) noted that illegal drug use by a minority of young people who spent much of their adolescent leisure with friends on street corners in their home estates was partly a consequence of the long-term unemployment and poverty that characterized the region, and the material and social circumstances that characterize their engagement in other forms of leisure (MacDonald and Shildrick 2007). MacDonald and Shildrick (2007) concluded that the pursuit of exciting, masculinising and status-enhancing forms of leisure among some males led them to engage in long-term commitment to local, street-based networks where crime, drug use and social exclusion characterized their emergent leisure careers and identities. For many other young people, drug use did not become an established feature of their later leisure careers. This led the authors to conclude that the use of illegal drugs (in common with many other forms of leisure) can only be adequately understood in the context of young people's 'shifting and differentiated leisure experiences and associations' (MacDonald and Shildrick, 2007: 350) that accompany their transitions from childhood to youth and into adulthood (Aldridge *et al.*, 2011).

Whether in relation to drug use or other activities including sport participation, investigations of youth leisure careers help identify how childhood and youth are significant life-stages when young people typically experiment with uses of leisure, most often in the company of peer groups, and for various reasons including the construction and development of their leisure tastes, skills and interests, which provide the foundations for adult leisure (Hendry *et al.* 1993; Roberts and Brodie, 1992; Roberts *et al.*, 2009). In this regard, studies of youth leisure that incorporate a longitudinal and biographical dimension in their research designs can assist in the investigation of young people's participation in activities that are finely age graded, while shedding light on their often experimental uses of leisure. As Roberts *et al.* (2009: 262) have noted 'mature 16–17-year-olds do not wish to hang around with 13–14-year-old kids, while 19–20-year-old young adults do not seek membership of crowds dominated by the 16–17-year-olds. Also, we know that young people's leisure is chronically unstable, more so than the leisure of any other age group. Young people are the experimenters and dabblers. They take up and drop activities in quick succession. Thereafter, in adulthood, leisure tastes and behaviour tend to stabilize.'

Adopting a biographical and career approach also helps capture some of the ways in which uses of leisure 'contribute to any progressive widening or narrowing of social divisions between the sexes, ethnic groups and social classes' (Roberts *et al.*, 2009: 262) as young people grow up and their future destinations become clearer. As MacDonald and Shildrick (2007) have demonstrated in their work with socially excluded youth, this research approach has been shown to be particularly useful in identifying how various leisure practices (such as the use of illegal drugs) may contribute to narrowing or widening the social distance between groups of young people from different social classes as they make the transition towards adulthood. More recent work by the authors – conducted with twenty families in Glasgow (Scotland), Middlesbrough (north-east England) – has also revealed very clearly the persistent (and often corrosive) impact of social class on the lives of those in some of the most deprived communities in the UK (e.g. Shildrick and MacDonald, 2013; Shildrick *et al.*, 2012). The present-day experiences of poverty and work recalled by the participants (especially those aged 21 and over) were intimately connected to experiences when they were young and growing up in families living in similar circumstances (e.g. Shildrick and MacDonald, 2013; Shildrick *et al.*, 2012). Becoming 'entrapped in long-term churning between insecure, low paid jobs and unemployment' (Shildrick and MacDonald, 2013: 286), otherwise known as the 'low-pay, no-pay cycle' (Shildrick and MacDonald, 2013: 286), was to a large extent structured by their social position and had a significant impact on how the participants spent their leisure. How social divisions such as social class can help explain variations in leisure (and related) behaviour in individual life stages, and between successive life-stages over the life course (e.g. from childhood to youth, and into young adulthood and later life), are thus among the additional advantages of the career-oriented and biography-focused approach to leisure research.

Youth sport careers and biographies

Youth as a key life-stage

Other studies in which leisure biographies and careers have been investigated have included those of sport participation, most usually among adults (Birchwood *et al.*, 2008; Lunn, 2010; Lunn *et al.*, 2013; Roberts and Brodie, 1992; Roberts *et al.*, 1991) and, to an extent, young people (Haycock, 2015; Wright *et al.*, 2003). One of the most significant longitudinal studies that has examined the sport and leisure careers of adults was Roberts' and Brodie's (1992) *Inner-City Sport*, a four-year investigation that began in 1986 and involved 4,354 adult sport participants (age 16 and over) who participated in seven sports (badminton, indoor bowls, keep fit, martial arts, snooker, football, and weights) at forty-six indoor centres in six United Kingdom cities. As part of its panel design, the study incorporated over three rounds of fieldwork in which a variety of methods (including health and fitness measurements, questionnaires, and interviews) were deployed to generate data on each participant's social background, including their sport participation, education, employment, diet, smoking and alcohol consumption, and engagement in other leisure activities (Roberts 2014; Roberts and Brodie, 1992).

As Roberts (2014: 151) has noted, the advantages of employing a panel design in social science research (such as *Inner-City Sport*) 'usually lie not so much in the longitudinal character of the evidence that can be collected as in the sheer quantity of information that can be obtained from each respondent'. In the case of *Inner-City Sport*, the information gathered shed new light on the long-term construction of adults' sport careers, on how adult sport careers were based upon foundations laid during youth, and on how engagement in sport up to the participants' mid-30s could be understood with reference to changes occurring in the youth life-stage and in other uses of leisure (Roberts, 2014; Roberts and Brodie, 1992). In each of these regards, the panel design employed in the study not only enabled the researchers to identify the well-known impacts of social divisions (especially gender and social class) on participation, but it also enabled them to report a number of unanticipated findings that perhaps would have otherwise remained unknown had other research designs been used, and had such detailed information of sport biographies not been collected. For example, the panel design employed in *Inner-City Sport* enabled the researchers to identify the many varied and complex changes that occurred in sport participation between 1987 and 1988, and 'revealed far more volatility in people's sporting lives than had previously been indicated' (Roberts 2014: 151). Such volatility was observed not only in relation to the frequency of participation, but also the mixes and numbers of sports that people played and how these served to effectively lock people into, or away from, sport participation as they were negotiating the transitions towards adulthood (Roberts, 2014; Roberts and Brodie, 1992). As Roberts has noted:

> The starkest conclusion to be drawn was that by their late 20s most people were either locked in or locked out of sport. Virtually everyone had played some sport regularly while they were at secondary school. Afterwards there was a steady and steep drop-out which leveled off among those who were still playing in their mid-20s. They were most likely to remain regular players for many more years. Those who had dropped out, in contrast, were unlikely to return and resume playing on a regular basis.
>
> *(Roberts, 2014: 151)*

As other studies have since indicated (e.g. Birchwood *et al.*, 2008; Lunn *et al.*, 2013; Pot *et al.*, 2014; Scheerder *et al.*, 2005; Stuij, 2015), the findings of *Inner-City Sport* revealed that drop-out from sport participation during leisure occurs in all age groups but that the heaviest drop-out is often in youth and young adulthood, and many people fail to participate at all, or on a regular basis, thereafter. Although there are important socio-cultural exceptions to this general trend which have been identified in countries such as Norway (e.g. Green *et al.*, 2013), youth-based drop-out from sport, the changing nature of participation, and the activities undertaken during the transition from youth to young adulthood were strongly related to the individualization of people's overall lifestyles and to their current life stages (Roberts, 2014; Roberts and Brodie, 1992). Indeed, as Green (2014a: 162) has noted, the findings of *Inner-City Sport* were particularly significant because they began to hint at what has since 'become recognized as the individualization of young people's lives and their leisure and sporting biographies in particular'. The individualization of sporting and leisure biographies, which occurs in the context of their increasing interdependence with many other people as their lives unfold, often finds particular expression in the mixes of sports that people play during youth and, in particular, adulthood. For many participants in Roberts' and Brodie's study (1992), engagement in full versions of team games (such as football and hockey) remained popular until the end of statutory schooling when these highly structured activities became less organizationally convenient than their derivatives (e.g. 5-a-side football), and less prominent features of their adult sport careers (Haycock and Smith 2014a, 2014b; Lunn *et al.*, 2013). Many adults whose sport careers were longer running were also more likely to begin engaging in more flexible, partner and individually orientated sports (e.g. squash and badminton) and 'lifestyle activities' (e.g. swimming and multi-gym) that could be accommodated within broader changes in their leisure lifestyles and were more likely to survive the transition into young adulthood (Haycock and Smith, 2014a, 2014b; Roberts, 2014; Roberts and Brodie, 1992). These adults' sport careers, it should be noted, remained relatively undisrupted 'largely as a result of experiences in sport during childhood and youth' (Roberts and Brodie, 1992: 41), and particularly the range and experience of sports they played regularly during the course of early sport socialization. We shall return to the significance of early socialization experiences for the construction of sport and leisure careers later, but it is first worth briefly exploring two significant predictors of sport participation associated with social class which help explain unequal propensities in levels, rates and patterns of sport participation during adulthood: education and income.

Education, income and social class

Income and education have been shown internationally to have a significant impact on sport participation (absolutely and relatively), and those from the higher socio-economic groups and those who have higher educational qualifications were more likely to be present-day and future sport participants than those who leave education once they reach the minimum school-leaving age (e.g. Coalter, 2007, 2013; Farrell *et al.*, 2014; Lunn *et al.*, 2013; van Tuyckom and Scheerder, 2010). Commenting on the importance of educational experience for sport participation and the construction of sport careers in Ireland, Lunn *et al.* (2013: ix) have argued that whether 'people remain active across their lifetimes is not primarily determined by whether they are active as children, but by transitions that occur as they grow up, mature and progress through adulthood'. In other words, as Lunn *et al.*, (2013: ix) have noted, 'the overall level of participation in sport and physical exercise among the population of Ireland is not determined by how active our children are, important though that is, but by what happens to them as they progress through life'. For Lunn *et al.* (2013: 97), there is said to be a 'sporting advantage associated with staying on longer in full-time education', and that educational transitions (particularly to HE) have an enduring impact on sport participation so that higher participation rates are consistently reported by the most highly educated from late adolescence onwards.

The links between levels of income, standards of education and other privileges associated with belonging to the higher social classes are well established, and can be effectively demonstrated when a longitudinal, biographical dimension is injected into studies of youth sport careers which employ the retrospective method. This is because, as Roberts (2003: 27) has noted, youth research 'needs to be longitudinal in perspective even when the methods are snapshot. Youth is an inherently transitional life stage, so all studies need to engage with how their subjects' lives are changing'. When examined in this way, however, it has been tentatively suggested that while educational experiences and class-related income (among other social divisions) are important predictors of youth (and adult) sport participation, the degree to which they impact on the construction of sport careers may to a large extent depend on other experiences obtained during childhood. For example, in their study of thirty-one- to thirty-seven-year-olds' sport careers in the three South Caucasus countries, Birchwood *et al.* (2008: 284) have suggested that although social class and length of time spent in education are thought to make an independent differ-ence to present-day participation rates and the construction of longer-term sport careers, the extent to which they do so may 'depend on predispositions that have been formed earlier in life, and the standard predisposition within a sociodemographic group will explain the rate change – whether overall this is upwards or downwards'. In this regard, Birchwood *et al.* (2008: 291) argued that although experiences of HE may be important, the higher rates of pre-university sport participation reported among HE students compared to non-university students meant that the length of time spent in education (at least at university) could not adequately explain present-day differences in sport participation. In fact, as students progressed through HE, the difference between their sport participation and those of non-graduates narrowed, rather than widened, as might be expected while participation among graduates declined more steeply from age sixteen than non-graduates (Birchwood *et al.*, 2008). These observations led Birchwood *et al.* to hypothesize that

> unlike in the South Caucasus, there will be a direct higher education effect on sport participation in countries where sport provisions in universities are more generous, of a higher standard, and where sport plays a more prominent role in student lifestyles than in Eastern Europe and the former Soviet Union, where students have remained home-based whenever possible and where universities have been and remain more narrowly academic institutions than in most western countries, especially the UK and North America.
>
> *(Birchwood* et al.*, 2008: 291)*

In addition, they commented that although 'more generous western provisions may trigger higher sport participation' (Birchwood *et al.*, 2008: 291), the major source of differences in participation was related to 'a distinct and enduring propensity to play sport [that] is acquired during childhood via a culture transmitted by the family', which is relatively independent of the social class of families, and that the propensity to play sport is similar to the propensity acquired to progress through HE. It was the cultural dimensions of family environments that were identified as being the crucial source of young adults' predispositions to take part in sport, and which helped sustain the unequal propensities to participate over the life course (Birchwood *et al.* 2008). These predispositions, they argued, were relatively fixed by age sixteen, were relatively independent of the social class of families and were largely 'a product of childhood socialization in the family' (Birchwood *et al.*, 2008: 293). Thus, it was concluded that even though more generous university sports provisions may generate independent effects on rates of participation, this is only likely to be observed among students who are appropriately predisposed to do so and who benefitted from childhood sport socialization during family leisure (Birchwood *et al.*, 2008).

A similar and more recent study was conducted in England by Haycock (2015) who investigated the development of 124 twenty- to twenty-five-year-old undergraduate students' present-day sport and leisure participation via a retrospective analysis of their sport and leisure careers. The study employed a cross-sectional, mixed-methods research design incorporating structured and semi-structured interviews held at two universities in England between March and July 2011. In light of the foregoing discussion about the significance of HE for helping to generate unequal propensities for sport participation during youth and adulthood, the study sought to explain why, in Britain, the rates of sport participation among the general population, including young people, have remained relatively static despite significant government policy and financial investment in interventions designed to boost youth sport participation alongside other favourable trends (Roberts, this volume; Rowe, 2015), including a doubling in the proportion of students entering HE since the 1980s (Haycock, 2015). More particularly, the study argued that if attending HE does indeed help explain why university students are more likely to become present-day sport participants and remain sports-active into later life, then one might have expected to observe increases in participation by young people and adults over the last three decades or so. Since this has not happened, however, it was argued that definitive conclusions about whether there is a HE effect on sport participation and, if so, what this effect/these effects are, cannot yet be drawn despite the prevailing and commonly accepted view that attending HE boosts sport participation (Haycock, 2015).

The findings of Haycock's (2015) study indicated that the two clearest predictors of differences in the present-day sport participation and sport careers of university students were subject of study and sex, with sport students and males being the most likely participants over the life course and while at university. These differences first emerged during childhood, widened from age twelve or thirteen-years old, and remained relatively set from age sixteen onwards. The differences in the present-day sport participation of university students, and the richness of their overall sport careers, could thus not be attributed to an *HE effect* as previous research has suggested. Indeed, the findings of the study suggested that the assumed contribution attending HE has previously been expected to make to students' current and future sport participation appears to have been over-stated, and in so doing diverted attention from other processes associated with the inequalities that underlie students' differential engagement in sport. These inequalities, and the preconditions required for constructing short- or longer-term sport (and leisure) careers, first emerged during childhood, rather than youth. This led Haycock (2015) to conclude that it was the differential childhood socialization practices students' experienced that played a crucial role in the unequal development of their sporting habituses and dispositions, and which provided the foundations upon which present-day inequalities in participation were based. We shall elaborate on the process of habitus formation and significance of childhood sport socialization for understanding students' (and other participants') sport and leisure careers next.

Explaining youth sport and leisure careers: figurations, habitus and capital

The biographical and career-oriented approach adopted in Haycock's (2015) study helped identify childhood and youth as important life stages in the construction of students' sport and leisure careers, and drew particular attention to the dynamic and processual character of sporting habituses and capitals which were most rapidly formed during childhood. The study adopted an explicitly Eliasian conceptualization of habitus which was viewed as a person's 'second nature' or 'embodied social learning' acting as an 'automatic, blindly functioning apparatus of self-control' (Elias, 2000: 368) that develops within the historically produced and reproduced relational networks (or human figurations) of which they are a part, and which stretch across generations. It was Elias's (2000) contention that each person develops their own individual and unique habitus as well as a series of social or group habituses – such as gender habituses – that are shared with others who have been habituated through similar experiences. As with conceptions of habitus more commonly associated with other sociological theorists (Bourdieu, 1984), Elias also noted that habitus formation was a process that develops most rapidly during the most impressionable life stages of childhood and youth (Elias, 2000). As in other studies (e.g. Nielsen *et al.*, 2012; Pot *et al.*, 2014; Quarmby and Dagkas, 2010, 2013; Stuij 2015), this was especially true for the participants in Haycock's (2015) study since it was childhood, rather than youth, which was the most critical life-stage in which the foundations for subsequent sport participation were laid, and in which some of the more impressionable phases of habitus formation took place (Elias, 2000; Engström, 2008; Stuij, 2015).

The organization of students' psychological make-up into an embodied habitus was a dynamic process that begun at birth and continued to develop as the changing figurations in which they were bound-up became more or less complex, and perceived as more-or-less compelling (Elias, 2000; Stuij, 2015). As students' habituses developed during childhood, their predispositions for sport participation were continually constructed and reconstructed in the context of their complex, historically produced and reproduced, networks of interdependencies which comprised, among other groups, their parents, siblings, other family members, and peers. As Engström (2008: 325) has noted, these significant others (especially parents) were 'important value transferors' of sporting tastes, preferences and predispositions during childhood. More particularly, while partly related to family socio-economic status, during childhood students' individual habitus was developed most impressionably within the cultural dimension of family environments where parents, in particular, helped transmit different propensities among their offspring towards present-day sport participation (Birchwood *et al.*, 2008; Neilsen *et al.*, 2012; Stuij, 2015). Students who were the most sports-active (sport students and males) currently were those who, from an early age, were brought up in families in which sport participation was highly valued and normalized by parents. For these students, sport participation appeared to become 'a deep anchorage in the personality structure' (Elias and Scotson, 1994: 103), or habitus, which developed during the course of being socialized more intensely and extensively than other students during childhood. These typically included traditional team sports (e.g. football and netball) alongside individual activities (e.g. swimming and running) that laid the foundations for future engagement in other sports that were undertaken by students as made the transition from childhood to youth.

The process of habitus formation during childhood, and the development of wide sporting repertoires (Engström, 2008; Roberts and Brodie, 1992), was closely associated with the 'amounts of material, social and educational capitals' (Neilsen *et al.*, 2012: 15) students acquired and was underpinned by their parents' concern with engendering in them a positive attitude towards the intrinsic value of sport (Engström, 2008; Haycock and Smith, 2014; Neilsen *et al.*, 2012; Stuij, 2015). The least active students were less likely to discuss experiences of this kind and acquired less 'knowledge, experience and competencies . . . from a childhood environment . . . [necessary] for participation in the fields of sports or other physical activities later in life' (Neilsen *et al.*, 2012: 4). The major differences between the most and least active students in the study, therefore, were generated in part by the unequal distribution of family capital between them and the associated differences in individual habitus formation, which helped generate the observed differences in present-day participation (Quarmby and Dagkas, 2010, 2013).

It was through encouraging their offspring to participate in a range of sports that students' family environments operated as social contexts where the accumulation of cultural and social capital was accomplished, initially through the transmission of parental values and preferences during primary socialization (Green, 2010; Lareau, 2011; Stuij, 2015). The kinds of primary socialization practices students recalled in relation to their childhood experiences of sport typically incorporated a number of features and often resembled what Lareau (2011) calls 'concerted cultivation'. Confirming the findings of previous studies (e.g. Haycock and Smith, 2014; Neilsen *et al.*, 2012; Pot *et al.*, 2014; Scheerder *et al.*, 2005), these features of family-based leisure were: having two sports active parents who encouraged them to participate in sport, often for enjoyment and the love of sport, and who experienced fewer financial and transport constraints than other parents (Haycock, 2015). Parents of the more frequent present-day participants were also better able to reinvest their offspring with symbolically significant forms of social, cultural, physical and economic capital to support the construction of their short- and longer-term sport careers (Evans and Davies, 2010; Green, 2010; Haycock and Smith, 2014). These parental investments in students' childhood sport appeared particularly efficacious for transmitting the kinds of values and norms of sport-supportive cultures that provided the foundations of their dominant cultural practices (Birchwood *et al.*, 2008; Stuij, 2015). Growing up with active parents who valued sport and who purposively fostered participation by developing students' repertoire of skills, interests and predispositions – which collectively comprised sporting capital (Nielsen *et al.*, 2012; Pot *et al.*, 2014; Rowe, 2015) – thus appeared to help maximize higher levels of present-day participation among the most sports-active.

As significant as parents and family were in the primary socialization of students into sport during childhood, it was also clear that friends and peers became especially significant to students' increasingly complex interdependency networks during the transition from childhood to youth in a dynamic, reciprocal and contingent process of secondary socialization (Green, 2010; Lareau, 2011; Stuij, 2015). For the most active students, being part of sport-oriented peer networks during the course of growing up strengthened the predispositions, tastes and skills they acquired as part of normative family practices to which they had been exposed during childhood (Quarmby and Dagkas, 2010, 2013; Stuij, 2015). During leisure, in particular, peers became significant agents in the on-going socialization of students in sport and to the continued 'internalisation of sporting capital' (Stuij, 2015: 785) that characterized this process, whether in formal settings such as sports clubs or in more informal leisure contexts where sport was being played. In these leisure sites, the most active students 'both influenced and were influenced by their peers' (Stuij 2015: 788) towards engaging in sport on a regular basis, often for intrinsic purposes, and almost always in the company of their peers who occupied significant positions within their developing networks of interdependence. The reproduction of interdependency networks in which predispositions towards sport participation were constructed thus helped the more active students to develop group habituses (Elias, 2000; Stuij, 2015) with other sporty people who had been, and continued to be, habituated through similar experiences (Nielsen *et al.*, 2012). In this regard, it became apparent that while many of the preconditions and predispositions for students' engagement in sport at university appeared to be relatively fixed by age sixteen, childhood socialization 'was still making a difference, that is, having additional effects' (Birchwood *et al.* 2008: 292) on their present-day participation in the peer-oriented networks which were playing a significant role in students' lives.

Recognizing the centrality of habitus construction and capital development to childhood sport socialization practices is also a vital pre-requisite for understanding young people's leisure careers, especially from mid-adolescence, and the threats this poses to sport participation (Haycock, 2015; Hendry *et al.*, 1993; Roberts, this volume). As we noted earlier, although childhood and youth are the life stages in which sport participation is usually highest, they are also the periods in the life course when participation gradually drops off and when some young people begin to drop-out altogether. The age-related declines in sport participation that are observed in many countries, and which often begin around mid-adolescence, are not necessarily evidence that young people begin to turn their backs on sport, or become less interested in it as they get older (Roberts, this volume). Rather, during the course of negotiating the opportunities and challenges encountered during the transitional youth life stage, sport becomes one among many other leisure activities that may be incorporated within young people's unfolding, and increasingly individualized, lifestyles (Green, 2014b; Haycock and Smith, 2014a,

2014b; Roberts, this volume). For some young people, peer-oriented activities such as eating out of the home, consuming alcohol and other drugs, shopping, and engaging in sedentary leisure activities (including social media use) come to dominate their leisure lives at the expense of sport and absorb more of their time, money and attention (Roberts, this volume). For many others, engaging in popular commercial leisure and home-centred activities are not undertaken at the expense of sport: they can and often are accommodated within busy leisure lifestyles that feature sport participation (Roberts, this volume). Thus, in order to adequately understand the sport careers of young people, it is essential also to recognize the increased appeal of other leisure activities during the youth life-stage, since doing so will reveal how sport participation comes to compete with many other activities within an already busy leisure market-place in which young people's competing leisure careers are simultaneously constructed (Roberts, this volume).

Conclusions

In this chapter, we have been centrally concerned with understanding young people's sport and leisure careers and how these might be researched to examine the realities, rather than simply supporting the myths surrounding, youth participation in sport and leisure. In doing so, we have argued that notwithstanding the advantages of panel designs to permit the detailed investigation of sport and leisure careers, their use remains rare by comparison to other approaches to researching young people's lives. As Roberts *et al.* (2009: 262) have noted, however, the benefits of injecting a longitudinal dimension into the study of young people's lives 'are potentially enormous in terms of both pure theory building and extracting policy implications'. This is especially true in relation to the study of sport and leisure careers, which as we noted earlier, need to be simultaneously understood if we are to provide a more adequate understanding of young people's lives and of the contribution childhood sports socialization makes to present-day inequalities in sport and leisure participation. Central to the explanation of youth sport and leisure careers would appear to be the differential contribution made by the construction of young people's habituses and capitals (acquired especially during childhood), and how these provide the foundations upon which the necessary predispositions and tastes for sport in later life are based. If this is indeed true, then it is clear that there is 'a need for more longitudinal and biographical, as well as qualitative alongside quantitative, research exploring sports careers and the sporting habituses of young people' (Green, 2014b: 371). Whether or not researchers will be inclined to engage in more longitudinal and biographical investigations is a moot point, but an appropriate starting point for future investigations might be the suggestion that the most appropriate focal point for policy interventions concerned with boosting longer-term sport participation is not with youth, but with children (Roberts, this volume).

References

Aldridge, J., Measham, F. and Williams, L. (2011). *Illegal leisure revisited*. London: Routledge.
Birchwood, D., Roberts, K. and Pollock, G. (2008). Explaining differences in sport participation rates among young adults: evidence from the South Caucasus. *European Physical Education Review, 14(3)*, 283–98.
Booker, C., Skew, A., Kelly, Y. and Sacker, A. (2015). Media use, sports participation, and well-being in adolescence: cross-sectional findings from the UK Household Longitudinal Study. *American Journal of Public Health, 105(1)*, 173–79.
Bourdieu, P. (1984). *Distinction*. London: Routledge.
Centre for Longitudinal Studies (2015a). *1970 British Cohort Study*. Available online at: www.cls.ioe.ac.uk/ page.aspx?andsitesectionid=795andsitesectiontitle=Welcome+to+the+1970+British+Cohort+Study+ per cent28BCS70 per cent29

Centre for Longitudinal Studies (2015b). *Next Steps*. Available online at: www.cls.ioe.ac.uk/page.aspx? andsitesectionid=1246andsitesectiontitle=Welcome+to+Next+Steps+ per cent28LSYPE per cent29

Centre for Longitudinal Studies (2015c). *Welcome to the Millennium Cohort Study*. Available online at: www.cls.ioe.ac.uk/page.aspx?andsitesectionid=851

Coalter, F. (2007). *A wider social role for sport*. London: Routledge.

Coalter, F. (2013). Game plan and the Spirit Level: the class ceiling and the limits of sports policy? *International Journal of Sport Policy and Politics*, 5(1), 3–19.

Department for Education (2011). *Youth cohort study and longitudinal study of young people in England: The activities and experiences of 19-year-olds: England 2010*. London: Department for Education.

Elias, N. (2000). *The civilizing process*. Oxford: Basil Blackwell.

Elias, N. and Scotson, J. (1994). *The established and the outsiders*. London: Sage.

Engström, L.-M. (2008). Who is physically active? Cultural capital and sports participation from adolescence to middle age – a 38-year follow-up study. *Physical Education and Sport Pedagogy*, 13(4), 319–43.

Evans, J. and Davies, B. (2010). Family, class and embodiment: why school physical education makes so little difference to post-school participation patterns in physical activity. *International Journal of Qualitative Studies in Education*, 23(7), 765–84.

Farrell, L., Hollingsworth, B., Propper, C. and Shields, M. (2014). The socioeconomic gradient in physical inactivity: evidence from one million adults in England. *Social Science and Medicine*, 123(1), 55–63.

Furlong, A. (2013). *Youth studies: an introduction*. London: Routledge.

Green, K. (2010). *Key themes in youth sport*. London: Routledge.

Green, K., Thurston, M., Vaage, O. and Roberts, K. (2013). '[We're on the right track, baby], we were born this way'! Exploring sports participation in Norway. *Sport, Education and Society*, DOI: 10.1080/ 13573322.2013.769947

Green, K. (2014a). Roberts' and Brodie's *Inner-city sport*: an undiscovered gem?; in A. Smith and I. Waddington (eds) *Doing Real World Research in Sports Studies*. London: Routledge.

Green, K. (2014b). Mission impossible? Reflecting upon the relationship between physical education, youth sport and lifelong participation. *Sport, Education and Society*, 19, 357–75.

Haycock, D. (2015). *University students' sport participation: the significance of sport and leisure careers*. Unpublished PhD thesis. Chester: University of Chester.

Haycock, D. and Smith, A. (2014a). A family affair? Exploring the influence of childhood sports socialisation on young adults' leisure-sport careers in north-west England. *Leisure Studies*, 33(3), 285–304.

Haycock, D. and Smith, A. (2014b). Sports participation and health during periods of educational transition: a study of 30–35-year-olds in north-west England. *Sport, Education and Society*, 19(2), 168–85.

Hendry, L., Shucksmith, J., Lowe, J. and Glendinning, A. (1993). *Young people's leisure and lifestyles*. London: Routledge.

Hendry, L., Kloep, M., Espnes, G., Ingebrigtsen, J., Glendinning, A. and Wood, S. (2002). Leisure transitions–a rural perspective. *Leisure Studies*, 21(1), 1–14.

Institute for Social and Economic Research (2015). *Understanding society*. Available online at: www.under standingsociety.ac.uk/

Lareau, A. (2011). *Unequal childhoods. Class, race, and family life*. (2nd ed). California: University of California Press.

Lunn, P. (2010). The sports and exercise life-course: a survival analysis of recall data from Ireland. *Social Science and Medicine*, 70(5), 711–19.

Lunn, P., Kelly, E. and Fitzpatrick, N. (2013). *Keeping them in the game: Taking up and dropping out of sport and exercise in Ireland*. Dublin: Economic and Social Research Institute.

MacDonald, R. and Shildrick, T. (2007). Street corner society: leisure careers, youth (sub)culture and social exclusion. *Leisure Studies*, 26(3), 339–55.

Neilsen, G., Grønfeldt, V., Toftegaard-Støckel, J. and Andersen, L. B. (2012). Predisposed to participate? The influence of family socio-economic background on children's sports participation and daily amount of physical activity. *Sport in Society*, 15(1), 1–27.

Parker, H., Aldridge, J. and Measham, F. (1998). *Illegal leisure*. London: Routledge.

Parker, H., Williams, L. and Aldridge, J. (2002). The normalization of 'sensible' recreational drug use: further evidence from the north west longitudinal study. *Sociology*, 36(4), 941–64.

Pot, N., Verbeek, J., van der Zwan, J. and van Hilvoorde, I. (2014). Socialisation into organised sports of young adolescents with a lower socio-economic status. *Sport, Education and Society*. DOI: 10.1080/ 13573322.2014.914901

Quarmby, T. and Dagkas, S. (2010). Children's engagement in leisure time physical activity: exploring family structure as a determinant. *Leisure Studies, 29(1)*, 53–66.

Quarmby, T. and Dagkas, S. (2013). Locating the place and meaning of physical activity in the lives of young people from low-income, lone-parent families. *Physical Education and Sport Pedagogy, 18(5)*, 459–74.

Roberts, K. (2003) Problems and priorities for the sociology of youth; in A. Bennett, C. Cieslik and S. Miles (eds) *Researching youth: Issues, themes, controversies* (pp. 13–28). Basingstoke: Palgrave Macmillan.

Roberts, K. (2014). Researching inner-city sport: who plays, and what are the benefits?; in A. Smith and I. Waddington (eds) *Doing real world research in sports studies*. London: Routledge.

Roberts, K. (2016). Youth leisure as the context for youth sport in K. Green and A. Smith (eds) *The Routledge handbook of youth sport* (pp. 18–25). London: Routledge.

Roberts, K. and Brodie, D. (1992). *Inner-city sport: who plays, and what are the benefits?* Culemborg: Giordano Bruno.

Roberts, K., Minten, J., Chadwick, C., Lamb, K. and Brodie, D. (1991). Sporting lives: a case study of leisure careers. *Society and Leisure, 14(1)*, 261–84.

Roberts, K., Pollock, G., Tholen, J. and Tarkhnishvili, L. (2009). Youth leisure careers during post-communist transitions in the South Caucasus. *Leisure Studies, 28(3)*, 261–77.

Rowe, N. (2015). Sporting capital: a theoretical and empirical analysis of sport participation determinants and its application to sports development policy and practice. *International Journal of Sport Policy and Politics, 7(1)*, 43–61.

Scheerder, J., Taks, M., Vanreusel, B. and Renson, R. (2005). Social changes in youth sports participation styles 1969–1999: the case of Flanders (Belgium). *Sport, Education and Society, 10(3)*, 321–41.

Shildrick, T. and MacDonald, R. (2013). Poverty talk: how people experiencing poverty deny their poverty and why they blame 'the poor'. *The Sociological Review, 61(2)*, 285–303.

Shildrick, T., MacDonald, R., Furlong, A., Roden, J. and Crow, R. (2012). *Are 'cultures of worklessness' passed down the generations?* York: Joseph Rowntree Foundation.

Stuij, M. (2015). Habitus and social class: a case study on socialisation into sports and exercise. *Sport, Education and Society, 20(6)*, 780–98.

van Tuyckom, C. and Scheerder, J. (2010). Sport for all? Insight into stratification and compensation mechanisms of sporting activity in the EU-27. *Sport, Education and Society, 15(4)*, 495–513.

Wright, J. and Macdonald, D. (2010). Young people, physical activity and the everyday: the *Life Activity Project*; in J. Wright and D. MacDonald (eds) *Young people, physical activity and the everyday*. London: Routledge.

Wright, J., Macdonald, D. and Groom, L. (2003). Physical activity and young people: beyond participation. *Sport, Education and Society, 8(1)*, 17–34.

SECTION 2

Youth sport around the world

6

INTRODUCTION

Andy Smith

In the last two decades, a number of book-length attempts have been made to understand the major patterns and trends in sport participation across the world, whether among whole populations (e.g. Da Costa and Miragaya 2002), or among distinct groups of national populations such as young people (e.g. De Knop *et al.* 1996). Nicholson *et al.* (2011) have also provided an important corrective to the dominance in the literature of analyses of elite sport policy by examining the relative success of national sport participation policies. To these can be added countless journal articles that have examined sport participation in a myriad of local, national and international contexts, and which have focused on different target groups, on individual and combinations of sports, and on a whole range of predictors of sport participation. The focus of Section 2 in this Handbook, however, is on youth and the major patterns and trends that are identifiable from their engagement in sport and physical activity in various countries around the world.

As in preceding attempts, the selection of material presented in this section is necessarily selective and reflective of our attempts to include chapters from authors who focus on youth sport participation in a reasonably broad range of geographical contexts. To this end, we have been able to include contributions on youth sport participation in specific regions (Western Europe [the European Union], Australasia and the Middle East), and in individual countries (Norway, the United States, Japan and China). For a variety of reasons, we were unable to secure other chapters that examined young people's engagement in sport and physical activity in other geographical locations, and as a consequence what is provided in Section 2 cannot be held to be representative of the diverse institutional, political and historical contexts in which youth sport participation around the world is enacted. This having been said, as readers will see from each of the contributions, there are important insights to be gleaned from the analyses that we have been able to include here and which shed new light on, among other things, the major levels, forms and kinds of participation identifiable in existing data sets. The major trends in youth sport that require careful examination are then considered in more detail in Section 3.

The first chapter in this section is by Charlotte van Tuyckom, and is entitled *Youth sport participation: a comparison between European member states*. Drawing on data from the 2014 Eurobarometer, van Tuyckom examines the frequency and levels of engagement of young people who exercise or play sport or other physical activities in the European member states. Perhaps unsurprisingly, the data reveal widespread differences in the frequency and levels of sport participation among young people across Europe, with those living in the Nordic countries being more likely to exercise or play sport regularly. Just under one in five European youth are identified as never exercising or engaging in sport, with the highest propositions being observed in Malta and Portugal. The contexts in which European youth participate in sport were diverse and often informal, with parks, being outdoors and the home being among the most popular settings reported by young people. Other popular locations included health and fitness centres and sports clubs. Membership of sports clubs varied widely among the member states however, with membership being highest in Sweden, Luxembourg and the Netherland: six in ten Europeans were not members of any club. The chapter concludes by reviewing some of the major motivations and barriers for engaging in sport and physical activity all of which will be familiar to readers.

In his chapter entitled *Youth sport in Norway*, Ken Green analyzes the relatively high rates of sport participation among young people living in the Nordic countries identified by van Tuyckom. In doing so, Green discusses what 'often appears as a kind of Nordic or, at least, Scandinavian, exceptionalism in the field of youth sport' and draws upon survey data to identify some of the major developments in youth sport in recent decades. More particularly, Green argues that in Norway there has been a trend toward: more young people (especially females) doing more sport more often; a later peak in sports participation than typically found outside Nordic countries alongside what he describes as a 'bounce-back' phenomenon identifiable among older adults; convergence in participation between the sexes; and, a shift towards engaging in lifestyle sports, which come to dominate the sporting biographies of Norwegian youth. These processes, Green suggests, can be explained by a configuration of interrelated process, including the relatively high levels of economic prosperity and class and gender parity that can be observed in Norwegian society, the cultural traction of sport in the country, the central role played by parents in the cultivation of sporting capital among youth during early sports socialization and the activities of schools and sports clubs that strengthen the propensity among Norwegian youth for engaging in sport. For these reasons, young Norwegians, Green concludes, are 'the quintessential sporting omnivores'.

In the next chapter, Jay Coakley focuses on the organization of *Youth sport in the United States*. Coakley notes that in the United States there is no interconnected youth sport system because programmes that organize and promote youth sport are not governed by any national, state or local plans. The picture of youth sport participation is thus complex and characterized by an admixture of programmes that are sponsored by a variety of agencies, ranging from private-for-profit businesses to local public agencies alongside a similarly diverse set of non-profit organizations (including local churches, regional and national faith-based organizations, and youth service organizations). In this regard, Coakley argues that youth sport in the United States resembles 'a disjointed collection of programmes that reflect the goals and perspectives of the adults who organize, manage, and coach them', and which attract participants from a particular social class or ethnic population due to combinations of cost and residential segregation.

In *Youth sport in Australasia*, Doune Macdonald and Clifford Mallett provide an equally fascinating and insightful analysis of the organization of, and major trends in, sport participation among Australasian youth. Six so-called sporting megatrends trends are identified:

- a growth in health-oriented (or 'lifestyle') physical activities alongside participation in organized sport for health benefit;
- an increase in the popularity of so-called extreme activities including skating, freestyle BMX cycling and rock climbing;

- the use of sport by government to achieve a variety health and other social outcomes;
- a shift in the sporting preferences of Australasian citizens amid the increasing cultural diversity that characterizes the region;
- the increased emphasis that is coming to be placed on wealth creation via sport and the attraction of sporting talent and media interest supported by business-oriented approaches to sport.

Despite these major trends, Macdonald and Mallett note that little reliable data exists on sport participation patterns for Australasian youth, but that in the absence of these data there are signs that 'traditional organized sport' is losing its participant base as new forms of physical activity participation emerge for youth with the appeal of being more flexible, accessible, cheaper, quicker and suited to the construction of personal identities.

Data from a 2013 nationwide research survey conducted by the private research institution Sasakawa Sports Foundation provides the starting point for the analysis of the next chapter, *Youth sport in Japan*, which is written by Atsushi Nakazawa and Aaron L. Miller. Based on data derived from 3,000 young people aged 19 years old, Nakazawa and Miller note that 87 per cent of Japanese young people play sport, and more than half of all young people do so more than five days a week. The sporting biographies of Japanese youth, it is claimed, feature team sports such as football and basketball alongside partner sports (e.g. badminton and table tennis) and more individualized activities, among which swimming and running/jogging are most popular. In contrast to some of their European counterparts, much of the sport participation reported by Japanese youth occurs in educational institutions such as schools (especially junior high and high schools) as well as in local parks and open spaces. Participation in extra-curricular clubs affiliated with schools is also especially common and this infrastructure, it is held, has helped provide 'a center of youth sports in Japan'.

The final two chapters in this section explore youth sport in the Middle East and China. In *Youth sport in the Middle East*, Nida Ahmed and Holly Thorpe first provide an historical sketch of sport participation in the Middle East and North Africa (MENA) region which, as in many other countries, is a history in which sport has commonly been regarded as a vehicle to 'integrate citizens, promote healthy behaviour, cultivate local and international partnerships and generate economic growth'. Following a discussion of the place of sport in physical education in schools, Ahmed and Thorpe demonstrate how currently popular sports among youth (mainly males, on whom most data are typically reported) in the Middle East include a variety of traditional and western sports, such as football (which is especially popular in North Africa, and in the Levant and Gulf countries) and swimming. However, as Ahmed and Thorpe note, sports that were traditionally popular in the region are now 'taking a back-seat among the younger generation, while sports of Western origin, such as football, basketball, boxing, bodybuilding, capiora, and parkour, are gaining popularity'. This popularity, they claim, has been supported by the various transformations associated with the growth of new social media, a political willingness to use sport as a tool for broader political goals, processes of glocalization and an increased commitment by governments to hosting and staging major elite sports competitions.

In the final chapter of this section, entitled *Youth sport in China*, Chen XueDong and Shushu Chen provide readers with a rare insight into the participation of young people in sport and physical activity in the world's fast growing economy. They note that, in China, there is a tendency for state sport policy to focus on elite and mass sport, rather than on youth sport, and that by comparison to other school subjects, sport is frequently left on the margins of educational curricula. This is shown to be related to the longstanding perception that sport is less important than other activities considered essential to the development of a good academic and work career, a view that permeates and is supported by other features of Chinese culture. Among these features, the authors note, are the traditional values and ideology which underpin social life in China and the social construction of the Chinese family, which has often been largely patriarchal in structure and one where parents typically encourage their children to prioritize academic achievement (rather than sport participation) as a means of achieving social status. In addition, they point out that despite its tendency to focus on elite and to an extent mass sport, the Chinese government nevertheless continues to adopt a very centralized approach to the organization and delivery of youth sport, much of which, as in Japan, is linked to the provision of physical education in schools. However, it is concluded that while youth sport is becoming an increasingly prominent feature of sport policy and practice in China, 'the current structure and system of school sport has made the development of a national sports development strategy problematic and particularly ineffective in responding to the social and health problems facing young people'.

References

Da Costa, L. and Miragaya, A. (2002). *Worldwide experiences and trends in sport for all.* Oxford: Meyer and Meyer.

De Knop, P., Engström, L.-M., Skirstad, B. and Weiss, M. (1996). *Worldwide trends in youth sport.* Champaign, Illinois: Human Kinetics.

Nicholson, M., Hoye, R. and Houlihan, B. (2011). *Participation in sport: international policy perspectives.* London: Routledge.

7

YOUTH SPORT PARTICIPATION

A comparison between European member states

Charlotte van Tuyckom

Introduction

Sport and Europe share a strong connection (Scheerder, van Tuyckom and Vermeersch, 2007). Not only is Europe the birthplace of modern sport, which originated in the British public schools in the eighteenth and nineteenth centuries (Renson, 1992), but Olympism and the 'Sport for All' movement also have their roots in European soil. Several European governments have contributed to the development of the current European sport sphere. After World War II, many (Western) European countries developed a noticeably active government policy with regard to sport and physical activity. An important aim of this policy was to inspire as many citizens as possible to get involved in sportive action and to take part in physical activities. In 1966, the Council of Europe had already launched the Sport for All idea, as a result of which Sport for All achieved a pioneer role in the advancement of sportive body movement among European citizens (Husting, 2003). In 1975, government actions with respect to recreational sport became institutionalized in the form of the European Sport for All Charter (Council of Europe, 1975). Inspired by the Universal Declaration of Human Rights, this Charter endorses the right to active sport participation for every citizen. All Council of Europe member-country ministers responsible for sport signed the Charter, and it still acts as a democratic counterbalance for the ideology of top level sport (Vanreusel, 2001).

It is evident that societal interest in sport has increased in past decennia, and that active sport participation has become one of the most common forms of leisure activity. Crum summarized this trend as the 'sportization of society' (1991, p. 15). However, despite the popularization of sport, more than half of the adult population in Europe is overweight or obese, and childhood obesity is of particular concern (van Tuyckom and Scheerder, 2010). The European Commission believes, therefore, that the European Union (EU) and its member states must take proactive steps to reverse the decline in physical activity that has occurred over the past several decades. In 2012, the Council adopted conclusions on promoting health-enhancing physical activity and on strengthening the evidence-base for sport policy making, both calling on the Commission to issue regular surveys on sport and physical activity. The Eurobarometer survey of 2014, which follows on from comparable surveys conducted in 2002 and 2009, contributes to providing some of the data to support the developing policy framework for promoting sport and physical activity.

Despite the growing importance attached to the promotion of physical activity in EU member states, the previous Eurobarometer surveys identified alarmingly high rates of inactivity in the EU among different age groups, and found that the vast majority of Europeans never exercise or play sport (Hartmann-Tews, 2006; van Bottenburg, Rijnen and van Sterkenburg, 2005; van Tuyckom and Scheerder, 2010; van Tuyckom, 2011; van Tuyckom, Scheerder and Bracke, 2010). The purpose of this chapter is to discuss the most recent Eurobarometer data (from 2014), thereby focusing explicitly on youth sport participation levels. The structure of the chapter is identical to that of the Special Eurobarometer 412 report (European Commission, 2014).

The first section looks at the *frequency* and levels of engagement of European youth who exercise or play sport or other physical activities. The second section focuses on *where* European youth engage in sport and other physical activity, and also examines club membership. The third section looks at the *reasons* why people engage in sport and other physical activity, as well as the *barriers* to practicing sport more regularly.

Research material

The most recent Eurobarometer survey was carried out by TNS Opinion and Social network in the twenty-eight member states of the EU between November and December 2013. Some 27,919 respondents (of which 2,888 aged between 15 and 24) from different social and demographic groups were interviewed face-to-face at home in their mother tongue on behalf of the Directorate-General for Education and Culture (Sport unit). The methodology used is that of Eurobarometer surveys (see http://ec.europa.eu/public_opinion/index_en.htm) as carried out by the Directorate-General for Communication. The findings are purely descriptive, and focus on general country differences. No associations with gender or socio-economic status are discussed here.

Frequency of sport participation and levels of engagement: '18 per cent of European youth never exercises or plays sport'

When looking at the frequency of engagement in sport and other physical activities, more than 50 per cent of the youth surveyed exercise or play sport a few times a week, with 13 per cent who even exercise or play sport almost daily (Table 7.1). The findings for the different countries show that respondents in the Nordic countries (Green, this volume) are the most likely to exercise or play sport on a regular basis. The proportion that exercises or plays sport at least a few times a week is 81 per cent in Finland and Denmark. Sweden also has a high proportion (79 per cent) of respondents who exercise or play sport regularly, with high figures also seen in Luxembourg (79 per cent), the Netherlands (75 per cent), Belgium (72.5 per cent) and Slovenia (72 per cent).

At the other end of the scale, Malta (58 per cent) and Portugal (42 per cent) have large proportions of youth who never exercise or play sport at all. The proportion of respondents who never exercise or play sport at all is also high in Cyprus (38 per cent), Bulgaria (37 per cent), Italy (34 per cent) and Romania (27 per cent). Moreover, Malta (34 per cent), Bulgaria (43 per cent) and Romania (46 per cent) also have the fewest youth citizens who exercise or play sport on a regular basis.

On average, still almost one in five of the European youth indicate that they never exercise or play sport (Figure 7.1).

Table 7.1 Levels of youth engagement in sport and other physical activity for all EU–28 member states (2014)

	Almost daily	A few times a week	Occasionally	Never	No answer
Total	12,9%	50,8%	18,2%	17,8%	0,3%
Austria	13,4%	54,6%	23,7%	8,2%	0,0%
Belgium	9,7%	62,8%	18,6%	8,8%	0,0%
Bulgaria	9,5%	33,7%	18,9%	36,8%	1,1%
Cyprus (Republic)	12,0%	38,0%	12,0%	38,0%	0,0%
Czech Republic	7,8%	58,8%	22,5%	10,8%	0,0%
Germany	7,8%	53,5%	21,0%	17,3%	0,5%
Denmark	18,1%	62,5%	13,9%	5,6%	0,0%
Estonia	12,9%	57,4%	20,8%	8,9%	0,0%
Spain	19,7%	47,9%	10,3%	21,4%	0,9%
Finland	8,0%	72,7%	9,1%	9,1%	1,1%
France	8,0%	57,1%	17,9%	17,0%	0,0%
United Kingdom	14,0%	46,3%	21,4%	18,4%	0,0%
Greece	15,3%	51,7%	13,6%	19,5%	0,0%
Croatia	5,7%	50,0%	32,3%	11,4%	0,6%
Hungary	30,4%	39,1%	14,1%	16,3%	0,0%
Ireland	19,8%	51,0%	13,5%	14,6%	1,0%
Italy	4,5%	55,7%	4,5%	34,1%	1,1%
Lithuania	19,9%	46,4%	12,7%	21,0%	0,0%
Luxembourg	18,2%	60,6%	6,1%	15,2%	0,0%
Latvia	8,4%	45,8%	35,2%	10,6%	0,0%
Malta	13,2%	21,1%	7,9%	57,9%	0,0%
The Netherlands	9,3%	66,0%	7,2%	17,5%	0,0%
Poland	7,8%	48,5%	22,3%	20,4%	1,0%
Portugal	16,7%	36,3%	4,9%	42,2%	0,0%
Romania	10,6%	35,6%	25,0%	26,9%	1,9%
Sweden	25,6%	53,5%	16,3%	4,7%	0,0%
Slovenia	18,3%	53,8%	23,7%	4,3%	0,0%
Slovakia	13,4%	51,8%	19,6%	15,2%	0,0%

Settings of sport participation: 'most of the activity takes place in informal settings, such as parks and outdoors or at home'

Among respondents who exercise or play sport, most of the activity takes place in informal settings, such as parks and outdoors (33.5 per cent of youth engage in sport or physical activity here), or at home (33 per cent). Activity also takes place at school or university (24 per cent), at a health or fitness centre (20.5 per cent), sport clubs (20 per cent) and sport centres (10 per cent).

The country-level data reveals very different preferences for the settings in which youth in the different countries choose to engage in sport or physical activity (Table 7.2). In the EU overall, the most common setting is a park or outdoors. The proportion of youth engaging in sport or physical activity in a park or outdoors is particularly high in Finland (67 per cent), Slovenia (50 per cent), Sweden (50 per cent), Austria (49.5 per cent), Denmark (42 per cent) and Spain (42 per cent). The lowest proportions are in Hungary (13 per cent) and Luxembourg (17 per cent). Sport or physical activity at home is popular among youth in Sweden (52 per cent) and

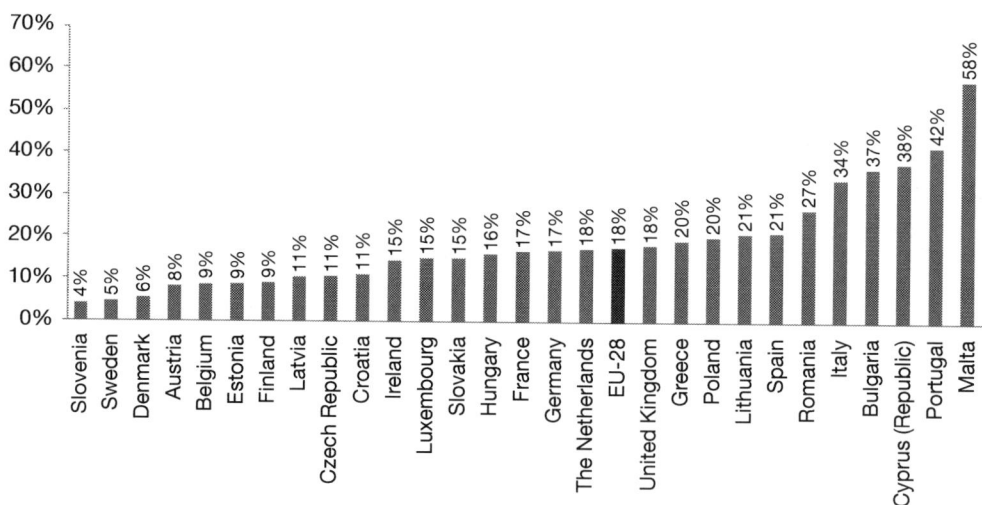

Figure 7.1 Youth sporting inactivity for all EU–28 member states (2014)

Eastern European countries. High figures are in Lithuania (52 per cent), Slovenia (48 per cent) and Romania (47 per cent). It is much less common in Southern European countries, specifically Spain (4 per cent), Malta (4 per cent), Portugal (5 per cent) and Cyprus (6 per cent). Respondents are more likely to engage in sport or physical activity in a health or fitness centre in Sweden (52 per cent), Denmark (41 per cent), Finland (34 per cent), Greece (32 per cent), Austria (31 per cent), Czech Republic (31 per cent) and Bulgaria (30 per cent). Sweden (36 per cent) also has a high proportion of youth who engages in sport or physical activity at a sport club (36 per cent), and this is also the case in the Netherlands (40 per cent), Belgium (31 per cent), France (30 per cent) and Luxembourg (30 per cent). Use of sport centres is the most common among youth in Italy (37 per cent) and Malta (21 per cent). The lowest figures for use of health or fitness centres are in Lithuania (2 per cent) and Latvia (9 per cent). Similarly, the figures for the use of sport centres are also low in Lithuania (5 per cent) as well as in Portugal (3 per cent), Hungary (3.5 per cent) and Romania (4 per cent). Romania also has the lowest figure for use of sport clubs (5 per cent), with similarly low figures also in Cyprus (6 per cent) and Latvia (7 per cent).

Club membership: 'six out of ten EU youth are not members of any club'

Sixty per cent of EU youth citizens say that they are not a member of any club (Table 7.3). Conversely, almost 20 per cent of respondents are members of a sport club, while 17 per cent belong to a health or fitness centre. In addition, 6 per cent are members of socio–cultural clubs that include sport in its activities, such as a youth club or a club related to school or university. The proportion of respondents who are members of a club varies across countries. The highest proportions for youth memberships at a sport club are in Sweden (39.5 per cent), Luxembourg (39 per cent) and the Netherlands (38 per cent), while respondents in Denmark (46 per cent) and Sweden (42 per cent) are the most likely to be members at a healthy or fitness centre. Conversely, the lowest figures for youth memberships at a sport club are in Romania (1 per cent), Bulgaria (6 per cent), Poland (7 per cent), Latvia (8 per cent), Portugal (10 per cent) and Finland (10 per cent), while respondents in Lithuania (2 per cent), Latvia (4.5 per cent), and Estonia (6 per cent) are less likely to be members at a health of fitness centre. Membership of a

Table 7.2 Settings of youth engagement in sport and other physical activity for all EU–28 member states (2014)

	At a health or fitness centre	At a sports club	At a sports centre	At school or university	At home	In a park, outdoors, etc.
Total	20,5%	19,8%	10,3%	24,4%	33,1%	33,5%
Austria	31,2%	21,5%	9,7%	26,9%	33,3%	49,5%
Belgium	10,3%	30,8%	10,3%	32,7%	22,4%	21,5%
Bulgaria	30,0%	12,9%	8,6%	27,1%	27,1%	28,6%
Cyprus (Republic)	25,0%	5,6%	5,6%	25,0%	36,1%	27,8%
Czech Republic	31,2%	22,6%	19,4%	26,9%	33,3%	29,0%
Germany East	22,8%	22,8%	7,6%	25,0%	34,4%	33,5%
Denmark	40,8%	26,8%	7,0%	32,4%	32,4%	42,3%
Estonia	20,2%	24,2%	9,1%	28,3%	22,2%	26,3%
Spain	24,0%	16,0%	16,0%	8,0%	6,0%	42,0%
Finland	33,7%	10,5%	14,0%	26,7%	41,9%	67,4%
France	11,0%	30,0%	10,0%	25,0%	29,0%	36,0%
United Kingdom	25,8%	20,0%	15,4%	15,0%	44,8%	31,5%
Greece	32,3%	22,2%	11,1%	13,1%	19,2%	29,3%
Croatia	19,7%	13,8%	7,9%	11,8%	37,5%	28,9%
Hungary	14,0%	14,0%	3,5%	24,4%	36,0%	12,8%
Ireland	19,3%	26,1%	8,0%	22,7%	25,0%	33,0%
Italy	23,8%	12,7%	36,5%	12,7%	4,8%	27,0%
Lithuania	2,4%	26,2%	5,4%	31,0%	51,8%	30,4%
Luxembourg	23,3%	30,0%	10,0%	50,0%	23,3%	16,7%
Latvia	8,6%	6,9%	11,5%	27,0%	40,2%	38,5%
Malta	25,0%	16,7%	20,8%	16,7%	25,0%	25,0%
The Netherlands	24,0%	39,6%	10,4%	30,2%	34,4%	28,1%
Poland	13,6%	11,4%	10,2%	27,3%	34,1%	23,9%
Portugal	24,6%	13,8%	3,1%	23,1%	12,3%	35,4%
Romania	12,0%	4,8%	3,6%	26,5%	47,0%	26,5%
Sweden	52,4%	35,7%	9,5%	45,2%	52,4%	50,0%
Slovenia	12,1%	22,0%	9,9%	16,5%	48,4%	50,5%
Slovakia	17,3%	16,3%	11,5%	29,8%	39,4%	36,5%

Note: the total of the percentages may exceed 100%, since the respondent had the possibility of giving several answers to the question.

social–cultural club is relatively high in Belgium (12 per cent), Sweden (12 per cent), Germany (10 per cent) and the Netherlands (10 per cent). The proportion of respondents not members at any club is the highest in Latvia (83 per cent), Bulgaria (79 per cent), Portugal (77.5 per cent), Romania (77 per cent), Poland (77 per cent) and Cyprus (76 per cent).

Motivators and barriers to sport participation

Motivators

Health is the main consideration for European youth when it comes to sport or physical activity, followed by a wide range of other factors.

Table 7.3 Youth club membership for all EU–28 member states (2014)

	Health or fitness centre	Sports club	Socio-cultural club that includes sport in its act	No, not a member of any club (SPONTANEOUS)
Total	16,7%	19,7%	6,0%	60,0%
Austria	25,8%	23,7%	7,2%	48,5%
Belgium	14,2%	32,7%	12,4%	46,9%
Bulgaria	10,5%	6,3%	4,2%	78,9%
Cyprus (Republic)	14,0%	12,0%	0,0%	76,0%
Czech Republic	24,5%	21,6%	2,0%	52,9%
Germany	18,6%	24,3%	10,4%	50,8%
Denmark	45,8%	25,0%	4,2%	38,9%
Estonia	5,9%	25,7%	7,9%	55,4%
Spain	16,2%	19,7%	5,1%	62,4%
Finland	23,9%	10,2%	5,7%	62,5%
France	8,9%	30,4%	5,4%	58,0%
United Kingdom	26,6%	19,1%	4,7%	57,8%
Greece	28,0%	20,3%	3,4%	53,4%
Croatia	15,8%	16,5%	3,2%	62,7%
Hungary	8,7%	13,0%	7,6%	72,8%
Ireland	22,9%	31,3%	7,3%	46,9%
Italy	12,5%	22,7%	0,0%	63,6%
Lithuania	2,2%	20,4%	8,3%	60,8%
Luxembourg	24,2%	39,4%	6,1%	39,4%
Latvia	4,5%	8,4%	3,9%	83,2%
Malta	13,2%	15,8%	2,6%	71,1%
The Netherlands	27,8%	38,1%	10,3%	36,1%
Poland	9,7%	6,8%	4,9%	76,7%
Portugal	10,8%	9,8%	5,9%	77,5%
Romania	12,5%	1,0%	5,8%	76,9%
Sweden	41,9%	39,5%	11,6%	34,9%
Slovenia	11,8%	23,7%	5,4%	58,1%
Slovakia	19,6%	19,6%	8,9%	54,5%

Note: the total of the percentages may exceed 100%, since the respondent had the possibility of giving several answers to the question.

This section reveals the wide range of personal motivations that individual respondents have for deciding whether to engage in sport or physical activity (Table 7.4). The most common reason for engaging in sport or physical activity for youth is to improve health (57 per cent), with more than 40 per cent of respondents also mentioning improving fitness and having fun. The other commonly cited reasons for engaging in sport or physical activity are to improve your physical appearance (37 per cent), to relax (37 per cent), to be with friends (32 per cent), to improve physical appearance (29.5 per cent) and to control weight (22.5 per cent). Respondents from several countries describe health considerations as heavily influencing their decision: Sweden (74 per cent), Denmark (67 per cent), Slovenia (67 per cent) and Cyprus (67 per cent). However, a lower proportion of youth in Bulgaria (41 per cent) and Hungary

(44 per cent) say they are motivated to improve their health. Improving one's fitness as a motivator is the most common in Sweden (71 per cent), Denmark (68 per cent) and the Netherlands (63.5 per cent). A much lower proportion of respondents cite this as their motivation in Romania (22 per cent), Portugal (23 per cent, Poland (25 per cent) and Spain (25 per cent). Sport and physical activity is generally viewed as being a fun activity in some EU member states, but not in others. In the Netherlands, 66 per cent of respondents say they do it for fun. However, a much smaller number of respondents in Romania (20.5 per cent) and Hungary (21 per cent) say they engage in sport or physical activity for fun. Improving physical appearance is a very common motivating factor for youth in some countries, especially Sweden (52 per cent), Italy (51 per cent) and Denmark (50 per cent). However, this is much less important in Ireland (24 per cent), the Netherlands (25 per cent) and Belgium (25 per cent). Relaxation emerges as a particularly compelling reason in the Netherlands (66 per cent), Slovenia (64 per cent) and Belgium (56 per cent). However, this is less of a factor in Poland (10 per cent) and Slovakia (14 per cent). Engaging in sport or physical activity as a way of spending time with friends is relatively common among youth in: Austria (53 per cent), Ireland (47 per cent) and Slovenia (46 per cent). In other countries, especially Romania (16 per cent), Poland (16 per cent) and Lithuania (17 per cent), this is less of a factor. Improving physical performance is a common motivating factor in some countries, especially Sweden (52 per cent), Austria (46 per cent) and Slovenia (45 per cent). However, this is much less important in Bulgaria (14 per cent) and Romania (17 per cent). Respondents in Denmark (48 per cent) and Malta (42 per cent) commonly cite 'controlling your weight' as a motivating factor, unlike those in Hungary (8 per cent). Other factors are generally viewed as being comparatively less important across the EU. However, 45 per cent of respondents in Sweden say they engage in sport or physical activity in order to improve their self-esteem and to develop new skills.

Barriers

Lack of time is the main reason given for not practicing sport

All respondents were asked about the main reasons that currently prevent them from practicing sport more regularly (Table 7.5). Lack of time is the main reason that youth in the EU give for not practicing sport more regularly (mentioned by 47 per cent). Other factors include a lack of motivation or interest (18 per cent) or the fact that it is too expensive (13 per cent). A small minority of respondents give other reasons: 6 per cent cite lack of suitable or accessible sport infrastructure close to where they live, 5 per cent do not like competitive activities, and 4.5 per cent do not have friends to do sport with.

Lack of time is the most common reasons for not practicing sport across the EU. On a country level, the proportions of youth giving this answer are the highest in Malta (68 per cent), Denmark (64 per cent), Sweden (63 per cent) and Luxembourg (61 per cent). The lowest proportions are in Italy (30 per cent) and Portugal (33 per cent). Lack of interest or motivation is mentioned by a large proportion of youth in Sweden (37 per cent), Denmark (31 per cent), France (29 per cent) and Croatia (27 per cent). Youth in Hungary (8 per cent), Italy (9 per cent), Latvia (11 per cent) and Romania (11.5 per cent) are least likely to see this as a problem. The cost of practicing sport is mentioned most frequently in Portugal (27 per cent), whereas only 3 per cent in Malta and Ireland say that it is too expensive. Other barriers are viewed as less important across the EU.

Table 7.4 Motivations of youth to participate in sport and physcial activity for all EU-28 member states (2014)

	To improve your health	To improve your physical appearance	To have fun	To relax	To be with friends	To make new acquaintances	To improve physical performance	To improve fitness	To control your weight	To improve your self-esteem	To develop new skills	For the spirit of competition
Total	56,9%	37,4%	42,4%	37,4%	32,2%	7,8%	29,5%	44,4%	22,5%	13,6%	14,0%	11,7%
Austria	61,3%	38,7%	51,6%	28,0%	52,7%	18,3%	46,2%	50,5%	29,0%	18,3%	17,2%	17,2%
Belgium	48,6%	25,2%	55,1%	56,1%	40,2%	10,3%	23,4%	53,3%	15,9%	12,1%	10,3%	17,8%
Bulgaria	41,4%	40,0%	34,3%	28,6%	28,6%	5,7%	14,3%	27,1%	28,6%	20,0%	5,7%	11,4%
Cyprus (Republic)	66,7%	36,1%	36,1%	30,6%	19,4%	2,8%	19,4%	44,4%	27,8%	16,7%	13,9%	2,8%
Czech Republic	46,2%	35,5%	48,4%	21,5%	40,9%	14,0%	19,4%	43,0%	15,1%	6,5%	5,4%	8,6%
Germany	62,3%	41,8%	50,3%	33,0%	41,7%	8,7%	43,1%	54,1%	27,1%	19,8%	17,6%	12,5%
Denmark	69,0%	49,3%	49,3%	33,8%	45,1%	16,9%	39,4%	67,6%	47,9%	32,4%	31,0%	22,5%
Estonia	50,5%	26,3%	34,3%	41,4%	23,2%	5,1%	24,2%	46,5%	32,3%	22,2%	25,3%	11,1%
Spain	51,0%	42,0%	45,0%	41,0%	26,0%	5,0%	31,0%	25,0%	13,0%	9,0%	11,0%	11,0%
Finland	64,0%	36,0%	39,5%	48,8%	38,4%	9,3%	43,0%	55,8%	32,6%	23,3%	19,8%	12,8%
France	61,0%	43,0%	34,0%	46,0%	36,0%	10,0%	28,0%	60,0%	29,0%	10,0%	13,0%	18,0%
Great Britain	64,5%	26,9%	52,4%	21,7%	32,4%	6,2%	25,4%	56,2%	33,5%	10,4%	17,1%	8,3%
Greece	50,5%	36,4%	37,4%	42,4%	36,4%	3,0%	29,3%	60,6%	22,2%	8,1%	7,1%	10,1%
Croatia	57,2%	44,7%	40,8%	48,7%	23,7%	5,9%	21,1%	34,2%	15,1%	7,2%	10,5%	6,6%
Hungary	44,2%	39,5%	20,9%	29,1%	29,1%	5,8%	34,9%	32,6%	8,1%	8,1%	7,0%	9,3%
Ireland	65,9%	23,9%	44,3%	31,8%	46,6%	4,5%	21,6%	44,3%	20,5%	8,0%	13,6%	14,8%
Italy	49,2%	50,8%	39,7%	44,4%	31,7%	4,8%	17,5%	34,9%	19,0%	11,1%	1,6%	3,2%
Lithuania	47,6%	36,9%	58,9%	36,3%	16,7%	3,6%	31,0%	30,4%	17,9%	7,1%	6,5%	4,2%
Luxembourg	53,3%	33,3%	46,7%	40,0%	36,7%	6,7%	33,3%	43,3%	26,7%	20,0%	10,0%	13,3%
Latvia	61,5%	45,4%	31,0%	34,5%	29,3%	9,2%	20,7%	46,6%	12,6%	12,6%	19,0%	10,9%
Malta	58,3%	37,5%	37,5%	54,2%	25,0%	8,3%	29,2%	41,7%	41,7%	16,7%	20,8%	29,2%
The Netherlands	56,3%	25,0%	65,6%	65,6%	33,3%	10,4%	34,4%	63,5%	28,1%	9,4%	22,9%	13,5%
Poland	52,3%	30,7%	36,4%	10,2%	15,9%	4,5%	31,8%	25,0%	13,6%	12,5%	5,7%	4,5%
Portugal	60,0%	43,1%	32,3%	32,3%	32,3%	4,6%	20,0%	23,1%	16,9%	10,8%	13,8%	7,7%
Romania	63,9%	34,9%	20,5%	41,0%	15,7%	3,6%	16,9%	21,7%	22,9%	9,6%	7,2%	6,0%
Sweden	73,8%	52,4%	54,8%	42,9%	38,1%	19,0%	52,4%	71,4%	35,7%	45,2%	45,2%	38,1%
Slovenia	67,0%	33,0%	42,9%	63,7%	46,2%	11,0%	45,1%	45,1%	27,5%	16,5%	18,7%	15,4%
Slovakia	52,9%	43,3%	33,7%	13,5%	35,6%	6,7%	31,7%	45,2%	16,3%	14,4%	12,5%	13,5%

Note: the total of the percentages may exceed 100%, since the respondent had the possibility of giving several answers to the question.

Table 7.5 Barriers of youth to participate in sport and physical activity for all EU–28 member states (2014)

	You do not have the time	It is too expensive	You do not like competitive activities	There is no suitable or accessible sport infrastructure	You have a disability or illness	You do not have friends to do sports with	You feel discriminated against by other participants	You lack motivation or are not interested	You are afraid of the risk of injuries
Total	47,2%	12,9%	4,7%	6,3%	3,6%	4,5%	0,7%	17,9%	2,5%
Austria	36,1%	6,2%	8,2%	1,0%	3,1%	1,0%	0,0%	18,6%	4,1%
Belgium	45,1%	11,5%	8,0%	4,4%	3,5%	8,0%	1,8%	15,9%	0,9%
Bulgaria	37,9%	12,6%	4,2%	6,3%	1,1%	5,3%	0,0%	15,8%	3,2%
Cyprus (Republic)	54,0%	18,0%	2,0%	6,0%	0,0%	6,0%	2,0%	18,0%	4,0%
Czech Republic	54,9%	19,6%	6,9%	7,8%	5,9%	2,9%	2,0%	21,6%	2,9%
Germany	37,2%	10,5%	3,5%	6,8%	5,0%	3,2%	0,5%	22,4%	1,8%
Denmark	63,9%	20,8%	1,4%	4,2%	6,9%	5,6%	0,0%	30,6%	5,6%
Estonia	46,5%	11,9%	3,0%	6,9%	6,9%	3,0%	0,0%	14,9%	4,0%
Spain	50,4%	7,7%	3,4%	0,0%	5,1%	2,6%	1,7%	17,1%	1,7%
Finland	40,9%	10,2%	6,8%	8,0%	6,8%	9,1%	0,0%	22,7%	2,3%
France	56,3%	6,3%	4,5%	4,5%	3,6%	2,7%	0,0%	28,6%	3,6%
United Kingdom	50,2%	18,5%	3,1%	6,5%	6,3%	4,2%	1,8%	20,5%	2,5%
Greece	43,2%	12,7%	5,1%	5,9%	0,8%	6,8%	0,0%	15,3%	0,0%
Croatia	47,5%	17,7%	3,8%	8,9%	3,2%	3,8%	1,3%	26,6%	1,9%
Hungary	48,9%	13,0%	8,7%	6,5%	4,3%	5,4%	2,2%	7,6%	2,2%
Ireland	40,6%	3,1%	5,2%	1,0%	3,1%	3,1%	0,0%	13,5%	1,0%
Italy	29,5%	13,6%	11,4%	5,7%	0,0%	2,3%	1,1%	9,1%	2,3%
Lithuania	49,7%	16,6%	5,0%	12,2%	1,1%	5,0%	1,1%	18,8%	0,6%
Luxembourg	60,6%	9,1%	3,0%	0,0%	6,1%	3,0%	0,0%	21,2%	3,0%
Latvia	58,1%	9,5%	5,0%	9,5%	2,2%	2,8%	0,0%	11,2%	0,6%
Malta	68,4%	2,6%	7,9%	2,6%	0,0%	2,6%	0,0%	21,1%	2,6%
The Netherlands	38,1%	9,3%	3,1%	2,1%	2,1%	2,1%	0,0%	13,4%	2,1%
Poland	53,4%	10,7%	1,0%	5,8%	3,9%	4,9%	0,0%	13,6%	5,8%
Portugal	33,3%	26,5%	5,9%	5,9%	1,0%	3,9%	0,0%	17,6%	2,0%
Romania	50,0%	12,5%	0,0%	11,5%	3,8%	3,8%	0,0%	11,5%	0,0%
Sweden	62,8%	11,6%	2,3%	4,7%	14,0%	7,0%	0,0%	37,2%	2,3%
Slovenia	50,5%	18,3%	4,3%	10,8%	5,4%	6,5%	0,0%	14,0%	6,5%
Slovakia	42,0%	15,2%	7,1%	7,1%	2,7%	9,8%	1,8%	17,9%	4,5%

Note: the total of the percentages may exceed 100%, since the respondent had the possibility of giving several answers to the question.

Conclusion

The main findings of the Eurobarometer survey on youth sport participation can be summarized as follows:

More than 50 per cent of European youth exercise or play sport regularly, while 18 per cent of them never do so.

Generally speaking, youth in the Northern part of Europe are the most physically active. The proportion that exercises or plays sport regularly is 81 per cent in Finland and Denmark. The lowest levels of youth participation are clustered in the Southern European countries. Most respondents who never exercise or play sport can be found in Malta (58 per cent) and Portugal (42 per cent).

Sport or physical activity takes place in a wide range of locations, most commonly in parks and outdoor (33.5 per cent) and at home (33 per cent).

Sixty per cent of European youth say that they are not members of any club.

The most common reason for engaging in sport or physical activity among European youth is to improve health (57 per cent). Other popular reasons include improving fitness and having fun (40 per cent), improve physical appearance (37 per cent), relaxing (37 per cent) and be with friends (32 per cent).

A shortage of time is by far the main reason given for not practicing sport more regularly (47 per cent). Other factors mentioned are a lack of motivation or interest (18 per cent) and that is too expensive (13 per cent).

Annex: questions asked

Frequency of sport participation and levels of engagement

How often do you exercise or play sport? By exercise, we mean any form of physical activity which you do in a sport context or sport-related setting, such as swimming, training in a fitness centre or sport club, running in the park, etc.

Possible responses: 5 times a week or more; 3–4 times a week; 1–2 times a week; 1–3 times a month; less often; never; don't know.

Settings of sport participation

Earlier, you said you engage in sport or other physical activity. Where do you engage in sport or physical activity?

Possible responses discussed here are: at a health or fitness centre; at a sport club; at a sport centre; at school or university; at home; in a park, outdoors, etc.; elsewhere.

Are you a member of any of the following clubs where you participate in sport or recreational physical activity?

Possible responses are: health or fitness centre; sport club; socio-cultural club that includes sport in its activities (e.g. youth club, school- and university-related club); other; no, I am not a member of any club.

Motivations and barriers to sport participation

Why do you engage in sport or physical activity?

Possible responses: to improve your health; to improve your physical appearance; to counteract the effects of ageing; to have fun; to relax; to be with friends; to make new acquaintances; to meet people from other cultures; to improve physical performance; to improve fitness; to control your weight; to improve your self-esteem; to develop new skills; for the spirit of competition; to better integrate into society; other.

What are the main reasons currently preventing you from practicing sport more regularly?

Possible responses: you do not have the time; it is too expensive; you do not like competitive activities; there is no suitable sport infrastructure close to where you live; you have a disability or illness; you do not have friends to do sports with; you feel discriminated against by other participants; you lack motivation or are not interested; you are afraid of the risk of injuries; you are already doing sports regularly.

References

Council of Europe (1975). *The European Sport for All Charter.* Strasbourg: Council of Europe.

Crum, B. (1991). *Over versporting van de samenleving. Reflecties over de bewegingsculturele ontwikkelingen met het oog op sportbeleid* [Sportification of society. Reflections for policy]. Rijswijk: Ministerie van Welzijn, Volksgezondheid en Cultuur.

European Commission (2014). *Special Eurobarometer 412. Sport and physical activity.* Brussels: Directorate-General for Education and Culture.

Hartmann-Tews, I. (2006). Social stratification in sport and sport policy in the European Union. *European Journal for Sport and Society, 3,* 109–124.

Husting, A. (2003). De Raad van Europa en sport [The council of Europe and sport] in K. Geeraerts (ed), *Praktijkgids Sportmanagement* (pp. 1–46). Antwerpen: F&G Partners.

Renson, R. (1992). *Geschiedenis van de sport in de oudheid* [History of sport in ancient times]. Leuven: Acco.

Scheerder, J., van Tuyckom, C. and Vermeersch, A. (2007). *Europa in beweging. Sport vanuit Europees perspectief* [Europe on the move. A European perspective on sport]. Gent: Academia Press.

van Bottenburg, M., Rijnen, B. and van Sterkenburg, J. (2005). *Sports participation in the European Union: Trends and differences.* Nieuwegein: Arko Sports Media.

van Tuyckom, C. and Scheerder, J. (2010). A multilevel analysis of social stratification patterns of leisure time physical activity among Europeans. *Science Sports, 25,* 304–311.

van Tuyckom, C. (2011). Modernization and sport participation in 27 European member states in the light of Beck's individualization these. In: Scheerder, J., Vandermeerschen, H., van Tuyckom, C., Hoekman, R., Breedveld, K. and Vos, S., *Sport participation in Europe.* From facts to sheets (Sport, Policy and Management 10). Leuven: KULeuven/Research Unit of Social Kinesiology and Sport Management).

van Tuyckom, C., Scheerder, J. and Bracke, P. (2010). Gender and age inequalities in regular sport participation. A cross-national study of 25 European countries. *Journal of Sports Sciences, 28(10),* 1077–1084.

Vanreusel, B. (2001). *Sport: bewegingscultuur tussen idealisering en degradering* [Sport: movement culture between idealizing and downgrading]. In: Raeymaekers, B. (ed), Moeten, mogen, kunnen. Ethiek en wetenschap (pp. 70–86). Leuven: Universitaire Pers.

8

YOUTH SPORT IN NORWAY

Ken Green

Introduction

In any investigation of sports participation, Norway, like its Nordic neighbours (fellow Scandinavian countries Denmark and Sweden together with Finland and Iceland), makes an interesting case study. In this chapter, I seek to shed light on what often appears as a kind of Nordic or, at least, Scandinavian, exceptionalism in the field of youth sport.[1] In the first instance, I offer an outline of relatively recent developments within youth sport in Norway followed by an attempt to provide a plausible explanation for the developments depicted. The data upon which the chapter is based is derived from two major and ongoing surveys.[2]

A few basic facts

At the outset, it is worth keeping in mind a few basic facts about sport around the world. The first of these is that sport tends *not* to be a central feature of adult leisure lives even if it *is* a significant feature for some. The next basic fact is that unlike some major uses of leisure (e.g. watching TV and consuming alcohol), sports participation declines with age – especially around significant life-stage transitions (coinciding roughly with ages 16, 45 and 70). When compared with other uses of leisure, loyalty rates in sport are not good. This is not necessarily because young people become less interested in sport. Nor is it because young people have simply become slothful – in other words, over-weight or obese screen-obsessed couch potatoes – although some may have. Rather, it is because they acquire wider ranges of leisure options and, for some, these are more appealing. These basic facts do not appear, however, to apply quite so readily to Nordic countries such as Norway. As van Tuyckom (this volume) points out, Eurobarometer findings confirm that those 'in the Nordic countries are the most likely to exercise or play sport on a regular basis'. In Finland and Denmark, for example, 81 per cent of people exercise or play sport 'at least a few times a week' while Sweden also boasts a high proportion (79 per cent) who exercise or play sport regularly.

Amid the generally high levels of sports participation alluded to in Eurobarometer, among other studies, surveys of sports participation in Norway reveal several interesting developments in youth sport in recent decades. These can be summarized as more young people doing more sport (including substantial increases among young females, in particular) more often; a later peak in sports participation than typically found outside Nordic countries (i.e. in the later teenage years) – alongside a phenomena I will refer to as 'bounce-back' among older adults, convergence between the sexes (towards sporting parity) and a shift towards lifestyle sports. It is worth saying a little more about each of these in turn.

Increases in sports participation

The first point of note is that unlike most Western European countries such as the UK – where participation grew in the 1970s and then more or less plateaued from the 1990s – participation in leisure-sport (on annual, monthly and weekly bases) in Norway increased from 1985, and from 2001 in particular. In addition, the increases in Norway occurred across most if not all social groups – among both children and youngsters (6–15 years) and adults (16–79 years) in general and females and early youth (16–19 years) especially (Dalen, 2013; Statistics Norway, 2014; Synovate, 2009; Vaage, 2009).

While sports participation has tended in very many countries to be normally distributed along a bell-shaped curve, in Norway participation has become asymmetrical – that is, negatively skewed (in statistical terms) towards the higher rates and frequencies (bouts) (Figure 8.1). More adults (including youth) were playing more sport more often in 2007 in Norway than only a decade earlier. Alongside the relatively large and increased majority at the active or regular participant pole (i.e. three to four times per week or almost daily), relatively smaller and steadily declining numbers were found at the rarely/never (inactive) end of the continuum. Indeed, the most marked increases in the period 2001–2007 were among those who exercised a lot. Interestingly, while there were increases in the proportions participating regularly across all age groups between 2001 and 2007, the greatest changes occurred in the 16–19 year age group. This points to the next development: the age at which sports participation peaks in Norway.

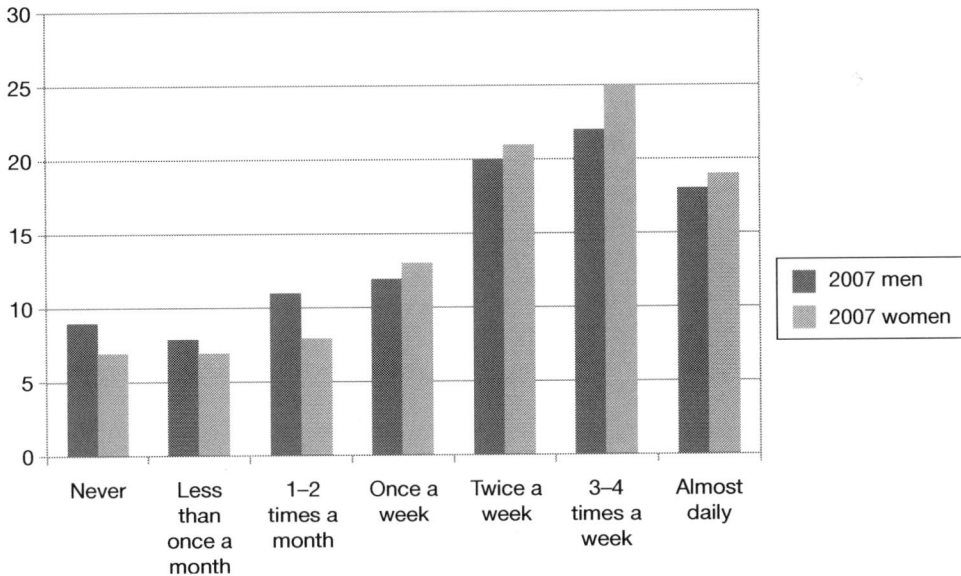

Figure 8.1 Frequency (per cent) of sport and physical activity participation for training or exercise by 16–79-year-olds (2007). Based on Vaage (2009)

A later peak in sports participation

In terms of participation, it is worth remembering that 'the youth life stage begins at a high point' (Roberts, this volume): that is, the peak age for sports participation in most countries is between 12 and 14 years of age. Thereafter, Roberts (this volume) argues that the overall trend is for young people to do progressively less. This leads towards the first point where substantial drop-off (doing less) and drop-out (stopping completely) occurs – around age 16, or the end of compulsory schooling. Although young people may spend more time playing, and play more sports than adults, youth tends to be the life stage when drop-off and drop-out from sport takes hold. But not so much in Nordic countries such as Norway it seems.

In Norway, between 1997 and 2007, the proportions of regular participants (three to four times per week or more) more than doubled (16 per cent to 39 per cent) between the age groups 6–8 and 9–12; climbed again, by one-quarter (39 per cent to 50 per cent), between those aged 9–12 and 13–15; and rose once more, by one-fifth (50 per cent to 60 per cent), among the 16–19-year-olds (Table 8.1). In 2007, nearly two-thirds (60 per cent) of 16–19-year-olds were taking part three to four times a week or more, of which 27 per cent exercised almost every day. Thus, the proportions of young Norwegians participating 'regularly' increased among older teenagers to peak among the 16–19 years age group; that is to say, several years later than generally assumed to be the case elsewhere in the world, beyond the Nordic countries.

Convergence between the sexes

The third big difference has to do with convergence between the sexes. Although they have lessened in recent decades, sex differences tend to be wider in sport than in any other area of leisure and can be stark. Males, whether young or old, have tended to participate in sport in greater numbers, more frequently, for longer periods and in more competitive and combative forms. As well as being less likely to devote themselves to sports than their male counterparts, females remain more likely to drop out of sport sooner and in greater numbers. Differences in participation between the sexes, coupled with the manner in which sport is said to inculcate, perpetuate and celebrate a type of physical, competitive, even aggressive masculine identity has led to its depiction as a male preserve. That said, and as Wright (this volume) observes, there have been some marked changes in females' relationships with sport in recent decades. In addition to their increased rates of participation, females now tend to take part in a wider array of sports

Table 8.1 Frequency (per cent) physical activity participation for training or exercise by 6–15-year-olds (2007)

	never	less than month	1-2x per month	1x per week	2x per week	3-4x per week	about daily
Boys 6–8yrs	17	6	5	25	30	15	2
Girls 6–8yrs	10	4	6	36	30	13	2
Boys 9–12yrs	5	2	2	15	32	32	12
Girls 9–12yrs	6	4	6	18	32	28	6
Boys 13–15yrs	3	4	6[13]	13	20[33]	27	25[52%]
Girls 13–15yrs	4	6	4[14]	9	29[38]	34	14[48%]

Source: based on Vaage (2009).

than hitherto, including those stereotypically associated with males and masculinity. While over-represented in body-management-type activities – especially those concerned with appearance – girls and young women are increasingly involved in sporting activities once associated almost entirely with males, such as football, martial arts and outdoor and adventurous activities. Despite the narrowing of sex differences in sports participation in recent decades, sport across the globe remains gendered. Once again, however, this is not so true of Norway.

In Norway, during the first decade of the twenty-first century, the skewed pattern of partici-pation – towards higher rates and more frequent bouts of participation – was especially pro-nounced among young women. Taken together, the two main large-scale studies of Norwegian sports participation (Dalen, 2013; Synovate, 2009; Vaage, 2009) indicate that towards the end of the first decade of the twenty-first century, sex differences in sports participation had reversed in Norway – Norwegian females had overtaken males as the more regular participants while males had become the group most likely to participate infrequently.

The situation among girls and young women in Norway in the 2000s appeared an exaggerated version of that of adult females. *Norsk Monitor* revealed that while sports participation was slightly higher among males in most of the younger age groups, the differences between the sexes in rates of participation steadily diminished between 1985 and 2009, such that by 2009 there were no major differences between boys and girls. According to Statistics Norway (Vaage, 2009), in 2007, by the time youngsters approached upper secondary school (15 years of age), the levels of participation among the sexes had converged. Although 13–15-year-old boys were almost twice as likely as girls to participate on an almost daily basis (25 per cent boys: 14 per cent girls), girls were more likely to take part three to four times each week (27 per cent: 34 per cent). When aggregated, therefore, similar proportions of girls (48 per cent) and boys (52 per cent) participated regularly in sport (three to four times each week or more). The convergence between Norwegian boys and girls involved not simply rates of participation but also bouts or frequency.

A shift away from games and towards lifestyle sports

The final transformation in sports participation in Norway is one that is not peculiar to Norway or, for that matter, the Nordic countries more generally (Gilchrist and Wheaton, this volume); that is, the increasing popularity of lifestyle sports – both absolutely and in relation to more traditional activities, such as team games. Big increases in participation in lifestyle sports – such as organized walking (which nearly doubled from, 48 per cent to 87 per cent), weight training (up by half, from 24 per cent to 36 per cent), jogging (up by approximately one-third, from 34 per cent to 45 per cent) and cross-country skiing (up by more than a quarter, from 38 per cent to 51 per cent) – was one of two major developments in the forms of sport young Norwegians engaged in during the first decade of the new millennium. The second major change in forms of sports participation involved team sports. Although young people (and 16–19-year-olds in particular) were the most active age group as far as team sports were concerned, the popularity of major games (such as football) and traditional games (such as handball), as well as relatively modern games (such as basketball and volleyball), declined among young Norwegians during this period.

Thus, despite the fact that sports clubs remain important social and sporting institutions in Nordic countries – and the bedrock of much sports participation among children and early youth – organized sport has not been primarily responsible for the increased levels of participa-tion in Norway and the Nordic countries. Rather, lifestyle sports have become the driver of increased participation among youth (Borgers, Seghers and Scheerder, this volume), and especi-ally among young women. The situation is very similar elsewhere in Scandinavia. Inevitably, very few of those participating in outdoor sports were associated with sports clubs (i.e. sports such as such as mountain-biking, boarding and blading of all kinds, downhill and cross-country skiing and snowboarding).

The shift towards lifestyle sports notwithstanding, it is apparent that a substantial minority of youth and young adults continued to take part in sport via sports clubs: almost half (44 per cent) of 16–19-year-olds, just under one-third of 20–24-year-olds (29 per cent) and one-quarter (24 per cent) of 25–34-year-olds did so in 2007. In this regard, and by way of emphasizing the point that the growing popularity of lifestyle sports has not led to an abandonment of team sports, in the first decade of the twenty-first century the numbers of children and early youth (and girls especially) who were members of sports teams grew substantially (Statistics Norway, 2014). Between 2001 and 2011, the proportion of boys aged 12 or younger who were members of sports teams increased by approximately 35 per cent (214,000 to 290,000) while the pro-portion of teenagers aged 13–19 years grew by around 24 per cent (152,000 to 188,000). Team membership among girls had grown even more rapidly: from 162,000 girls aged 0–12 years in 2001 to 240,000 by 2011 (an increase of 48 per cent) and from 105,000 13–19-year-old girls in 2001 to 139,000 by 2011 (an increase of 32 per cent). Thus, in the decade leading up to 2011, there was both substantial growth alongside convergence between the sexes in terms of membership of sports teams. The stagnation in traditional sports and games that Fridberg (2010) has identified in Denmark and, for that matter, Scandinavia as a whole, does not appear to have occurred, however, among children and youth in Norway.

While trends in forms of participation were by no means clear-cut, it was apparent that within the particular mix of conventional and lifestyle sports adopted by individual youngsters, lifestyle sports had become substantially more prominent in 2007 than they had been only a decade earlier. As with forms of participation, it seems that the trend towards less formal, less organized venues for participation has not, however, resulted in an abandonment of sports clubs as vehicles for participation. Rather, it represents a (seemingly significant) shift in the blend of traditional and lifestyle sports and club-based and informal venues as sports clubs and team games become less important generally for children moving into youth and young adulthood.

It seems likely that the growing popularity of lifestyle sports has played a significant part in shifting the peak of sports participation to a later point (an older age) in childhood and youth in Norway than hitherto and, for that matter, elsewhere in Europe.[3] This is, in part, because the typical peak ages for participation in individual sports (and, by extension, lifestyle sports) represents not so much a peak as a plateau.[4] Indeed, while participation in sports generally (and in team sports in particular) peaks in the early teenage years, the plateau in individual sports seems to postpone drop-off and drop-out to the late teens/early 20s.

It may be that some of the aforementioned developments in youth sport (perhaps in combination) in recent decades have played a part in a bounce-back effect. Having peaked among the 16–19 years age group, regular participation rates in sport in Norway then begin to decline, starting with the 20–24-year-olds. Nonetheless, having dipped during early adulthood through to middle-age (20–44 years) – the main years of economic and child rearing activity – rates of regular participation returned to virtually the same level as that for 20–24-year-olds (43 per cent) from the age of 45 through to retirement and beyond (25–34 years: 39 per cent; 35–44 years: 37 per cent; 45–54 years: 44 per cent; 55–66 years: 40 per cent; 67–79 years: 42 per cent) (Figure 8.2). This is markedly different from what tends to happen in very many countries beyond the Nordic region, where the mid-40s is the next major point of drop-out. Thus, in terms of what is variously called *lifelong participation* in, *adherence* to, and/or the *tracking* of sports participation (Scheerder and Vanreusel, this volume), in Norway late youth/early adulthood does not appear to mark the beginning of the end for sports participation usually associated

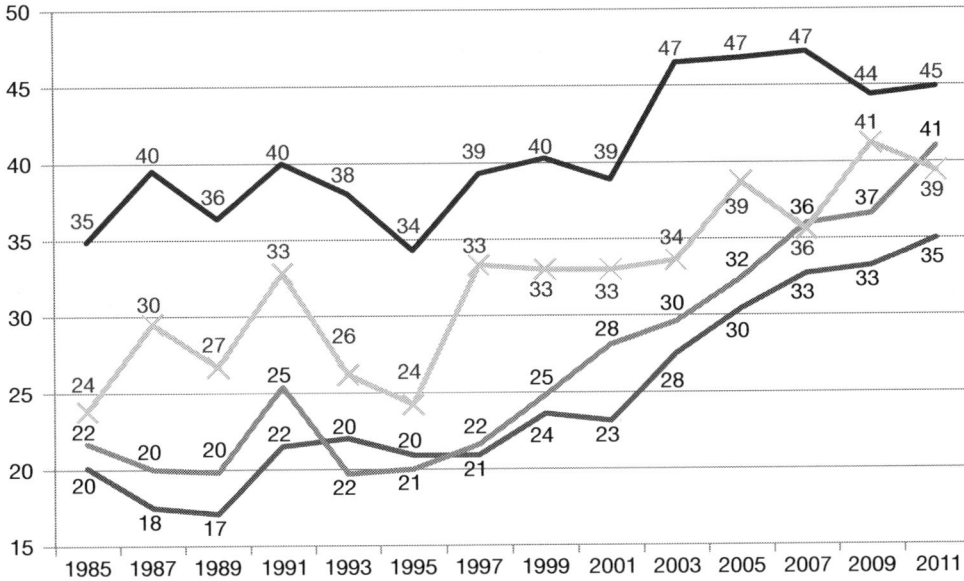

Figure 8.2 Norsk Monitor (2013): Age and participation. How often would you say you are doing physical activity in the form of training or exercise? 3x a week or more

with growing older. It seems plausible to suggest that this bounce-back is likely to have its roots in the kinds of sporting habituses and repertoires that sustained engagement with sport into youth facilitates among Norwegians.

All in all, the main trends in youths' sports participation in Norway in recent decades have been: more youth doing more sport, more often; a later peak in sports participation in the age group 16–19 years; convergence between the sexes; and, a shift towards lifestyle sports, especially among youth. So, how might these trends be explained?

Making sense of sports participation in Norway

In making sense of the trends in sports participation in Norway countries, I want to speculate on the causes, in other words, the main drivers and mechanisms. I provide an explanation based upon the context in which Norwegian youth develop their initial relationships with sport and point to the attitudes and predispositions to sport – what some sociologists would refer to as their individual and group habituses. I point, in particular, to three contexts: the economic and political context, the socio-cultural context and the socio-geographic context. From within these contexts, I pick out three tried and tested themes: namely, social class, gender and the family for particular attention.

The economic and political context

First, it is necessary to say something about the significance of economic and political developments in Norway for the creation of what others have referred to as the propitious or favourable circumstances (Birchwood *et al.*, 2008) for the seeming good news story that is sports participation in Norway. Three-quarters (75 per cent) of Norwegians aged 15–64 are in paid employment, well above the Organisation for Economic Co-operation and Development (OECD) average of 66 per cent (OECD, 2012). During roughly the same period (1999–2007) as substantial increases in sports participation occurred in Norway, average monthly earnings increased by approximately 50 per cent (from 23,176 Norwegian Kroner [NOK] per month in 1999 to 33,394 NOK per month in 2007) – almost 50 per cent higher than the OECD average. In addition, while Norwegian women's pay tended, as in all developed countries, to be lower than that of Norwegian men, there had been greater convergence by 2007 (with women earning 87 per cent that of men) in Norway than pretty much anywhere else beyond the Nordic countries (Statistics Norway, 2011). The apparent rise in economic *in*equalities in Nordic countries in the 1980s and 1990s notwithstanding, income distribution continues to be more equitable in Norway than in most other countries and, more significantly perhaps, levels of economic inequality [between top and bottom] are relatively compressed (Chan, Birkelund, Aas and Wiberg, 2010). This is, in no small measure, due to the fact that in the second half of the twentieth century, Norway and other Nordic countries built and retained the world's strongest state welfare regimes (Roberts, 2012). All-in-all, Norway, like the Nordic countries in general, performs exceptionally well against a variety of measures of economic and social well-being, and this is reflected in their rankings among the top countries in the the the *Legatum Prosperity Index*[5] (The Legatum Institute, 2013) and the OECD (2012) *Better Life Index.*

Gender and class in Norway

The improved position of Norwegian females in socio-economic terms is particularly striking. The *Global Gender Gap Index* (Hausmann *et al.*, 2012) revealed that, in 2012, the Nordic countries of Iceland, Finland, Norway and Sweden occupied the top four positions – having done so each year since 2006. While no country has yet achieved complete gender equality, almost all of the Nordic countries 'have closed over 80 per cent of the gender gap' (Hausmann *et al.*, 2012: 18). For many Nordic females, the significance of ascribed status has diminished as that of achieved status has increased markedly.

The significance of social mobility is particularly pertinent in the case of girls' and women's participation in sport. All countries recording high levels of sports participation, by definition, also record high levels of female participation (Coalter, 2013) and convergence between the sexes has, as indicated earlier, been a feature of participation trends in Norway. Few countries can boast the levels of sports participation among women (young and old) of Norway and it is unlikely to be a coincidence that nowhere is women's social status (as indicated by the percentage of women in legislatures and senior positions in business; the proximity of male/female incomes; and the percentage of women completing higher education [Coalter, 2013]) of a similar standing to that of their male counterparts than in Scandinavia in general and Norway in particular. It seems reasonable to posit, therefore, that such developments are likely to have had an impact on the general outlook and self-efficacy of girls and young women as well as their mothers while, more specifically, facilitating not only parents' own involvement in sport (with the concomitant role-modelling effects) but also that of their off-spring (both female and male). Put another way, the female parental role model for children (and girls especially) in Norway is increasingly likely to be a financially independent, working, and sporty mother. In this regard, the evidence suggests that gender has been re-shaped and is less significant for sports participation in Norway than it was as recently as the late 1990s.

It seems, then, that the growth of sports participation between 1997 and 2007 (from a high base in relation to many other non-Scandinavian countries) coincided with substantial increases in income across all age groups and both sexes. Being wealthier is likely to have contributed to the substantial growth in sports participation among Norwegian youth. Money makes it possible for people to do more during leisure of the things people already do or that those around them (or that they aspire to be among) do. Money facilitates sport, especially in the form of transport, equipment, coaching, club memberships and so on. It saves time and enables sovereignty. The growth in sports participation is unlikely, however, to have been a consequence of merely economic capital. While money is necessary for much sports participation, it is by no means sufficient: contact with (sporty) people who can facilitate youngsters' access to particular sporting experiences (so-called 'social capital') and possessing the necessary skills and knowledge ('cultural' or 'sporting capital') tend to be additional pre-requisites for sports participation.

The socio-cultural context

The likely significance for sports participation of far greater levels of economic and gender parity in Norway than many countries notwithstanding, it is unlikely that these have been the sole contributory factors to the high levels and increasingly varied forms of sports participation. Sports participation is multi-dimensional and the causal explanation is probably, therefore, multi-factorial. Thus, it seems likely that improvements in the general political, economic and social conditions of Norwegians, and females in particular, have created and reinforced already favourable conditions for sports participation – not least of which are the cultural traction of sport and the centrality of the family to Nordic sporting life. It is worth saying a little more about each of these.

The cultural traction of sport in Norway

Perhaps the most striking particularity of the Nordic cultural context is the enormous cultural traction (Roberts, 2014) of sport. Cultural traction refers to the rootedness of sport in what sociologists might call the group habitus or natural attitude; in other words, those aspects of physical culture deeply embedded in the everyday attitudes and practices of individuals and groups in particular societies and nations – the habits acquired (via socialization) by Norwegian youngsters as a consequence of growing up and living in a culture within which sport is so common-place and so highly valued.

Nordic countries make a particularly interesting case study of the rootedness of sport not least because their (sporting) cultures contain within them in the form of *friluftsliv* what, historically, has amounted to an almost ideal-type of cultural traction: that is, those lifestyle activities that take place in so-called nature-based settings and have a long and deeply rooted tradition. Friluftsliv has hitherto encompassed such activities as cross-country skiing, walking and camping as well as those historically associated with the etymological roots of the term sport – hunting, fishing and shooting. Nonetheless, the metaphorical ground is evidently shifting under frilufsliv, both in terms of forms and styles of participation, as well as context. In Norway, for example, between 1970 and 1997 there was an especially sharp decline in the proportion of youth (16–24-year-olds) who undertook traditional friluftsliv activities, such as long walks in the woods and longer skiing in the woods and mountains in the course of a year. It was noticeable that young Norwegians tended to be most active in physically demanding and often adventurous outdoor activities such as skiing, skating, climbing mountains and ice, rafting and kayaking. It was also the young as well as younger adults who participated to the greatest extent in mountain-biking and snowmobiling in their spare time. 'Berry and mushroom trips', on the other hand, are nowadays the preserve of older adults (Statistics Norway, 2014). These changes may well reflect a shift among Norwegian youth towards sports that offer alternative forms, as well as types, of participation to conventional sports (albeit still outdoors): put simply, more outdoor *adventure*, less outdoor *life*.

The significance of parents and family

As indicated above, the significance of the political and economic context notwithstanding, sports participation is not economically predetermined. We know this because of the differences within, as well as between, differing socio-economic strata. There are, in other words, some middle-class children and youth that do little in sporting terms and some working-class youngsters that do a lot. So what might the other factors be? The main mechanism for the continued cultural traction of sport is, first and foremost, primary socialization via the family (Quarmby, this volume): 'Childhood is the life stage when there is mass recruitment into sport' (Roberts, this volume), and while the vast majority of young people enter the post-child life stage with foundations in sport already laid, 'these foundations are not all equally strong' (Roberts, this volume). What makes them more or less strong can be experiences during school physical education, in sports clubs and so forth but, first and foremost, it tends to be parental and family support. This may take the form of modelling participation, encouraging and supporting, as well as facilitation in the form, for example, of transportation to and from sports locations – something that is particularly positively related to girls' participation. In particular, it takes the form of middle-class parents' tendency to pro-actively and strategically engage in the 'concerted cultivation' of their children's sporting capital (Wheeler, 2014). In other words, parents invest in their children's cultural capital (the things they know and can do), in general, and their sporting capital, in particular.

As intimated above, in Norway, parental involvement in their children's sporting lives appears to be made more likely by favourable socio-economic conditions; for example, the ways in which Nordic countries 'have made it possible for parents to combine work and family' (Hausmann *et al.*, 2012, p. 20), resulting in more shared participation in childcare including leisure among families. The hypothesized pivotal role of parents in the increases in sports participation may have been reinforced by demographic developments. Over the past two decades or more, Norway has been a relatively young society populated by couples who have tended to have children during a concentrated period around their late-20s to mid-30s.[6]

The centrality of the family to Norwegian youngsters' sports participation is marked, as are the ways in which families form a kind of virtuous sporting circle with sports clubs and elementary schools. Parents tend to be centrally involved in the sports club scene in Norway, spending a large amount of time facilitating their children's involvement in sport as well as coaching, organizing and administrating activities (Toftegaard Støckel *et al.*, 2010). Parents also tend to be intimately involved (once again, in a voluntary capacity) with their children's elementary schools. The role of parents in the (potentially) mutually reinforcing trinity of parents, school and sports club is in keeping with the strong sense of community and high levels of civic participation that the OECD (2012) views as characteristic of Norway. This sporting trinity is said to have been bolstered in recent years by a strengthening of cooperation between schools (especially elementary) and sports clubs (Toftegaard Støckel *et al.*, 2010). The close relationships between the three institutions and the interdependencies generated is likely to provide youngsters with a foundation for sports participation not just in terms of physical competencies and physical/ sporting capital, but also in terms of social and cultural capital – all the building blocks, in fact, for ongoing participation in sport.

The significance of parents' notwithstanding, 'by age 14, 13, 12 or even earlier, young people begin escaping into their own worlds. Adults begin to lose control. Children begin to express independent desires. They begin choosing their own friends and meeting unsupervised, or subject to looser and less obtrusive adult supervision than formerly' (Roberts, this volume). When coupled with increased disposable wealth, the growing independence of young people begins to explain the growth of lifestyle sports.

The socio-geographic context

The generally positive socio-political context and cultural traction of sport in Norway is reflected in the fact that approximately 60 per cent of state funding for sport is spent on developing sports facilities. The upshot is that there are between 10,000–12,000 sports centres in Norway (from the most modest local ground to large stadiums and indoor sports halls). Alongside a plentiful supply of human-made sports facilities and venues are an abundance of natural resources[7] for the increasingly popular lifestyle and adventurous sports (such as mountain-biking, kayaking, all forms of skiing and snow sports, mountaineering, orienteering and so forth). Thus, a wealth of natural and artificial outdoor and indoor sporting facilities alongside a well-established voluntary sports club sector and an elementary school system that emphasizes physical exercise and recreation and outdoor life as well as sport, together with high levels of parental involvement, add to the favourable socio-economic conditions to create seemingly optimal circumstances for sports participation. All these reinforce the sporting and physical recreation cultures deeply embedded in Norwegian society and embodied by the very many middle-class parents in a country that, for the time being at least, remains relatively young in demographic terms.

Conclusion

In this chapter, I have explored recent developments in sports participation in a country, Norway, in which participation has tended to be markedly higher than anywhere other than fellow Scandinavian and Nordic countries. Among other things, I have noted substantial increases in participation (among young people and females especially), a shift in the peak of participation to the late teenage years and a growth in lifestyle sports.

In making sense (or exploring the causes) of these developments, I have taken as my starting point Coalter's (2013, p. 18) observation that sport should be considered as largely epi-phenomenal: 'a secondary set of social practices [largely] dependent on and reflecting more fundamental structures, values and processes'. The structures are socio-economic, the values lie in the cultural traction of sport in Norway and the processes involve, among other things, parental cultivation of their children's sporting capital. The upshot is that youths in Norway grow up with sport as a deep-seated aspect of the Norwegian way of life, such that it has become an established part of the group habitus. Such predispositions appear to be intimately related to – even exacerbated by – relatively high levels of economic prosperity as well as class and gender parity. Sporting dispositions also seem to owe something to the especially central role of parents in early sports socialization in Norway in conjunction with schools and sports clubs. All-in-all, it seems that young Norwegians are the quintessential sporting omnivores.

Notes

1   In this chapter, the term *sport* will be used in a manner consistent with the General Introduction to this book; that is, to incorporate not only competitive game-contests (that is to say, conventional sports such as football, hockey, basketball and badminton) but also less competitive, less organized, recreational versions of these sports as well as more recreationally-oriented physical activities and exercise (aerobics, cycling, skateboarding, health and fitness gyms, surfing, cheerleading, dance, parkour and so forth)

variously referred to as lifestyle, lifetime and adventure sports and activities. On a handful of occasions, specific use will be made of terms such as lifestyle sport and physical recreation. The latter term will also be employed, where necessary, in order to obviate the importance of the aforementioned recreationally oriented activities to the point being made.

2   *Sports and Outdoor Activities, Survey on Living Conditions* is carried out by Statistics Norway [Statistisk Sentralbyrå] and *Norwegian (Norsk) Monitor* is currently delivered by Ipsos-mmi.no.

3   Indeed, among those who exercise a lot, there appears to be *no* gradual decline in participation.

4   An escarpment may be a better metaphor than a plateau insofar as participation levels out before beginning a slow but steady decline from the late teens, flattening out somewhat around middle age.

5   The *Legatum Prosperity Index* is an annual ranking of 110 countries developed by the Legatum Institute, a privately funded think tank. Based on 79 variables, it includes a number that is likely to be conducive to sports participation such as economic fundamentals, health, social capital, education, safety and security, personal freedom and democratic institutions.

6   The average age of Norwegian mothers and fathers at first birth and all births, for example, was between 28 years and 33 years in 2010 (Statistics Norway, 2011).

7   Everyone in Norway has a right-of-access (allemannsrett) and passage through, uncultivated land in the countryside under the 1957 Outdoor Recreation Act. Canoeing, kayaking, rowing and sailing are allowed in rivers and lakes. Swimming is only restricted in reservoirs used for drinking water. Foraging for mushrooms and berries is also part of allemannsrett.

Acknowledgement

I am grateful to the editors of the *International Journal of Sport Policy and Politics*, *Leisure Studies* and *Sport, Education and Society* for permission to use material from the following articles published in their journals as a basis for this chapter:

Green, K., Thurston, M. and Vaage, O. (2014). Isn't it good, Norwegian wood? Lifestyle and adventure sports participation among Norwegian youth. *Leisure Studies*, DOI: 10.1080/02614367.2014

Green, K., Thurston, M., Vaage, O. and Mordal-Moen, K. (2015). Girls, young women and sport in Norway: A case study of sporting convergence amid favourable socio–economic conditions. *International Journal of Sport Policy and Politics*, DOI: 10.1080/19406940.2015.1031812.

Green, K., Thurston, M., Vaage, O. and Roberts, K. (2015). "[We're on the right track, baby], we were born that way!" Exploring sports participation in Norway. *Sport, Education and Society*, 20(3), 285–303.

References

Birchwood, D., Roberts, K. and Pollock, G. (2008). Explaining differences in sport participation rates among young adults: Evidence from the South Caucasus. *European Physical Education Review, 14(3),* 283–300.

Borgers, J., Seghers, J. and Scheerder, J. (2016). Dropping out from clubs, dropping in to sport light? Organizational settings for youth sports participation; in K. Green and A. Smith (eds) *The Routledge handbook of youth sport* (pp. 158–174). London: Routledge.

Chan, T.W., Birkelund, G.E., Aas, K.A. and Wiberg, Ø. (2010). *Social status in Norway*. Available at: http://users.ox.ac.uk/~sfos0006/papers/status3.pdf. [Accessed 1 August 2012].

Coalter, F. (2013). Game plan and the Spirit Level: the class ceiling and the limits of sports policy? *International Journal of Sport Policy and Politics, 5(1),* 3–19.

Dalen, E. (2013). *Norsk monitor [Norwegian Monitor] 2012–13*. Presentation at Hedmark University College, Elverum, Norway, 13 April 2013.

Fridberg, T. (2010). Sport and exercise in Denmark, Scandinavia and Europe. *Sport in Society, 13(4),* 583–592.

Hausmann, R., Tyson, L.D. and Zahidi, S. (2012). *The global gender gap index 2012*. Geneva: World Economic Forum.

The Legatum Institute. (2013). *The Legatum prosperity index*. London: The Legatum Institute.

Office for Economic Cooperation and Development (OECD) (2012). *OECD Economic Surveys: Norway 2012*. Paris: OECD Publishing.

Quarmby, T. (2016). Parenting and youth sport. In K. Green and A. Smith (eds), *The Routledge handbook of youth sport* (pp. 209–217). London: Routledge.

Roberts, K. (2012). *Sociology: An introduction*. Cheltenham: Edward Elgar.

Roberts, K. (2014). Researching inner-city sport in A. Smith and I. Waddington (eds) *Doing real world research in sports studies*. London: Routledge.

Roberts, K. (2016). Young people and social change. In K. Green and A. Smith (eds), *The Routledge handbook of youth sport* (pp. 10–17). London: Routledge.

Roberts, K. (2016). Youth leisure as the context for youth sport. In K. Green and A. Smith (eds), *The Routledge handbook of youth sport* (pp. 18–25). London: Routledge.

Statistics Norway [Statistisk Sentralbyrå] (2011). *Statistical yearbook of Norway. 130th Issue*. Oslo-Kongsvinger: Statistics Norway.

Statistics Norway [Statistisk Sentralbyrå] (2014). *Sports and Outdoor Activities, Survey on Living Conditions, 2014*. Available at: www.ssb.no/en/sok?sok=sport. [Accessed 12 January 2015].

Synovate (2009) *Rapport barn og ungdom 2009* [Report on Children and Youth 2009]. Oslo: Synovate.

Toftegaard Støckel, J., Strandbu, Å., Solenes, O., Jørgensen, P. and Fransson, K. (2010). Sport for children and youth in the Scandinavian countries. *Sport in Society, 13(4)*, 625–642.

Vaage, O.F. (2009). *Mosjon, friluftsliv og kulturaktiviteter. resultater fra levekarsundersøkelsene fra 1997–2007. Rapport 2009/15 [Exercise, outdoor life and cultural activities. Results from a survey of living conditions from 1997–2007. Report 2009/15]*. Oslo-Kongsvinger: Statistics Norway.

van Tuyckom, C. (2016). Youth sport participation: A comparison between European member states; in K. Green and A. Smith (eds), *Routledge Handbook of Youth Sport* (pp. 61–71). London: Routledge.

Wheeler, S. (2014). *Patterns of parenting, class relations and inequalities in education and leisure: A grounded theory*. Unpublished PhD thesis. Chester: University of Chester.

9

YOUTH SPORT IN THE UNITED STATES

Jay Coakley

As of 2014, there were about 41 million 5–14-year-old boys and girls living in the United States. They constituted about 13 per cent of the total population. According to Sports Marketing Surveys, about half of those young people play sports, either organized or casual, during a given year, and it is estimated that 10–12 million play sports regularly or frequently.

Despite these numbers and the significance of youth sports as a cultural phenomenon, few scholars in the sociology of sport have studied the sport experiences of children under 14 years old. Michael Messner and Michela Musto from the University of Southern California recently reported that between 2003 and 2013, there were only eight articles that focused on children in the three major journals in the field: the *Sociology of Sport Journal*, the *Journal of Sport and Social Issues* and the *International Review for the Sociology of Sport*. Only three of these studies focused on children under 10 years old, and only one of those dealt with children in the United States (Messner and Musto, 2014). This means that since 2003 little knowledge has been produced about the experiences of young people under 14 years old in a wide variety of youth sport programmes across the country.

Data from an ESPN-commissioned survey of a nationally representative sample of parents in the United States indicated that 70 per cent of the parents were concerned about the time commitments and costs required for their children to play sport, and over 80 per cent of parents with children old enough to play organized sports were concerned with the quality or behaviour of youth sport coaches (Farrey, 2014). Additionally, a study that rated fifteen countries on nine factors related to physical activity among children and youth gave the United States a grade D– (where Grade A is the highest and F is the lowest) on overall physical activity (Tremblay *et al.*, 2014). Other grades included an F on *active transportation* (the 'percentage of children and youth who use active transportation to get to and from places'), a D on sedentary behaviours, a C– on organized sport participation and activity at school, a B– on community and built environment, and *incompletes* on active play, family and peers who facilitate physical activity opportunities, and government strategies and investments.

Although it has become difficult to obtain the multiple permissions required to collect data related to children in the United States, this record of neglect among researchers in the sociology of sport is glaring given the social importance of youth sports in United States (Champaign, Illinois) culture and the relatively low rates of physical activity among young people. The added fact that youth sport programmes are extraordinarily diverse makes it even more important to learn about the range of experiences that occur in youth sports and the ways that young people perceive those experiences.

For this reason, my discussion will focus on the organization of youth sports in the United States along with the challenging issues associated with existing programmes.

A general description of youth sports in the United States

Youth sports in the United States are fragmented with little or no continuity from programme to programme. The programmes are not governed by any national, state or local plans, so there is no interconnected youth sports system. The philosophy and organization of each programme is based on the perspectives and goals of its sponsoring organization and/or the adults who manage it. This means that there are thousands of diverse programmes with a few here and there linked by a single governing body or sponsoring organization, such as Pop Warner Football; Amateur Athletic Union (AAU) basketball; Little League, Incorporated; or local park and recreation departments.

Programmes are sponsored by a wide array of organizations ranging from private-for-profit businesses to local public agencies. Sponsors also include non-profit organizations such as local churches, regional and national faith-based organizations, local affiliates of national sport federations, youth service organizations such as the YMCA and Boys and Girls Clubs, and local civic and service organizations such as the Rotary or Kiwanis clubs. Increasingly popular are private-non-profit programmes created by sport entrepreneurs who manage them for paying participants. A number of these have become successful enough to expand across states and regions. In the process, they gain power based in their ability to sponsor large tournaments that often attract college coaches scouting for young talent in a particular sport.

This wide variation in programmes makes it difficult to describe or analyze youth sports in the United States. Even when research is done, it generally focuses on a particular type of programme and provides little basis for generalizing to others, which makes publication difficult. Additionally, many programmes attract participants from a particular social class or ethnic population due to combinations of cost and residential segregation. Programmes with participants from upper-middle-class families are often described with a rhetoric that emphasizes personal development and overall excellence along with a career- or academically-focused achievement orientation. Those that involve young people from lower income and ethnic minority populations are often described with a rhetoric emphasizing deficit reduction and social control along with benefits assumed to exist because they keep young people off the streets in adult supervised settings (Coakley, 2002). Regardless of the rhetoric used to describe them, most programmes are also touted with clichés about building teamwork, discipline and character.

Beginning in the 1980s, youth sports, which had often been provided locally as a public service, became increasingly privatized and exclusive in many U.S. communities. As a result, they were marketed and consumed as commodities linked with potential payoffs in terms of instrumental outcomes for participants and their families. This trend has intensified over subsequent decades.

Although stated programme goals may take into account the age of participants, the likelihood that programmes are organized to reflect research-based knowledge about age-related physical and psychosocial development is slim or incidental. Exceptions to this have emerged in recent years as some programmes, such as those associated with a few progressive national sport federations, have used selective sport science knowledge to guide parents and coaches and provide age-appropriate experiences for children (USA hockey approach, www.admkids.com; Kanters *et al.*, 2014). In some cases, these changes were made in an attempt to reduce drop-out rates that threatened the viability of certain youth sport programmes.

Youth sports in the United States, like youth sports in many countries, are organized around the values and experiences of men who see competition as an important social and cultural process that mediates personal and collective success. This means that the cultures of most programmes appeal more directly to boys and young men than to girls and young women. As this becomes apparent to young women during early adolescence, they drop out of organized programmes at rates that far exceed drop-out rates among their male peers (Sabo and Veliz, 2008). Those young women who remain in sports do so for a variety of reasons yet to be thoroughly identified by research.

Despite, or possibly because of their importance in U.S. culture, youth sports have never been governed or regulated at the national level. There is no central ministry of sport or public agency that controls sports on a state-by-state basis. Local and state agencies may regulate where, when and under what conditions certain sports can be played, but they have focused more on the treatment of dogs, horses, and bulls than children. Therefore, there has never been a national model of youth sports nor have there been institutional structures through which such a model could be developed and implemented. The goals of youth sport programmes vary with the specific interests and orientations of the adults and organizations that sponsor them. Organizational sponsors usually fall into one of the following four categories (adapted from Coakley, 2015a):

1 *Public, tax-supported community recreation organizations.* These include local park and recreation departments and community centres, which traditionally offer free or low-cost sport programmes for children. The programmes are usually inclusive and emphasize overall participation, health, general skill development and enjoyment.
2 *Public-interest, nonprofit community organizations.* These include the YMCA, Boys and Girls Clubs, the Police Athletic League (PAL) and other community-based organizations, which have provided a limited range of free or low-fee sport programmes for children, especially those living in inner cities where facilities are scarce. The goals of these programmes are diverse, including everything from providing a 'wholesome, Christian atmosphere' for playing sports to providing 'at-risk children' with opportunities to play sports and keep them off the streets.
3 *Private-interest, non-profit sport organizations.* These include organizations such as the nationwide Little League, Inc. (www.littleleague.org/Little_League_Online.htm), Rush Soccer (http://rushsoccer.com/club-profile), Pop Warner Football and Cheerleading www.popwarner.com/About_Us.htm) and local organizations operating independently or through connections with larger sport organizations, such as USA Swimming and other national federations. These organizations usually offer more exclusive opportunities to selective groups of children, generally those with special skills from families who can afford relatively costly participation fees.
4 *Private commercial clubs.* These include gymnastics, tennis, skating, golf, soccer, lacrosse, swimming and other sport clubs and training programmes. These organizations have costly membership and participation fees, and some emphasize intense training, progressive and specialized skill development and elite competition.

Because each of these sponsors has a different mission, the sports programmes they fund are likely to offer different types of experiences for children and families. This makes it difficult to draw general conclusions about what happens in organized programmes and how participation affects child development, family dynamics, community integration and public health.

When public funds are scarce, support for the youth sport programmes in category 1 (above) fades. This limits opportunities for children from low-income families and funnels them into one or two sports that may survive the cuts or are formally offered in their schools—a prospect that has become less and less likely in recent years. A lack of publicly funded programmes also creates a demand for youth sports in the remaining three sponsorship categories. But sponsors in categories 3 and 4 thrive only when they serve families with the resources to pay fees and arrange personal transportation for their children.

Overall, this means that the opportunities and experiences available to young people are influenced by local, state and national politics, especially those related to taxation and public spending. At present, youth sport opportunities and experiences are strongly influenced by voters and political representatives who make decisions about taxes and how they are used in local communities. Current neoliberal approaches shape the overall organization of youth sports in the United States.

Disparate origins of youth sports in the United States

U.S. culture is known for being oriented toward the future rather than the past. But to explain youth sports today requires a brief review of their historical origins during the progressive era of the late-eighteenth and early nineteenth centuries. The period of 1880–1920 was a vibrant and exciting time of rapid change riddled by diversity and cultural contradictions (Cavallo, 1981; Goodman, 1979; Mrozek, 1983). There was a strong emphasis on nation-building and a general concern with the role of the United States in world affairs and how to expand its political and economic power as it dealt with internal social diversity and a rapidly expanding population driven by immigration and a high birth rate.

Prior to the progressive era, sports were seen as recreational activities that were ends in themselves. They were not seen as instrumental activities that produced certain outcomes in individuals and communities. Additionally, it was not until the early 1900s that people in the United States began to realize that the behavior and character of children were strongly influenced by their social environment and everyday experiences.

This Darwin-inspired belief that the environment influenced a person's overall development was encouraging to progressives and reformers with varying motives. It caused them to think about how they might control the experiences of young people so that they would grow up to be responsible and productive adults in a society where citizenship and work were highly valued. Leaders in various institutional spheres knew that democracy depended on responsibility, and a growing capitalist economy depended on productivity.

Progressive reformers in the United States during the early twentieth century were influenced by educators in England who saw sports as ideal activities for molding the characters of boys in exclusive private schools. Playing sports, thought the headmasters at these schools, would help the sons of wealthy and powerful people in British society become future leaders in business, government, and the military.

Reform-oriented adults in the United States took the notion that sports built character and used it as a basis for organizing youth sports, especially team sports for boys, in schools, on playgrounds, in church groups and through service organizations. Their hope was that team sports would teach boys from working-class and immigrant families values about work, cooperation, productivity and obedience to authority in the pursuit of competitive success. It was also hoped that sports would turn boys from middle- and upper-class households into strong, assertive, competitive men who would become leaders in industry, government and the military.

Teaching privileged boys to be tough, competitive men was important to many reformers because they worried that these boys were learning too many feminine values while being raised exclusively by mothers. Fathers worked long hours and were seldom home, so there was a fear that boys had few chances to learn about manhood in positive terms. Sports were seen as activities that would turn them into productive men. At the same time, other activities were organized to help girls learn about motherhood and homemaking (Cavallo, 1981; Goodman, 1979; Mrozek, 1983).

The historical context in which youth sports emerged in the United States was characterized by unregulated industrialization, a high rate of immigration, rapid economic expansion, local and national political turmoil, escalating militarization, institutional employment discrimination and exploitation, and social disorganization. At the same time, there were emerging ideas about individualism and individual development, the social significance of religion, the use of science to guide social and material progress, and an array of social movements focused on social reform, rescuing children from the perils of urbanization, Puritan conceptions of morality, universal suffrage based on new and contentious definitions of gender and femininity, and various racial ideologies that supported segregation in housing, work and social activities.

Within this context, people with divergent and conflicting ideas about the organization of social life began to see youth sports as a vehicle for creating a nation that fit their ideas and interests. Industrialists saw them as a means of turning undisciplined working-class boys into productive workers familiar with teamwork and goal achievement. Nation builders saw youth sports as a tool for acculturating immigrant boys and creating a large pool of patriotic young men who would serve as soldiers as well as loyal workers. Social reformers, child savers, and law enforcement officials saw them as a means of controlling and/or building character in unsupervised boys who used urban streets as play areas and battle grounds. Muscular Christians saw youth sports as contexts in which boys would learn *god-based* morality, self-discipline and self-control. Educators, including physical educators, saw them as learning activities that fostered overall development. And the founders of the playground movement saw them as a means of providing boys with breathing space in parks and natural environments and a respite from suffocating urban neighbourhoods.

During this time, youth sports were sponsored by a range of public and private agencies and organizations, philanthropists, schools, businesses and others wanting to prepare boys and young men to live productive and controlled lives as adults. As a result, youth sports emerged in fragmented and disconnected manner. There were a wide range of different ideas about the organization and goals of youth sports and there was little interest in minimizing those differences for the sake of unifying programmes or creating a system characterized by continuity and agreed upon rational guidelines.

The Baby Boom and youth sports

As the first wave of the Baby Boom generation (born between 1946 and 1964) moved through childhood during the 1950s and 1960s, it spurred rapid growth of community-based youth sports in the United States. The programmes were funded by a combination of public and private sponsors. Inspired by the belief that playing organized competitive sports would develop the kind of character that led to occupational success, fathers entered the scene as volunteer coaches, managers, administrators, referees and local lobbyists for organized youth sport programmes. Mothers with discretionary time played behind-the-scene support roles by doing laundry and becoming chauffeurs and short-order cooks so their sons were always ready and properly suited up for practices and games.

Most organized youth sports through the mid-1970s were for boys 8–14 years old. Although there were girls and young women who managed to play sports and develop respectable skills, it was not until the mid-1970s that the women's movement, the health and fitness movement and government legislation (*Title IX*) prohibiting sex discrimination in public school programs all came together to stimulate more widespread development of youth sports for girls.

Young people with a disability were ignored by those creating youth sport programmes during the 1950s through the 1970s. Efforts to be inclusive were practically non-existent, and programmes that offered regular participation opportunities in adapted sports were rare at best. There were occasional one-off events that enabled young people to sample one or more sports, but these did not lead to regular participation in organized programmes. In 1968, the International Olympic Committee granted Eunice Kennedy Shriver, the sister of President John F. Kennedy, permission to use the word *Olympics* for a sporting event that would offer adults and children with intellectual disabilities year-round training and competitions (Foote and Collins, 2011). Although the Special Olympics would receive stinging criticism in subsequent years, people in many U.S. communities formed local programmes that provided sport participation opportunities for children and adults with intellectual disabilities. Volunteers in these programmes often had their eyes opened to access barriers, prevailing stereotypes and patronizing attitudes that ran deep in the structure and culture of the United States.

Despite cultural and structural constraints, playing youth sports become an accepted part of growing up for many children by the end of the 1970s. Children generally played in local, neighboorhood-based, public programmes that were free or low cost. Public parks and playing fields were used by the programmes, which were coached by volunteers – mostly fathers – and administered by paid staff in local park and recreation departments.

The neoliberal shift in youth sports: 1980s to the present

Partly in reaction to transformational social movements and economic recessions during the 1960s and 1970s, there was an increased emphasis on individualism and a laissez-faire approach in government during the 1980s. President Ronald Reagan and his administration tapped into the emerging cultural belief that *government was the problem, not the solution* to whatever was ailing the United States and the rest of the world. About the same time, Reagan's closest political ally, Margaret Thatcher, then Prime Minister in England, declared that the only way to solve contemporary national and global problems was to assume that society was a figment of liberal imagination, and that in reality, there were only individuals and their families.

These two ideas – *government is the problem* and *there is no society* – served as the basis for a neo-liberal policy orientation that re-shaped everyday life throughout the United States during the 1980s. Decision making in both public and private spheres increasingly reflected the ideological assumptions that: (i) the sole foundation of social order was personal responsibility; (ii) the most effective source of economic growth was unregulated self-interest; (iii) people were motivated by observable inequalities of income and wealth and (iv) competitive reward structures were the only effective way to allocate rewards in society (Bourdieu, 1998; Harvey, 2005).

As a result, public funding for local park and recreation departments was drastically reduced, which made it difficult to maintain free and low-cost youth sport programmes. Instead of maintaining and managing those programmes, park and recreation departments became brokers of public sport spaces and began to issue permits to emerging private programmes created by parents with resources and by youth sport entrepreneurs seeking full-time careers.

The outcome of these changes was the emergence and growth of privatized youth sports organized to promote progressive skill development through training and competition in a single sport through most of the year. Some of these programmes used public fields and facilities, and others, especially in upper-middle-income areas, built their own. Commercial programmes also entered the scene with gymnastics facilities, indoor tennis, indoor soccer, specialized high performance training venues and other youth sports that were costly and increasingly exclusive.

Youth sports became sites for adult careers. Most coaches/managers/administrators were well intentioned but knew little about child development. They also needed year-round income to feed their families and pay bills twelve months a year. This led them to convince paying parents that year-round participation in a singlesport was important for the future success of their children. The resulting marketing spin that surrounded this selling of year-round specialization was in part legitimized by the successful international performances of East German and Soviet athletes who were widely thought to have specialized in a particular sport from a very early age. Additionally, some youth sport entrepreneurs received media attention for producing high performance athletes in specialized sport academies where daily training regimes were intense and highly regulated.

At the same time, there were others who founded competitive-tournament-based programmes that were promoted as community, state, regional and national championships to attract the attention and participation of parents, coaches, and athletes. The Disney-owned ESPN Wide World of Sports facility in Orlando, Florida, continues to be the classic corporate example of this approach (see www.espnwwos.com). By labelling their youth sport events and tournaments as 'national championships' or something similar, they attract many thousands of 'sport tourists' to Orlando and then to neighbouring Disney World and other holiday destinations in the area. Other communities have followed the Disney example on a much smaller scale by hosting glamorously named tournaments to attract sport-family tourists who stay in local hotels and motels, eat in restaurants and visit leisure attractions in the area.

The success of youth-sport entrepreneurs and the extent to which they have influenced private youth sport programmes nationwide is noteworthy and deserving of research. Early childhood specialization and year-round participation in a single sport has become common. Practice and competition schedules have become more demanding, there is an increase in long distance travel to regular and special contests and games and parents now see their sponsorship of a child's sport participation as an investment in the child's future. 'Keeping up with the Jones's kids' has become a preoccupation of both coaches and parents.

Overall, youth sports in the United States were transformed in the course of a generation. New foundational philosophies and new goals were established and pursued by many coaches, parents, and players. These changes had an impact on the everyday rhythm of family life as well as family relationships, budgets and discretionary expenditures. There were also significant changes in children's play patterns and priorities, and a new, exclusive focus on the family rather than the local neighbourhood or community as the primary sponsors of youth sport participation. Local communities became less relevant as teams were increasingly composed of young people from geographically disparate neighbourhoods and as parents were willing to drive significant distances to obtain the best sport training for their children. Coaches and managers in these programmes depended on competitive success and year-round participation to insure a steady income and to successfully recruit more parents and young people as paying members of their teams and clubs.

These organizers and entrepreneurs did not make changes in youth sports by themselves. Their success depended on cultural timing and compatibility with the larger social context. That is, their programmes had to provide participation opportunities that resonated with parents and attracted children. Resonance during the 1980s was facilitated by the growing cultural emphasis on neoliberal ideology as an organizing platform for political, economic and social life. As parental moral worth was linked with the success of their children in visible and culturally valued activities, the stakes associated with youth sports increased significantly (Coakley, 2006, 2010). When a child became an age group champion or participated on a highly successful team, parents were seen as being responsible. For example, the cash prize received by Tiger Woods when he won his first Masters tournament in 1997 was less than what his father made that year on proceeds from his book, *Training a Tiger: A Father's Guide to Raising a Winner in Both Golf and Life* (Woods, 1997).

This tendency to see child athletes as the creations of their parents has become a central feature of neoliberal culture in the United States. Its influence is powerful, often leading parents to become strongly dedicated to nurturing the sport dreams of their children, despite heavy costs in time, energy and money. Sports are culturally valued and youth sports are organized with an emphasis on progressive skill development and a hierarchical structure that sorts young people by skill and rewards them in public ways. Parents may list a litany of sacrifices they make to sponsor their children's sport participation, but rather than complaints, these are presented in the process of claiming parental moral worth. At the same time, parents unwilling or unable to nurture the sport dreams of their children risk being defined as morally flawed.

Youth sports today: issues and controversies

Apart from mandatory schooling, youth sports are the most popular adult supervised activities for children and young people in the United States. But they remain diverse, fragmented, unregulated, and inaccessible to significant segments of the population. There are, however, important patterns and trends that can be identified. These include the following:

1   Near disappearance of informal player-controlled games due to

   (a)   a decline in public spaces perceived to be safe;
   (b)   a cultural emphasis on organized sport participation as a valuable developmental experience and
   (c)   the constraints imposed by parents who fear what might happen if their children engaged in spontaneous, unsupervised collective activities outside the home (Echeverría *et al.*, 2014).

   The era of informal player-controlled games in various sports has faded away among children and young people generally (Farrey, 2015; Medcalf and O'Neil, 2014). Parents now seek for their children various adult-controlled, formally organized activities, and organized, competitive sports are perceived favorably by nearly all parents (Farrey, 2015; Project Play, 2014a). As a result, children have few opportunities to participate in unstructured, player-controlled physical activities and games, despite their developmental benefits (Bowers and Green, 2013; Bowers *et al.*, 2014). An exception to this pattern exists in certain neighbourhoods with a critical mass of similarly aged children who have immediate access to safe play areas by their homes (Hochschild, Jr., 2013).

2   Lack of publicly funded youth sport programmes due to budget cuts and a general unwillingness among voters to support taxation at any level of government. Additionally, there have been dramatic cuts in federal matching funds that municipalities have previously used to maintain urban parks and sport venues (www.outdoorindustry.org). Low-cost, public, neighborhood-based youth sports have therefore been replaced by more expensive private programmes, which survive and prosper by recruiting children from families with resources

to support year-round participation dedicated to achieving excellence and competitive success, and 'moving to the next level' in a particular sport. This undermines any semblance of 'sport for all' at the same time that children from wealthy families receive the best technical training in sport programmes that compete with each other for paying members.

3   Rising costs of participation due to the privatization and rationalization of youth sports programmes (Holland, 2014; Hyman, 2009, 2011). Private programmes, even those that are explicitly non-profit, depend on year-round revenue streams to support coaches, administrators, and venues. To recruit members, programmes are marketed as goal-oriented and professionalized, although there is an underlying commitment to sport development over child development. As this trend has increased the cost of youth sport programmes (Project Play, 2014a, 2014b), it has also intensified socioeconomic, racial and ethnic segregation as it has raised the stakes associated with participation. Because of the money and time required to sponsor the participation of a child, youth sports have become increasingly serious activities for parents, coaches and children. This has led to the development of high cost supplementary training programmes and private coaches dedicated to enhancing personal skills, performance and competitive success at increasingly elite levels of competition. Additionally, research has shown that as family expenditures for a child's sport participation increase, children feel additional pressure and express less satisfaction with their participation (King and Rothlisberger, 2014).

4   Increased parental involvement due to changing definitions of what constitutes a good parent. As parental moral worth has become linked with the achievements of their children, parents expect more from and for their children. They become more concerned about the quality of sport programmes, the competitive success of their children's teams, the decisions of coaches and referees that impact their children's experiences, the performances of their children's teammates and their children's performances. Parents generally feel that they have a moral obligation to challenge anyone or any decision that interferes with their children's success in sports. This has turned many parents into insistent advocates for their children and active managers of their children's sport experiences. They believe that if this is done effectively, their children will reap external rewards such as college scholarships and professional contracts or prize money. At the same time, parents and children often have different goals related to participation as well as participation outcomes (Schwab, Wells and Arthur-Banning, 2010).

5   Inequities and lack of inclusion due to the high cost of participation and a lack of public provision in traditionally underserved neighbourhoods and poor rural areas (Holland, 2014; Kelley and Carchia, 2013; Sabo and Veliz, 2008). Girls, especially girls of colour in these areas, lack access to youth sports because public and family resources are scarce or more often used to support boys' programmes. Similarly, children from low-income or single-parent homes are regularly priced out of youth sports (Project Play, 2014a, 2014b). The formal and informal emphasis on competition and competitive success in youth sports also limits and discourages participation among awkward or obese children, late bloomers and children with a disability or a chronic condition that creates special needs (Krieger, 2012). Data clearly show that the rate of youth sport participation in the United States is directly related to family income. Households reporting less than $25,000 in income during 2013 accounted for about 25 per cent of all households but only 15 per cent of youth sport participants and only 11 per cent of soccer participants, according to a study by the Sports and Fitness Industry Association (Holland, 2014). Households with annual incomes over $100,000 constituted 20 per cent of all households, but accounted for 33 per cent of youth sport participants and 37 per cent of soccer participants.

6   Year-round specialization in a single sport due to a full-time need for income among sport entrepreneurs who operate and coach private youth sport programmes. Parents buy into this arrangement because they fear that their children will be selected out of the mobility pipeline in a sport if they opt out of a program for season or decide to sample another sport. Even though this emphasis on specialization often restricts overall physical and social development, undermines motivation, increases overuse injuries and burnout rates, parents and young people see it as important for achieving success. Some parents, often those who are highly educated, ascribe to the '10,000-Hour Rule' as described by Malcolm Gladwell in his best-selling book, *Outliers* (Gladwell, 2008). Logging 10,000 hours of focused practice in a field was described by Gladwell as a prerequisite for success. This further promoted specialization in a single sport year-round.

7   Injuries due to overuse and repetitive movements in a single sport played for long duration by preteen children, and due to the increased perceived stakes and intense training associated with youth sport participation (American Academy of Pediatrics, 2014; DiFiori *et al.*, 2014). Researchers and surgeons at major children's hospitals in the United States have reported dramatic increases in the number of ligament tears, joint injuries and concussions among child athletes (Tsai, 2014). Although exact numbers are difficult to verify, parents have become increasingly concerned about the safety of their children in competitive youth sport programmes. In heavy contact sports such as football and hockey, there have been decreases in the number of participants due to injury fears on the part of parents and young athletes themselves. The cost of treating acute injuries now and related chronic problems in later life has not been calculated, but it is certain that the certain forms of sport participation are not decreasing health care costs or contributing to the long-term physical well-being of many young people playing competitive youth sports.

8   Untrained coaches due to the lack of requirements for coach education, especially in the case of volunteer coaches who lack time resources, and (mostly) male coaches who feel that they already understand sports and do not need training to work with children. As a result, many youth sport programmes consist of structures and standards imposed by adults unfamiliar with age-based developmental preferences, abilities and orientations of children. Child athletes are regularly treated as adults despite lacking the physical and psychosocial skills to participate in complex competitive activities. This contributes to retention problems as children are turned off activities that offer them little fun in terms of action and controlled challenges faced with friends. It also contributes to parental dissatisfaction with youth sport programmes (Project Play, 2014b; Smith, Smoll and Cumming, 2007).

9   Declining participation rates due to

(i)   everyday mobility constraints imposed by parents who feel compelled control the whereabouts of their children 24/7;

(ii)   pervasive access among children to home-based entertainment technologies that they enjoy and

(iii) an unwillingness of children to play sports that emphasize performance and competitive success rather than enjoyment on their terms.

Parents fear that children will cause trouble or be exploited by others if unsupervised. As children see that organized youth sports are often organized around their most talented and well-supported peers, they lose interest and gravitate toward video games that are more exciting and diverse than organized sports and can be done in the safety of their homes with at least passive approval from parents. According to the Sports and Fitness Industry

Association's annual survey in 2013, the proportion of children that play at least one sport per year has declined from 59 per cent to 52 per cent in the five years between 2007 and 2012 (Project Play, 2014a).

10   Low physical activity rates due to a growing realization among children that they will never experience much success in highly competitive, performance-oriented youth sports. This begins at around 10 years old and continues through early adolescence. The result is that young people in the United States have declining physical activity rates (Dentro *et al.*, 2014a, 2014b), and those rates are lower than their European peers (Tremblay *et al.*, 2014) and peers in other nations (Nike, Inc., 2014). Unfortunately, this pattern of being sedentary carries over into adulthood and is associated with obesity and related health problems.

11   Attraction to alternative sports due to the desire among some young people to engage in physical activities that provide joy, spontaneity, autonomy and participant control. The adult imposed pressures to seek constant improvement and competitive success in the organized youth sport industry have fuelled an increase in a wide range of unstructured activities that young people claim as their own. Although this attraction is not as strong among pre-teen children as it is among teens, participation in alternative sports has impacted on participation rates in organized youth sports. Parents initially disapproved of these sports due to their association with non-conformist youth subcultures, but there are recent indications that parents are changing their opinions and supporting their children to the point of accompanying them to skate parks, BMX tracks and other sites at which alternative sports are played (Atencio *et al.*, 2014).

Conclusion

This critical description is not intended as a condemnation of youth sports in the United States. There are programmes that provide supportive and responsive contexts for children whose parents have permitted or sponsored their participation. Some of those children are strongly attracted to organized sports, others are sampling them and some are personally resistant yet temporarily bending to encouragement or pressure from parents or peers. But none of this changes the fact that youth sports in the United States remain a disjointed collection of programmes that reflect the goals and perspectives of the adults who organize, manage and coach them. Nor does it change the fact that participants in those programmes have a wide range of experiences to which they give meaning and integrate into their lives in various ways, depending heavily on the social context in which participation takes place. It is this process of meaning making and integration that requires much further research (Fraser-Thomas and Côté, 2009; Swanson, 2009).

The problems in youth sports have attracted considerable attention from individuals and organizations. However, it is difficult to make changes and it is impossible to create what might be called a system in which programmes in the United States would conform to general guidelines related to science-based knowledge about growth, development and the constructive integration of sport participation into the lives of young people. Youth sports have become an industry, and many people have vested interests in preserving them as they are. A growing number of people depend on them for their income; youth sport travel is a rapidly growing segment of the tourism industry and parents depend on them to occupy the time of their children.

The most encouraging recent development related to youth sports is that a growing number of national governing bodies (NGBs) are adopting new guidelines that focus on providing age-appropriate experiences for children in their youth development programmes. Although the stated goal on which these guidelines are based stresses that all children should have opportunities to play sports organized to fit their stage of development, it remains to be seen if the actual programmes will do this rather than focusing on producing elite sport performers at all ages. Additionally, the programmes maintained by the NGBs constitute a small minority of youth sport programmes in the country.

Experience worldwide suggests that focusing on overall development while producing young elite athletes is difficult even when resources are plentiful. In the face of limited resources, it appears to be beyond reach. In the meantime, increasing rates of childhood obesity and related health problems in the United States have created a growing awareness that the current organization of youth sports may be seriously deficient. But converting this awareness into transformational actions will require strategies endorsed and implemented by influential people at the local, state and national federal levels – something vigorously resisted by many people in the United States.

References

American Academy of Pediatrics (2000). Intensive training and sports specialization in young athletes. *Pediatrics, 106(01)*, 154–57.

American Academy of Pediatrics (2014). American Academy of Pediatrics recommends training programs to reduce risk of ACL tears in young athletes. American Academy of Pediatrics Available online at: www.aap.org/en-us/about-the-aap/aap-press-room/Pages/American-Academy-of-Pediatrics-Recommends-Training-Programs-to-Reduce-Risk-of-ACL-Tears-in-Young-Athletes.aspx [Accessed 28 April 2014].

Atencio, M., Beal, B., McClain, Z. and Wright, M. (2014). *The Symbolic Field of Skateboarding in the San Francisco Bay Area: Social Logics of Parenting and Youth Engagement.* Paper presented at the annual conference of the North American Society for the Sociology of Sport (Portland, 5–9 November 2014).

Bowers, M.T. and Green, B.C. (2013). Reconstructing the community-based youth sport experience: How children derive meaning from unstructured and organized settings. *Journal of Sport Management, 27(6)*, 422–38.

Bowers, M.T., Green, B.C., Hemme, F. and Chalip, L. (2014). Assessing the relationship between youth sport participation settings and creativity in adulthood. *Creativity Research Journal, 26(3)*, 314–27.

Cavallo, D. (1981). *Muscles and morals: Organized playgrounds and urban reform, 1880–1920.* Philadelphia: University of Pennsylvania Press.

Coakley, J. (2002). Using sports to control deviance and violence among youths: Let's be critical and cautious' in M. Gatz, M.A. Messner and S.J. Ball-Rokeach (eds), *Paradoxes of youth and sport.* Albany, NY: State University of New York Press, 13–30.

Coakley, J. (2006). The good father: Parental expectations and youth sports. *Leisure Studies 25(2)*, 153–64.

Coakley, J. (2010). The "logic" of specialization: Using children for adult purposes. *Journal of Physical Education, Recreation and Dance*, 81(8), 16–18, 25.

Coakley, J. (2015a). *Sports in society: Issues and controversies* (11th edition). New York: McGraw-Hill.

Coakley, J. (2015b). Assessing the sociology of sport: On cultural sensibilities and the great sport myth. *International Review for the Sociology of Sport, 50(1)*, in press.

Côté, J. Lidor, R. and Hackfort, D. (2009). ISSP Position Stand: To sample or to specialize? Seven postulates about youth sport activities that lead to continued participation and elite performance. *International Journal of Sport and Exercise Psychology, 7(1)*, 7–17.

Dentro, K.N., Beals, K., Crouter, S.E., Eisenmann, J.C., McKenzie, T.L., Pate, R.R., Saelens, B.E., Sisson, S.B., Spruijt, D., Sothern, M.S. and Katzmarzyk, P.T. (2014a). The 2014 United States report card on physical activity for children and youth. Columbia, SC: National Physical Activity Plan. www.physicalactivityplan.org/reportcard/NationalReportCard_longform_final per cent20for per cent20web.pdf

Dentro K.N., Beals, K., Crouter, S.E., Eisenmann, J.C., McKenzie, T.L., Pate, R.R., Saelens, B.E., Sisson, S.B., Spruijt, D., Sothern, M.S. and Katzmarzyk, P.T. (2014b). Results from the United States' 2014 Report Card on Physical Activity for Children and Youth *Journal of Physical Activity and Health, 11 (Supplement 1)*, S105–S112.

DiFiori, J.P. Benjamin, H.J., Brenner, J. S., Gregory, A., Jayanthi, N., Landry, G.L. and Luke, A. (2014). Overuse injuries and burnout in youth sports: A position statement from the American Medical Society for Sports Medicine. *Clinical Journal of Sport Medicine, 24(1)*, 3–20.

Echeverría, S.E., Kang, A.L., Isasi, C.R., Johnson–Diaz, J. and Pacquiao, D. (2014). A community survey on neighborhood violence, park use, and physical activity among urban youth. *Journal of Physical Activity and Health, 11(1)*, 186–194.

Farrey, T. (2008). *Game on: The all-American race to make champions of our children.* New York: ESPN Books.

Farrey, T. (2015). *Project Play report.* Washington, DC: The Aspen Institute (forthcoming).

Fraser-Thomas, J. and Côté, J. (2009). Understanding adolescents' positive and negative developmental experiences in sport. *Sport Psychologist, 23(1)*, 3–23.

Goodman, C. (1979). *Choosing sides: Playground and street life on the lower east side.* New York: Schocken Books.

Hochschild, Jr, T.R. (2013). Cul-de-sac kids. *Childhood, 20(2)*, 229–243.

Holland, K. (2014). Lower-income students getting shut out of sports. *NBCNews.com* (July 27): www.nbcnews.com/business/consumer/lower-income-students-getting-shut-out-sports-n164941

Hyman, M. (2009). *Until it hurts: America's obsession with youth sports and how it harms our kids.* Boston: Beacon Press.

Hyman, M. (2011). *The most expensive game in town.* Boston. Beacon Press.

Kanters, M., McKenzie, T., Edwards, M., Bocarro, J., Mahar, M. and Hodge, C. (2014). Youth sport practice model gets more kids active with more time practicing skills. Research Brief (March). Available at: http://activelivingresearch.org/blog/2014/04/youth-sport-practice-model-gets-kids-active-more-time-practicing-skills. [Accessed 17 November 2014].

Kelley, B. and Carchia, C. (2013). 'Hey, data data – swing!' The hidden demographics of youth sports. *ESPN The Magazine* (July 11): http://espn.go.com/espn/story/_/id/9469252/hidden-demographics-youth-sports-espn-magazine.

King, M. and Rothlisberger, K. (2014). Family financial investment in organized youth sport. *Research on the Hill (Salt Lake City).* Paper 17; http://digitalcommons.usu.edu/poth_slc/17.

Krieger, J. (2012). Fastest, highest, youngest? Analysing the athlete's experience of the Singapore Youth Olympic Games. *International Review for the Sociology of Sport, 48(6)*, 706–19.

Medcalf, M. and O'Neil, D. (2014). Playground basketball is dying. *ESPN.go.com* (July 23): http://espn.go.com/espn/feature/story/_/id/11216972/playground-basketball-dying

Messner, M.A. and Musto, M. (2014). Where are the kids? *Sociology of Sport Journal*, 31(1), 102–22.

Mrozek, D.J. (1983). *Sport and American mentality, 1880–1920.* Knoxville: University of Tennessee Press.

NASPE (2010). *Guidelines for participation in youth sport programs: Specialization versus multiple-sport participation* (Position Statement). Reston, VA: National Association for Sport and Physical Education.

Nike Inc. 2014. *Designed to move: A physical activity action agenda.* Available online at: http://s3.nikecdn.com/dtm/live/en_US/DesignedToMove_FullReport.pdf [Accessed 17 November 2014].

Physical Activity Council. (2012). *2012 participation report: The Physical Activity Council's annual study tracking sports, fitness and recreation participation in the USA.* Jupiter, FL: Sports Marketing Surveys USA.

Project Play. (2014a). *espnW/Aspen Institute Project Play survey of parents on youth sport issues.* Washington, DC: Aspen Institute. Available online at: http://espn.go.com/espnw/w-in-action/article/11675649/parents-concern-grows-kids-participation-sports.

Project Play. (2014b). *Facts: Sports activity and children.* Washington, DC: The Aspen Institute. Online, www.aspenprojectplay.org/the-facts.

Sabo, D. and Veliz, P. (2008). *Go out and play: Youth sports in America.* East Meadow, NY: Women's Sports Foundation.

Schwab, K.A., Wells, M.S. and Arthur–Banning, S. (2010). Experiences in youth sports: A comparison between players' and parents' perspectives. *Journal of Sport Administration and Supervision, 2(1)*, 41–51.

Smith, R., Smoll, F.L. and Cumming, S.P. (2007). Effects of a motivational climate intervention for coaches on young athletes' sport performance anxiety. *Journal of Sport and Exercise Psychology, 29(1)*, 39–59.

Swanson, L. (2009). Soccer fields of cultural [re]production: Creating good boys in suburban America. *Sociology of Sport Journal, 26(3)*, 404–424.

Tremblay, M.S., Gray, C.E., Akinroye, K., Harrington, D.M., Katzmarzyk, P.T., Lambert, E.V., Liukkonen, J., Maddison, R., Ocansey, R.T., Onywera, V.O., Prista, A., Reilly, J.J., Rodríguez Martínez, M., Sarmiento Duenas, O.L., Standage, M. and Tomkinson, G. (2014). Physical activity of children: A global matrix of grades comparing 15 countries. *Journal of Physical Activity and Health, 11(Supp 1)*, S113–S125.

Tsai, J. (2014). Acute sports injuries up: Pediatricians report rise in severe 'adult' injuries in children. *The Berkshire Eagle* (Pittsfield, Massachusetts). Available online at: www.berkshireeagle.com/health/ci_26625415/tommy-john-surgery-kids-cute-sports-injuries-up [Accessed 29 September 2014].

Weiss, M.R. and Wiese-Bjornstal, D.M. (2009). Promoting positive youth development through physical activity. *Research Digest* (of the President's Council on Physical Fitness and Sports), *10(3)*, September.

Woods, E. (1997) *Training a tiger: A father's guide to raising a winner in both golf and life.* London: HarperCollins.

10

YOUTH SPORT IN AUSTRALASIA

Doune Macdonald and Clifford Mallett

Introduction

For Australia and its geographical neighbours, sport is integral to our national identity. Australia's newly elected Prime Minister in 2013 said in response to the country's political and sporting challenges, 'happy the country (such as Australia) which is more interested in sport than politics'. As this chapter will outline, while sport is a significant institution for Australasian youth, the participation patterns in, and practices and purposes of, sport are changing.

We start with the future by introducing a comprehensive report, *The Future of Australian Sport* (Hajkowicz *et al.*, 2013). This far-reaching report provides a backdrop for discussion on the participation patterns of youth in sport and what quantitative and qualitative research tells us shapes these patterns. Schools, and less so, universities, continue to provide important access for young people to sport. For those considered at risk, there are programmes that seek to use sport as a medium for rehabilitation and/or positive pathways and across the Asia-Pacific sport is increasingly recruited as a medium for community development. Cross-cutting the place and purposes of sport in Australasia are social and political movements, elaborated upon elsewhere in this book, that include globalisation, neoliberalism, equity and positive youth development. In Australia and New Zealand, possibly the most significant movement is the thinking of neoliberalism that prioritizes decreased government provision, increased outsourcing of what might have been a government program or service, market-driven solutions, new partnerships/networks and increased individual responsibility (Macdonald, 2011).

Megatrends in sport

A 2013 report compiled by Australia's leading scientific (Commonwealth Scientific and Industrial Research Organisation – CSIRO) and sporting (Australian Sports Commission – ASC) organisations examined the sporting megatrends in Australia (Hajkowicz *et al.*, 2013). We introduce the trends early in the chapter as they help to situate some of the significant aspects of youth sport upon which we elaborate. While the report does not solely focus on youth, the data sets upon which they draw are particularly relevant to young people. The six trends can be summarised as follows:

- A perfect fit: with an increased awareness of the relationship between physical activity and health, health-oriented physical activities are on the rise. These activities include individualised, lifelong activities such as jogging, yoga or aerobics that allow for flexible participation in busy lives. Where participation in organised sport continues, Australians are 'increasingly playing sport to get fit, rather than getting fit to play sport' (Hajkowicz *et al.*, 2013, p. 1) (see also Robert's earlier discussion on individualisation).

- From extreme to mainstream: what were once sports on the margins such as inline skating, freestyle BMX cycling, and rock climbing are increasingly popular with young people. They are attracted to the identity, self-expression, adventure and risk associated with these activities that sit in contrast to their sedentary educational or work sites.

- More than sport: sport is increasingly being recruited by governments to meet extrinsic goals such as health outcomes (e.g. reduction in metabolic disease: see Malina *et al.*, in this volume) and social outcomes (e.g. community development, crime reduction, international relations).

- Everybody's game: as Australia (and New Zealand) becomes increasingly culturally diverse, different sporting and recreation preferences are shifting the sporting landscape as exemplified with the rise of soccer. This trend also accounts for our ageing populations and their demand for suitable lifelong physical activity opportunities.

- New wealth, new talent: throughout Asia, investment in sport is growing bringing with it increasing pressure for Australia and New Zealand to perform successfully in international competition but also opportunities for sport-related business, know-how and entertainment.

- Tracksuits to business suits: pressure on organised sports to attract highly talented players, media rights, advertising and audiences means that many sports will formalise and diversify their business models to compete nationally and internationally, including engaging with new media. This trend also identifies the decline in volunteering, a trend that is particularly impactful on child and youth sport.

These trends have implications for young people's physical activity engagement, identities and employment opportunities both as participants and spectators. As concluded in a Sport and Recreation New Zealand report *It's All About the Children and Young People*, the trends suggest that sport may need to plan and practice differently in order to adapt to an uncertain future:

> In many instances sport and recreation services and opportunities are being delivered to children and young people in much the same as they always have been. However, society, including youth culture, is changing constantly and the challenge for sport and recreation is to remain relevant in a changing world.
>
> *(Sport and Recreation New Zealand, 2007, p. 17)*

Participation patterns in Australasian sport

Sport for children and young people boomed in Australia after World War II as it coincided with a number of social trends such as: dual employment in nuclear families, perceptions of good parenting, safe occupation of children's time, interest in high performance sporting success, and individuals' responsibility for their health and leisure management (Phillips and Macdonald, 2013). That said, there is no national data set collected regularly in Australia that maps details of participation in sport, particularly in the age bracket 16–25 years. A summary of these findings by Trost (2013) provides an overview of sporting patterns largely for 6–16-year-olds: two out of three students participate in an organised sport with participation remaining relatively stable over the last fifteen years; boys have higher participation than girls; participation declines with age (peaking between 9 and 11); with participation lower for those from non-English speaking and low socio-economic backgrounds and those who are obese and overweight.

In a national study, in the adolescent age group (defined in Olds, Dollman and Maher's 2009 study as 9–16 years), sport was found to be an important contributor to the daily energy expenditure of Australian adolescents (approximately 17 per cent) and that schools provide important access to sport for many young people. 'The most common sports were soccer, Australia Rules football, dance, basketball, netball, rugby league football, tennis, cricket, hockey and swimming' (Olds *et al.*, 2009, p. 11). The *Healthy Kids Queensland* study (Abbott *et al.*, 2007) collected data for children aged approximately 6, 10 and 15 years and followed similar patterns to that described above. For boys in Year 10 (approximately 15 years of age), their top ten physical activities/sports recorded in minutes in the previous week were (in descending order) physical education (PE)/school sport, bike riding, soccer, rugby league, running around/jogging, touch football, tennis, walking, basketball and surfing. The girls' participation was highest in PE/school sport followed by walking, dancing, running around/jogging, netball, touch football, athletics, soccer and swimming. In Western Australia, the most popular sports for the senior school students were Australian Rules, soccer, basketball, tennis and cricket for boys, and dancing, netball, swimming, soccer and basketball for girls (Hands *et al.*, 2004).

The Australian Bureau of Statistics (ABS) provides further insight into participation patterns, even though the 15–24 years cohort data is not always separated from other adults. The youth cohort has the highest participation rate in sport and physical activity compared to all other adult age groups and within this males have higher participation rates than females. The 15–17-year-olds have the highest participation rate in traditional organised sports and, from 15–24, fitness or gym activities were particularly popular. For a similar age cohort in New Zealand, 53.1 per cent are reported participating in organised sporting competitions or events and their preferred activities were swimming, walking, equipment-based activities, jogging/running, dance, cycling, basketball, rugby union, touch and tennis (Sport and Recreation New Zealand, 2008). Although somewhat dated, Hamlin and Ross's (2005) New Zealand study suggested that 17–25-year-olds were maintaining their levels of physical activity participation, although females and some ethnic minorities participated less than males and European New Zealanders. This contrasts with the findings of Sinclair, Hamlin and Steel (2005) who reported that in the transition from secondary school to university, students substantially reduce their levels of physical activity. Taken together, the Australian and New Zealand data could be interpreted as revealing a post-school dip in participation before young people find avenues to resume participation.

Youth sports participation data in other Australasian countries is sparse, although low levels of physical activity are reported and these underpin many health interventions. Phongsavan *et al.* (2005) found that over half the 15-year-olds surveyed in three Pacific Island populations (Pohnpei, Tonga and Vanuatu) engaged in less than two hours of physical activity weekly, with girls engaging substantially less than boys. In Tonga, a country that rates fifth in the world for obesity, Fotu *et al.* (2011) conducted a community-based project that included a range of informal physical activities and organised sports requested by the community (e.g. aerobics, walks for health, volleyball, tennis, soccer, hip hop, cultural dancing, fun runs and sports competitions). The physical activities proved to be unsustainable and the evaluation concluded that, in order to promote longer-term engagement, physical activity and sport needed to be more tightly connected to existing community structures and secondary schooling.

Many policies to promote sport participation are frequently driven by health authorities interested in increasing population-level physical activity. That said, in 2001, Australia released its *Backing Australia's Sporting Ability* (BASA) policy (ASC, 2001) with a twofold objective: to assist athletes to even higher levels of performance and to broaden the talent pool by having more widespread children and youth sport participation. This is one of several policy documents released over recent years intended to boost participation and success in sport. Very much focused on athletes' success (many of whom are 16–25 years) is the more recent *Winning Edge* (ASC, 2012) policy that outlines a restructuring of elite sport support in Australia. It emphasises a partnership model across the Australian Institute of Sport, national sporting organisations and state/territory high performance sport academies, good sport governance, and evidence-based practices.

Facilitators, barriers and pathways to participation

Stories from school-leavers in Australia, collected as part of the *Life Activity Project* (Wright and Macdonald, 2010), revealed how busy young people were, with significant commitments to casual and part-time work being a higher priority for many than physical activity and sport (Wright *et al.*, 2005). However, the sporting stories were diverse and complex as the voices of cohorts (varying with geographical location, socio-economic status, gender, ethnicity and so on) revealed different relationships with physical activity and sport as young adults. Common patterns that enabled or motivated participation in sport included available time, no or little cost, sense of competence and confidence, sociability and proximity. Not having sufficient time or money was identified as a barrier for all cohorts, as were factors such as not having the prerequisite skills or body shape, lack of transport, an overly competitive environment and stereotyping youth's interest or potential (manifested, for example, as sexism and racism). A New Zealand study of young people (13–17 years) reinforced the importance of sociability in sport for participants, with key motivations being 'it's fun' and 'to hang out with friends' (Utter *et al.*, 2006). Cost of sports participation is repeatedly reported as a barrier to participation. Hoye (2013) concludes that despite data being limited, the costs can be prohibitive particularly given the rising costs to the sporting organisation of providing its services (e.g. insurance, legal costs, water charges and local government pricing) and the decline in volunteerism that has traditionally contained costs.

Despite increasing issues associated with access and recruitment, community sports clubs have been integral to sport participation in Australasia as well as valued for the role they play in creating and building a sense of community, particularly in non-urban areas. The above-mentioned BASA policy positions clubs as sites for: managing youth alienation and preventing social dislocation; increasing club membership and building school–club partnerships; providing clearer pathways from club to high performance sport; and community development and cohesion (Light, Harvey and Memmert, 2011). That said, community clubs, commercial clubs and school sport programmes, while each providing pathways to participation, can also compete for participants, facility access, volunteer labour and the modest financial support that may be available. In Australia and elsewhere, governments, schools, universities and sports clubs are continually seeking ways to build partnerships that optimise the use of resources and streamline access.

As outlined above, transitions from school into university or the workforce trigger reduced sports participation for many. A transition is usually associated with life events that produce a change in how one views oneself (Schlossberg, 1981) as well as one's social context (i.e. social disequilibrium; Wapner and Craig-Bay, 1992). From the *Australian Longitudinal Study on Women's Health*, Brown, Heesch and Miller (2009) reported that for young women aged 22–27 years life events such as starting work, getting married and having children tended to decrease participation in physical activity in relation to decreases in discretionary time. This type of data reminds us of the importance of educating young people about life-stage transitions and giving them the skills and interest in lifelong physical activities as well as sport providers being attuned to the impact of transitions and how they can work more effectively with youth.

Focusing on facilitators and barriers for high-performing athletes, Gulbin *et al.* (2010) published a comprehensive study of the Australian sports system. Data from their survey of 673 Australian high performance athletes (including fifty-one Olympians) from thirty-four sports revealed that their pathway to expertise was characterised by engagement in a range of sports prior to specialisation in their representative sport (early specialisation), and a significant investment in deliberate practice as competition level increased. This supports Côté's (1999) model of sports participation in which sampling sports and engaging in play-based activities during childhood tends to lead to the development of sporting expertise. Most athletes commenced their senior competition between 15 and 16 years of age and achieved national representations around 19–20 years, on average. Typically, a further eight years of experience was required to reach the Olympic level of competition. Other emergent themes for promoting engagement and success included: access to high quality coaching, significant parental support, passion for the sport at an early age and resilience. Similarly, other Australian studies have also reported that elite players in invasion games (e.g. all kinds of football) had unstructured activity pathways prior to committing to an elite focus (Baker, Côté and Abernethy, 2003; Berry, Abernethy and Côté, 2008).

The abovementioned *Winning Edge* (ASC, 2012) document also provides insights into how to best support elite athletes. Its revised model suggests that prioritised investment in those athletes likely to be successful at major championships will provide the best return on investment. Specifically, national sporting organisations (NSOs) will have increased autonomy to appropriately resource and ensure optimal daily training environments are created for successful athlete pathways to the podium. The National Institute Network will provide high performance services and support to the NSOs. Indeed, NSOs will be held accountable for appropriate performance outcomes that are tied to future funding.

Sport and educational institutions

For many young people, schools provide a route into sport that may be unavailable elsewhere; although this can vary across government and private (independent, fee-paying) schools. Sport has a strong history in Australia's school system, with its functions said to include contributing to health for work, health for war, the promotion of (gendered and classed) citizenship, or indeed, the marketing of the school itself (Georgakis, 2011; Kirk, 1998; Lennox, 2008).

Most secondary schools in Australia and New Zealand offer access to sport and physical recreation in the senior years of schooling through intra- and inter-school sporting competitions: school-based teams entering community club sport competitions, optional curricula choices (e.g. senior PE) or informal recreational pursuits (e.g. school weights room). The private school systems often make significant investment in their sporting facilities and senior sporting teams and athletes with, for example, the employment of specialised coaches. In the highly competitive school market, success in sport is used in school marketing as a signifier of the quality of the school and the strategies that schools may adopt to be successful, such as offering sporting scholarships, are under constant scrutiny.

Those schools that do not have access to specialist sporting facilities have a stronger reliance on school-community partnerships. These community-school partnerships have focused on sport club and industry links and therefore have mostly engaged secondary schools. There are typically loose networks of mostly self-nominated specialist sport schools across Australia and New Zealand. Once again, with the marketisation of education (Macdonald, 2011), schools can establish themselves as a hub for elite athletes where these students are supported with specialist teachers/coaches and flexible school attendance. Recently, there has been interest in some regional enclaves of Australian primary and secondary schools partnering with community sporting organisation to share resources (e.g. coaches, facilities). These evolving partnerships have been designed to increase engagement in physical activity, community sport participation, and potential talent identification and development. The need for access to off-campus facilities for schools exacerbates their use of private providers to deliver aspects of the PE and school sport programmes, in turn, raising interesting questions about cost, programme coherence, expertise and the role of the (PE) teacher (Williams, Hay and Macdonald, 2011).

In Australia, it is anticipated that by 2015 all students up to the age of 16 will participate in a new national Health and Physical Education (HPE) curriculum that includes a range of physical activities informed by futures/predictive research such as that conducted by Hajkowicz *et al.* (2013). The physical activity focus areas (active play and minor games; challenge and adventure activities; fundamental movement skills; games and sports; lifelong physical activities; and rhythmic and expressive activities) are intended to provide a foundation in which students develop competence and confidence in 'traditional' and emerging activities with an aspiration that they will adopt a commitment to lifelong physical activity. In many schools, the HPE curriculum will require students to engage in physical activity in later years of schooling than they may have previously thereby increasing the likelihood that they will stay engaged as they transition from schooling.

As indicated above, the transition from school to work or university may be a critical point of declining participation. For those who enrol at university, the opportunities to be active at university will vary from established facilities and playing fields in often older universities to relatively little provision. Increasingly, universities are using their sporting facilities, scholarships for elite athletes and the sporting successes of their students as integral to their branding. However, unlike the United States, Japan, South Korea and increasingly the UK, Australia and New Zealand's elite athlete development programmes are not embedded in university sport. Nevertheless, several universities in Australasia are contractually linked with professional sporting organisations in order to share resources (e.g. expertise, facilities), provide scholarships, undertake research and test athletes. There is an Elite Athlete Friendly University (EAFU) Network in which signatories agree to support student athletes to maintain both their academic studies and elite participation through special arrangements when required. The EAFU Network was established in response to the specific needs of student-athletes engaged in high performance sport. The EAFU Network has developed policies and procedures to assist these student-athletes balance the collective demands of both academic and sporting goals.

Sport, risk and positive youth development

As suggested by the *more than sport* megatrend, sport is increasingly being recruited as a medium for the education, guidance or encouragement of pro-social behaviours. More specifically, government, philanthropic and sporting organisations invest in sport programmes to prevent crime and anti-social behaviours, and promote school attendance and educational aspirations. As introduced by Roberts earlier in this Handbook, 'Sport has always been recommended as a way of keeping young people out of trouble and saving those deemed "at risk"' (p. 22). The notion of 'at risk' is approached with caution by many scholars who are loathe to segment and label particular sub-groups of youth and who recognise that risk can be subjective. The positive youth development literature (Côté, Turnnidge and Vierimaa, this volume) is persuasive in arguing against the risk/deficit orientation. However, whereas reducing or eliminating health-compromising behaviours is clearly important, defining everything in terms of problem reduction is limiting: we should assess youth not in terms of their problems, or lack of problems, but in terms of their potential (Danish *et al.*, 2004; Sport and Recreation New Zealand, 2007). Holt's (2008) edited collection on *Positive Youth Development Through Sport* provides an international overview of the global interest in positive youth development through the medium of sport. The text draws on Roth *et al.*'s (1998) definition of positive youth development where 'positive development is defined as the engagement in prosocial behaviors and avoidance of health compromising behaviors and future jeopardizing behaviors' (p. 426).

The Hokowhitu programme – designed by New Zealand Maori for New Zealand Maori – sought to use sport as a medium to 'teach life skills such as decision-making, time management, task-related discipline and goal setting' (Danish *et al.*, 2004, p. 43) against a backdrop of Maori's relatively poor education and health profiles. The rationale was to 'take an area of natural strength (sporting pride) and build a program around these attributes as a way to connect with the culture' (Danish *et al.*, 2004, p. 44). The programme has reportedly been effective in developing life skills for the participants (10–18 years) and seen as a model for how to create a positive learning environment that does not position Maori as a minority 'at risk' (Theokas *et al.*, 2010). As Theokas *et al.* conclude, 'Being told what not to do is common fodder for youth . . . and the message often has a limited impact' (p. 78–79). Sporting activities have been shown to provide opportunities for adaptive personal development (Larson, 2000) that foster 'healthy, satisfying, and productive lives as youth and later as adults' (Hamilton, Hamilton and Pittman, 2004, p. 3)

Australia's football codes are particularly engaged in working with Indigenous youth development. While the programmes do not necessarily align themselves with a particular theoretical position, they do frequently share several characteristics of positive youth development and strength-based approaches. For example, the Australian Football League's (AFL) *Kickstart* programme has the aims of providing developmental pathways in sport as well as life-skills (i.e. expectations of school attendance, no substance abuse and no violence). An evaluation of *Kickstart* with Indigenous students in a Cape York community reported the programme as providing positive life experiences, pro-social behaviours and regular school attendance (Dinan-Thompson, Sellwood and Carless, 2008).

Rynne and Rossi's (2012) recent study with Indigenous youth and surfing, in collaboration with the Laureus Sport for Good Foundation and the ASC, suggests that researchers should embrace theoretical positions that allow them to adopt a strengths-based approach rather than a deficit-focused starting point. Their subsequent suggestion is that this permits cultural assets to be highlighted rather than obscured.

Development-through-sport

As outlined in the *Future of Australian Sport* (Hajkowicz *et al.*, 2013), Australia (and New Zealand) draws on sport as a vehicle for providing aid and promoting international relationships in the Oceania region. In a joint strategy between the ASC and AusAID (2013–2017) outline development-through-sport on the premise that sport has unique attributes that enable it to contribute to development processes. Its popularity, its capacity as a communication platform, its role in reducing risk of non-communicable diseases and its potential to set the foundation for healthy child development, together with its ability to connect people, make it a tool that can be used to meet a range of developmental objectives (p. 3). In turn, the *A Outreach Program* (ASOP) supports development-through-sport in communities including Vanuatu, Kiribati, Tonga, Solomon Islands, Nauru, Fiji and Samoa. Three outcomes it seeks to address are:

1   an increase in healthy behaviours across the Pacific;
2   an improvement in social cohesion outcomes for youth, people with disabilities and women;
3   an improvement in social cohesion.

Each international partnership is tailored to meet the priorities and build on the capacities of the communities. For example, the ASOP in Fiji focuses on a partnership with the Fiji Paralympic Committee to develop inclusive sport programmes in the country. In the Solomon Islands, the ASOP partnership with Save the Children and the Solomon Islands Football Federation focuses on young people's leadership and health behaviours, whereas in Tonga the priority is the promotion of healthy body weight for women through netball. National and international sport organisations, such as the International Cricket Council and the International Rugby Board, also are active in leading development-through-sport across Australasia, often in tandem with the ASOP. It is important to note that these multi-organisational projects are subject to fluctuations in the quantity and quality of administrative and financial support from key organisations due to changing priorities and economic trends. Integral to all programmes is the intention to develop local capacity for sports leadership and establish a network of support and partnerships that increase the likelihood of sustainability as well as capacity for programme monitoring and evaluation. To date, the evaluation of projects has been problematic and ways forward highlight the need for post-colonial methodologies that reflect relationship-building between the researched and researchers, inclusive data collection strategies and recognising the cultural wealth of those with whom we are working (Rossi, Rynne and Nelson, 2010).

Conclusion

Participation data for Australasian youth who are transitioning from school to post-school options is sparse and fragmented. Little reliable data exists on participation patterns for youth as defined in this text, and this is an impediment to being able to discuss with any certainty participation trends, facilitators and barriers and thereby arrive at robust strategies for building or maintaining participation. However, signs are that traditional organised sport is losing its participant base as new forms of physical activity participation emerge for youth with the appeal of being more flexible, accessible, cheaper, quicker and suited to the construction of personal identities. At the same time, educational institutions are struggling with how they should invest in youth sport while government and non-government agencies are using sport as a medium for individual and community capacity building. Consequently, ways of understanding and promoting engagement in sport, and physical activity more broadly, are increasingly using models that shift the emphasis from the individual and 'deficit' to ecological (e.g. Utter *et al.*, 2006), positive youth development (e.g. Côté and Mallett, 2013) and strengths-based approaches (e.g. Macdonald, 2013; Sport and Recreation New Zealand, 2007). Therefore, it is a particularly significant time in Australasia to ponder the future of youth sport.

In the Australian context, there has been a steady decline in the number of gold medals and overall medals since the 2004 (*Winning Edge*, ASC, 2012). Furthermore, the number of world champions in priority sports has also declined since that time (ASC, 2012). This decline coincides with greater government investment in both developing and developed countries for international success in the sporting arena. Hence, a key concern is the sustainability of Australia at least maintaining (and preferably improving) its world ranking in the Olympics, Paralympics and in other professional sports in the foreseeable future. How will previously successful countries on the international stage, such as Australia, continue to compete with the rise of organised sport in other countries (notably Asia) combined with the decline in participation in Australia? Are conventional models of team sport anachronistic? If so, how should organised sport change its product and promise in order to attract and retain young, busy, health-conscious Australasians? Can schools play a pivotal role here in educating young people for physical activity futures with the competence, confidence and interest to be lifelong participants? And what of elite sport? Will our appetite for international sporting success continue, with its high investment, when global competition continues to increase?

References

Australian Sports Commission. (2012). *Australia's Winning Edge: Our Game Plan for Moving from World Class to World Best*. Canberra: Australian Government.

Australian Sports Commission. (2001). *Backing Australia's Sporting Ability: A More Active Australia*. Canberra: Australian Government.

Australian Sports Commission and AusAID (2013). *Development-Through-Sport 2013–2107*. Canberra: Australian Government.

Berry, J., Abernethy, B. and Côté, J. (2008). The contribution of structured activity and deliberate play to the development of expert perceptual and decision-making skill. *Journal of Sport and Exercise Psychology, 30*, 685–708.

Brown, W.J. Heesch, K.C. and Miller, Y.D. (2009). Life events and changing physical activity patterns in women at different life stages. *Annals of Behavioural Medicine, 37*, 294–305.

Côté, J. (1999). The influence of the family in the development of talent in sport. *The Sport Psychologist, 13*, 395–417.

Côté, J. Baker, J. and Abernethy, B. (2003). From play to practice: A developmental framework for the acquisition of expertise in team sports, in J.L. Starkes and K.A. Ericsson (eds) *Expert Performance in Sports: Advances in Research on Sport Expertise* (89–113), Champaign, Illinois: Human Kinetics.

Côté, J. and Mallett, C.J. (2013). *Review of Junior Sport Framework Briefing Paper: Positive Youth Development Through Sport*. Canberra: Australian Sports Commission.

Côté, J., Turnnidge, J. and Vierimaa, M. (2016). A personal assets approach to youth sport, in K. Green and A. Smith (eds) *Routledge Handbook of Youth Sport*. London: Routledge.

Danish, S., Forneris, T., Hodge, K. and Heke, I. (2004). *Enhancing youth development through sport*. World Leisure Journal, *46*, 38–49.

DinanThompson, M., Sellwood, J. and Carless, F. (2008). A kickstart to life: Australian football league as a medium for promoting lifeskills in Cape York Indigenous communities. *Australian Journal of Indigenous Education, 37*, 152–64.

Fotu, K., Moodie, M., Mavoa, H., Pomana, S., Schultz, J. and Swinburn, B. (2011). Process evaluation of a community-based adolescent obesity prevention project in Tonga. *BMC Public Health, 11*, 284–295.

Gulbin, J., Oldenziel, K.,Weissensteiner, J. and Gagné, F. (2010). A look through the rear view mirror: Developmental experiences and insights of high performance athletes. *Talent Development and Excellence, 2*, 149–164.

Hajkowicz, S., Cook, H., Wilhelmseder, L. and Boughen, N. (2013). *The Future of Australian Sport: Megatrends Shaping the Sports Sector over Coming Decades. A Consultancy Report for the Australian Sports Commission.* Canberra: CSIRO, Australia.

Hamilton, S.F., Hamilton, M.A. and Pittman, K. (2004). Principles for youth development', in S.F. Hamilton and M.A. Hamilton (eds). *The Youth Development Handbook: Coming of Age in American Communities (3–22)*, Thousand Oaks: Sage Publications.

Hamlin, M.J. and Ross, J.J. (2005). Barriers to physical activity in young New Zealanders. *Youth Studies Australia, 24*, 31–37.

Hands, B., Parker, H., Glasson, C., Brinkman, S. and Read, H. (2004). *Physical Activity and Nutrition Levels in Western Australian Children and Adolescents: Report*. Perth: Western Australian Government.

Holt, N.L. (2008). *Positive Youth Development Through Sport*. London: Routledge.

Hoye, R. (2013). *Review of Junior Sport Framework Briefing Paper: Cost of participation*. Canberra: Australian Sports Commission.

Kirk, D. (1998) *Schooling Bodies: School Practice and Public Discourse, 1880–1950*. London: Leicester University Press.

Light, R.L., Harvey, S. and Memmert, D. (2011). Why children join and stay in sports clubs: case studies in Australian, French and German swimming clubs. *Sport, Education and Society*, *18*, 550–566.

Macdonald, D. (2013) The new Australian Health and Physical Education Curriculum: a case of/for gradualism in curriculum reform? *Asia–Pacific Journal of Health, Sport and Physical Education*, *4(2)*, 95–108.

Macdonald, D. (2011). Like a fish in water: Physical education policy and practice in the era of neoliberal globalization. *Quest*, *63*, 36–45.

Olds, T., Dollman, J. and Maher, C. (2009). Adolescent sport in Australia: who, when, where and what? *ACHPER Australia Healthy Lifestyles Journal*, *56*, 11–16.

Phillips, M. and Macdonald, D. (2013). *Review of Junior Sport Framework Briefing Paper: Historical, Cultural, and Social Perspectives*. Canberra: Australian Sports Commission.

Phongsavan, P., Olatunbosun-Alalkija, A., Havea, D., Bauman, A., Smith, B., Galea, G., Chen, J. and members of the Health Behaviour and Lifestyle of Pacific Youth Survey Collaborating Group and Core Survey Teams. (2005). Health behaviour and lifestyle of pacific youth surveys: a resource for capacity building, *Health Promotion International*, *20(3)*, 238–248.

Rossi, A., Rynne, S. and Nelson, A. (2013). Doing whitefella research in blackfella communities in Australia: Decolonizing method in sports related research. *Quest*, *65*, 116–131.

Roberts, K. (2016). Youth leisure as the context for youth sport, in Green, K. and Smith, A. (eds) *Routledge Handbook of Youth Sport*. London: Routledge.

Rynne, S. and Rossi, T. (2012). *The Impact of Indigenous Community Sports Programs: The Case of Surfing*. Canberra: Australian Sports Commission.

Schlossberg, N.K. (1981). Major contributions. *Counseling Psychologist*, *9*, 2–15.

Sinclair, K.M., Hamlin, M.J. and Steel, G. (2005). Physical activity levels of first-year New Zealand university students: a pilot study. *Youth Studies Australia*, *24*, 38–42.

Sport and Recreation New Zealand (2007). *It's All About the Children and Young People*. Wellington: New Zealand.

Sport and Recreation New Zealand (2008). *Sport, Recreation and Physical Activity Participation among New Zealand Adults: Key results of the 2007/08 Active NZ Survey*. Wellington: SPARC.

Trost, S.G. (2013) *Review of Junior Sport Framework Briefing Paper: Trends in Sport and Physical Activity Participation in Australian Children and Youth*. Canberra: Australian Sports Commission.

Utter, J., Denny, S., Robinson, E. M., Ameratunga, S. and Watson, P. (2006). Perceived access to community facilities, social motivation, and physical activity among New Zealand youth. *Journal of Adolescent Health*, *39*, 770–773.

Williams, B.J., Hay, P.J. and Macdonald, D. (2011). The outsourcing of health, sport and physical educational work: A state of play. *Physical Education and Sport Pedagogy*, *16*, 399–415.

11

YOUTH SPORT IN JAPAN

Atsushi Nakazawa and Aaron L. Miller

Introduction

In this chapter, we describe youth sport in Japan by analyzing various statistical data, exploring its socio-cultural background and examining several contemporary controversial issues found within it. First, we describe several general trends of youth sport in Japan by using nation wide statistical data, focusing on how frequently sports are played, which sports are played most and least, where play occurs, which clubs are most popular, why youth play sports, who coaches them and how many injuries occur. Second, we describe the current state of affairs in Japanese school sport, chiefly because it is the most important centre for Japanese youth sport. In particular, we try to understand the role of teachers in school sport and their challenges by using nation wide survey data. Third, we offer a brief history of Japanese youth sport. Fourth, and finally, we consider the kinds of problems that currently exist in contemporary youth sport, focusing on two serious issues as case studies: judo accidents and corporal punishment (*taibatsu*).

General trends

First, let us examine some general quantitative trends in Japanese youth sport. Let's use statistical data derived from a 2013 nationwide research survey conducted by the private research institution Sasakawa Sports Foundation (SSF), in which the sporting lives of 3,000 randomly selected young people aged 10–19-years old, including elementary school students (10–12), junior high school students (12–15), high school students (15–18), university and college students (18–19) and workers (15–19) were examined. This survey (Sasakawa Sports Foundation, 2013) answers the following questions.

How frequently do Japanese young people play sports in a year?

Thirteen per cent of young people never play, 10.3 per cent play less than once a week (1–51 times a year), 6.3 per cent play more than once a week but less than twice a week (52–103 times a year), 5.0 per cent play more than twice a week but less than three times a week (104–155 times a year), 4.9 per cent play more than three times a week but less than four times a week (156–207 times a year), 4.7 per cent play more than four times a week but less than five times a week (208–259 times a year), 6.5 per cent play more than five times a week but less than six times a week (260–311 times a year), 10.7 per cent play more than six times a week but less than seven times a week (312–363 times a year), and 38.6 per cent play more than seven times a week (more than 364 times a year). As a whole, 87.0 per cent of young Japanese play sports, and more than half of all young people play sports more than five days a week.

When they play, what sports interest them most?

According to the SSF, the top twenty most popular sports are as follows: soccer (31.1 per cent), followed by tag (30.0 per cent), jogging/running (26.4 per cent), basketball (25.9 per cent), swimming (25.3 per cent), dodge ball (24.0 per cent), skipping rope (23.1 per cent), badminton (22.3 per cent), muscle training (20.7 per cent), swing (20.2 per cent), playing catch (18.9 per cent), baseball (18.7 per cent), table tennis (18.5 per cent), riding bicycles (17.2 per cent), walking (16.6 per cent), volleyball (16.5 per cent), bowling (16.5 per cent), hide-and-seek (15.7 per cent), gymnastics (15.3 per cent) and horizontal bar (15.3 per cent).

Where do Japanese youth play sports?

Most of all they play in schools (73.4 per cent), followed by parks, open spaces and vacant land (42.1 per cent). They also play in gymnasia and on grounds not affiliated with schools (29.5 per cent), in private homes (22.1 per cent), on the road (7.6 per cent), at bowling alleys (6.5 per cent), by the sea, coast, or port (6.3 per cent), in the pool (5.8 per cent), on ski slopes (5.6 per cent) and around the house (4.5 per cent). As you can see, Japanese youth mostly play sports at schools or other public institutions.

Which sports clubs are the most popular among Japanese youth?

According to the SSF, 50.5 per cent of all young Japanese people have participated in a sports club at some time, 21.5 per cent have never participated in club and 28.1 per cent had participated in club but have quit it for some reason. Among the young Japanese who have participated, more than half have done so as a member of an extracurricular sport club in a junior high or high school (54.7 per cent). Meanwhile, a smaller percentage of Japanese youth have participated in a community-based club outside the school (19.0 per cent), in a private club outside the school (16.6 per cent), in an extracurricular sport club in an elementary school (10.9 per cent), in an intramural (*sākuru*) club during university (3.2 per cent) or in an extracurricular sport club during university (2.0 per cent).

Why do young people play?

The top ten reasons were the following: to have fun (64.1 per cent), to become physically active (49.9 per cent), to develop physical strength (45.9 per cent), to improve skills (45.3 per cent), to be a member of club (43.0 per cent), to win (31.2 per cent), to make new friends (28.6 per cent), to be asked by friends (27.6 per cent), to play with friends (26.8 per cent) and to be healthy (25.1 per cent). Japanese youth clearly play sports for various reasons.

Who coaches Japanese youth in sport?

First of all, it should be noted that many Japanese youngsters do not have a coach at all. According to the SSF in 2013, 45.7 per cent of young people did not have a coach, while 54.3 per cent did. In some sports, coaches are more common. For example, in soft tennis (85.4 per cent), baseball (80.6 per cent), volleyball (78.0 per cent), table tennis (76.3 per cent), basketball (67.4 per cent), soccer (62.9 per cent) and badminton (55.3 per cent), more than half of all Japanese youth have a coach. Yet in cases such as jogging/running (21.1 per cent) or dodge ball (10.9 per cent), a very small percentage of youth enjoy the guidance of a coach. Of course, few youth who play tag ever have a coach.

How many young people suffer injuries?

According to the SSF, the percentage of young people who were injured while playing sport was 15.2 per cent. If we further investigate this rate by age category, we find that 14.6 per cent occurred among elementary school students, 18.2 per cent occurred among junior high school students, 16.9 per cent occurred among high school students, 8.3 per cent occurred among university and college students and 1.8 per cent occurred among corporate athletes (many Japanese companies support after work sports clubs for their employees). These injuries include sprains (29.6 per cent), fractures (18.0 per cent), bruises (6.0 per cent), pulled muscles (4.7 per cent), ligament damage (4.3 per cent) and fatigue induced fractures (3.9 per cent).

School sport: a major centre for Japanese youth sport activities

As the aforementioned SSF survey reveals, youth sport, especially during junior high and high school, is largely dependent upon the institution of school sport in Japan. While in many countries youth sports revolve around community clubs outside the school, Japanese youth sports mostly revolve around extracurricular sports activities affiliated with schools. Therefore, Japanese schools not only offer formal classroom curricula in line with the Ministry of Education, Culture, Sports, Science and Technology's Course of Study, but they also set the informal agenda for extracurricular sports activities. Accordingly, Japanese teachers not only teach students inside the classroom, but also manage extracurricular sports activities outside the classroom. These are two distinct aspects of youth sports in Japan, compared with youth sports in other countries.

What is the current state of affairs in school sport in contemporary Japan? In 2001, the Ministry of Education, Culture, Sports, Science and Technology convened the *Undō bukatsudō no jittai ni kansuru chōsa kenkyū kyōryokusha kaigi* [Supporter's conference for an investigation regarding the actual situation of extracurricular sports activities] in order to conduct a nation wide survey regarding extracurricular sports activities in junior high schools and high schools. Based on the results of this survey, we can summarize the following seven points regarding the current state of school sports in Japan (Undō bukatsudō no jittai ni kansuru chōsa kenkyū kyōryokusha kaigi, 2002):

1   Overall trends. Almost all Japanese schools offered extracurricular sports activities in line with school educational activities. On average, the number of clubs each school offered was 19.2 clubs for junior high school and 29.0 clubs for high school. The participation rate of students was 73.0 per cent in junior high school and 52.1 per cent in high school. On average, the number of students in each club was 24.5 for junior high school and 18.3 students for high school. On average, the number of teachers who coached students in extracurricular sports activities was 18.1 teachers (66.8 per cent of all teachers) for junior high school and 35.8 teachers (62.6 per cent of all teachers) for high school. Clearly, extracurricular sports activities play a large role in the lives of both Japanese students and teachers.

2   Types of clubs. Regarding participation rate, junior high school students preferred the following sports in this order: basketball (13.4 per cent), soft tennis (13.4 per cent), rubber baseball (11.7 per cent), volleyball (11.4 per cent), table tennis (10.3 per cent), track and field (8.8 per cent), soccer (8.5 per cent), *kendo* [fencing] (5.6 per cent), badminton (4.5 per cent) and tennis (4.3 per cent).

Meanwhile, in the case of high school students, the top ten was the following: basketball (12.8 per cent), soccer (11.3 per cent), volleyball (9.4 per cent), baseball (8.2 per cent), track and field (8.2 per cent), tennis (7.5 per cent), soft tennis (5.5 per cent), badminton (4.5 per cent), table tennis (4.4 per cent) and *kyudo* [archery] (4.0 per cent).

3   Amount of activity. During the academic term, most junior high school students participated in sports activities six days a week (34.5 per cent). A slightly fewer number participated seven days a week (29.3 per cent), and even fewer participated five days a week (19.2 per cent). On average, junior high school students participated 5.5 days a week. In terms of how long each student participated in their sport each time, 46.7 per cent participated more than 2 hours but less than 3 hours, 34.5 per cent participated more than an hour but less than 2 hours and 11.2 per cent participated more than 3 hours but less than 4 hours. At the high school level, more than a third of all students participated in their sport six days (36.6 per cent), followed by seven days (34.5 per cent) and five days (11.3 per cent). On average, high school students participated 5.6 days in a week. As for how long they participated each time, more than half participated for more than 2 hours but less than 3 hours (50.3 per cent), less than a quarter participated for more than an hour but less than 2 hours (23.8 per cent) and less than a fifth participated for more than 3 hours but less than 4 hours (17.3 per cent).

4   Student worries. Students who participate in school sport have various worries. For example, junior high school students worry that they enjoy too few holidays (20.9 per cent), experience routine fatigue (19.0 per cent), have no time to play or study (18.2 per cent), don't have a chance to improve skills (18.0 per cent), narrow space (17.4 per cent), friendship among students (14.3 per cent), not enough instruction (13.9 per cent) and 23.7 per cent of all students had no worry. On the other hand, high school students also worry that they enjoy too few holidays (22.6 per cent), experience routine fatigue (22.5 per cent), have no time to play and study (21.5 per cent), don't have a chance to improve skills (20.9 per cent), do not get enough instruction (17.1 per cent), narrow space (16.0 per cent), friendship among students (11.7 per cent) and 19.6 per cent of all students had no worry. As you can see, the trends found in junior high school are similar to those found at the high school level.

5   School sport educators. Almost all instructors and coaches of extracurricular sport activities are school teachers, not professional coaches. This research asked teachers why and how they instruct and manage school sport. Most of these educators aim to help students learn co-operation and sociability (51.1 per cent of junior high school teachers, 46.0 per cent of high school teachers), seek to develop mental strength and a sense of responsibility (36.3 per cent of junior high school teachers, 35.3 per cent of high school teachers), strive to foster students' attitude for enjoying sports throughout their lifetimes (31.0 per cent of junior high school teachers, 23.9 per cent of high school teachers), try to improve their competitiveness and achieve better scores (26.5 per cent of junior high school teachers, 40.5 per cent of high school teachers) and to exercise students' body and to help them live active lives in the future (20.1 per cent of junior high school teachers, 14.2 per cent of high school teachers). As you can see, most Japanese school teachers aim to use sports for educational purposes first and foremost, rather than focusing on attaining victory. In this

survey, Japanese school teachers were also asked how many days in a week they instructed students in extracurricular sport activities. On average, each junior high school teacher instructed their sport 4.7 days a week, and each high school teacher instructed 3.9 days a week. As a result, though teachers willingly and voluntarily coach school sports with a broad sense of education in mind, they must bear a heavy burden to do so.

6   Teacher worries. Teachers who coach school sport also have various worries. For example, many teachers worry that they will be unable to instruct satisfactorily because of their other school duties (51.2 per cent of junior high school teachers, 48.9 per cent of high school teachers). Many also worry that they might have a shortage of professional instruction ability (42.9 per cent of junior high school teachers, 39.7 per cent of high school teachers), that they might have to eliminate their free time for research (22.3 per cent of junior high school teachers, 17.4 per cent of high school teachers), that they have a shortage of institutional facilities or equipment (19.7 per cent of junior high school teachers, 22.6 per cent of high school teachers), that only a small number of students participate in the club (16.4 per cent of junior high school teachers, 24.8 per cent of high school teachers), that they have budget shortages (10.6 per cent of junior high school teachers; 13.3 per cent of high school teachers) and that they cannot maintain a relationship of friendship among students (10.1 per cent of junior high school teachers, 6.8 per cent of high school teachers). Only 2.5 per cent of all junior high school teachers and 3.6 per cent of high school teachers have no worries at all.

Socio-cultural background: a brief history of youth sport in Japan

As mentioned above, youth sport in Japan is largely dependent on school sports. In order to understand why and how school sports have become the centre of youth sport in Japan, we will briefly describe the history of youth sport in Japan, especially focusing on the post World War II history of school sport (for further details, please see Nakazawa, 2014a, 2014b).

In the latter part of nineteenth century, and until 1945, Japan became a modern nation-state, rising from the pre-modern Edo period (1603–1868) to the modern Meiji period (1868–1912). During this modernizing process, Japan learned and absorbed much European and American knowledge, technology and culture, including sport culture. This foreign sport culture was initially introduced through the school system, especially through Japanese universities. Extracurricular sports clubs were later established within higher education in the latter part of the nineteenth century. These sports spread to secondary education, beginning in the early twentieth century (Guttmann and Thompson, 2001). In short, Japanese sports, including youth sports, were from the early years of Japan's modernization associated with school sport. However, extracurricular sports activities before World War II did not generally depend on the assistance of teachers, schools and educational policies, but rather depended a great deal on students' voluntary participation. As a result, students' participation rates were not as high at the time as they became after World War II.

Between 1945 and the 1950s, the structure of Japanese youth sport became largely dependent on school sport. In August 1945, Japan accepted the Potsdam Declaration and removed 'all obstacles to the survival and strengthening of democratic tendencies among the Japanese people. Freedom of speech, religion, and of thought, as well as respect for fundamental rights shall be established' (Anderson, 1975, p. 61). World War II was over, Japan was a defeated nation, and she had lost her sovereignty to determine her own political system. The General Headquarters (GHQ) of the United Nations began a period known as the Occupation and promoted postwar education reforms. Twenty-seven distinguished educators, known as the United States Education

Mission to Japan, were invited from the United States to investigate Japanese education and produce a report suggesting a vision of postwar educational reform. In line with the report's recommendations, a set of postwar educational reforms were implemented, shifting Japanese school physical education away from the militaristic mindset that had guided them before the war and toward democratic values. Students' participation rates in extracurricular sports activities grew in the early postwar period as a result.

Between the 1960s and early 1970s, school sport in Japan changed, especially around 1964, when the Tokyo Olympics became the first Olympics ever to be held in Asia. In the run-up to these Olympics, Japan's sport policy was characterized by elitism. For example, in 1959 and 1960, the *Hoken taiiku shingikai* [Health and Physical Education Council], which at the time was the most influential council on national policy regarding physical education and sport, emphasized improving sports skills and increasing body strength in order to win at the Olympic games. However, after a decrease in students' participation rates in extracurricular sports activities, policymakers reconsidered these elitist policies. After 1964, the focus of policy shifted to popularization. For example, in 1972 the *Hoken taiiku shingikai* (Health and Physical Education Council) reconsidered their previous emphasis on elitism and began to champion the 'sports for all' cause. Before 1964, Japan's sporting discourse had primarily revolved around the question of how to train elite athletes. At the time, some physical education experts wanted to use physical education to train adolescents who exhibited higher than average potential to contribute to Japan's victories at the Olympic Games. However, this philosophy was criticized by others who spoke from an egalitarian perspective. After 1964, Japan's sporting discourse shifted to the issue of how to engage everyone in sports, not just elites. Japanese physical educators thereafter criticized the prioritization of training of elite athletes, and they argued that extracurricular activities must be inclusive school educational activities offered to all students. After 1964, the focus of sports policy and discourse thus shifted toward popularization and equal opportunity. As a result, students' participation rates began to increase again.

Between the late 1970s and the 1980s, participation in school sports continued to expand. Participation in school itself also expanded during this time; in the late 1970s, the percentage of students who chose to attend high school after compulsory junior high school exceeded 90 per cent. Schooling until the age of 18 became the standard for almost all Japanese adolescents during this era. Schools and teachers were forced to handle a broad range of students and to face many problems with students' misbehaviour (e.g. alcohol and tobacco use, violence). As a result, they began using extracurricular sports activities to eliminate these problems. For example, a junior high school teacher said that extracurricular activities were very useful in preventing delinquency because they let students break a sweat, helped them release their frustrations and deprived them of time necessary to be involved in misconduct (Hayashi, 1980). While there are no statistically significant studies that show whether such extracurricular sports activities actually prevented or rehabilitated delinquent students of the day, nevertheless, there were many people who believed that extracurricular sports activities had such power. Moreover, discipline was increasingly emphasized in the discourse regarding extracurricular sports activities during this period.

Throughout Japan's postwar history, extracurricular sports activities have expanded, and Japanese schools have used sports as tools to promote democracy, equality and discipline. Japanese schools have therefore regarded sports as an integral part of Japanese education, so Japan's system of extracurricular sport activities has become the main centre of youth sports in Japan.

Recently, however, neo-liberal educational reforms, which aimed at downsizing the school, have been put in place. Hence, at the policy level, there is currently an attempt to shift extracurricular sports clubs from the school to the community. For example, in 1997 the *Hoken taiiku shingikai* (Health and Physical Education Council) mentioned the possibility of shifting all extracurricular sport activities away from the school and toward community organizations. Still, at the practice level, Japanese teachers continue to use sports for educational purposes, and many are unwilling to let this work be completely taken over by community sports clubs.

Contemporary issues: towards the safeguarding of youth in Japanese sport

Youth sports are played widely in contemporary Japan and in public institutionary spaces, including schools, raising the issue of how Japanese youth are safeguarded in sport. Recently, accidents in judo have become an important national issue, as has the issue of *taibatsu* (corporal punishment). Both threaten the bodies, minds and lives of youth playing sport.

Judo accidents

On 17 April 2013, *The New York Times* reported that over the past thirty years, 118 children have died, and nearly 300 have ended up disabled or comatose while practicing judo in Japan. Such shocking news was based on the statistical studies of Uchida Ryo, a sociologist of education, who researches school safety. Although the Japanese government and the national judo association have generally ignored these incidents, Uchida has gathered school accident records from the Japan Sport Council and tracked 118 fatal incidents in judo practice since 1983. Uchida's published studies have had a great impact on youth sport in Japan and have forced authorities, including judo coaches, teachers and officials to reflect on their instructional style and to pay closer attention to children's safety.

On the other hand, some parents whose children have been involved in judo accidents have made their voices heard and have taken action. For example, Murakawa Yoshihiro, whose son suffered a head injury in 2009 and died a month later, and Kobayashi Yasuhiko, whose son had been badly hurt doing judo at school, together created the Japan Judo Accident Victims Association in March 2010, and they started helping other victims who also suffered from judo accidents. Their goal is to prevent such terrible accidents from ever happening again.

Meanwhile, in 2013 Uchida published a new book entitled *Jūdo jiko* [Judo accidents], aiming at 'reducing serious accidents in judo as significantly as possible so as to save children lives' (Uchida, 2013, p. 227). It seems that his work has stimulated some progress. Since 2012, when judo accidents became better known among the Japanese public, there have been no recorded deaths. Can Japan continue this trend in the future? That depends upon Japan's ability to remember these terrible accidents and work toward preventing them from happening again.

Taibatsu

Corporal punishment is another controversial issue in Japanese youth sports. In December 2012, a second-year high school student of Sakuranomiya High School in Osaka committed suicide after his basketball coach, Komura Hajime, repeatedly beat him. After the incident, Komura admitted to having injured the 17-year-old team captain when the boy 'failed to meet his expectations' (Japan Daily Press, 2013). Komura told authorities that he had used corporal punishment, known as *taibatsu* in Japanese, to 'guide his pupil strictly', in large part because he was the team captain and thought he could handle it (Osaka Board of Education, 2013). This incident, along with Uchida's research of judo accidents, brought the issue of safeguarding children in Japanese sport into the public consciousness.

Tragically, corporal punishment remains a widely used disciplinary practice throughout the world (Lang, Harthill and Rulofs, this volume), most commonly used by parents at home but also by teachers at school, and it represents an important crossroads at which the policies of schools and sports meet (Donnelly and Straus, 2005; Miller, 2013). The issue also raises important issues regarding power, the body and human rights. The physical discipline of children has been used in Japan for centuries, and many incidents of corporal punishment in Japan today follow a strikingly similar pattern, especially in the case of fatal or severe incidents. The perpetrator of the punishment, whether coach or teacher, commonly argues that the victim is actually not a victim at all but rather a specially chosen pupil who must be strictly trained to maximize their potential. Such educators do not regard corporal punishment as problematic, and they use it to set an example to the team of steadfast perseverance in the face of hardship, absolute obedience to authority and constant loyalty to the team. Japanese coaches like Komura believe this teaches athletes a powerful lesson that the team comes before the individual – a mantra they hope athletes will carry with them into their adult life. For example, Komura told the Osaka Board of Education, 'I have often hit my students for their own sake . . . I thought I could hit them without incident because we had a good relationship' (quoted in Osaka Board of Education, 2013). Athletes, meanwhile, are expected to accept corporal punishment without complaint, accepting it for their own growth and for the growth of unity of the group.

Ultimately, Komura was fired for his involvement in the boy's death, was tried and found guilty by the Osaka District Court and sentenced to three years in prison (Asahi Shimbun, 2013). However, while Komura was held responsible for playing a direct in the student's death, he never served jail time, because his sentence was suspended. (Japan Times, 2013). If coaches like Komura are not proportionately punished for their excessive violence, who will be? More importantly, who is responsible for safeguarding the Japanese youth athlete from such abuse? This is a question that the Japanese people have yet to answer.

Conclusion

This chapter has described the current state of youth sport in Japan as well as two controversial issues that exist with it today. First, we examined general quantitative trends in youth sport using nation wide statistical data, which showed that Japanese youth play a variety of sports actively, especially as members of extracurricular clubs affiliated with their schools. Second, we described the current state of affairs of Japanese school sport as a centre of Japanese youth sport, demonstrating that there is a large system of extracurricular sport activities sanctioned by the state. These sports are coached by volunteer teachers, but both these teachers and the students they guide have their own particular worries. Third, we delineated a brief history of youth sport in Japan by focusing on the postwar history of school sport, showing how this large system of extracurricular sport activities became a centre of youth sports in Japan. Finally, we considered two serious issues, judo accidents and corporal punishment, as a way to better understand the current challenges facing youth sport in Japan. We must address such problems so as to save and safeguard youth lives, and to make sure that in the future all Japanese youth can truly enjoy their sporting experiences.

References

Anderson, R.S. (1975) *Education in Japan*, US Government Printing Office.

Asahi Shimbun (2013). *Guilty verdict handed down in case of corporal punishment at Sakuranomiya High School.* 11th October.

Donnelly, M. and Straus, M. (2005). *Corporal Punishment of Children in Theoretical Perspective*, New Haven: Yale University Press.

Guttmann, A. and Thompson, L. (2001). *Japanese Sports*, University of Hawai'i Press.

Hayashi, M. (1980). *Bukatsudō koso hikōka no hadome* [Extracurricular activities are stopping delinquency], *Taiikuka kyoiku [Physical education pedagogy]*, *28(2)*, 42–43.

Japan Daily Press (2013). *Osaka Basketball Coach who Bullied Student to Suicide to Face Criminal Prosecution.* 6th July.

Japan Times (2013). *No jail for hoops coach who triggered suicide in Osaka.* 26th September.

Miller, A. (2013). *Discourses of Discipline: An Anthropology of Corporal Punishment in Japan's Schools and Sports*, Berkeley, CA: Institute for East Asian Studies.

Nakazawa, A. (2014a). Seeing sports as educational activities: A postwar history of extracurricular sports activities in Japan, *Hitotsubashi Journal of Social Sciences*, *45 (1)*, 1–14.

Nakazawa, A. (2014b). *Undō bukatsudō no sengo to genzai: Naze supōtsu wa gakkō kyōiku ni musubi tsuke rarerunoka* [A postwar history and current state of extracurricular sports activities in Japan: Why are sports connected to schooling?], Tokyo: Seikyūsha.

New York Times (2013). *Japan Confronts Hazards of Judo.* 17th April.

Osaka Board of Education (2013). Board of Education Response Regarding the Death of a Student at Osaka Sakuranomiya High School. Osaka: Author Publisher. Online. Retrieved from www.city.osaka.lg.jp/contents/wdu020/english/residents/parenting_education/2013_sakuranomiya_info.html on 2nd September 2015.

Sasakawa Sports Foundation (2013). *Seishōnen no supōtsu raifu dēta 2013 [The 2013 SSF national sports–life survey of young people]*, Sasakawa Sports Foundation.

Uchida, R. (2013). *Jūdo jiko* [Judo accident], Kawade shobō shinsha.

Undō bukatsudō no jittai ni kansuru chōsa kenkyū kyōryokusha kaigi [*Supporter conference for an investigation regarding actual situation of extracurricular sports activities*](2002). *Undō bukatsudō no jittai ni kansuru chōsa kenkyū hōkokusho* [Report of investigation regarding actual situation of extracurricular sports activities].

12

YOUTH SPORT IN THE MIDDLE EAST

Nida Ahmed and Holly Thorpe

Introduction

The Middle East and North Africa (MENA) region includes Algeria, Bahrain, Egypt, Iran, Iraq, Jordan, Kuwait, Lebanon, Libya, Morocco, Oman, Palestinian Territory, Qatar, Saudi Arabia, Syria, Tunisia, Turkey, the United Arab Emirates and Yemen. The MENA has been a site of much discussion and debate over the past three decades. The region is faced with 'declining productivity . . . decreasing school enrolment, and high illiteracy, and with health conditions lagging behind comparable nations' such that they seem 'richer than they are developed' (Bayat, 2010, p. 1). The recent political and social movements in this region have damaged infrastructures and displaced many people, especially youth.

Arab youth play an integral role in the social, cultural and economic development of their societies. For example, many youth are critical income earners for their families but are also viewed as particularly susceptible to processes of modernization, including the rise of new technologies. While many of the older generation express concerns over youth access to new technologies and exposure to global media, others suggest that these technologies enable young people to forge new relationships and develop greater autonomy and mobility. Yet not all young people in the MENA region have access to these resources. For many children and youth in the Middle East, sport is an important space to experience the social and physical pleasures of movement, to (temporarily) escape the harsh realities of their everyday lives and/or to express their frustrations in their present conditions.

History of sports in the MENA region from the nineteenth to twentieth century

Sports are not a new phenomenon in MENA. In fact, the MENA countries have a long history of using sports and physical activity to integrate citizens, promote healthy behaviour, cultivate local and international partnerships and generate economic growth (Fizel, 2006; Levermore, 2011; Madichie, 2009; Wagner, 1989). Traditional sports in the Middle East were motivated primarily by organized ceremonial activities that tended to be based on everyday tasks (e.g. hunting or trading), festive or religious ceremonies, and tribal wars (Struna, 2000). Since the nineteenth century, archery, equestrian (horse and camel racing), shooting and fencing became part of the traditional sport culture for the majority of Middle East countries (Wagner, 1989). Camel racing, in particular, remains widely popular in the United Arab Emirates, Oman, Jordan, Egypt, Kuwait, Qatar and Saudi Arabia.

During the nineteenth century, at the height of British colonialism, many MENA countries were introduced to contemporary Western sports. Sports such as football, basketball and handball were first introduced on British military bases, and then quickly spread to the streets of cities and villages (Amara, 2012a, 2012b). Due to the popularity of some Western sports, local clubs were formed which later promoted the creation of national teams across the different nations. Some sports were embraced more readily in some MENA countries than others. Basketball, for example, gained popularity in Lebanon and Israel around the 1900s and resulted in the development of numerous basketball clubs, which thrived until Lebanon faced political unrest during the 1970s, 1980s and 1990s. While civil unrest crippled the country, the Lebanese basketball team achieved much success, including winning several International Basketball Federation (FIBA) championships. Such successes stimulated large investments in the sport by corporations and prompted the government to finance youth basketball programmes, which contributed to further successes both nationally and internationally (Nassif, 2012).

In Iran, basketball, taekwondo, motor racing and volleyball were popular during the 1980s and 1990s. However, gymnastics and wrestling were the most successful sports in Iran. These two sports became an important bridge between the older and younger generations (Fozooni, 2012). During the late 1990s and early 2000s, football also gained significance in Iran, primarily as a result of when Iran beat the United States in the group stage of the 1998 FIFA World Cup. This game has been declared 'the most politically charged game in World Cup history' due to the long-standing political tensions between the two countries (Billingham, 2014, p. 1). As a result of this event, football surged in popularity in Iran making it more popular than basketball and wrestling, which until that point had dominated the nation's attention.

In Iraq, bodybuilding gained popularity in the 1980s primarily due to the global visibility of international movie stars such as Arnold Schwarzenegger and Sylvester Stallone, who were well regarded in the region for their physical attributes (Londoño and Al-Izzi, 2008). The interest in bodybuilding continued even with the ongoing Iraq war, which created employment opportunities for bodybuilders in the security sector (Londoño and Al-Izzi, 2008). At the same time, gymnasiums started opening throughout Baghdad and other cities across the country to support the growing body building community in Iraq.

In Oman, sports were originally limited to exercise groups and schoolyard activities. During the 1970s, however, the Omani government became increasingly interested in the physical health and wellbeing of their younger populations and integrated physical education (PE) into the curriculum. Football was the preferred activity for young males, while volleyball became a popular option for girls and young women. Further, the local geography of the region with its high mountain ranges and coastal plains fostered a growing interest in climbing and sailing activities. In 2010, Khalid Al-Siyabi became the first Omani to reach the summit of Mount Everest (Collins, 2011). Another successful Omani was Mohsin Al-Busaidi, who became the first Arab to sail around the world non-stop in 2009 (Al-Maskari, 2012). The success of athletes such as Al-Siyabi and Al-Busaidi helped gain global recognition of Oman as a sporting nation, and reignited the country's maritime heritage, and increased awareness of hiking and climbing as popular activities.

Sports in the physical education curriculum

In the early 1970s, the majority of Arab states developed Ministries of Youth and Sports, which then worked to PE policies and programmes into school curricular. According to Wagner (1989), such processes were one of the many impacts of colonialism in the region. The colonial era had introduced the British or French education model that, in contrast to previous educational approaches, was not taught through the medium of religious texts, and instead emphasized the teaching of secular subjects. During the post-colonial period, many of the Arab states continued to incorporate Western and traditional subjects into their curriculum. Some regions advanced more quickly when developing PE programmes in schools, and there was some communication between Arab States as they too incorporated these programmes into the school curricular. For example, it was not until the 1970s that Oman – under the influence of the Sultan (King) who highly valued education – first developed a state education system. In 1976, the same Sultan supported the implementation of a physical education system. To respect Islamic requirements, grades 1–4 were mixed gender and grades 5–10 were segregated (Al–Sinani, 2012). The objective of the early PE programme was to enable individuals to acquire knowledge of body and mind (Al–Sinani, 2012). To incorporate PE into Oman's school curriculum, assistance was sought from other Arab states that had already integrated PE into their curriculum. Interestingly, the Ministry of Education in Jordan designed the original national PE curriculum for Oman, with further consultation with Egypt in 1983. The programme was initially based on Jordan's curriculum, which incorporated games, gymnastics and athletics. The Egyptian consultant then integrated exercise as part of Oman's curriculum and further changes were made to incorporate age-appropriate activities. The curriculum for younger students, for example, focused on activities that developed basic motor abilities such as throwing and catching the ball. The PE programme in Oman continues to evolve with ongoing participation in global dialogues related to health, sport and PE.

Oman's neighbour, Saudi Arabia also implemented a physical education curriculum, but omitted girls and women from all levels. In 2013, however, the Saudi Arabian government ruled that female students attending private schools may participate in sports, but only under the supervision of a female instructor and they must abide by the cultural dress code (Human Rights Watch, 2013). More recently, in the spring of 2014, the government voted to be inclusive of girls and women's sports participation, primarily as a response to health concerns among the female population. With more than 51 per cent of Saudi Arabian women classified as obese, such concerns are gaining increasing governmental attention (Human Rights Watch, 2014). A country known for its strict policies that prohibit girls and women from participating in sports, such changes suggest the potential for new opportunities for female participation in physical activity, albeit still constrained by strict cultural and religious value systems.

Contemporary state of sports in MENA

Popular sports in the Middle East today include an array of traditional and western sports. Football became popular in the region during and following the period of colonialization, and its popularity continues. For example, in North Africa, 33 per cent of the population participates in football, 11 per cent in swimming and 6 per cent in mixed martial arts. In the Levant countries (Israel, Jordan, Lebanon, Palestine, Syria), 24 per cent participate in football, 12 per cent swimming and 6 per cent in basketball, and in the Gulf countries (GCC) 26 per cent participate in football, 9 per cent in swimming and 4 per cent in volleyball (SMG YouGov, 2011). It is important to note, however, that these numbers relate primarily to male participation rates.

The Gulf countries, and particularly the United Arab Emirates (UAE), Bahrain and Qatar, have established themselves as international arenas for hosting major sporting events such as horse and motor racing, tennis, golf and rugby tournaments. Their effort in generating high-level sporting events has attracted large financial investments in sponsorship events and world-class sporting facilities (also known as sport cities) such as Aspire Sports facility in Qatar, and the Formula 1 circuit in Bahrain (Bromber *et al.*, 2013). In 2022, Qatar will become the first Arab state to host the FIFA World Cup. However, Qatar is currently facing bribery allegations in winning the bid to host the major event (Pielke, 2013). The significant efforts by Gulf countries to write themselves into the global mega sport events industry are a result of recognition of the value of sports as a potentially valuable investment in future post-oil economy (Amara, 2012a).

There have been major societal changes in many of the MENA countries, in which policies and politics have been transformed in the Arab world, which impact the role of sport and physical activity in the lives of children and youth. According to Amara (2012a, p. 7), many of those in power understood well the 'multiple uses of sport as an element of political, social and cultural recognition' and thus the 'western dominant model of sport' was 'accepted by the newly independent countries with little criticism or adaptation to local particularism'. Many MENA countries are increasingly embracing the 'strategy of development through sport in the bidding for, and staging [of], mega-sport events' as a 'scheme for urban regeneration, for strengthening internal and external political legitimacy and for integrating the commercial values of sport' (Amara, 2012a, p. 14). Through deeply political relationships with international sporting bodies such as FIFA and the IOC, sport in the Arab world 'came to be regarded in general as an effective arena for future international treaties and conventions between North and South, East and West' (Amara, 2012a, p. 7). However, as Amara (2012a, p. 17) is careful to point out, 'the adoption of democratic or popular practices' in the Arabic world 'are always fragmentary and deceiving'. Indeed, despite recognition among the Arabic elite of the potential of sport, some cultural and religious differences between the West and the Arab world continue to pose difficulties, particularly regarding women's participation in sport, and youths' participation in unorganized, non-competitive sports that celebrate fun, creativity and self-expression.

Youth sport participation in MENA

The MENA region has the largest youth cohort in current history. The youth population (15–24-year-olds) is one of the fastest growing in the region with more than 100 million youth comprising approximately 30 per cent of the MENA region population (Dhillon and Yousef, 2009). Between the 1970s and 1990s, there was a rise of Ministries of Youth and Sport across various MENA countries. These ministries were responsible for creating, managing and regulating programmes and policies related to sports and youth development (Sowers and Toensing, 2012). The policies instituted by some Ministries of Youth and Sport focused on utilizing traditional sports along with western sports (e.g. football) to engage children and youth. In Yemen, for example, the government recognized the potential of sports to unify its increasingly diverse population, so the Supreme Council of Youth and Sport was established with the objective to bring together and unite citizens from different countries by preserving traditional sports (i.e. horse and camel racing) while simultaneously incorporating new sports (e.g. football) (Wagner, 1989). In Egypt, the Supreme Council for Youth Welfare and Sport (SCYS) was established in 1979 with the focus on promoting healthier youth and developing national pride. The Council implemented sporting programmes, such as football and basketball, into Egyptian schools. Similar initiatives developed across many other MENA countries. Local governments are continuing to modify existing programmes and implement new programmes to encourage children and youth sport participation. Such programmes are particularly important as youth obesity rates continue to rise in many MENA countries (Abraham, 2011; Behbehani and Beales, 2013).

While young men and women in the MENA countries are, according to Chaaban (2008, p. 6), encountering 'increased social exclusion and marginalization . . . rising unemployment rates, higher exposure to health issues, and a precarious education system', they are also demonstrating forms of agency and political engagement that should not be overlooked. Many social commentators and researchers have identified the large number of unemployed youth in Arab nations as a major cause of recent political unrest. According to Mohammad (2011, p. 159), unemployed youths' political frustrations were 'aggravated by their inability to express themselves in tightly controlled police state', combined with 'political corruption and the incapability of the state to deal with social and economic problems'. Simultaneously, youth were also gaining access to new media, which not only exposed them to other ways of knowing the world, but also facilitated greater communication and organization across groups. As a result of access to new media, many of those sports traditionally popular in the MENA region are taking a back-seat among the younger generation, while sports of Western origin, such as football, basketball, boxing, bodybuilding, capiora and parkour, are gaining popularity. In the following section, we briefly discuss the recent popularity of newer, action sports and the significance of social media on trends in youth sport participation. It is important to note, however, that youth in the MENA region are not simply uncritically adopting Western sports, but rather reappropriating them in local contexts. Such processes are a unique form of 'glocalization', which involves youth in local contexts adapting and redefining the global product of sport to 'suit their particular needs, beliefs and customs' (Giulianotti and Robertson, 2004, p. 546; see also Robertson, 1992, 1995; Robertson and White, 2003; Thorpe and Ahmad, 2013).

Trends in youth participation: reclaiming space with action sports

For many years, action sports (e.g. BMX, kite-surfing, skateboarding, surfing, snowboarding) were thought to be the exclusive domain of privileged, white, narcissistic western youth (Booth and Thorpe, 2007; Kusz, 2007; Wheaton, 2004a 2010). However, due to the rapid expansion of the internet and the global reach of transnational action sport companies, media and events, combined with the increasingly exotic travel patterns of action sport athletes and enthusiasts (Thorpe, 2014a), children and youth throughout the eastern world are also exposed to action sports. While some reject action sports as crazy American sports, others have adopted and re-appropriated these activities in relation to their local physical and social environments. In the Muslim world, for example, surfing is gaining popularity in Iran and Bangladesh; Pakistani youth are taking up skateboarding in growing numbers; and sand boarding is a popular activity among privileged youth (and ex pats) in Saudi Arabia.

As suggested above, the appropriation of the predominantly western phenomenon of action sports by local groups in the Middle East raises interesting questions about the complex and multi-faceted nature of global flows of sport and physical culture in the twenty-first century. Recently we built upon recent scholarship on the globalization of youth culture and sport (Giulianotti, 2004; Giulianotti and Robertson, 2004; Henseler, 2012; Thorpe, 2011; Wheaton, 2004b) to shed light on the development of action sports in the Middle East, and in so doing, reveal the agency of youth to negotiate space for themselves within complex networks of power in global, local and virtual geographies (Thorpe and Ahmed, 2013). We focused specifically on the grassroots development of parkour (also known as free running) – the act of running, jumping, leaping through an urban environment as fluidly, efficiently and creatively as possible – in the Middle East at a unique historical conjuncture in which youth have (to varying degrees) gained greater access to global information and opportunities to virtually communicate beyond their local environments, yet continue to live with the everyday realities (or threats) of war, poverty and political upheaval.

121

Youth in the Middle East are some of the world's most active users of the internet and new social media. Youth make up around 70 per cent of the 45 million Facebook users in the Arab world, and Arabic is the fastest growing language in Twitter history (Facebook in the Arab region, 2012). It is perhaps not surprising then that the internet and social media have been integral to the development of new sports in Middle Eastern countries. In contrast to the historical movement of sports across countries – in which colonizers often imposed their sports on the local peoples who adopted, appropriated or rejected the activities – young men in the Middle East were first exposed to parkour via cable television and the internet in the early 2000s. Parkour had been popular among western youth for almost a decade before it reached the Middle East in the new millennium. According to photojournalist David Denger, parkour 'migrated to Egypt without direct contact but through iconic movies such as District 13 and homemade YouTube videos' (personal communication, January 2013). Nasser Al-Refaei – a PE graduate – was among the first to start practising parkour in Egypt in 2003. In his own words, he had 'always been in love with extreme sports', and was quickly impressed by the maneuvers he saw on YouTube: 'I started to analyze the moves based on my background studies and then applied that to myself. Then I shot a small clip of my trainings and posted it on YouTube' (cited in Against Gravity, 2012). Al-Refaei then went on to become the primary trainer for Parkour Egypt, the first official parkour group in the Middle East. Since its establishment in 2005, Parkour Egypt has grown to include more than 200 members. Virtual media continue to play an integral role in the daily organization, and local and international communications, of the group. As Mahmoud explained, 'the social networking websites are helping us to spread the art and keep all our fans and students updated with anything we do. internet has an essential role making the parkour spreading in Egypt, and for communication with many groups from different Arabic states' (personal communication, January 2013). Shortly after the development of parkour in Egypt, the activity also drew the attention of young men in Kuwait who went on to found PK Jaguars in 2006. The primary goal of this group is to 'spread Parkour's way of life to the Middle East any way possible and make the youth and community realize how important Parkour and movement is to our daily lives' (PK Jaguars Facebook page). As with Parkour Egypt, the PK Jaguars are very active in their use of online media.

Groups of (mostly young male) traceurs and free runners can today be found in Bahrain, Doha, Egypt, Israel, Kuwait, Libya, Morocco, Oman, Palestine, Saudi Arabia and UAE. Many of the early participants tended to be young men in their late teens and early 20s, and often university graduates unable to find full-time employment. As coaching sessions have been made available, however, the groups are becoming more diverse with younger boys increasingly taking up the activity. Almost all have Facebook pages with the number of followers ranging from 300 (Parkour Libya Free) to 42,000 (Parkour Egypt). These pages feature short edited videos with group members performing parkour or free running in various environments, news of upcoming training sessions and performances, or reviews of events, mostly written in Arabic. Some parkour groups are relatively small, informal groups of young men who train together, whereas others have grown into highly organized, hierarchical and commercial organizations with hired training facilities and coaches. Key members of some groups are travelling inter-nationally to compete and perform, and make regular appearances in movies and commercials (e.g. Chevrolet, Vodafone, Pepsi). For example, members of the PK Kuwait and Bahrain Parkour teams performed together on the beach at the Qatar National Day celebration in December 2011. Both Parkour Egypt and PK Jaguars have featured in the Arab's Got Talent television programme, and in 2011 Kuwait hosted the Red Bull Art of Motion international competition, including some of the top free runners and parkour athletes from Kuwait and around the world (Thorpe and Ahmed, 2013).

As the case of parkour illustrates, new social media has been influential in the introduction and adoption of newer, action sports in the MENA region. Of particular interest here is the agency being demonstrated by youth. Through the consumption of global media, some young men became inspired by the athleticism and novelty of parkour and quickly adopted active roles in learning the sport, finding and creating their own spaces for participation, training others and establishing their own media (e.g. videos, websites, newsletters). Some groups, such as PK Gaza, are consciously using their sport participation and transnational online platforms for political purposes and to raise awareness of the harsh realities of their lives in war-torn communities (Thorpe and Ahmad, 2013).

Female sport participation

The MENA region is known for its pervasive gender-based discrimination perpetuated by cultural and family values, and political laws. In a study by the Global Gender Gap conducted in 2010, the majority of the MENA countries ranked at the bottom of the global gender gap index (Roudi-Fahimi and El-Feki, 2011). While structural constraints are very slow to change, there have been some notable improvements throughout the region in regards to girls' and women's participation in sport and physical activity.

Research surrounding Muslim women in sports is limited (Benn, Pfister, and Jawad, 2010; Pfister, 2010; Samie and Schlikaglu, 2015), yet it is important to note that Muslim women are not new to the sporting world. Origins date to the time of the Prophet Mohammad, who is said to have encouraged women's participation in sports. Records show that his wife often competed in horseraces (Walseth and Fasting, 2003). Furthermore, a few women have competed in sporting events at the international level since the early 1960s. Iran and Turkey were the first to send women to the Olympic Games, with female athletes competing in the 1964 Summer Olympics in Tokyo, Japan. During the 1980s, a number of other Arab states, including Algeria, Libya, and Syria, followed suit. In 1984, Nawal El-Moutawakel from Morocco was the first female from the region to win a gold medal at the Olympics; her success was in the inaugural 400m hurdling event (Baker, 2012). Further, several Arab women competed in the 1985 Pan-Arab (MENA) Games. The inaugural Women Islamic Games were then held in 1993. The annual event was held in Tehran, Iran, and provided opportunities for both able-bodied and disabled women to compete in an array of sporting events (Walseth, 2012). The initial Games were open only to Muslim women, but non-Muslim women from all nationalities were welcomed in 2005. Women could choose to compete in their hijabs, and men were only allowed to participate as spectators, coaches or referees. Ten countries and 407 athletes competed in the first Women Islamic Games, and by 2005 the numbers had increased to 1,316 female athletes representing 44 countries (Islamic Games, 2005). Unfortunately, due to unpaid finances, the Women Islamic Games were discontinued in 2005 (Sehlikoglu, 2010). While the Women Islamic Games appeared to be gaining increasing popularity, they remained highly controversial. Indeed, some Arab states still did not allow women to compete due to the presence of some men in the arena. Whereas many MENA women proclaimed the value of this inclusive female-only event, a common Western view was that such events reinforce gender inequality through the ongoing separation of male and female participants. Such a perspective, however, does not take into consideration the unique cultural and religious value systems inherent in many Arab states that continue to limit girls' and women's sport participation.

Barriers to girls' and young women's sport participation

Islam does seem to suggest that both men and women can participate in sports (Sfeir, 1985; Walseth and Fasting, 2003), yet many girls and women continue to be discouraged from sport and physical activity participation in most MENA countries. Moreover, many women who do pursue such opportunities experience strong social and cultural discrimination and marginalization. It is important to note, however, that there is considerable variation in Muslim women's sport participation across the MENA states. Indeed, the opportunities for female sport participation, and the social and cultural responses to this participation, vary across and within the MENA states and depends on various factors, including the gender relations and regimes within the particular societies in which they live, as well as girls' and women's age and social position, and obligations (religious or cultural). For instance, Muslim women are not allowed to engage in mixed-gender sports, and their sporting participation is often strongly discouraged by family and/or community pressures (Benn *et al.*, 2010). Saudi Arabian climber Raha Moharrak discussed her barriers to participation, explaining that 'convincing [my family] to let [me] climb was as great a challenge as the mountain itself' (Jones, 2013, p. 1). According to one young Kuwaiti male parkour participant, 'a lot of women want to join [participate in sports], but our religion doesn't allow it. In Islamic [tradition], man can't touch the woman, so captains [coaches] can't catch them during training' (personal communication, 2013). A young Egyptian male participant made similar comments:

> We don't train girls due to religious and traditional reasons. In Islam it is not allowed to touch women at certain sensitive body parts, as parkour training requires the trainer to hold and catch the student in specific positions, this makes training impossible. Also . . . for a girl it will be dangerous and more risky than a boy to have an injury. In Egypt people criticize boys who do parkour and always mock them in streets, imagine a girl doing parkour in the streets, she would get negative feedback.
>
> *(Mahmoud, personal communication)*

While some physically and socially dangerous sports such as parkour may remain out of limits for girls and young women in most MENA countries, a few sports are deemed more socially appropriate. According to Erhart (2011, p. 84), those girls whose families do allow them to participate in sports are encouraged to practice 'proper sports for girls' such as ballet, swimming or gymnastics. The dress code of particular sports such as swimming, however, can also hinder participation since it is important to some Muslim women, and particularly their families and the broader society, that women dress modestly and do not reveal their flesh (Yuka, 2002).

Women's sport participation and the wearing of the hijab is highly controversial and has gained global media attention over the past few years, particularly in response to FIFA's decision to ban Muslim women from wearing Islamic headdress. While a common Western perception is that the hijab is an ongoing form of female oppression, several Muslim women have argued that the hijab allows them autonomy, control of their body and protects them from the male gaze (Hong and Abingdon, 2014). Some women choose sports such as fencing and archery, which are not limited by the hijab, while others argue that such headwear does not interfere with their performance or safety. In 2001, an online clothing store, Capsters, was launched, which produces a range of sports hijabs to support various sporting activities (i.e. aerobics, running, football and swimming) (Capsters, 2001). Moreover, some women refuse to accept limits placed upon them by international sports organizations such as Fédération Internationale de Football Association (FIFA). For example, Jordan national football team players, Farah Al-Badarneh and Reema Ramoniah, created a Facebook page 'Let Us Play' in response to FIFA's ban on all political and religious symbols on the pitch, including the hijab. Within two weeks their webpage received almost 70,000 'likes' from around the world, but when their page was unexplainably removed they engaged in a global campaign. In their own words:

For one and a half years we started to contact people around the globe and convinced them on our cause . . . we contacted researchers who . . . started to design [a] special kind [of] safe hijabs . . . Prince Ali Bin Al-Hussein's [of Jordan] support was essential and . . . once we had him on our side the pressure was on. Organizations such as the International Working Group on Women and Sport, UN agencies and women's rights organizations started to support our case and sent their own statements to FIFA.

(cited in Toroi, 2012)

Their efforts helped raise global awareness of the voices and arguments of Muslim female athletes who want to be allowed to wear the hijab on the field. In 2012, following a request from the Asian Football Confederation, the International Football Association Board (IFAB) allowed the newly designed hijabs to be tested out over a two-year period. As a result of the successful trial and the strong campaigning of women such as Al-Badarneh and Ramoniah, FIFA lifted the ban on religious head covers in March 2014. According to FIFA Secretary-General Jérôme Valcke, the hosting of the 2016 women's under-17 World Cup by the Arab kingdom of Jordan also played a part in the authorization being introduced: 'It was a plus for them to have authorization from the IFAB for women to be able to play (wearing head covers). It was a request from these (Muslim) countries that said it would help support women's football there' (cited in FIFA Lifts, 2014, para. 8). As this example suggests, although social and cultural barriers to girls' and women's sport participation are prevalent both within and outside the MENA region, they are certainly not insurmountable, particularly for those politically and technologically savvy female athletes who are passionate about sport and willing to fight for their rights to (re)define the female sporting body.

Sports initiatives for girls and women

While religious and cultural obligations remain as significant barriers to many girls' and women's sport participation, they do not entirely prohibit Muslim women from participating recreationally and competing at local, national and international levels. The participation of Muslim women in the sports arena is gaining strength and effectiveness as policies change and programmes are being implemented that target female participation. Indeed, women in MENA countries are increasingly showing persistence to become athletes, coaches, educators and policymakers. For example, Sarah El-Hawary, daughter of a famous Egyptian soccer referee, organizes football workshops and trains women from her home since women are banned from competing in clubs (Parrish and Nauright, 2014). Sheikha Naima Al-Ahmad Al-Sabah, President of the Kuwait Women's Sports Federation, also uses her position to encourage sports in schools through facilitating workshops, conducting seminars and hosting conferences (Baker, 2012).

Since the early 1970s, women in Oman have increasingly held positions of leadership, such that today, women constitute 12 per cent of senior positions in government, 31 per cent in civil service and 56 per cent as teachers in schools (Hong and Abingdon, 2014). Women's participation in sport in Oman, however, does not reflect these changes. While women are participating as PE teachers in schools, they remain invisible in public spheres as coaches as the majority of sports clubs continue to be led by men with few opportunities for women. As previously discussed, Saudi Arabia recently changed their education policy so sports can be part of the educational curriculum for girls and young women. While the inclusion of sports in schools is an important development for girls, there is also a growing concern about the obesity of Saudi Arabian women such that there is an increased acknowledgement of the need to create facilities with adequate equipment and wellness information (trainers, nutrition) so women can achieve healthier lifestyles.

In Qatar, Aspire Academy incorporates sports science and development to promote healthy lifestyles and participation in sports such as the Multisport Skill Development Program (MSDP). This after school programme is offered from grade one to grade six and includes sports popular among the broader Qatari population including football, basketball, handball, volleyball, swimming, table tennis, golf, archery, fencing and shooting. The goal of the program is to identify talent among the Qatari population, and to train youth so they can compete at the club and international levels. A specialized programme is also offered to Qatari girls aged 6–16, whom are then divided into specific sports based on skill levels. According to programme director Melanie Longdill, the MSDP takes into account the cultural values and dress code, which can allow girls to easily participate in some sports such as archery, golf, fencing, equestrian and shooting. In contrast, while the sports of swimming, football and basketball are encouraged by the sports federations, they lack female participants due to concerns related to dress and difficulties of finding enough interested girls to create teams. Longdill described Qatar's recent and vast investment in sports programs targeting girls and women as stipulated by the country's desire to obtain highly lucrative mega sporting events. For Qatar to win such events, it is required to demonstrate significant investment in girls' and women's sport; however, current programmes have 'very little substance' due to ongoing cultural and social barriers (personal communication, June 2014).

Despite ongoing cultural and social barriers to girls' and women's sporting participation in MENA countries, the visibility of a few key role models is contributing to the slow process of change. For example, Amna Al-Haddad is a successful weight lifter from the United Arab of Emirates (Leigh, 2012), and Raha Moharrak made history by becoming the first female from Saudi Arabia, and the youngest Arab, to summit Mount Everest (Jones, 2013). Moreover, some international sporting organizations are increasingly putting pressure on MENA governments and sporting federations to create change in women's sporting opportunities. For example, Dalma Malhas, the first female equestrian from Saudi Arabia to qualify for the London 2012 Olympics, provided an empowering example for MENA women to participate in sports. While the Saudi government originally prohibited Malhas from competing in the 2012 Olympic Games in London, the International Olympics Committee (IOC) stepped in and pressured Saudi Arabia to allow Malhas to compete. While a select few Muslim women are accomplishing tasks by breaking barriers and setting examples for other women, everyday girls and women continue to face ongoing social and cultural constraints, barriers, and risks in local contexts. Some girls and women are willing to negotiate such risks for the opportunity to play sport, yet many others do not yet feel ready or willing to confront such strong barriers. As Longdill explained, the process of creating significant change in girls' and women's sport participation in the MENA region requires a slow and steady struggle by culturally sensitive female athletes, coaches and administrators.

Sport-for-Development (SDP) in the Middle East MENA

The long history of war, conflict and political unrest in the MENA region has seen radical political and social changes in the Middle East (i.e. Tunisia, Libya, Egypt, Syria, Yemen, Kuwait, Saudi Arabia, Morocco and Bahrain). This has seriously impacted their internal, regional and international relations along with displacement of populations and human right violations. In response to such events, local, national and international governments and organizations are increasingly implementing sporting initiatives for development (i.e. unemployment, health, gender inequality) in the region.

International non–profit organizations are also increasingly using sports to promote healthy behaviour, life skills, cultural understanding, and/or gender equity across the MENA region. A plethora of Sport-for-Development and Peace Building (SDP) organizations such as Peace

Players International, Skateistan, Right to Play, and Binda Capoeira are actively working in war-torn region in efforts to enhance the health, well-being and resilience of populations living in refugee camps and conflict zones, and to facilitate cultural exchanges between groups of different religious and cultural backgrounds (Bellotti, 2012; Sugden, 2006, 2008).

Since 2001, Peace Players International (PPI), a non-profit organization with funding from the U.S. government grants and donations, has used basketball to develop leadership skills and facilitate tolerance in Northern Ireland, South Africa, Cyprus and Israel and the Palestinian West Bank. The Middle East programme was founded in 2005 with the aim to promote peace between Jewish, Israeli Arab and Palestinian youth. The programme objective is to develop leadership skills, individual goals and create safe spaces for youth from communities in conflict to interact in positive ways.

In 2006, Australian skateboarder Oliver Percovich founded Skateistan, an Afghan-based NGO that provides skateboarding tuition, art and language learning to displaced youth in Afghanistan (Thorpe, 2014b). Using the three boards he had brought to Afghanistan, Percovich established a small school that provided free skate lessons to street children (Ramp it Up, 2010). In 2009, with just over $700,000USD in international donations and space provided by Afghanistan's Olympic Committee, Skateistan built a 19,000 square foot indoor skateboard park – Kabul's largest indoor sports facility. Since the opening of this skatepark, Skateistan has registered more than 1,100 Afghan children and youth (37 per cent female). In 2013, Skateistan's Kabul facility offered free weekly skateboarding and educational programming to 400 Afghan girls and boys aged 5–17, as well as a Back-to-School programme for street working and refugee youth. In December 2013 a second Skateistan facility in Afghanistan opened in Mazar-e-Sharif (northern Afghanistan), which can accommodate up to 1,000 children and youth each week for skateboarding, sports and educational activities. Skateistan has continued to expand, now offering similar skateboarding and educational programmes for children in Cambodia and Pakistan, and in 2014 is commencing work in South Africa. Skateistan won the 2009 Peace and Sport Non-Governmental Organization Award, for its efforts in educating urban and internally displaced children in Kabul (Afghanistan), as well as the 2012 Innovation Through Sport award at the Beyond Sport Forum. In 2013, Skateistan was also selected as a Top 100 NGO by *The Global Journal*, making it the highest ranking sport-related NGO.

Another example of an international non-profit organization using sport to promote peace and development is Binda Capoeira. Founded in 2007 in Syria, Binda Capoeira is funded through international grants and donations. The mission of the organization is to use capoeira (Brazilian martial arts) to provide psychological and social support youth living in areas of conflict and poverty. In 2011, they launched a program in Palestine to work with youth who are traumatized by daily violence and poverty in the settlements and refugee camps. Another example is the Real Madrid Foundation, which is supported by the legendary Spanish football league along with national and international corporations and donations from Real Madrid fans. Between 2011 and 2013, the Real Madrid Foundation has developed several sports initiatives throughout the Middle East with the aim to utilize sports to promote social and cultural awareness and assist at-risk youth populations. The programme employs both Spanish and local coaches to develop youth skills, and have established training camps with the aim of developing future professional football players. Such initiatives are also aimed at stimulating the local football industry, and in so doing, promoting development in the local community through the use of sports.

While such initiatives appear to promote positive development in the MENA region, a growing number of critical sport scholars have questioned the assumptions underpinning the SDP movement, with some arguing that some of these well-intended initiatives 'may not be serving the ends towards which they are directed, or are even having counterproductive results'

(Hartmann and Kwauk 2011, p. 286; also see Coakley 2011; Coalter 2007; Darnell 2010, 2012; Giulianotti 2011; Hartmann and Kwauk 2011). Coakley (2011, p. 314), for example, is concerned that too many sport for youth development programmes (many of which are in the MENA region) use sport as a 'hook on which to hang socializing experiences that promote forms of personal development valued by the sponsoring organization and its staff'. He argues that the current neoliberal approach to youth development 'uncritically supports[s] the evangelistic promise that sport produces positive development among young people' (Coakley, 2011, p. 306), before calling for more critical research and theory that 'identifies the processes through which sport participation is or is not linked with subsequent forms of civic engagement and efforts to produce progressive change transcending the lives of particular individuals' (p. 306).

Conclusion

Many social, cultural and religious barriers and constraints continue to limit the opportunities available to some youth in the MENA region. However, this chapter has also challenged assumptions (particularly by western audiences) that youth in the MENA region are victims, ideologues or fundamentalists (Barber, 2001; Bayat, 2010; Gregory, 2004; McEvoy-Levy, 2001; Spaaij, 2011). We have offered examples of MENA youth practicing forms of agency that we hope will contribute to resisting the orientalist tendencies among westerners to presume knowledge of youth in the Middle East in ways that fit with, or confirm, western goals, narratives and ideologies, but often overlook the actual experiences and voices of everyday young people. Further research into the lived, everyday sporting and physical activity experiences of children and youth in the MENA region is greatly needed and such work must create space for voices of youth themselves.

References

Ahmed Hamdi (26 December 2012). Against Gravity. *Al-Ahram*. Retrieved from http://weekly.ahram.org.eg/News/698/-/-.aspx

Al-Maskari, S. (2012). Sport in Oman. In J. Nauright and C. Parrish (ed). *Sports around the World: History, Culture, and Practice* (pp. 306–309) Santa Barbara, CA: ABC-CLIO.

Al-Sinani, Y. (2012). The establishment and development of the initial physical education teacher's training programme for women in Oman. *The International Journal of the History of Sport, 29(15)*, 2184–2199.

Amara, M. (2012a). *Sport, Politics and Society in the Arab World*. London: Palgrave Macmillan.

Amara, M. (2012b) Sports history, culture, and practice in the Middle East and North Africa, in J. Nauright and C. Parrish (ed). *Sports around the World: History, Culture, and Practice* (pp. 269–272) Santa Barbara, CA: ABC-CLIO.

Baker, R. (2012). Gender and sport, Middle East and North Africa, in J. Nauright and C. Parrish (ed). d*Sports around the World: History, Culture, and Practice* (pp. 290–291) Santa Barbara, CA: ABC-CLIO.

Barber, B. (2001). Political violence, social integration, and youth functioning: Palestinian youth from the Intifada. *Journal of Community Psychology, 29(3)*, 259–280.

Bayat, A. (2010). *Life as Politics: How Ordinary People Change the Middle East*. Stanford: Stanford University Press.

Behbehani, K. and Beales, P. F. (2013). New perspectives on health issues, research and innovation, in T. Andersson and A. Djeflat (eds) *The Real Issues of the Middle East and the Arab Spring* (pp. 259–273), New York: Springer.

Bellotti, J. A. (2012). Peace and sport: Challenging limitations across the sport for development and peace sector. Unpublished Masters thesis. Indiana University, Indiana.

Benn, T., Pfister, G. and Jawad, H. (eds). (2010). *Muslim Women and Sport*. Abingdon, Oxfordshire: Routledge.

Billingham, G. (6 June 2014). 98: The most politically charged game in World Cup history. *FourFourTwo*. Retrieved from www.fourfourtwo.com/features/98-most-politically-charged-game-world-cup-history

Booth, D. and Thorpe, H. (2007). The meaning of extreme, in D. Booth and H. Thorpe (eds), *The Berkshire Encyclopedia of Extreme Sports* (pp. 181–197). Great Barrington, MA: Berkshire Publishing.

Bromber, K., Krawietz, B. and Maguire, J. (eds) (2013). *Sport Across Asia: Politics, Cultures, and Identities: Politics, Cultures, and Identities.* London: Routledge.

Capsters (2001). Retrieved from www.capsters.com/background.jsp

Chaaban, J. (2008).The costs of youth exclusion in the Middle East. *Middle East Youth Initiative, working paper number 7.* Retrieved from www.shababinclusion.org/content/document/detail/983/

Coakley, J. (2011). Youth sports: What counts as 'positive development'? *Journal of Sport and Social Issues, 35*(3), 306–324.

Coalter, F. (2007). *A Wider Social Role for Sport: Who's Keeping the Score?* London: Routledge.

Collins, A. (2011, May 20). *Khalid Al Siyabi – Climbing for Oman, One Year On.* Retrieved from http://knowledgeoman.com/en/ko-interviews/khalid-al-siyabi-one-year-on-climbing-for-oman.html

Darnell, S. (2010). Power, politics and 'sport for development and peace': Investigating the utility of sport for international development. *Sociology of Sport Journal, 27(1)*, 54–75.

Darnell, S. (2012). *Sport for Development and Peace: A Critical Sociology.* New York: Bloomsbury Academic.

Dhillon, N. and Yousef, T. (eds) (2009). *Generation in Waiting: The Unfulfilled Promise of Young People in the Middle East.* Washington, DC: Brookings Institution Press.

Erhart, I. (2011). Ladies of Besiktas: A dismantling of male hegemony at Inönü Stadium. *International Review for the Sociology of Sport, 48(1)*, 83–98.

Facebook in the Arab region (2012) Arab social media report. Retrieved from www.arabsocialmediareport.com/Facebook/LineChart.aspx?and;PriMenuID=18andCatID=24andmnu=Cat

FIFA lifts ban on head covers. (1 March 2014). *Aljazeera.* Retrieved from www.aljazeera.com/sport/football/2014/03/fifa-allows-hijab-turban-players-20143113053667394.html

Fizel, J. (2006). *Handbook of Sports Economics Research.* New York: M.E. Sharp.

Fozooni, B. (2012). Iran and sport since the Islamic "revolution", in J. Nauright and C. Parrish (eds) *Sports around the World: History, Culture, and Practice* (pp. 293–295) Santa Barbara, CA: ABC-CLIO.

Giulianotti, R. (2004). Celtic, cultural identities and the globalization of football. *Scottish Affairs, 48*, 1–23.

Giulianotti, R. (2011). The sport, development and peace sector: A model of four social policy domains. *Journal of Social Policy, 40(4)*, 757–776.

Giulianotti, R. and Robertson, R. (2004). The globalization of football: A study in the glocalization of the 'serious life'. *British Journal of Sociology, 55(4)*, 545–568.

Gregory, D. (2004). *The Colonial Present.* Malden, MA: Blackwell.

Hartmann, D. and Kwauk, C. (2011). Sport and development: An overview, critique and reconstruction. *Journal of Sport and Social Issues, 35(3)*, 284–305.

Henseler, C. (ed.) (2012). *Generation X Goes Global: Mapping a Youth Culture in Motion.* New York: Routledge.

Hong, F. and Abingdon, O. (2014). *Sport in the Middle East: Power, Politics, Ideology and Religion.* New York: Routledge.

Islamic Games (2005). *The Women's Islamic Games*, Muslim Women's Sport Foundation. Retrieved from www.mwsf.org.uk/islamic_games.html

Jones, B. (20 May 2013). First Saudi woman summits Mount Everest. *CNN.* Retrieved from http://edition.cnn.com/2013/05/19/world/meast/first-saudi-woman-climbs-everest

Kusz, K. (2007). Whiteness and extreme sports, in D. Booth and H. Thorpe (eds) *Berkshire Encyclopedia of Extreme Sport* (pp. 357–361), Great Barrington, MA: Berkshire Publishing.

Leigh, K. (23 October 2012). Amid glares, female weight lifters compete. *New York Times.* Retrieved from www.nytimes.com/2012/10/24/sports/amid-glares-female-muslim-weightlifters-compete.html?_r=0.

Levermore, R. (2011). Sport in international development: facilitating improved standard of living, in B. Houlihan and M. Green (eds), *Routledge Handbook of Sports Development* (pp. 285–307), London: Routledge.

Londoño, E. and Al-Izzi, S. (10 June 2008). In Iraq, muscle is a growth industry. *Washington Post.* Retrieved from www.washingtonpost.com/wp-dyn/content/article/2008/06/09/AR2008060902624.html?sid=ST2008060902684

Madichie, N. O. (2009). Professional sports: A new "services" consumption mantra in the United Arab Emirates (UAE). *Marketing Review, 9(4)*, 301–318.

McEvoy-Levy, S. (2001). Youth as social and political agents: Issues in post-settlement peace building. Joan B. Kroc Institute for International Peace Studies, University of Notre Dame. Retrieved from www.unoy.org/downloads/resources/YandP/2001_McEnvoy-Levy.pdf

Nassif, N. (2012). Basketball, Lebanon, in J. Nauright and C. Parrish (eds) *Sports around the World: History, Culture, and Practice* (pp. 281–282). Santa Barbara, CA: ABC-CLIO.

Raspaud, M. (2012). Association Football, Egypt, in J. Nauright and C. Parrish (ed) *Sports around the World: History, Culture, and Practice* (pp. 273–274). Santa Barbara, CA: ABC-CLIO.

Parrish, C. and Nauright, J. (2014). *Soccer Around the World: A Cultural Guide to the World's Favorite Sport*. Santa Barbara, CA: ABC-CLIO.

Pfister, G. (2010). Outsiders: Muslim women and Olympic Games—barriers and opportunities. *The International Journal of the History of Sport* 27(16–18), 2925–2957.

Pielke Jr, R. (2013). How can FIFA be held accountable? *Sport Management Review, 16(3)*, 255–267.

Robertson, R. (1992). *Globalization: Social Theory and Global Culture*. London: SAGE.

Robertson, R. (1995). Glocalization: Time-space and homogeneity–heterogeneity, in M. Featherstone, S. Lash and R. Robertson (eds) *Global Modernities* (pp. 25–44). London: Sage.

Robertson, R. and White, K.E. (eds) (2003). *Globalization: Critical Concepts in Sociology*. London: Routledge.

Roudi-Fahimi, F. and El-Feki, S. (2011). Youth sexuality and reproductive health in the Middle East and North Africa, *Population Reference Bureau*. Retrieved from www.prb.org/pdf11/facts-of-life-youth-in-middle-east.pdf

Samie, S.F. & Sehlikoglu, S. (2015). Strange, incompetent and out-of-place: Media, Muslim sportswomen and London 2012. *Feminist Media Studies*, 15(3), 363–381.

Saudi Arabia: Accelerate reforms for girls' sport in state schools. (11 April 2014). *Human Rights Watch*. Retrieved from www.hrw.org/news/2014/04/11/saudi-arabia-accelerate-reforms-girls-sport-state-schools

Saudi Arabia: Let all girls play. (8 May 2013). *Human Rights Watch*. Retrieved from www.hrw.org/news/2013/05/07/saudi-arabia-let-all-girls-play-sports.

Sehlikoglu, S. (13 August 2010). The Islamic Federation of Women Sport (IFWS) is shut down due to budget cuts. [Blog] *Muslim Women in Sports*. Retrieved from http://muslimwomeninsports.blogspot.com/2010/08/islamic-federation-of-women-sport-ifws.html

Sfeir, L. (1985). The status of Muslim women in sport: conflict between cultural tradition and modernization. *International Review for the Sociology of Sport, 20(4)*, 283–306.

SMG YouGov (2011). *Popularity and Participation of Sports in the Middle East and North Africa*. Retrieved from www.revolutionsports.co.uk/news/wp-content/uploads/2011/11/SMGI-Middle-East-North-Africa-Report-180911final.pdf

Sowers, J. and Toensing, C. (2012). *The Journey to Tahrir: Revolution, Protest, and Social Change in Egypt*. London: Verso Books.

Spaaij, R. (2011). *Sport and Social Mobility*. London: Routledge.

Sugden, J. (2006). Teaching and playing sport for conflict resolution and co-existence in Israel. *International Review for the Sociology of Sport, 41(2)*, 221–240.

Sugden, J. (2008). Anyone for football for peace? The challenges of using sport in the service of co-existence in Israel. *Soccer and Society, 9(3)*, 405–415.

Thorpe, H. (2011). Have board, will travel: Global physical youth cultures and transnational mobility, in J. Maguire and M. Falcous (eds), *Sport and Migration: Borders, Boundaries and Crossings* (pp. 112–126). London: Routledge.

Thorpe, H. (2014a). *Transnational Mobilities in Action Sport Cultures*. Houndmills: Palgrave Macmillan.

Thorpe, H. (2014b). Action sports for youth development: Critical insights for the SDP community, *The International Journal of Sport Policy and Politics*, 1–26. Champaign: 10.1080/19406940.2014.925952.

Thorpe, H. and Ahmad, N. (2013). Youth, action sports and political agency in the Middle East: Lessons from a grassroots parkour group in Gaza, *International Review for the Sociology of Sport*, Champaign: 1012690213490521.

Toroi, N. (2012). Removing FIFA's hijab ban. Retrieved from www.iwg-gti.org/catalyst/february-2013/removing-fifa-s-hijab-ban/

Wagner, E.A. (1989). *Sport in Asia and Africa: A Comparative Handbook*. New York: Greenwood Press.

Walseth, K. and Fasting, K. (2003). Islam's view on physical activity and sport. Egyptian women interpreting Islam, *International Review for the Sociology of Sport, 38(1)*, 45–60.

Walseth, K. (2012). Women Islamic Games (Iran), in J. Nauright and C. Parrish (ed.) *Sports around the World: History, Culture, and Practice* (pp. 312–313) Santa Barbara, CA: ABC-CLIO.

Wheaton, B. (2004a). *Understanding Lifestyle Sports: Consumption, Identity and Difference*. Oxford: Routledge.

Wheaton, B. (2004b). Selling out? The globalization and commercialization of lifestyle Sports, in L. Allison (ed.) *The Global Politics of Sport: The Role of Global Institutions in Sport* (pp. 140–185). London: Routledge.

Wheaton, B. (2010). Introducing the consumption and representation of lifestyle sports, *Sport in Society, 13(7/8)*, 1057–1081.

Yuka, N. (2002). Beyond the hijab: Female muslims and physical activity, *Women in Sport and Physical Activity Journal, 17(1)*, 234–255.

13

YOUTH SPORT IN CHINA

Chen XueDong and Shushu Chen

Introduction

Mapping the territory of youth sport in China is extremely difficult, not only because of the relatively large numbers of young people in the Chinese population, but also because of the marginal position of sport in the school curriculum and the tendency for state sport policy to focus on elite and mass sport rather than youth sport. According to the Ministry of Education (MoE, 2014a), in 2014, there were more than 162 million school-aged children and young people (7–22-years old) in 316,166 schools based in 37 provinces and municipalities, with over 24 million graduate and undergraduate students attending 2,491 higher education institutions. Overall, school-aged young people constitute approximately 13.6 per cent of the total population.

While the Chinese government still adopts a very centralised approach to the organisation and delivery of youth sport, the General Administration of Sport (GAS) and MoE have joint responsibility for providing the majority of school facilities and a range of development programmes and services, and are the only legitimate and effective political bodies with an interest in sport for young people. The GAS has particular responsibility for organising national youth sport events and administering sports schools for young talented athletes, while the MoE develops policies related to school sport and physical education (PE). It is important to note, however, that nationally the GAS and MoE are primarily concerned with improving PE rather than youth sports per se (Liang *et al.*, 2012). Although some community-based sports clubs and sport centres exist for young people (General Administration of Sport of China, 2004), at the local level the organisation of youth sport is supported largely by the sporting infrastructure provided by schools (Ren, 1996). In this regard, youth sport in present-day China is linked, directly and indirectly, with the provision of sport and PE in schools on which the discussion of this chapter is based. In particular, the chapter:

1   discusses the value of sport and Chinese family culture;
2   provides a general description of youth sport development in China, particularly in relation to the history of government policies for school sport and PE;
3   reviews the available empirical evidence on the levels and patterns of young people's participation in sport and physical activity, and health more broadly and

4   concludes by reviewing some of the salient issues associated with youth sport in China and reflects upon its future.

National sport policy in China

In national sport policy, youth sport and school sport have typically been considered less important than elite sport and mass participation in sport (Lin, 1989). One indicator of the political prioritisation of elite and mass sport is the funding allocated to these two policy areas. The government publishes figures for funds and expenses generated by the government for sport each year, and in 2013, RMB 6.12 billion (1 billion USD) was allocated to elite sport (excluding funding for sports facilities) and RMB 2.76 billion (0.44 billion USD) to mass participation (China Ministry of Finance, 2013). In contrast, it is very difficult to determine the amount of funding and resources allocated to school sport and PE for young people. In 2014, the Chinese government reported a state financial expenditure of RMB 2448.8 billion on education (391.8 billion USD), which accounts for 4.3 per cent of GDP (China Ministry of Education, 2014b), but the report did not specify the amount spent on school sport and PE since the school budget is devolved to local level where schools can use their educational funding as they wish, but not necessarily for sport (Qui and Chen, 2004; Sun, 2006). The survey findings of one study, however, revealed that the average funding allocated to PE by 500 schools in ten provinces constituted just 2 per cent of the total funding received by schools (Yao, 2004).

The lack of political priority and funding allocated to school sport and PE is particularly notable for, as Dong (2008) has noted, since 1985 there has been a continuous decline in the health and fitness status of children and young people in China. Increased concern about the health of young people did eventually prompt the government (in 2000) to undertake a major review of education including the state of PE and sport in the curriculum. This resulted in the publication of the experimental PE guidelines and standards by the MoE (China Ministry of Education, 2001), which marked a watershed in the policy status of youth sport in China and placed increased emphasis on school sports development. The new educational standards require that elementary (ages 7–12) and middle schools (ages 13–15) offer at least three sessions of PE each week and that high schools (ages 16–18) provide at least two sessions of PE weekly. However, after more than ten years of implementation of the PE guidelines, findings from the 2014 National Physical Fitness and Health Investigation (General Administration of Sport of China, 2014) revealed that only three in ten (28.9 per cent) of children and young people from elementary and middle schools engaged in three sessions of PE per week, and just over one-half (51.6 per cent) had participated in two sessions.

In addition to state provision of PE and school sport, it is worth noting that the Youth Sports School – a specialised network of schools for training and fostering talented athletes from a very young age (normally 6–9-years old) – is also an important youth-focused feature of the Chinese sport system. Currently led by the GAS, the Youth Sports School system was established by the government in 1956 as part of its desire for international sporting success that would enhance China's international reputation and inspire national self-confidence (Wu, 1999). The most recent data indicate that, in 2013, there were over 41,128 young athletes training in more than 1,797 sports schools around China (National Bureau of Statisticas of China, 2014). It is clear, however, that preparation for sporting success dominates all other concerns, including the education of young people. Indeed, in 2010 it was reported that young athletes typically received one half day of normal academic education with the rest of the day spent engaging in training on a daily basis (General Administration of Sport of China, 2010; General Administration of Sport of China and Ministry of Education, 2011).

The value of sport and the Chinese family

As Jones (1999, p. 17) has noted, 'to understand the contextual position of sport in China – its "Chineseness" – demands a much fuller awareness of Chinese culture, conditions and values'. More particularly, to adequately understand youth sport in China, it is important to have some appreciation of the social construction of the Chinese family and especially the traditional values and ideology that underpin social life in China. Traditionally, the Chinese family has essentially been patriarchal in structure (Chow and Zhao, 1996) in which parents tend to have considerable power and influence over their offspring (Queen *et al.*, 1985) so that they determine, to a large extent, what their children should and should not do. The traditional ideology adopted by Chinese families is that the main objective for children is to get good academic results as a means of achieving social status – a concern that has become increasingly significant following the introduction of China's one-child policy. Accordingly, many parents typically regard participation in PE and sport more broadly as a component of play and leisure and not an intrinsic part of the educational process (Chan and Lo, 1992).

The Chinese family has also persisted in valuing '万般皆下品，唯有读书高'; that is to say 'All pursuits are of low values; only studying the books is high' (He, 2000). This has been exacerbated by the reform of the National College Entrance Exam, known as *Gaokao*, in which academic success and socio-economic upward mobility have been valued as extremely important for young people (Yu and Suen, 2005). Students would be admitted into different universities based solely on their *Gaokao* test scores. The subjects in which young people are tested include the three compulsory areas of Chinese language, mathematics and foreign languages, together with optional subjects (biology, chemistry, history, and physics and civil/politics science). One of the major criticisms of this high-stakes testing system is the limit it places on young people's experiences of the curriculum and the tendency for students to de-prioritise or ignore other subjects (including PE and sport) in which they are not tested (Yu and Suen, 2005). For example, sport and PE are commonly viewed as a 'distraction' from academic tests and has making little positive contribution to academic achievements (Ha *et al.*, 2010; Yates and Lee, 1996). According to Ji's (2013) study of twenty-five middle schools in HeBei, only 44 per cent of required PE sessions were delivered to final year students, one-third (32 per cent) delivered one-half of the required sessions, and in one-quarter (24 per cent) of schools PE lessons were cancelled completely. Thus, as Zhang (2015, p. 166) observed in relation to north China, 'While the academic results become the only critical for entrance to university, it is not surprising that other subjects, e.g. PE and culture, take second place to exams'.

A general description of youth sports in China

Although research on adults' participation in sport and physical activity has a relatively long history, comparatively little is known about young people's involvement (particularly in terms of the legitimacy of PE within the school system) (Wang, 2005). PE was officially included within the elementary schooling system in 1922 (Li and Yang, 2002), and was later made a compulsory subject in middle schools in 1931. Young people's participation in school-based sport most usually occurs in several contexts, including PE sessions, after-school sports activities, representing sports teams, sports day events, and morning and between-class physical exercise. Historically, sport participation in these domains has been justified as important because it plays a crucial role in 'cultivating students interests, attitude, skills, habit, knowledge and ability in sport, to assist students' physical and psychological development, to strengthen students' health and fitness condition, in order to make a contribution to building socialisation and defend the country' (China Ministry of Education, 2011, p. 2). In addition, as Houlihan (2011) argued, highly politicised school PE has been commonly considered as a vehicle for implanting nationalist and socialist values to the young, including in China. Since the establishment of the People's Republic of China in 1949, sport and PE became an important tool for building nationalist sentiment (Fan and Lu, 2011).

In the mid-1950s, sport and PE activities were officially conducted in cities, villages, schools and government institutions (Fan and Lu, 2011). At the same time, the initial development of the PE system was based on the Soviet Union's Labour Defence System and implemented in middle schools, vocational schools and universities, with a particular focus on promoting participation in track and field, gymnastics, weight lifting and other physical exercises (Fan and Lu, 2011). The level of students' performance was assessed and honoured with medals or certifications (Wu, 1999). After the termination of the Great Leap Forward – an economic and social campaign led by the Communist Party of China from 1958 to 1961, which caused three years of widespread famine, resulting more than 15 million famine victims (Ashton *et al.*, 1984) – the number of hours allocated to school PE were reduced. In some parts of China, physical classes were even cancelled as a result of the great famine and economic crisis (Fu, 2007). Together with mass sport, school PE recovered slowly after 1963. Replacing the Labour Defence System, the Training Standard for the Youth was introduced, together with a regulations including the Regulations on Cultural Revolution in Elementary and Middle Schools and the Regulations on Cultural Revolution in Colleges and Universities, both of which essentially required students to participate in compulsory military training in the curriculum for national defence purposes. School and university PE was also renamed as Military Physical Education (Fan and Lu, 2011) as particular focus was placed on exercising formation drills, grenade throwing, shooting, military hiking, camping and field training. In order to provide appropriate PE sessions, teachers were trained with basic military knowledge and skills, and veterans and soldiers were brought into school as PE instructors (Fu, 2007). However, from 1970 to 1976 (i.e. mainly during the Cultural Revolution period), the focus of school sport shifted from military exercise to encourage students to participate in sport for health benefits. Published guidance, including the Fifth Broadcast Gymnastics for Children, issued by the State Physical Cultural and Sports Commission (later known as the GAS) and the State Council, required students to take part in gymnastics for 15 minutes every school day in elementary schools to benefit students' health (State Council, 1973).

The benefits of youth sport participation, particularly in relation to health and fitness, were promoted strongly by the Sport Ministry (National Sport Commission, 1978). An announcement made jointly by the State Physical Culture and Sports Commission and the Ministry of Education in 1979 stated that school PE policy should be focused on fitness and health promotion (Hao, 2006). Since the mid-1970s, the policy focus on health and fitness in school PE has continued. For example, the 'Guidance for Physical Education in Higher Education', which was introduced in 1992, made explicit that a central purpose of delivering PE in schools was to cultivate students' awareness of sport, enhance their lifelong participation in sport and physical activity, and turn them into healthy citizens of socialist China (China Ministry of Education, 1992).

As we noted earlier, in 2000 the Chinese government undertook a major review of the curriculum that strengthened the position of PE in the curriculum. As a result, the requirement that PE is formally delivered in schools has been incorporated into official government policy (The Fundamental Law of Education, 2001), together with two syllabuses for school PE issued by the Ministry of Education (i.e. the Nine-year Compulsory Education Syllabus for PE and Health Education in Elementary Schools and Nine-year Compulsory Education Syllabus for PE and Health Education in Middle Schools), both of which are considered as two milestone documents for school sport in China (Ji, Wang, and Tang, 2011). According to the syllabuses, PE is mandatory for all students from elementary school to the first two years of university and is offered as an elective subject thereafter. The daily combined time for PE classes (including jumping, throwing, dance, ball games (football, volleyball and basketball), track and field, and gymnastics) and extra-curricular physical activity should be no less than one hour (China Ministry of Education, 2001; Ma, 2007).

In 2002, the positive development of children's health was identified as the fundamental goal of school-based PE by the revised syllabus Physical and Health Education Course Standards for Elementary and Middle Schools (China Ministry of Education, 2002a). The MoE (2011, p. 6) then published the second edition of physical education and health education guidelines and standards in 2011, which incorporated the following four standards:

- Standard 1. Physical activity participation – students participate in physical activities and are able to enjoy exercise and experience success.
- Standard 2. Mastery of knowledge, skills and safe exercise methods – students learn knowledge about exercise, perform physical skills, understand safe exercise principles and learn self-defence.
- Standard 3. Developing physical health – students learn and master knowledge and method of maintaining health, develop and sustain healthy posture and bodily shape, develop and maintain physical fitness, and improve adaptive ability in nature environments.
- Standard 4. Developing mental health – students learn to develop mental strength, control emotions, develop ability to collaborate and cooperate, and follow ethical norms of physical activity.

According to Wang *et al.* (2008, p. 61; emphases in the original), these standards emphasise a *health-first* approach to the delivery of PE, rather than a *sport-central* one. The promotion of children's health and fitness was emphasised as being not only to the development of the PE curriculum (Chinese Communist Party Central Committee and State Council of the Chinese Government, 2007), but also to the fitness development campaigns for youth (which is evidenced by the Sunshine Sport Movement programme, which will be discussed later), which emerged partly out of the deterioration of physical fitness in children and adolescents and increasing prevalence of overweight and obesity between 2000 and 2005 (General Administration of Sport of China, 2011). The alleged commitment to addressing the ill-health of children and youth was further reinforced by the 2011 guidelines and standards in which time allocated to PE was expected to constitute 10–11 per cent of the total teaching time in elementary and middle schools (between 135 and 180 minutes). High schools are also now expected to should offer at least two sessions of PE each week basis, while the education syllabus for PE and Health Education in Higher Education Institutions (China Ministry of Education, 2002b) states that it is compulsory for year 1 and 2 undergraduate students to complete a total of 144 sessions of PE within two years and for year 3 and final-year students PE is a selective module.

Youth sport and physical activity participation

Few data sources exist, with varying degrees of accessibility, to enable an accurate assessment of sport participation among young people in China. The latest available data on youth sport participation has been collected as part of a national study of Chinese citizens' *Ti Zhi* (fitness), namely the National Physical Fitness and Health Investigation (NPFHI). This national fitness database was established by the MoE, the GAS and Minister of Health in 1980, under the regulation of the Sport Law and National Health Regulations to monitor health-related physical fitness status for Chinese citizens (aged 3–69-years old) every five years. Overall, the 2010 NPFHI revealed that just over four-fifths (81.7 per cent) of children and young people (aged 6–19) taking part thirty minutes or more of moderate intensity sport and physical activity participation at least three times each week in school (General Administration of Sport of China, 2014). However, only three in ten (28.6 per cent) of children and young people have participated in moderate intensity sport and physical activity outside of school for more than thirty minutes three times a week. It was also reported that, among those who engaged in some physical exercises outside of schools, 78 per cent had played sports by themselves informally, without receiving any instructions from specialists.

A second data source on youth (6–18-year-olds) participation in physical activity is provided by the longitudinal China Health and Nutrition Survey. Data from the survey conducted between 1997 and 2011 indicated that more school children engaged in some moderate intensity physical exercises during school (93 per cent) in 2011 compared to 72 per cent in 1997 (Tudor-Locke *et al.*, 2003). Of those who participated in 2011, young people engaged in sport and physical exercise at school for an average of forty minutes more than four times per week. The most widely played sports were track and field and swimming (both 54 per cent), gymnastics and dance (48 per cent), ball games (football, basketball and tennis: 36 per cent), other activities such as Ping Pong (table tennis) and Tai Chi (28 per cent), badminton and volleyball (21 per cent), and martial arts (1.6 per cent). Another survey conducted by Song *et al.* (2012), which investigated sport participation in thirty provinces by 166,812 elementary and middle school students (aged 9 and above), indicated that just under one-quarter (22.7 per cent) of students engaged in sport and physical activity (including PE sessions and extra curricular PE) for more than one hour per day. The proportion of students engaging in sport and PA for more than one hour per day decreased with age from 32.8 per cent among 9–13-year-olds to 12.5 per cent for those aged 16–19. The opposite relationship was observed for those who participated for less than thirty minutes per day, with 18.6 per cent of those aged 9–13-year-olds and 46 per cent of 16–19-year-olds spending this amount of time participating (Song *et al.*, 2012). The increased tendency for young people to spend less time participating in sport and physical activity is not surprising given the increased pressure on them to engage in their academic studies as they get older and the *Gaokao* gets closer (Song *et al.*, 2012).

Overall, the findings of studies of the major trends in youth sport participation in China reveal that:

- PE continues to be the main form of sport participation for children and young people in China. Although there is some evidence of young people participating in sport outside of PE sessions, it appears to be shorter, less intensity and not well-organised.
- The development of PE and sport participation for young people is still constrained by traditional Chinese culture and values (especially for high school students), while sport continues to have a marginal role in Chinese family life.
- Although there has been a gradual increase in overall levels of sport and physical activity participation in recent decades, the proportion of young people who participate regularly (i.e. for more than three times per week), and who do so at least at moderate intensity level, are still low.
- Very little is known from existing studies about the types, levels, patterns and forms of typology of sport participation in China and how these are structured by social divisions. A lack of rigorous methodological research designs are adopted in published studies and there exists widespread variation in definitions of what constitutes physical activity, sport

and physical exercise. Some studies also fail to separate school-based participation from out of school participation, which further compounds the difficulties of comparing youth sport participation between studies.

In relation to the final point, it is clear that, as Shen and Fan (2012) point out, while most academic study of Chinese sport has focused on elite sport, mass sport and major sports event, there has been very few that examined PE in particular, and youth sport in general, in China. Within the rather limited number of published research articles in relation to PE, the quality of the evidence is sometimes problematic: according to a review of scholarly and research work in PE between 2000 and 2010 in top-tier Chinese kinesiology/sport and exercise/PE journals, Ding *et al.* (2014) note that there were only 169 (23 per cent) articles that reported original empirical data, and 562 articles (77 per cent) were dominated by non-empirical, theoretical discussions on policy, teaching, and content and instruction in PE curricular. Student learning, measurement and evaluation, and studies on after-school sport participation were rarely included.

The Sunshine Sports Campaign

Unlike a plethora of sports programmes in some western countries such as England (e.g. Phillpots, 2011), few sport programmes exist for young people in China. However, the Sunshine Sports Campaign (SSC) can be characterised as the best attempt by the government to provide a nationwide programme to increase youth sport participation and the physical fitness of young people. Following the announcement of the Decision on Launching a National-wide Sports Campaign for Hundreds of Millions by the MoE, GAS, and the Communist Youth League of China (China Ministry of Education, The General Administration of Sport, and The Communist Youth League of China, 2006), the SSC campaign was launched to improve physical fitness for youth and was implemented regionally through local schools and universities. In 2007, further details of the campaign were released by the State of Council, including a target of having at least 85 per cent of students engaging in physical exercise for at least one hour every day, and having 85 per cent passing the National Fitness and Health test (Chinese Communist Party Central Committee and State Council of the Chinese Government, 2007).

A case study of Civil Aviation University of China (CAUC) provides a useful means of understanding the impact of the SSC initiative. Located in Tianjin, the CAUC is directly under the jurisdiction of Civil Aviation Administration of China and has over 23,000 students. To facilitate the delivery of the SSC national initiative, CAUC has invested significantly in sport provision since 2008, including the introduction in 2010 of a RMB10 million (1.6 million USD) special fund for recruiting more teaching and research sport staff, and improving sport facilities and equipment, as well as adopting a revised school sport and PE integrated framework to provide good quality PE sessions and extra curricular activities. In order to monitor the progress being made with the SSC, physical and health well-being status has also been traced annually for year 1 and year 2 students. Since the launch of the SSC in CAUC in 2008, the proportion of students meeting the health and fitness standard has increased from 21.2 per cent to 98 per cent and 99 per cent in 2009 and 2011, respectively. In addition, in 2009 only 5.0 per cent of males and 1.5 per cent of females from a random sample of 4,601 students in the CAUC were classified as overweight, while 4.1 per cent of males and 1.3 of females were classified as obese. For both males and females, there was also an 11 per cent increase in the proportions defined as having a healthy weight between 2006 (46 per cent males; 39 per cent females) and 2009 (57 per cent males; 50 per cent females) (Chen, 2012; Zhao and Xue, 2011).

In 2010, surveys were completed by a sample of 500 year–one students to investigate how they used their leisure time. The findings revealed that the most popular uses of leisure were internet surfing (24.6 per cent), study (17.4 per cent), sleep (12.4 per cent), sport and physical exercise (11.8 per cent), general entertainment activities (8.8 per cent), social activity (7.2 per cent), part-time job (6.2 per cent), shopping (4.6 per cent) and others. In particular, while sport and physical exercise was reported as the second most popular leisure activity for male students (16.5 per cent), it was the least popular leisure activity for female students just 4.6 per cent of whom had spent their leisure time doing sport and physical exercise. As later identified from the interviews, there were several factors that prevented girls from sport and physical exercise participation (e.g. concern about sweating, getting dirty, and generally being reluctant to play sport).

Although there has been some improvement in the sport participation and health and fitness of students in CAUC, it is difficult to draw firm conclusions about whether these improvements can be directly attributable to the national SSC. For example, it is clear that some degree of displacement of sport participation has occurred as the CAUC simply added 'Sunshine Sports' into the names of some existing sports programmes, and reported the results of the 'new' sports programmes to central authorities, which distorts and questions the validity of the sport participation data reported above. Nonetheless, the role of sport and PE within the university's curriculum has certainly been regarded as being more important than previously, and has led to an increase in allocated funding for staff and facilities.

Conclusion

The current discourse on Chinese youth sport policy is still very much focused on the presumed health and physical benefits of sport participation, while other benefits (e.g. social, affective and cognitive) have not yet been expressed in the government's youth sport agenda. Of particular significance, however, are a number of processes associated with the provision of youth sports development in China that are worth considering.

First, the Chinese culture and citizen's traditional perspectives on the values of sport have a significant impact on young people's sport participation. Fundamentally, there has always been an emphasis on intellectual development at the expense of sport and physical activity in Chinese culture (Shuttleworth and Chan, 1998). School sport was, and currently still is, perceived to be less important than other activities considered essential to the development of a good academic and work career. When young people experience significant time constraints as a result of their heavy academic study load, the time they devote to participating in sport often diminishes.

Second, the school curriculum is generally more focused on the outcomes of economic development than promoting participating in sport and physical activity. Although the central government does have control over the curriculum, schools are operating in their own ways at a local level and are not necessarily penalised for not following government standards for PE and school sport. In addition, despite the new PE curriculum reform focusing on the promotion of health and fitness, specific health–related educational materials are yet to be embedded into the curricular.

Third, the centralising and decentralising pressures that school and PE teachers experience have had a significant impact on youth sport participation in schools. On the one hand, there is a strongly centralising curriculum development process that determines the standards for curriculum, while on the other hand, a decentralisation of decision making over school budgets, course content planning and management style at provincial, regional and local levels has led to a battle between PE and other core subjects fighting for funding, and a debate over the content organisation and implementation of school curricular. It is clear that in China the role of the state in providing PE and sport has been strongly contested. For example, the constitutional arrangements within which the delivery system operates are unclear, particularly in relation to the role and responsibility of state and local government, and between central government departments. Accordingly, while sport participation targets and fitness status objectives have been set by the national government, these regulations are rarely enforced.

Fourth, as Ding *et al.* (2014) have noted, it is the role of sport skill development in the health-first approach to PE. On the one hand, under the influence of the traditional, technocratic (in relation to sport skill/techniques) teacher education programmes, most PE teachers consider sport skills to be the primary content in PE, and therefore embedded skill development tasks into PE sessions (Ji *et al.*, 2011; Wang *et al.*, 2007). On the other hand, the technocratic view of the content of PE curricular stands in marked contrast to the humanistic view of PE with its focus on health where few skills are required to participate in specific fitness activities (Deng and Yange, 2002; Li, 2004).

Overall, although the promotion of participation in sport and physical activity among young people has become an increasingly prominent feature of sport policy and practice, the current structure and system of school sport has made the development of a national sports development strategy problematic and particularly ineffective in responding to the social and health problems facing young people. In other words, the question is not about whether the government has or not pay attention to the sport provision for young people; the real point of concern is the level of interest, involvement and investment being given to youth sport participation by the state for whom sport and physical activity below the elite level remains a marginal priority compared to other activities.

References

Ashton, B., Hill, K., Piazza, A. and Zeitz, R. (1984). Famine in China, 1958-61, *Population and Development Review*, 613–645.

Chan, P. and Lo, C. (1992). *Principals' Attitudes towards PE and Sport in Schools.* Hong Kong Baptist University: Hong Kong, Faculty of Social Sciences.

Chen, X. (2012). The Effectiveness of Sunshine Sports in Civil Aviation University of China. *Book of Campus Sunshine Sports Five Years, 8*, 193-196.

China Ministry of Education (1992). *Guidance for Physical Education in Higher Education Sectors.* Beijing: China.

China Ministry of Education (2001). *Physical and Health Education Course Standards for Elementary and Secondary Schools (Experimental Edition).* Beijing: China.

China Ministry of Education (2002a). *China Student Fitness Standards and Execution Methods.* Beijing: China.

China Ministry of Education (2002b). *The Education Syllabus for PE and Health Education in Higher Education Institutions.* Available at: www.moe.edu.cn/publicfiles/business/htmlfiles/moe/moe_28/201001/80824. html.

China Ministry of Education (2011). *Physical and Health Education Course Standards for Elementary and Secondary Schools* (2nd edition). Beijing: China.

China Ministry of Education (2014a). *Number of Schools, Educational Personnel and Full-time Teachers by Type and Level.* Available at: www.moe.gov.cn/publicfiles/business.

China Ministry of Education (2014b). *The Statistics Bulletin of National Education Implementation in 2013.* Available at: www.moe.gov.cn/publicfiles/business/htmlfiles/moe/s3040/201411/xxgk_178035. html [accessed 4 April 2015].

China Ministry of Education, The General Administration of Sport, & The Communist Youth League of China. (2006). *Decisions on Launching a Nationwide Hundreds of Millions Students Sunshine Sports Campaign.* Retrieved 24 March 2015. Available at: www.moe.gov.cn/publicfiles/business/htmlfiles/moe/moe_2530/201001/xxgk_80870.html.

China Ministry of Finance (2013). *The 2013 National Public Expenditure Balance Sheet.* Available at: http://yss.mof.gov.cn/2013qgczjs/201407/t20140711_1111874.html [accessed 30 April 2015].

Chinese Communist Party Central Committee, & State Council of the Chinese Government (2007). *Executive Recommendations for Improving Physical Fitness in Children and Adolescents*. Beijing: China.

Chow, E.N-l. and Zhao, S. M. (1996). The one-child policy and parent-child relationships: a comparison of one-child with multiple-child families in China, *International Journal of Sociology and Social Policy*, *16(12)*, 35–62.

Deng, X. and Yange, W. (2002). The academic basis on health first and school physical education in 21st century, *Journal of Physical Education*, *9*(1), 12–14.

Ding, H., Li, Y. and Wu, X. (2014). A review of scholarly and research work in physical education in China during the first decade of the 21st century, *Quest*, *66(1)*, 117–133.

Dong, J. (2008). Reasons and countermeasures of physique declining of Chinese teenagers, *Journal of Lianning University of Science and Technology*, *31*(3–4), 408–410.

Fan, H. and Lu, Z. (2011). *China*. London: Taylor & Francis.

Fu, Y. (2007). *The History of Sport in China: 1949–1979 (Vol. 5)*. Beijing: People's Sport Press.

General Administration of Sport of China (2004). *The Experimental Work Program of Community Sports Club*. Available at: www.sport.gov.cn/n16/n33193/n33208/n33418/n33598/127893.html.

General Administration of Sport of China. (2010). *The Instruction about Further Strengthen Athletes' Culture Education and Guarantee Work*. Available at: www.sport.gov.cn/n16/n1077/n1467/n1701156/n1701206/1809596.html.

General Administration of Sport of China. (2011). *National Report of Students' Physique and Health*. from www.gov.cn/test/2012-04/19/content_2ilable17320.htm

General Administration of Sport of China. (2014). *The Results of Sampling Surveys on Physical Activity and Fitness Condition for Ages 6–69 Population in China*. Available at: www.fitness.org.cn/news/201486/n7248668.html [accessed 24 March 2015].

General Administration of Sport of China, & Ministry of Education. (2011). *Regulations for the Administration of Secondary Sports School*. Available at: www.sport.gov.cn/n16/n1092/n16864/2653226.html [accessed 2 April 2015].

Ha, A.S., Macdonald, D. & Pang, B.O.H. (2010). Physical activity in the lives of Hong Kong Chinese children, *Sport, Education and Society*, *15(3)*, 331–346.

Hao, Q. (2006). *History of Sport*. Beijing: People's Sport Press.

He, J. M. (2000). *China Gaokao Report*. Beijing: Huaxia Publishing House.

Houlihan, B. (2011). Sports development and young people: introduction: socialisation through sport, in B. Houlihan & M. Green (eds) *Routledge Handbook of Sports Development* (pp. 127–129). London: Routledge Taylor & Francis Group.

Ji, L., Wang, X. and Tang, L. (2011). Ten year review on new physical education curriculum reform in elementary education in China, *The Journal of Shanghai University of Sport*, *35(2)*, 77–81.

Ji, Y. (2013). The examination and analysis of the sports participation level of high schools in Hebei Province. *Journal of Learning Weekly Magazine*, *12*, 81.

Jones, R. (1999). Sport in China, in J. Riordan and R. Jones (eds) *Sport and Physical Education in China*. London: E&FN SPON.

Li, C. (2004). Investigation and research on the enforcement and effect of delightful sports in the break time in Tangshan City, *Journal of Beijing Sport University*, *27*, 106–107.

Li, L. and Yang, B. (2002). China's history of physical education in schools & colleges: retrospection and reconsidered. *Journal of Physical Education*, *9(4)*, 130–132.

Liang, G., Lynn, H., Walls, R. and Yan, Z. (2012). Failure and revival: physical education and youth sport in China, *Asia Pacific Journal of Sport and Social Science*, *1(1)*, 48–59.

Lin, X.F. (1989). Understanding the conception of Ti Yu, *Journal of Beijing Teachers College of Physical Education*, *2*, 70–73.

Ma, L. (2007). *Investigation of Beijing Public Schools Students on The Implementation of One Hour Physical Activity Per Day – School Physical Education Reform*. Beijing: People's Education Press.

National Bureau of Statistics of China. (2014). *China Statistical Yearbook*, in N. o. I. a. E. P. o. P. E. S. (2013). Beijing: China.

National Sport Commission (1978). 1978 National Sport Conference. Paper presented at the *The Collected Compilation of Sport and Physical Education Documents of PRC* (1949–1981). Beijing.

Phillpots, L. (2011). Sports development and young people in England, in B. Houlihan & M. Green (eds) *Routledge Handbook of Sports Development*. London: Routledge, Taylor & Francis Group.

Queen, S., Habenstein, R. and Quadagno, J. (1985). *The Family in Various Cultures* (5th edition). New York: Harper & Row

Qui, S. and Chen, Q. (2004). Investigation on physical education in middle and primary school in rural areas in Shanxi Province, *Sport Science*, 24(7), 78–79.

Ren, H. (1996). China in P. De Knop, L.M. Engström, B. Skirstad and M. Weiss (eds). *Worldwide Trends in Youth Sport*. Leeds: Human Kinetics.

Shen, L. and Fan, H. (2012). Historical review of state policy for physical education in the People's Republic of China, *The International Journal of the History of Sport*, 29(4), 583–600.

Shuttleworth, J. and Chan, W.K. (1998). Youth sport education and development in Hong Kong: a conflict model social impact assessment, *Sport, Education and Society*, 3(1), 37–58.

Song, Y., Zhang, X., Yang, T.-b., Zhang, B., Dong, B. and Ma, J. (2012). Current situation and cause analysis of physical activity in Chinese primary and middle school students in 2010, *Journal of Peking University (Health Sciences)*, 44(3), 347–354.

State Council (1973). *Details of the 1973 national sports conference*. The Fundamental Law of Education: No.17 17 C.F.R. (2001). Retrieved [20 March 2015] from www.gov.cn/gongbao/content/2001/content_60920.htm. Beijing.

Sun, H. (2006). Research on the current situation and developing strategy of PE for primary and middle school in the west of China, *Journal of Beijing Sport University*, 29(7), 967–968.

The Fundamental Law of Education: No.17 17 C.F.R. (2001).

Tudor-Locke, C., Ainsworth, B., Adair, L., Du, S. and Popkin, B. (2003). Physical activity and inactivity in Chinese school-aged youth: the China Health and Nutrition Survey, *International Journal of Obesity*, 27(9), 1093–1099.

Wang, H. (2005). Evolvement and historical experience of the PE curriculum of elementary and middle schools in modern China, *Journal of Beijing Sport University*, 28, 941–943.

Wang, X., Ji, L., Huang, C., Liu, H. and Lin, P. (2008). School physical education reform and development in the People's Republic of China. In C. Haddad (ed.) *Innovative Practices in Physical Education and Sports in Asia* (pp. 59–71). Bangkok, Thailand: UNESCO Asia and Pacific Regional Bureau for Education.

Wang, X., Ji, L., & Jin, Y. (2007). Investigation on status quo of a new round of physical education curriculum reform in elementary and middle schools of our country, *Journal of Shanghai University of Sport*, 31(6), 62–68.

Wu, S. (1999). *The History of Sport of the PRC*. Beijing: China Books Press.

Yao, L. (2004). Consideration and current condition of city school sports in China, *Journal of Sport Science*, 24(12), 68–72.

Yates, J.F. and Lee, J.W. (1996). Chinese decision-making, in M. H. Bond (ed.) *The Handbook of Chinese Psychology*. Oxford: Oxford University Press.

Yu, L., & Suen, H.K. (2005). Historical and contemporary exam-driven education fever in China, *KEDI Journal of Educational Policy*, 2(1), 17–33.

Zhang, L. (2015). The strategic research on strengthening the adolescents' physiques – based on the reflection of physical education. *Journal of Northeast Normal University (Philosophy and Social Sciences)*, 2, 164–169.

Zhao, Q. and Xue, Y. (2011). An empirical study of the change of physical fitness condition among undergraduates, *Journal of Sports Culture Guide*, 4, 94–97.

SECTION 3

Trends in youth sport

14

INTRODUCTION

Ken Green

In Section 3, *Trends in youth sport*, the various contributions explore what amounts to change and transformation in youth sport. The section opens with a chapter entitled *Tracking and youth sport: the quest for lifelong adherence to sport and physical activity*, in which Bart Vanreusel and Jeroen Scheerder examine the potential for sporting experiences during youth to impact upon active involvement in sport during the later stages of the life course. Utilising the concept of 'tracking' (continuity or persistence of sports participation over time), they conclude that the empirical studies related to tracking provide support for the taken-for-granted assumption that participation during childhood and youth is one of the strongest predictors of adult involvement in sport. Indeed, adult involvement in sport and physical activity appear more strongly influenced by childhood and youth involvement than by social and economic constraints experienced during adulthood. In other words, people who are locked in to sport during childhood tend to be able to sustain their involvement almost (but not quite) irrespective of the cross-cutting effects of such social divisions as class, ethnicity and gender later on in life. Empirical support for the existence of tracking notwithstanding, Vanreusel and Scheerder also note that unstable patterns of sport involvement in youth and between youth and adulthood tend to be the norm, with stable patterns of participation from youth to adulthood more likely to be exceptional. Indeed, the tracking of *in*activity appears more deep-seated than that of activity *per se*: those who spend little or no time on sports during youth have, it seems, a much higher risk of continuing this pattern into adulthood and, subsequently, throughout the life course. While the extant research confirms some patterns of tracking in youth sport and between youth sport and later phases in life, Vanreusel and Scheerder are keen to insert several caveats. Perhaps the most significant of these is that no causal relationship between input and output can be established; not least because a number of other intervening variables may account for both youth sport and later life participation. Vanreusel and Scheerder also draw our attention to the fact that tracking has gender-specific features – the participatory patterns of females are more likely to be characterised by change, instability and drop-out. This latter observation makes sense of the findings in relation to lifestyle sports (Gilchrist and Wheaton, this volume) and trends in Nordic countries (Green, this volume) even more pertinent vis-à-vis youths' sports participation.

The topic of tracking dovetails neatly with the remaining three chapters in this section on the place of organised sports settings (such as sports clubs), the growing popularity of lifestyle sports and the shift of outdoor sports indoors. In the first of these, *Dropping out from clubs, dropping in to sport light?*, Julie Borgers, Jan Seghers and Jeroen Scheerder reflect upon the role of the organisational setting for youths' sports participation, including traditional sports and sports clubs as well as what they refer to as 'sport light' – the less organized/less structured modes of sports participation. We have known for a while that young people nowadays are less clubbable than hitherto (Roberts, 2008) and that when they cease actively participating in one sporting context (e.g. competitively) they sometimes take up the same or a similar activity in another, perhaps more recreational, setting (Coakley, 2007). In this regard, Borgers *et al.* investigate whether drop-out and drop-off from traditional/conventional sports participation in clubs during youth leads to drop-in to more recreational and informal forms of sport (sport light) – in effect, lifestyle sports – in late youth/early adulthood. In the process, the authors ask a number of questions regarding the organisational settings for sports participation in relation to life stage, the groups most involved in club-based sport, drop-out from clubs, and whether drop-out from clubs reflects decreasing patterns of sports participation in general as opposed to new ways of participation. Borgers *et al.* explore the popularity of different settings for sports participation among youth and why they choose particular contexts, as well as the appeal of sport light. Data derived from a large scale cross-sectional survey on sports participation in Flanders is utilised in order to develop profiles of sports participants in relation to the organisational setting of sports participation and preferences. In short, the findings of Borgers *et al.* suggest that whereas 15–18-year-old youths are more inclined to engage in the traditional club sports system, the life stage of youth is associated with drop-out from club-organised sport and, for some if not many, drop-in to sport light. Thus, Borgers and her colleagues conclude that the commonly reported issues of drop-out during youth should not be seen simply as drop-out from sport per se: moving away from sports clubs does not necessarily mean becoming inactive. In doing so, they remind us that youth should not be treated as a single participatory market – participation patterns differ not only with regard to sporting preferences but also in terms of the organisation of, and settings for, sporting practices.

The shift away from participation via sports clubs and traditional sports (towards sport light pehaps) during youth provides the background for exploration of another salient feature of trends in youth sport; namely the shift towards so-called 'lifestyle sports'. In their chapter entitled *Lifestyle and adventure sports among youth*, Paul Gilchrist and Belinda Wheaton chart what they refer to as an 'intensifying trend' toward increases in 'the range and diversity of sports practices, particularly more informal and individualistic activities', especially in Western societies. They point out that lifestyle sports have experienced unprecedented growth, drawing participants from increasingly diverse global geographic settings in the process. Although it is virtually impossible to accurately chart the size of the lifestyle sports phenomenon, the authors note how the rapid growth of lifestyle and adventure sports has outpaced the expansion of most traditional sports in many Western nations. In particular, Gilchrist and Wheaton reflect upon the growing popularity and significance of the various so-called extreme, alternative, adventure and whizz sports (brought together under the label 'lifestyle sports') and the impact of these on the contemporary sporting landscape. Gilchrist and Wheaton describe the ever-increasing and seemingly divergent body of lifestyle sports enthusiasts – ranging from the occasional participants to the hard core of committed practitioners for whom participation signals a particular way of life as well as style of participation. They also point to the diversity among participants – including increasing numbers of women and girls – and the expanding and diversified ways in which consumers can experience lifestyle sports, including the indoor variations subsequently discussed by Salome and van Bottenburg. Gilchrist and Wheaton present lifestyle sports as potentially significant sites for identity construction among youth (and, for that matter, adults). In the process, they explore the interrelationships between youth lifestyle sports subcultures, lifestyles and identities, wherein particular activities enable youths to feel like and be recognised as particular kinds of people on the basis of what they do, where they do it and who they do it with. Among other things, they argue that from the perspective of those youths involved in lifestyle sports, it is often the extra-sporting qualities that are significant, not least in terms of social interaction in spaces beyond the home, in adult-free zones. In this regard, the authors highlight the importance of lifestyle, identity and subculture to understanding the growing popularity and global cultural appeal of lifestyle sports among youth.

The manner in which the appeal of lifestyle sports has been fanned by globalising social media and commercial enterprise provides a suitable backdrop for Lotte Salome and Maarten van Bottenburg's chapter on the indoorisation of lifestyle sports. In *Indoorising the outdoors: tempting young people's interests in lifestyle sports*, Salome and van Bottenburg explore the trend for ostensibly adventurous, not to say dangerous, outdoor sporting activities to be brought indoors – into relatively safe and predictable but artificial settings and environments. These include some of the lifestyle sports mentioned by Gilchrist and Wheaton. Salome and van Bottenburg note the increasing popularity, not only among youth, of indoor variants of lifestyle sports, ranging from the now well-established indoor climbing, skiing and skateboarding venues to the more recent surfing and even sky-diving facilities. The authors explain the process of indoorisation in terms of an interplay of cultural trends among youth, technological advances and commercial enterprise; in other words, a twenty-first century example of technology-led innovations that commerce has pioneered as leisure industries (Roberts, 2004). Salome and van Bottenburg focus upon the complex relationship between lifestyle sports – and those with indoors variants, in particular – and commercialisation processes, including the rapid development of artificial sport environments for the safe and accessible, but still relatively exciting experience of adventure sports. Lifestyle sport participation in controlled indoor settings appear to be attracting increasing numbers of youth. Years of time, money and effort to master techniques are no longer required in order to experience some, but by no means all, of the sensations and thrills (in other words, the emotions) of adventurous sports. In effect, (young) people can take sporting risks while being protected from the more serious consequences of the real thing.

In examining the general direction in which youth sport has been travelling recently, it is noteworthy that trends reflect not only alternative forms of provision (from voluntary clubs and public facilities through to commercial gyms as well, increasingly, as looser, ad hoc, informal arrangements) but also alternative and distinct drivers or motivations, drawing in enthusiasts for conventional team sports, body sculptors, and fitness fanatics through to thrill seekers and recreational players. The relatively new provision of commercial gyms for individual health and fitness activities alongside the rapid growth of lifestyle sports more widely have not however, been at the expense of voluntary sports clubs and competitive team games, the ongoing boundary adjustments between organised and lifestyle sports notwithstanding. That said, commercial involvement in gyms and indoor–outdoor activities and the ingenuity of lifestyle players have not merely provided a wider range of sporting opportunities but also tended to change the character of some sports, such that additional variants have become specialist activities in their own right, attracting their own 'taste publics' among youth (e.g. indoor rock-climbing and mountain-biking). There is no sign that the broadening and diversification of sports participation among youth will abate any time soon.

References

Coakley, J. (2007). Socialization and sport, in George Ritzer (ed.) *The Blackwell Encyclopedia of Sociology* (pp. 4576–4580). Basingstoke: Basil Blackwell.

Roberts, K. (2004). *The Leisure Industries*. Basingstoke: Basil Blackwell.

Roberts, K. (2008). *Youth in Transition*. In Eastern Europe and the West. Basingstoke: Palgrave Macmillan

15

TRACKING AND YOUTH SPORT

The quest for lifelong adherence to sport and physical activity

Bart Vanreusel and Jeroen Scheerder

Introduction

Does youth sport affect active involvement in sport at later stages in life? Do young sport participants have better chances to remain physically active during adulthood? Is early socialization into sport related to continued sport participation in later life? What is the impact of early sport experiences in youth on future involvement in sport and physical activity? Can lifelong participation in sport and physical activity be promoted by youth sport programming? What is the longitudinal stability or instability over time of participation patterns in sport from youth into adulthood? These questions are raised throughout the literature on youth sport from a lifetime perspective. They reflect the expectations from various fields that youth sport contributes to a lasting physically active lifestyle.

The central concept in these questions and expectations on youth sport, shared by research, policy and pedagogical practice, is that of *tracking*. Tracking refers to patterns of continuity or stability over an observed period of time (Malina, 1996). It studies the changes in a relative position or the ranking in a group over time. The tracking concept is useful to study continuity or stability of participation in youth sport into later stages in life. In general, empirical findings of tracking would support the often assumed positive relationship between youth sport and adherence to sport and physical activity during adulthood.

The interest in tracking of youth sport comes from different angles. Socialization research, sport pedagogy, sport policy and public health each show a particular interest in youth sport and its expected contribution to a continued physically active lifestyle. Sport socialization research focuses on how young people are socialized into sport and a physically active lifestyle by adopting roles, norms, values and skills. But it also wants to reveal how the socialization process is continued or discontinued into later life. This involves processes of socialization, desocialization and even resocialization (Chapter 18). Socialization refers to the adoption of an active lifestyle with sport as a dominant cultural expression among young people. Desocialization is characterized by various forms of permanent or temporary drop-out from sport and physical activity, whereas resocialization encompasses forms of re-entry and renewed involvement in sport and physical activity. The study of these socialization processes over a period of time or between different life phases requires a longitudinal observation of the same subjects. Tracking data, collected by longitudinal observation, helps to understand these socialization processes.

Physical education and sport pedagogy are fundamentally based on the assumption of tracking. The objectives of physical education curricula often refer to its assumed contribution to a continued physically active lifestyle across the lifespan. In sport pedagogy, the image of youth sport as a preparatory field for later life is a classic and strong one. Physical education and youth sport base their position and values in an educational context on an outspoken belief in tracking of physical skills, but also of social competences and attitudes.

In recent decades, youth sport has become a focus for policy-making. Providers of youth sport programmes nowadays come from private, public and commercial sectors with objectives varying from elite sports to sport for all and to health-enhancing physical activities. All these initiatives count on the tracking qualities of youth sport for future continuation or performance.

From a public health perspective, the quest for continued physical activity from youth into further life is also evident. It is commonly accepted that moderate but continued physical activity in all stages of life is beneficial to health. Therefore, the public health sector is eager to know whether and how sport and physical activities in youth can be continued into adulthood.

In contrast to the high expectations and the firm belief in the tracking qualities of youth sport, knowledge on tracking is, however, rather limited. The number of studies is relatively small and results can hardly be generalized due to limitations of samples and research methods, and because of the complexity of the issue. Most empirical studies on tracking in and of youth sport inevitably represent a reduced and simplified perspective on the social reality of growing up as children and adolescents into adulthood. Furthermore, because of the longitudinal character of the process, empirical data on tracking is hard to collect.

The aim of this chapter is twofold. First, empirical findings in the literature on tracking of youth sport are summarized. We will illustrate the findings with results from the ongoing *Leuven Longitudinal Study on Lifestyle Fitness and Health* (hereafter referred to as the Leuven Longitudinal Study). The objective of the Leuven Longitudinal Study has been to detect tracking patterns in sport participation from youth into adulthood. Second, the tracking concept itself will be discussed in relation to youth sport. The specific methods of the Leuven Longitudinal Study or more general methodological issues concerning longitudinal research on tracking in sport participation will not be addressed in this chapter. They are covered in previous publications on tracking, such as Vanreusel *et al.* (1993; 1997), Malina (2001a; 2001b), Breuer (2003), Telama *et al.* (2005), Scheerder *et al.* (2006; 2008), Engström (2008) and Skille and Solbakken (2014).

Tracking and youth sport: what do we know?

Although the common interest in tracking of youth sport is high, there is no clear coherent theoretical perspective on tracking and its impact on adhesion to sport and physical activity. Tracking data is one element in a network of determinants and correlates of sport and physical activity in youth at the one hand, and between youth and adulthood at the other (Yang *et al.*, 1999). Social learning theory points out that youth experiences have an influence on ideas, attitudes and behaviour at adult age (Ormrod, 1999). Social roles and identities, for example, being a sport participant or a non-participant, adopted in youth may have a significant impact on lifestyle patterns in later life (Bandura, 1977; Bronfenbrenner, 1979). Tracking fits within such encompassing theoretical models on socialization that perceive adherence to physical activity from youth into adulthood as a result of complex interactions between personal factors, significant others and/or socializing agents and a socialization environment (Vanreusel *et al.*, 1997; Breuer, 2003; Telama *et al.*, 2005; Scheerder *et al.*, 2006; 2008). These factors may interact in a two-way direction. They may enhance tracking in and of youth sport, but they may also hamper tracking and continuity and provoke drop-out and discontinuity resulting in physical inactivity. This means that tracking data should not be interpreted in an isolated way and that tracking always needs to be contextualized by (de)socializing factors.

In general, the findings from tracking studies confirm that physical activity in early youth is significantly related to forms of physical activity in adolescence and young adulthood, with youth sport as a dominant form of physical activity. Furthermore, youth sport involvement shows significant relationships with adherence to physical activity in adulthood. These general patterns of tracking are confirmed in different longitudinal studies with a focus on tracking (Breuer, 2003; Engström, 2008; Malina, 2001a; 2001b; Scheerder, 2006; 2008; Telama *et al.*, 1997; Vanreusel *et al.*, 1997; Yang *et al.*, 1999). However, these general observations on tracking and youth sport need to be complemented by a more nuanced picture of research results and interpretations. The state of the art in tracking research demands a careful and preliminary interpretation of tracking data.

In a twenty-one-year longitudinal tracking study of Finnish subjects, analysed at various interval years, Telama *et al.* (2005; 2006) concluded that a high level of physical activity at ages 9 to 18, especially regular and persistent participation in youth sport, significantly predicted a high level of adult physical activity. This confirmed the findings from work on tracking of different samples in Belgium (Scheerder, 2006, 2008; Vanreusel *et al.*, 1997), in Sweden (Engström, 2008) and in a review publication on tracking research in youth sport and physical activity (Malina, 2001b). These studies share the observation that tracking correlations in youth, between 9 and 18 years, tend to be moderate to high and correlations between youth and adulthood tend to be low to moderate. Findings suggest that sport participation in late adolescence and adulthood is related to patterns of physical activity in youth. But many authors have pointed out that more and other variables intervene in the interval period between the observation of tracking. Tracking data in youth sport, although significant, only partially reveal the process of adherence or non-adherence to physical activity. Engström (2008), among others, suggested that a complex set of individual, social and environmental factors in youth influence adherence to sport and physical activity.

Based on their extensive study of tracking, Yang and colleagues (1999:125) concluded that 'early physical activity was one of the best predictors of adult physical activity'. They summarized their findings as follows:

> Previous studies have concerned either the influence of early socialization or current factors in adulthood. The important finding of this study is that adult physical activity appears to be more influenced by physical activity in childhood and in adolescence than by the current social and environmental factors in adulthood.
>
> *(Yang* et al.*, 1999: 125)*

Tracking data also explores the stability of patterns of sport involvement between youth and adulthood. Unstable patterns of sport involvement in youth and between youth and adulthood appear to be dominant, whereas stable patterns of participation from youth to adulthood are exceptional. In an analysis of tracking data on samples of youth sport participants in Germany, Breuer (2003) pointed out that the intra-individual stability of regular sport involvement in youth and between youth and adulthood is relatively small. Only one-third of a sample observed over seven years showed a stable pattern of regular physical activity. Two-thirds of the sample represented an unstable pattern of various changes in modes of physical activity, temporary drop-outs and restarts, periods of increasing and decreasing activity. Furthermore, the general stability over the seven years was primarily due to a relatively high stability from the age of 25 upwards. In contrast to this finding, the stability was low in the observed seven year interval between 16 and 24 years of age (Breuer, 2003).

These findings are consistent with our study on the stability of sport involvement over time in a sample of males between 13 and 35 years of age in Belgium (Vanreusel *et al.*, 1997). Unstable patterns of sport participation over these years accounted for 71 per cent of the sample. Only about one-third of the sample showed a stable pattern, including those with a stable pattern of low physical activity. Again, these results make clear that tracking of sport and physical activity is not as straightforward as often suggested and assumed. Tracking data compare input and output observations at both sides of a time interval. But somewhat hidden behind these input-output tracking data lies a more complex social reality of events that obviously influence continued participation from youth to adulthood.

In a longitudinal study of tracking on sport participation of women from youth to adulthood, Moyaert (2013) focused on the organizational context of sport participation. The study observed different interval periods in an overall interval period of 33 years, covering youth to adulthood. Participation in sport clubs, in so-called light communities and individual forms of involvement were distinguished as a social context of sport involvement. Sport in light communities is defined as self-organized sport with different ways of shared involvement, but without formal membership in a sport club. Autonomy and freedom of choice are essential but participants still prefer to be part of a larger community on a temporary basis (Duyvendak and Hurenkamp, 2004). Scheerder and Vos (2011) have pointed to the growth of sport in light communities as a most relevant way of involvement in sport and physical activity in today's societies. Light community sports may become the dominant pattern of sport involvement in actual generations (Scheerder and van Bottenburg, 2010).

Moyaert (2013) showed that women who participate in light community sport have equal chances for continued involvement than those who participate in more formal club organized sport compared to individualized ways of participation. The study suggests that being a member of a group, in a sport club but also in a light community context, endorses chances for a continued physically active lifestyle. Preliminary findings of tracking indicate that tracking qualities and capacities might be different for various ways and organizational forms of youth sport. Sport in light communities appears to have similar qualities compared to organized sport in clubs when it comes to its contribution to adherence to sport. Social environment matters, however more in depth studies are needed to understand tracking qualities in different social contexts of youth sport.

Studies suggest that tracking has gender-specific features. In general, tracking of sport involvement appears to be less stable for girls than for boys when observed from youth into adulthood. Scheerder and colleagues (2008) found slightly stronger tracking results for boys than for girls into adult sport participation. These results were linked with information on lifestyle changes in the period from youth (late adolescence) to adulthood, such as end of studies, start of working life, giving birth, moving and job changes. Both, men and women showed a high and similar level of lifestyle changes over the interval period. However, the pattern of sport participation of the men in that period remained more stable compared to that of the women. The sport pattern of the women was characterized by change, instability and drop-out. These results suggest that the impact of lifestyle changes is experienced more as an obstacle for continued involvement in sport for women than it is for men. Although the amount of lifestyle changes were similar for men and women, men appear to have privileged chances to continue their sport activities from youth into adulthood. Once again, these tentative conclusions need to be verified by further research.

Tracking of physical inactivity

The majority of studies on tracking have used the perspective of physical activity, as a generic concept for various forms of sport, as a starting point. Only a few studies have taken the opposite perspective and explored the tracking of physical *in*activity. Yet, the opposite focus on tracking of inactivity or low activity can be most relevant for knowledge on health-related physical activity. While a lack of physical activity is widely accepted as a health risk factor, little is known about tracking of low or even non-activity levels throughout the lifespan, particularly from youth to adulthood. The same socialization theories suggest that physical inactivity and non or low participation in sport can also be the result of a social learning process. Is a pattern of inactivity in youth determinant for inactivity in adulthood? Tracking research may provide new insights in this relatively unexplored relationship.

The Leuven Longitudinal Study (Scheerder, 2006; 2008; Vanreusel, 1993; 1997) studied tracking of sport inactivity between late adolescence (age 17 for male and age 15–18 for female subjects) and adulthood (age 30 for male and age 35–41 for female subjects). The study contrasted two groups with a different profile of sports participation in youth. The first group of inactive young subjects is presented in Figures 15.1 (boys) and 15.2 (girls). These inactive youngsters spent no or little time (less than one hour a week) on sport in late adolescence. Figures 15.3 and 15.4 present tracking data of very active young boys and girls at late adolescence. They practiced sport during six hours or more a week over a year of observation. All four figures show the level of (in)activity of the same individuals in adulthood at age 30 or more. Adult (non-)participation is presented in three categories: active, moderately active or inactive. The concept of sport is inclusive and covers recreational, individual as well as competitive sport, aggregated into time spent on sport activity. The data presented are based on sub-samples of the Leuven Longitudinal Study and are limited in scope and size. Therefore, the results are indicative and cannot be representative for larger populations.

Almost eight out of ten boys (78 per cent) in the inactive category at late adolescence also belong to the inactive category at 30 years of age. Only 4 per cent of inactive boys changed

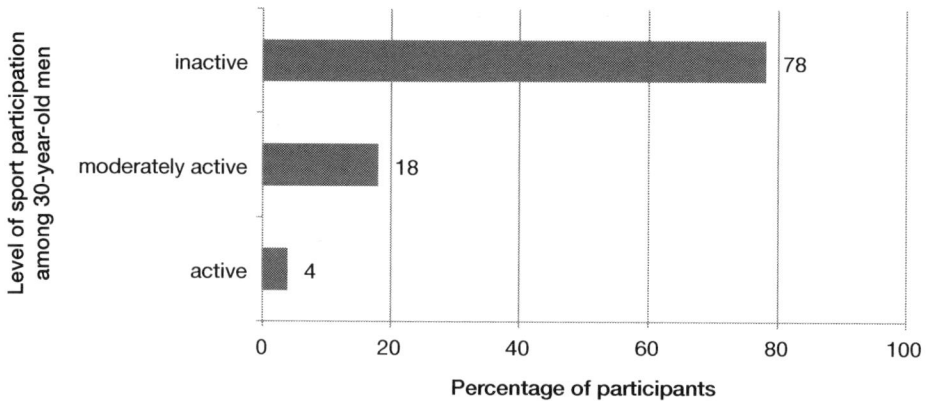

Figure 15.1 Level of sport participation among 30-year-old men who did not participate in sport at the age of 17

Source: Vanreusel *et al.*, 1997: 381.

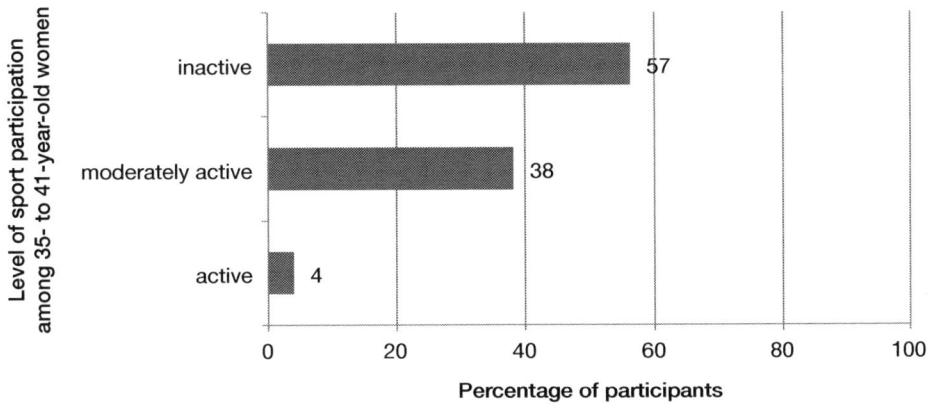

Figure 15.2 Level of sport participation among 35- to 41-year-old women who did not participate in sport at the age of 15, 16, 17 and/or 18

Source: Scheerder *et al.*, 2008: 35.

this pattern into an active lifestyle and belonged to the active category at age 30 (Figure 15.1). A similar but less obvious pattern is shown in the sample of females. Here, almost six out of ten inactive girls (57 per cent) at adolescence belong to the inactive group in adulthood. Once more, only 4 per cent of inactive girls moved into the category of active women in adulthood. Such data, although preliminary and non-representative for larger populations, indicate a relatively clear-cut pattern of tracking of physical inactivity and of low or non-participation in sport (Figure 15.2).

Figures 15.3 and 15.4 show a contrasting image. They present tracking data for boys and girls who were very active in late adolescence. Only 34 per cent of very active boys were still part of the active category in adulthood. On the other hand, 38 per cent of the very active young boys were moderately active in adulthood, whereas 28 per cent of the very active young boys ended up in the inactive category in adulthood (Figure 15.3). A similar pattern is apparent in the female sample. Here, 47 per cent of very active late adolescent girls remained active in adulthood, while 32 per cent had moved into the category of moderately active women and 21 per cent of them had become inactive in adulthood.

Together, these results, limited as they are, suggest that tracking of physical inactivity might be more deep-seated than tracking of physical activity. It can be provisionally concluded that adolescents who spend little or no time on sports during youth, have a much higher risk of continuing this pattern into adulthood and, as a consequence, to develop an inactive lifestyle throughout the lifespan. This pattern of learned and continued physical inactivity from youth into adulthood may contribute to the creation of at risk groups for the health consequences of a physically inactive lifestyle. However, more research is needed on representative samples with more sophisticated analyses of intervening variables in order to obtain a clear picture of tracking of physical inactivity and non-participation in sport. Nevertheless, the lack of research of more extensive and generalizable research in tracking of inactivity should not prevent policy-makers, practitioners and educators from developing intervention models for the low or non-physically active in youth. Given the sense of urgency on the consequences and on the scope of physical inactivity communicated by the health sector, research and practice need to make substantial progress on this issue.

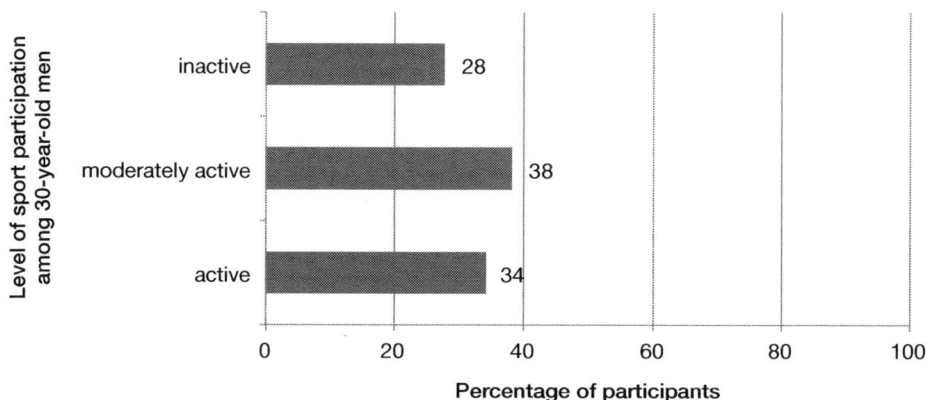

Figure 15.3 Level of sport participation among 30-year-old men who participate in sport at the age of 17 (> 6 hours/week)

Source: Vanreusel *et al.*, 1997: 381.

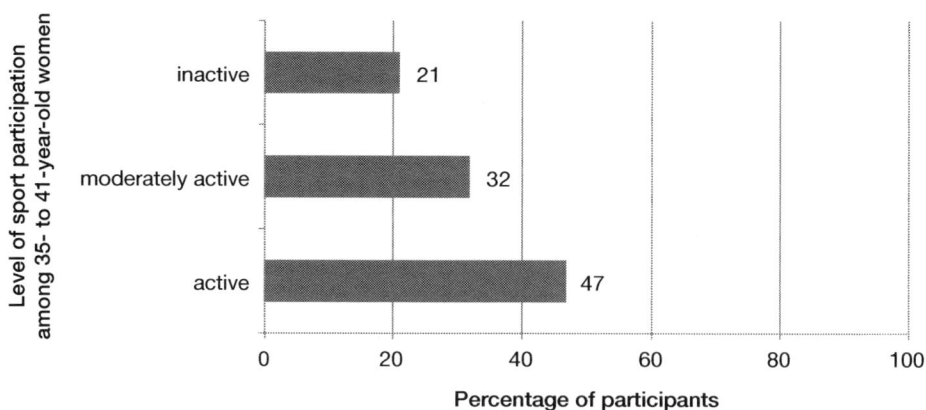

Figure 15.4 Level of sport participation among 35- to 41-year-old women who participate in sport at the age of 15, 16, 17 and/or 18 (> 6 hours/week)

Source: Scheerder *et al.*, 2008: 36.

Tracking in youth sport discussed

The quest for tracking in youth sport reveals a striking contrast. In applied fields of youth sport, continued patterns of behaviour are almost taken for granted as a natural feature of youth sport. Youth sport programmes and policies are partially legitimized on the assumption of their tracking qualities. The idea that youth sport is a premise for lifelong participation in sport and physical activity is reflected in the firm belief in tracking. This, however, is in contrast with the careful and moderate conclusions found in research on tracking. Research confirms some patterns of tracking in youth sport and between youth sport and later phases in life. But, at the same time, it is recognized that tracking is moderate, that no causal relationship between input and output moments can be established and that a number of other intervening variables may account for both youth sport participation and for continued participation.

Although tracking may provide useful insight in the relationship between youth sport and adherence to sport, the concept of tracking is debated. Several remarks can be formulated. First, tracking studies need longitudinal data covering years from youth to adulthood. Such data are scarce, hard to get, limited in scope and mostly unrepresentative of larger populations beyond the observed sample. This means that the available results in the literature tend not to be generalizable let alone translated into policy programmes or pedagogical practice in youth sport. Knowledge based on tracking data so far only offers exploratory and indicative insights into the quest for lifelong adherence to sport and physical activity.

A second weakness of the tracking concept is conceptual in its nature. Tracking studies can be labelled as black box research. This implies that tracking basically observes input and output data, but that it leaves what happens over or during the observed period of time unravelled, in a black box. Features of youth sport such as type, frequency, intensity or context of participation are input information on one end of the black box. Data of the same sample many years later, on involvement in sport and physical activity in adulthood, provide information at the other end – at the output side of the black box. Tracking studies relationships between the input and the output side. But what happens in between remains mostly unknown. Tracking studies hardly reveal information on the throughput processes, changes and intervening variables between the input and output observations. The life phase between youth and adulthood is particularly sensitive for lifestyle changes, related to age, parenthood, work, study, relationships, leisure, housing and so forth. Although these agents of change may have a considerable impact on continuity or discontinuity of participation in sports, they remain in the black box of most tracking studies on youth sport.

Third, the use of concepts of sport and physical activity in longitudinal studies is divergent between studies and lacks clarity. Some studies focus on competitive sport in youth while other studies adopt a broad definition of sports participation. Similarly, research definitions of physical activity, both in youth and in adulthood are often different, not clearly defined and even difficult to interpret. However, there is a growing consensus that involvement in sport and physical activity needs to be understood as a broader disposition, composed of various sub-features. Similarly, tracking of physical *in*activity and non-participation in sport may fit within similar umbrella concepts.

Finally, tracking from youth to adulthood does not proceed in a social vacuum. On the contrary, age, cohort and time-trend effects have an impact on longitudinal socialization processes (Breuer, 2003). Such effects are particularly true for sport and physical activity. It is well documented that participation in sport as a social practice is influenced by changing external conditions over time in society (Hoekman *et al.*, 2011). For example, it can be assumed that young people actually have a much wider choice in a broad repertoire of sport activities than former generations of young people. On the other hand, today's socioeconomic conditions can make it more difficult for youngsters to participate (Vandermeerschen *et al.*, 2013). With regard to tracking research, this means an extra difficulty in interpreting the changes in tracking data.

These limitations of tracking studies clearly indicate that youth sport data alone can neither explain nor predict participation in sport and physical activity during later stages in life. Various forms and modes of participation in youth sport are only an element of the complex and ongoing (de-)socialization process into and from sport and physical activity between youth and adulthood.

Conclusion

Skille and Solbakken (2014) recently reviewed and scrutinized the relationship between adolescent sport participation and lifelong participation in physical activity. They summarized tracking knowledge.

> Despite some divergences between studies, countries and genders, it seems that the relationship between adolescent sport participation and lifelong participation in physical activity depends on:
>
> 1 continuing with sport into the late teens (versus dropping out earlier);
> 2 having a wide repertoire (Roberts and Brodie, 1992) and a various experience;
> 3 perceiving self-control or self-governance in relation to one's leisure time.
>
> *(Skille and Solbakken, 2014: 36)*

The authors suggest, with reference to Bourdieu (1986), that participation in the field of sport, both in youth and in adulthood, requires a specific *habitus*. In their review of tracking research, Skille and Solbakken (2014) suggest that a habitus suitable for sport participation in late adolescence correlates with a habitus for physical activity in adulthood. A relatively specific habitus of personal, social and environmental features might explain both youth sport involvement and lifelong adherence to physical activity. Along the same line of thinking, and as a result of empirical research, Engström (2008) suggested that a combination of social position variables and sport involvement variables in teenage years are the best predictors for continued participation when taken together. Skille and Solbakken (2014: 42) conclude that 'There is little evidence to claim a causal relationship between adolescent sport participation and lifetime physical activity. However there seems to be an underlying mechanism that explains both, namely a habitus comprising accomplishments suited to both fields'.

These observations might guide future thinking and research on tracking and youth sport. We conclude that the quest for tracking in youth sport needs to be continued both as a policy debate and as a subject for theoretical and empirical research. The debate needs to move on from beliefs and claims on the tracking qualities of youth sport towards evidence-based knowledge and implementation. Research needs to be continued, including sound theoretical models and empirical observation beyond the black box approach and including encompassing explaining variables. A well-needed match between the public claims and research findings on tracking and youth sport will be a major step forward, both for sport pedagogy and for sport policy.

References

Bandura, A. (1977). *Social Learning Theory* (Prentice-Hall Series in Social Learning Theory). Englewood-Cliffs, NJ: Prentice-Hall.

Bourdieu, P. (1986). *Distinction. A Social Critique of the Judgment of Taste.* London: Routledge.

Breuer, C. (2003). Entwicklung und Stabilität sportlicher Aktivität im Lebensverlauf, zur Rolle von Alters-, Perioden- und Kohorteneffekten, *Sportwissenschaft 33 (3)*, 263–279.

Bronfenbrenner, U. (1979). *The Ecology of Human Development. Experiments by Nature and Design.* Cambridge, MA: Harvard University Press.

Duyvendak, J.W. and Hurenkamp, M. (eds) (2004). *Kiezen voor de kudde. Lichte gemeenschappen en de nieuwe meerderheid* (Kennis, Openbare mening en Politiek). Amsterdam: Van Gennep.

Engström, L.-M. (1990). Exercise adherence in sport for all, from youth to adulthood, in P. Oja and R. Telama (eds) *Sport for All (Proceedings of the World Congress on Sport for All; Tampere, June 3–7, 1990).* (pp. 473–483). Amsterdam: Elsevier.

Engström, L.-M. (2008). Who is physically active? Cultural capital and sports participation from adolescence to middle age. A 38-year follow-up study, *Physical Education and Sport Pedagogy 13(4)*, 319–343.

Hoekman, R., Breedveld, K. and Scheerder, J. (eds) (2011). Special Issue on sports participation in Europe, *European Journal for Sport and Society (Special Issue) 8(1+2)*, 7–13.

Malina, R.M. (1996). Tracking of physical activity and physical fitness across the lifespan, *Research Quarterly for Exercise and Sport 67(3, Supplement)*, 48–57.

Malina, R.M. (2001a). Physical activity and fitness. Pathways from childhood to adulthood, *American Journal of Human Biology 13*, 162–172.

Malina, R.M. (2001b). Adherence to physical activity from childhood to adulthood. A perspective from tracking studies, *Quest 53(3)*, 346–355.

Moyaert, W. (2013). *Levenslang light? Lichte organisatievormen van sport vanuit een longitudinaal perspectief. Longitudinale studie naar de stabiliteit in de sportloopbaan van 12 tot 51-jarige vrouwen uit Vlaanderen: bijdrage tot de Leuvense Longitudinale Studie naar Levensstijl, Fysieke Fitheid en Gezondheid* (p. 52). Leuven: KU Leuven, Masters thesis).

Ormrod, J.E. (1999). *Human Learning*. 3rd edition. Upper Saddle River, NJ: Prentice Hall.

Roberts, K. and Brodie, D.A. (1992). *Inner-City Sport: Who Plays and What are the Benefits?* Culemborg: Giordano Bruno.

Scheerder, J., Thomis, M., Vanreusel, B., Lefevre, J., Renson, R., Vanden Eynde, B. and Beunen, G.P. (2006). Sports participation among females from adolescence to adulthood. A longitudinal study, *International Review for the Sociology of Sport*. DOI: 41(3/4): 413–430.

Scheerder, J. and van Bottenburg, M. (2010). Sport light. De opkomst van lichte organisaties in de sport, in B. Pattyn and B. Raymaekers (eds) *In gesprek met morgen (Lessen voor de eenentwintigste eeuw 16)*. (pp. 89–120). Leuven: Universitaire Pers Leuven.

Scheerder, J., Vanreusel, B., Beunen, G., Claessens, A., Renson, R., Thomis, M., Vanden Eynde, B. and Lefevre, J. (2008). Lifetime adherence to sport and physical activity as a goal in physical education. In search of evidence from longitudinal data, in J. Seghers and H. Vangrunderbeek (eds) *Physical Education Research. What's the Evidence?* (pp. 29–40). Leuven: Acco.

Scheerder, J. and Vos, S. (2011). Social stratification in adults' sports participation from a time-trend perspective. Results from a 40-year household study, *European Journal for Sport and Society 8(1+2)*: 31–44.

Skille, E.A. and Solbakken, T. (2014). The relationship between adolescent sport participation and lifelong participation in physical activity in Norway. A critical analysis, *Scandinavian Sport Studies Forum 5*, 25–45. (www.sportstudies.org)

Telama, R., Yang, X., Hirvensalo, M. and Raitakari, O. (2006). Participation in organized youth sport as a predictor of adult physical activity. A 21-year longitudinal study, *Pediatric Exercise Science 17*, 76–88.

Telama, R., Yang, X., Laakso, L. and Viikari, J. (1997). Physical activity in childhood and adolescence as predictors of physical activity in young adulthood, *American Journal of Preventive Medicine 13*, 317–323.

Telama, R., Yang, X., Viikari, J., Välimäki, I., Wanne, O. and Raitakari, O. (2005). Physical activity from childhood to adulthood. A 21-year tracking study, *American Journal of Preventive Medicine 28(3)*, 267–273.

Vandermeerschen, H., Vos, S. and Scheerder, J. (2013). Who's joining the club? Participation of socially vulnerable children and adolescents in club-organised sports, *Sport, Education and Society*. DOI: 10.1080/13573322.2013.856293

Vanreusel, B., Renson, R., Beunen, G., Claessens, A., Lefevre, J., Lysens, R., Maes, H., Simons, J. and Vanden Eynde, B. (1993). Involvement in physical activity from youth to adulthood. A longitudinal analysis, in A.L. Claessens, J. Lefevre and B. Vanden Eynde (eds) *World-wide variation in physical fitness (proceedings of the 1992 Symposium of the ICPAFR, Leuven, July 1992)* (pp. 187–195). Leuven: Institute of Physical Education.

Vanreusel, B., Renson, R., Beunen, G., Claessens, A.L., Lefevre, J., Lysens, R. and Vanden Eynde, B. (1997). A longitudinal study of youth sport participation and adherence to sport in adulthood, *International Review for the Sociology of Sport 32(4)*, 373–387.

Yang, X., Telama, R., Leino, M. and Viikari, J. (1999). Factors explaining the physical activity of young adults. The importance of early socialization, *Scandinavian Journal of Medicine and Science in Sports 9*: 120–127.

16

DROPPING OUT FROM CLUBS, DROPPING IN TO SPORT LIGHT?

Organizational settings for youth sports participation

Julie Borgers, Jan Seghers and Jeroen Scheerder

Introduction

This chapter addresses patterns of sports participation over the life-course from an organizational perspective. In the frame of this handbook on youth sport, the transition stage from youth to adulthood will be addressed in more detail. Studies on sports participation among youngsters are often restricted to traditionally organized sport, defined alike structured and competitive, ludic forms of physical activity that typically take place in a club (Coakley, 2008; McPherson *et al.*, 1989). However, sociological research on sports participation shows an increasing share of informal modalities for organizing sporting practice, which do not fit with such a traditional approach (e.g. Eime *et al.*, 2013; Pilgaard, 2012; Scheerder and van Bottenburg, 2010). In particular, the transition from adolescence to adulthood comes along with changes in daily life patterns of young people, such as entering university, creating new social networks, leaving the parental environment or starting to work, where youngsters have to make decisions regarding conflicting time-occupations. Therefore, it is likely that this new stage relates to changes in values and logics in the experience of leisure-time activities like sport and physical exercise, and may lead to a decreasing interest in club-organized activities (Balish *et al.*, 2014; Jakobsson *et al.*, 2012; Pilgaard, 2013). This chapter investigates which organizational settings 15–25-year-old youngsters engage with in practising sport. Youth will be divided into two groups:

1   adolescents (aged 15–18 years); and
2   young adults (aged 19–25 years).

Besides outlining participation rates in different organizational settings over the life-course, a more detailed picture is elaborated on the reasons for choosing particular organizational settings, sports preferences and, lastly, the profile of participants in different organizational settings; that is to say, as suggested by Taks and Scheerder (2006), the context of participation (organized versus non-organized) and types and diversity of sports preferences are useful components to take into account when examining participation styles.

As in other chapters of this book, we will adopt a broad definition of sports participation, including people's voluntary participation in conventional, structured sports, as well as in recreational, non-organized and/or sporadic sports activities. This will allow for a discussion of the role of traditional sports providers, such as sports clubs, in relation to issues of drop-out and new, lighter, ways of active involvement in sport. The main question for exploration is whether dropping out of organized sports in adolescence and early adulthood leads to a decrease or a shift in sports participation. In the first part of this chapter, the rationale and research context is outlined before empirical evidence is presented and discussed.

Traditional sports clubs versus sport light

Repeated cross-sectional studies have shown that club sports participation is, in many western countries, the most popular setting for sports participation among children and youngsters (Jakobsson *et al.*, 2012; Scheerder *et al.*, 2013; Vandermeerschen *et al.*, 2014). Sports clubs traditionally offer structured/fixed training sessions under the supervision of a coach, as well as facilities, competitions and social activities established for and adapted to specific age groups or stages of development. Being often voluntarily run, sports clubs have for long been the focus of grassroots sports policies in western countries and, from this perspective, gained a major position in the sports landscape, both for recreational and competitive purposes (Vos *et al.*, 2013). From a longitudinal perspective, benefits of participation in club-organized sports are found in terms of lifelong and sustained participation: people who engaged in club-organized or competitive sport at a young age are more likely to engage in sport or lead an active lifestyle in adulthood as compared to those who never practiced sport (De Montes *et al.*, 2011; Kjønniksen *et al.*, 2009; Scheerder *et al.*, 2006, 2008; Telama *et al.*, 2005; Wichstrom *et al.*, 2013). A study by Seghers *et al.* (2015) revealed that youngsters staying in a sports club between 11 and 15 years of age are more independent and self-motivated to practice sport during leisure time as compared with peers who left the club. The authors also found that feeling socially and/or physically safe in the living environment positively predicted continued club membership during adolescence. Moreover, sports clubs are found to be an important site to create and cultivate a supportive environment for health promotion (Geidne *et al.*, 2013; Meganck *et al.*, 2014; Scheerder *et al.*, 2015a, 2015b), as well as for the development of social skills and attitudes, like cooperation, responsibility, empathy, leadership and building positive peer relations (e.g. Engström, 1996; Fraser-Thomas *et al.*, 2005; Mahoney and Stattin, 2000). Seghers *et al.* (2015) detected that youngsters with continued club sports participation between 11 and 15 years of age referred to both personal factors (e.g. enjoyment of the provided activities), social factors (e.g. motivation by other friends), but also structural factors (e.g. quality and accessibility of sports facilities) as important correlates of staying in a club during adolescence. The reported advantages of sports clubs may, for many researchers, be an important argument to focus on organized sport in youth sports research.

Nevertheless, due to societal trends and changes, sports clubs no longer possess a monopoly position in sports provision. Trend research in Flanders has shown that, over a ten-year period, club membership rates of youngsters decreased from 57 per cent to 52 per cent (Scheerder and Seghers, 2011). However, clubs are increasingly challenged by new, less formal ways of practising and organizing sport (Eime *et al.*, 2014; Pilgaard, 2013; Scheerder and van Bottenburg, 2010). A pluralized structure of sports providers has come into existence since the 1970s with the implementation of (local) sport for all policies, by which municipalities increasingly provide and facilitate sport. In more recent years, many commercially driven health and fitness centres have also been established, and market-oriented mass sports events have entered the sporting arena (Scheerder and van Bottenburg, 2010; Vos *et al.*, 2013). In addition, people have increasingly tended to organize sports by themselves, in informal groups or alone (Eime *et al.*, 2014; Klostermann and Nagel, 2014; Scheerder *et al.*, 2011; Scheerder and Vos, 2011). As Green *et al.* (2014, p. 13) observe, 'shifts are underway in the manner in which youngsters [in his study, among Norwegian youth] participate in sport (not only *what* they do, *how*, *where* and with *whom* they do it, but also *why* they do it)'. This was also observed in surveys in the Flemish context, where participation styles seem to diversify and expand from traditional ways of practising sport (i.e. typically club-organized, competitive), towards an increased interest for alternative popular action sports, exclusive glide sports or lifestyle sports, which are newer on the scene and/or do not necessarily take place within a club-organized structure. Such sports are favoured to be practiced with peers and/or individually (Borgers *et al.*, 2015; Scheerder *et al.*, 2005; Taks and Scheerder, 2006).

It is suggested that such new ways of sports participation particularly emerge among adults, as they may be an answer to a need for more flexible arrangements when entering new stages of life (Pilgaard, 2013; Scheerder and Vos, 2011). Taks and Scheerder (2006) found that among/within 6–18-year-old youngsters, the group of late-adolescents were most likely to practise sport in a non-organized context. Therefore, such generational and life-stage effects are important to consider when explaining patterns of participation among 15–25-year-old youngsters, a group facing significant changes in the transition to adulthood. That is, after leaving the secondary school system, young adults enter a more independent stage of life where they put a focus on education and career building before the parent phase and where schedules are more changeable and flexible than in the traditional school system (Pilgaard, 2013). For this reason, the current study will distinguish between adolescents (15–18-years old) and young adults (19–25-years old). Generally, little is known about patterns of sports participation among youngsters in the transition period from adolescence to young adulthood. Overall, there is consensus in the literature that many adolescents quit club-organized and competitive sport in the late teenage years (Berger *et al.*, 2008; Crane and Temple, 2015; Jakobsson *et al.*, 2012; Pilgaard, 2013; Scheerder *et al.*, 2006, 2008; Taks and Scheerder, 2006; Vandermeerschen *et al.*, 2014). However, there is a lack of evidence to state whether they quit sports in general, or if they move away from clubs to other settings of participatory sport. In this regard, recent studies on drop-out among children and youth revealed that reasons and determinants for drop-out are mainly located on the intrapersonal and interpersonal level (Balish *et al.*, 2014; Crane and Temple, 2015). Crane and Temple classified major reasons for quitting organized sport in five categories:

1   lack of enjoyment
2   perceptions of (in)competence
3   social pressures
4   competing priorities
5   physical factors (maturation and injuries).

According to Balish *et al.* (2014), the main correlates for sport-specific attrition are age, autonomy, perceptions of (in)competence, a lack of social attachment (relatedness) and the task climate. In a study by Seghers *et al.* (2015), however, these reasons were preceded by time-constraints (e.g. the hours do not fit with patterns of daily life) as the most reported reason to drop out from a club. When considering life-stage effects, however, one should also be aware of potential conflicting interests between young adults' programmes and the fixed course offers of sports clubs (Pilgaard, 2013). Whereas clubs in their traditional approach expect regular attendance in order to engage in competition and social activities, more 'light' self-organized or commercially organized activities may better suit the demands for flexibility and sports preferences of young adults (e.g. Pilgaard, 2013).

Research materials and methods

Data

The study conducted in light of this contribution builds on a large-scale cross-sectional participation survey regarding the domains of culture, youth, sport and media in Flanders (Belgium). This survey was carried out in 2014 by the Flemish Policy Research Centre on Culture, Youth, Sports and Media (supported by the Flemish government) among a representative sample of 15–86-year-old people (n=3,951). For the purpose of this study, we will mainly focus on patterns of sports participation in 15–25-year-old adolescents and young adults (n=594), of whom 81.3 per cent participated in sport.

Sports participation in this survey was defined as active participation in sport during leisure-time, whether for competitive or recreational purposes, at least once during the past twelve months. Sports and physical activities for merely utilitarian purposes (e.g. transport to work or shopping) were not included. For the purpose of this study, organizational settings for sports participation were classified as follows:

- Sports clubs. Conventional (non-profit, often voluntarily ran) community based and non-governmental sports associations with scheduled trainings, offering at least one sports activity. Membership is required to be able to use the facilities and/or offers provided by the club. Activities often take place at fixed times and places, where attendance is expected as part of the team, in preparation of an event or competition, and so forth;
- Alternative organizations. Organizations that provide sports activities without long-term membership requirements. The activities take place at a designated place and/or time, but participants are free to come and go when they want or engage for a short-term package (e.g. 10-hours card, one-day event, etc.). Generally speaking, alternative organizations are more flexible to engage in than sports clubs. Examples are health and fitness centres, programmes or summer camps offered by (local) sports authorities, optional after-school sports activities, mass sports events and organized sports holidays or sports tourism;
- Informal groups. Self-organized groups of friends, family members, colleagues or other kinds of sports *buddies* that gather to practise sport independently from a formal organization with an active sports supply; and
- Individual sports participation. Self- or non-organized sports participation where the participant is alone and independent from a formal organization with an active sports supply.

The concept of 'sport light' (Scheerder and van Bottenburg, 2010) captures all settings beyond and within the traditional structures of a sports club, which allows for a more flexible experience of the sporting practice (i.e. alternative organizations, informal groups, individual practices).

Statistical procedures

First, descriptive (bivariate) analyses were carried out to map the popularity of distinct organizational settings for sports participation over the life-course (age 15–86), reasons to choose for certain organizational settings and the popularity of sports activities in different organizational settings. Second, the profile of adolescents and young adults engaging in *club* and/or *light* settings is investigated using multinomial regression analysis. The dependent variable consists of three categories, representing adolescents and young adults that engage in sport:

- only in a club
- only in sport light
- both in a club and a light setting.

The latter category was constructed because active adolescents and young adults may participate in multiple sports activities, albeit in various organizational settings (Taks and Scheerder, 2006). The independent variables include demographic and socioeconomic variables, sporting capital, characteristics of the current sports activity and perceptions on the availability of leisure-time. Demographic and socioeconomic variables, as well as sporting capital, were included because they are found to play an important role in explaining sports participation among youngsters (e.g. Kraaykamp *et al.*, 2013; Nielsen *et al.*, 2012; Taks and Scheerder, 2006; Scheerder *et al.*, 2005; Vandermeerschen *et al.*, 2013, 2014). Demographics control for age, gender, level of education (still studying or not) and level of urbanization (living area). Socioeconomic variables include the parental socioeconomic status (SES, based on level of education of the parents) and financial status (i.e. a subjective measure of how easy/difficult it was to financially sustain the household). The sporting capital of the adolescents and young adults was based on whether or not the parents practiced sport at the respondent's age of 12–14-years old. The inclusion of sports related factors such as current sports activity (type of main sport), sports diversity, the average time spent on sport per week and travel distance, as well as motives for sports participation, were included to enhance understanding of the background of club-organized and light sports participants. Also one's perception on the availability of leisure-time is included. According to studies that found that people experiencing time constraints spend less time on sport (e.g. Downward, 2007; Ruseski *et al.*, 2011; Wicker, Breuer and Pawlowski, 2009), this may help to explain whether or not – among sports participants – time-perceptions relate to the way of organizing the sporting practice. The diversity of background variables included in the multivariate model also allows for exploring which factors contribute more or less to explaining patterns of sports participation among youngsters.

A life-course perspective on organizational settings for sports participation

Figure 16.1 provides a life-course perspective on club sports participation and participation in light forms of sport among 15–86-year-old Flemish people. It shows that sports participation is the highest among adolescents aged 15–18 years, and participation rates decrease gradually thereafter (see also Breedveld and Hoekman, 2011; Breuer and Wicker, 2009; Gratton *et al.*, 2011; Scheerder *et al.*, 2006, 2008; Stamm and Lamprecht, 2005; van Bottenburg *et al.*, 2005). Even though general participation rates do not differ substantially between adolescents (82.9 per cent) and young adults aged 19–25 years (80.1 per cent), club sports participation shows a significant drop (-23 per cent) in the transition to adulthood. Contrary, the graphic line shows a substantial rise in individual (i.e. non-organized) sports participation in this stage. Alternative organizations are most popular among the 19–25-year-old age group and lose share in later stages of life. The popularity of these alternative organizations is mainly attributed to participation in fitness centres that attract significantly more young adults (age 19–25 years) as compared to adolescents (age 15–18). Table 16.1 confirms that the age-related differences regarding club-organized sport and alternative organizations are significantly different between adolescents and young adults. The age-effect for individual sports participation, however, is only significant for the total number of people practicing sport individually per age group. Informal groups show a relatively stable share of participants over the total course of life.

Overall, we can conclude that general sports participation keeps stable between adolescents and young adults, but the organizational setting changes. As such, drop-out rates in sports clubs around the age of 18 rather imply a shift in participation (drop in to sport light) than patterns of inactivity. However, to adequately address the relation between patterns of drop-out and drop-in, longitudinal research would be more appropriate to look at shifts on an individual level.

Sports preferences and reasons to engage in organizational settings

Tables 16.2a and 16.2b present reasons to engage in sport in a particular setting. This may help to understand why sports participants in different age groups choose for different types of organization. For each sport practised, respondents indicated the main setting to practise that sport, and why this was used the most. About half (53 per cent) of the respondents indicated to mainly engage in a sports club for a particular sport, whereas 64 per cent mainly practised at least one sport in a light setting.

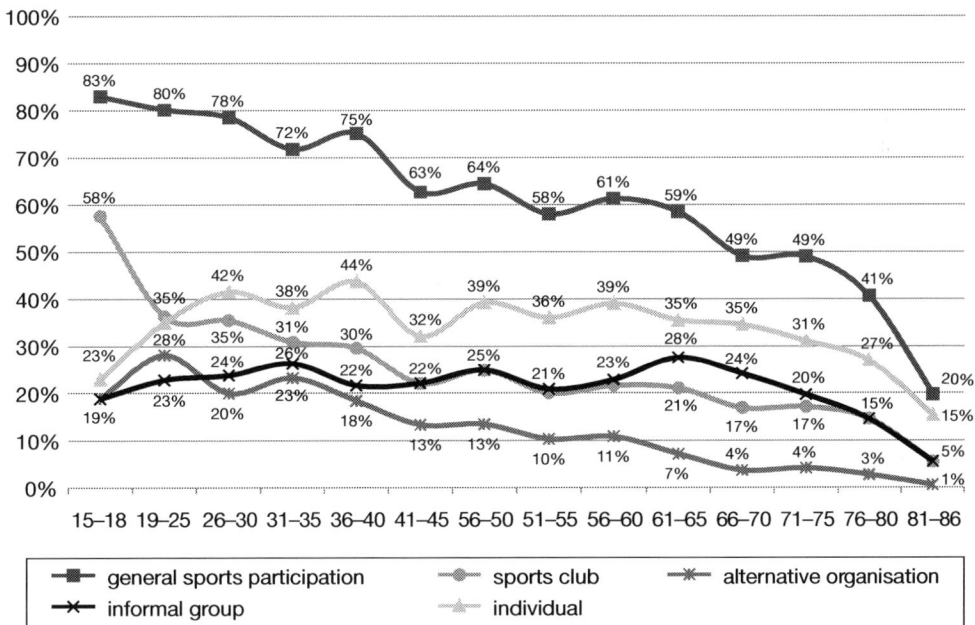

Figure 16.1 Organizational settings of sports participation over the life-course (general sports participation, club-organized sport, alternative organization, informal group, individual participation); cross-sectional data of 15- to 86-year-old people in Flanders; percentages of population (n=3,951)

163

Table 16.1 Overview of popularity of organizational settings for sports participation among 15- to 18-year-old (n=180) versus 19- to 25-year-old (n=303) youngsters; percentages of sports participants

	15–18 yrs (n=180)		19–25 yrs (n=303)		Significant age difference?	
	at least one sport in . . .	only in . . .	at least one sport in . . .	only in . . .	at least one sport in . . .	only in . . .
Sports club	57.6	41.7	36.3	18.8	★★★	★★★
Alternative organization	18.9	5.0	28.1	15.2	★★	★★★
Informal group	18.8	9.4	22.8	8.9	NS	NS
Individual	22.9	10.0	35.0	14.5	★★★	NS

Note: *p<.05, **p<.01, ***p<.001, NS=not significant.

From the results it appears that sports clubs were mostly used for the social context (26.0 per cent) or because they were perceived as the only possible way to practice the sport (24.6 per cent). The social environment was also an important reason for sport light (24.3 per cent). Furthermore, 'light' settings were chosen because it was the easiest way (37.5 per cent) or without a particular reason (24.4 per cent). The ease of organization is mostly reported by the oldest age group, whereas adolescents more often mention that sport light is the only way to practice a sport, or that they do not have a particular reason. Such arguments may refer to a limited knowledge on the availability of other facilities and opportunities to practice the sport, because in the Flemish context most sports are offered by a federation and/or sports clubs.

The popularity of sports activities in general and over different organizational settings is presented in Table 16.2b. This includes a top fifteen of all sports that were reported by the respondents. One sport could be practiced in one or more settings. It is possible to identify more or less typically club-based or light sports activities. The list is led by light activities such as fitness (25.4 per cent), running (22.2 per cent) and recreational swimming (14.6 per cent), for which only about one third of the participants engaged in a club. Soccer (20.7 per cent) was the third most popular sport, represented by about 81 per cent of participants that play in a club. Other typically club-based sports (i.e. at least 50 per cent participate in a club) included racket sports, dancing, other team ball sports, horse riding and martial arts. Consistent with previous findings, it was observed that age differences carried over in the type of sports practiced: typically club-based sports were more popular among adolescents, whereas light activities were preferred by young adults (Green et al., 2014).

Profiles of youngsters in club-organized sport versus 'sport light'

Tables 16.4 and 16.5 display frequencies and odds rates (Exp(β)), respectively, of background variables in relation to the organizational setting for sports participation. For the purpose of the current contribution, three categories are compared in the dependent variable (organizational setting for sports participation):

1   *only club* sports participants (27.4 per cent)
2   *only light* sports participants (45.7 per cent)
3   *club and light* sports participants (26.9 per cent)

Table 16.2a Reasons for participating in club and light settings among 15- to 25-year-old sports participants, per sport; percentages of sports participants

Reason for participation in context . . .	Club (n=255)	Light (n=316)
Because of the social environment (friends, family)	26.0	24.3
Because it is the only way to practice this sport	24.6	10.6
Because this is the easiest way to organize the sporting practice	14.0	37.5
No particular reason	13.5	24.4
Because it is the closest to home	10.5	9.6
Because I don't know another way	9.6	4.3
Because it is the cheapest opportunity	1.1	4.2
Due to bad experiences in other settings	0.8	0.9

Table 16.2b Reasons for participating in club and light settings among 15- to 25-year-old sports participants, per age group (15–18 vs. 19–25), per sport; percentages of sports participants

Reason for participation in context . . .	Club			Light		
	Age 15–18	Age 19–25	Sign.	Age 15–18	Age 19–25	Sign.
Because of the social environment (friends, family)	22.4	29.8	NS	19.6	26.3	NS
Because it is the only way to practice this sport	24.2	24.6	NS	16.3	8.0	★
Because this is the easiest way to organize the sporting practice	10.4	17.6	NS	23.1	43.3	★★★
No particular reason	16.0	10.8	NS	33.7	20.5	★
Because it is the closest to home	12.9	8.4	NS	9.8	9.4	NS
Because I don't know another way	12.1	6.9	NS	5.4	4.0	NS
Because it is the cheapest opportunity	0.8	1.5	NS	4.3	4.5	NS
Due to bad experiences in other settings	1.6	0.0	NS	0.0	1.3	NS

Note: ★$p<.05$, ★★$p<.01$, ★★★$p<.001$, NS=not significant.

In the multivariate model (Table 16.3b), the first group (*only club* sports participants) was used as the reference category in order to be able to compare and discuss new profiles of participants. The odds rates (Exp(β)) for practicing sport in *only light* or *combi club+light* are to be interpreted in relation to the reference variable, i.e. *only club* sports participants. The overall model explains 51.2 per cent of the total variance in the dependent variable (i.e. organizational setting for sports participation). Generally, the sports related variables appear to contribute to the largest part (39 per cent) of the explanation in the dependent variable. The variance explained by each block (pseudo Nagelkerke R^2) is presented in the model.

From the multinomial regression analysis, it appears that age remains a significant predictor for the organizational setting of sports participation even when other controlling variables are taken into account: 19- to 25-year-old sports participants were about twice as likely than 15- to 18-year-old youngsters to practice sport *only* in a light setting (p<.05). This concurs with findings from other studies stating that the likelihood of active involvement in club-based sport decreases with age (Pilgaard, 2013; Vandermeerschen, 2014). To practice sport only in a club or in both a club and a light setting, however, was not influenced by age. In the current model, the latter was only affected by sports diversity (i.e. the number of sports activities one currently

Table 16.3a Top fifteen sports preferences among adolescents (aged 15 to 18 years) and young adults (aged 19 to 25 years) in Flanders; percentages of sports participants (n=483), per sport

		Total sample n=483	Age	
			15 to 18 (n=180)	19 to 25 (n=303)
1.	fitness	25.4	13.3	32.7
2.	running	22.2	17.2	25.2
3.	soccer (i.e. field soccer, soccer, futsal, street soccer)	20.7	21.1	20.4
4.	recreational swimming (not in a club)	14.6	7.1	19.1
5.	racket sports (tennis, table tennis, squash, badminton)	10.4	12.2	9.4
6.	dancing	9.9	18.5	4.8
7.	traditional team ball sports (basketball, (beach)volleyball, handball)	5.6	7.8	4.3
8.	recreational cycling	5.4	3.5	6.5
9.	horse riding, equestrianism	4.6	5.8	3.9
10.	winter sports (e.g. skiing, snowboarding, cross-country skiing, ice skating)	3.9	4.5	3.5
11.	martial arts	2.9	3.6	2.4
12.	swimming (club)	2.7	2.9	2.6
13.	recreational walking	2.4	1.1	3.1
14.	aerobics	2.3	1.0	3.0
15.	road cycling	2.0	1.1	2.6

practices): logically, one is more likely to engage in both club and light settings if at least two different sports are practiced (p<.001). Furthermore, in the overall model, boys are more likely than girls to engage only in a light setting than only in a club ($Exp(\beta)$=3.862, p<.01). It should be noted that the significant effect of gender only appeared when including sports related variables, which explained the majority of variance in the current model (cf. supra). This may partially explain the seemingly contradicting findings regarding the frequencies displayed in Table 3.3.3a, where a 50–50 distribution of boys and girls in light settings is observed.

Youngsters from higher social strata (high SES) were less likely to engage in sport light than in club-organized sport ($Exp(\beta)$=.382, p<.05). This opens up opportunities for groups of lower social strata, who have been found to be out of reach of organized sports activities (e.g. Vandermeerschen, 2013). Consistently, there was also a trend for sport light to involve more people with financial constraints; although this effect was not found to be significant in the multivariate model. According to previous research, parental sporting capital may be an important factor to consider when explaining sports participation in general (e.g. Kraaykamp *et al.*, 2013; Scheerder *et al.*, 2007; Taks and Scheerder, 2006), but does not appear to influence whether or not participants engage in a club or in sport light.

Participation in solo sports (i.e. sports that can be practised alone on recreational purposes) was more likely to predict light sports participation as compared to participation in duo and team sports, where one depends on one or more team mates or opponents for the sport to be practiced. This concurs with findings on sports preferences, where sports such as running, cycling, swimming or fitness were observed to be more favourable for practicing outside of a club.

With regard to consumer characteristics of sports participants, the results show that youngsters spending more time on sport were less likely to engage in sport light than in a club. This suggested

Table 16.3b Top fifteen sports preferences among adolescents (aged 15 to 18 years) and young adults (aged 19 to 25 years) in Flanders; row percentages of participants per sport in different organizational settings

	Organizational settings (100 per cent)					
	Only club	Only alternative organization	Only informal group	Only individual	Combi light settings	Combi club and light
1. fitness	7.2	35.4	2.2	3.5	21.9	29.8
2. running	1.7	1.4	7.0	28.8	27.8	33.2
3. soccer (i.e. field soccer, soccer, futsal, street soccer)	47.5	0.8	10.3	1.9	6.2	33.3
4. recreational swimming (not in a club)	0.0	3.8	25.8	28.1	19.4	23.0
5. racket sports (tennis, table tennis, squash, badminton)	24.2	6.0	0.0	3.7	7.6	58.5
6. dancing	47.8	7.9	1.1	1.5	0.0	41.8
7. traditional team ball sports (basketball, (beach)volleyball, handball)	23.8	0.0	0.0	4.3	15.4	56.6
8. recreational cycling	0.0	0.0	10.9	7.3	52.5	29.3
9. horse riding, equestrianism	35.2	0.0	0.0	12.9	15.9	36.0
10. winter sports (e.g. skiing, snowboarding, cross-country skiing, ice skating)	17.7	2.7	11.8	0.0	31.6	36.2
11. martial arts	55.6	0.0	10.9	0.0	0.0	33.6
12. swimming (club)	43.1	0.0	0.0	0.0	0.0	56.9
13. recreational walking	0.0	10.1	40.6	6.3	35.8	7.3
14. aerobics	32.6	13.8	0.0	4.6	20.2	28.8
15. road cycling	16.9	0.0	0.0	0.0	0.0	83.1

Note: light settings = settings outside of a club (i.e. alternative, informal groups and/or individual).

that sports clubs have the ability to build more time-intensive, thus sustainable, patterns of participation for youngsters as compared to more flexible settings. Even though the time people spend on sport might still be influenced by other factors (e.g. age, gender, etc.), on this view, sports clubs could be considered as health promoting settings to contribute to reaching guidelines for sport and physical activity (Geidne *et al.*, 2013). On the other hand, neither the distance people cover to reach facilities for practicing sport, nor the living environment, differs significantly between club and light sports participants. Also, even though other authors (e.g. Pilgaard, 2012; Scheerder and van Bottenburg, 2010) often intuitively refer to issues of time-pressure when it concerns sport light, the experience of time-availability does not affect the context to participate in sport for youngsters.

Lastly we point to the reasons for sports participation. Participants reporting health- and body-related motives for sports participation (i.e. weight loss, appearance, improving health and physical condition) were more likely to engage in light settings as compared to club-based sport ($Exp(\beta)$=3.244, p<.01). This was also reflected in the character of typical light sports activities, which were mainly keep-fit activities such as fitness, swimming, running and cycling. On the other hand, club sports participation was predicted by higher scale scores on motives related to sociability and competitiveness.

Table 16.4 Background characteristics of sports participants in different organizational settings, age 15 to 25; percentages of sports participants in 'only club', 'only light', 'combi club+light'

		Only club (n=132)	Only light (n=221)	Combi club+light (n=130)	Sign.
	Demographic variables				
age	15 to 18 years old	56.8	25.0	38.5	★★★
	19 to 25 years old	43.2	75.0	61.5	
gender	girls	49.2	50.7	43.8	NS
	boys	50.8	49.3	56.2	
education	no full-time education	27.1	43.0	35.4	★
	full-time education	72.9	57.0	64.6	
living environment	big city (Brussels, Antwerp, Ghent)	11.5	12.3	12.3	NS
	suburb around big city	8.4	10.0	6.9	
	middle-sized city (centre city)	10.7	12.7	10.0	
	suburb around middle-sized city, small city	29.0	21.4	33.1	
	transition area	28.2	25.9	21.5	
	rural area	12.2	17.7	16.2	
	Socioeconomic variables				
SES parents	low	5.3	7.2	3.8	NS
	medium	20.5	26.7	15.4	
	high	74.2	66.1	80.8	
financial situation	difficult	1.6	3.8	0.8	NS
	medium	34.4	41.1	33.6	
	easy	64.0	55.0	65.6	
	Sporting capital				
parental sports participation at respondent's age 12 to 14	none of the parents practiced sport	35.4	53.9	35.4	★★
	one of the parents practiced sport	41.5	27.4	36.9	
	both parents practiced sport	23.1	18.7	27.7	
	Current sports participation				
type of main sports activity	solo	49.6	88.7	50.0	★★★
	duo	11.5	2.3	19.2	
	team	38.9	9.0	30.8	
sports diversity	1 sport	77.3	67.9	14.6	★★★
	at least 2 sports	22.7	32.1	85.4	
average time spent on sport per week	≤1 hour per week	18.9	51.1	10.0	★★★
	>1 up to 3 hours per week	31.1	24.9	31.5	
	>3 up to 5 hours per week	21.2	11.8	20.0	
	>5 hours per week	28.8	12.2	38.5	
travel distance for sports participation	0 – 3 km	32.3	42.7	28.0	★
	>3 up to 7 km	26.2	27.2	32.3	
	>7 up to 20 km	31.5	23.8	32.3	
	>20 up to 100 km	10.0	4.9	3.2	
	> 100 km	0.0	1.2	4.3	

Note: ★*p*<.05, ★★*p*<.01, ★★★*p*<.001, NS=not significant.

continued . . .

Table 16.4 Continued

		Only club (n=132)	Only light (n=221)	Combi club+light (n=130)	Sign.
	Motives for sports participation				
social	not important	22.9	68.8	36.2	★★★
	important	77.1	31.2	63.8	
health & body	not important	25.0	12.7	11.5	★★
	important	75.0	87.3	88.5	
competition	not important	56.8	91.8	63.1	★★★
	important	43.2	8.2	36.9	
stress release	not important	31.1	43.4	35.4	NS
	important	68.9	56.6	64.6	
fun	not important	0.8	5.0	1.5	★
	important	99.2	95.0	98.5	
	Perceptions on leisure-time availability				
perceived	few	25.6	33.0	33.1	NS
availability of	sufficient	55.6	46.6	50.0	
leisure time	many	18.8	20.4	16.1	

Note: ★*p*<.05, ★★*p*<.01, ★★★*p*<.001, NS=not significant.

Table 16.5 Multinomial regression analysis of organizational settings for sports participation among 15- to 25-years old youngsters in Flanders (n=483); reference variable = 'only club'

	only light Exp(β)	combi club+light Exp(β)
Demographic variables (Nagelkerke R^2 = .108)		
age (15 to 18 years old = ref.)		
19 to 25 years old	2.315★	1.426
gender (girls = ref.)		
boys	3.862★★	1.811
education (no full-time education = ref.)		
full-time education	.952	.931
living environment (rural area = ref.)		
big city (Brussels, Antwerp, Ghent)	.656	.356
suburb around big city	1.580	.456
middle-sized city (centre city)	1.572	.878
suburb around middle-sized city, small city	.380	.557
transition area	.514	.505
Socioeconomic variables (Nagelkerke R^2 = .46)		
SES parents (medium = ref.)		
low	.588	.570
high	.382★	1.167

Note: ★*p*<.05, ★★*p*<.01, ★★★*p*<.001, NS=not significant.

continued . . .

Table 16.5 Continued

	only light Exp(β)	*combi club+light* Exp(β)
financial situation (medium = ref.)		
difficult	4.764	.819
easy	1.037	.898
Sporting capital (Nagelkerke R^2 = .29)		
Parental sports participation at respondent's age 12 to 14 (none of the parents practiced sport = ref.)		
one of the parents practiced sport	.483	.823
both parents practiced sport	.572	.644
Current sports participation (Nagelkerke R^2 = .39)		
type of main sports activity (solo = ref.)		
duo	.126★★	.983
team	.135★★★	.448
sports diversity (at least 2 sports = ref.)		
1 sport	.517	.068★★★
average time spent on sports per week (≤1 hour per week = ref.)		
>1 up to 3 hours per week	.520	1.,740
>3 up to 5 hours per week	.258★	.806
>5 hours per week	.303★	1.489
travel distance for sports participation (0 - 3 km = ref.)		
>3 up to 7 km	1.583	1.662
>7 up to 20 km	.654	1.043
>20 up to 100 km	.452	.480
>100 km	5.721	6.301
Motives for sports participation (Nagelkerke R^2 = .41)		
reason sport: social (not important = ref.)		
reason sport: social (important)	.283★★★	.619
reason sport: health, body (not important = ref.)		
reason sport: health, body (important)	3.244★★	1.636
reason sport: competition (not important = ref.)		
reason sport: competition (important)	.324★	.702
reason sport: stress release (not important = ref.)		
reason sport: stress release (important)	.865	1.060
reason sport: fun (not important = ref.)		
reason sport: fun (important)	.323	.867
Perceptions on leisure-time availability (Nagelkerke R^2 = .03)		
perceived availability of leisure-time (sufficient = ref.)		
few	1.715	1.366
many	1.450	.880

Notes: Pseudo R^2 = .617 (Nagelkerke); Model $\chi^2(62)$=288.344. ★$p<.05$, ★★$p<.01$, ★★★$p<.001$, NS=not significant.

Conclusion

The goal of this chapter was to outline patterns of sports participation in youth from a social-organizational perspective. More particularly, a focus was put on 15- to 18-year-old adolescents and 19- to 25-year-old young adults to detect whether and how patterns of sports participation change in the transition stage from youth to adulthood. For the purpose of this study, data were used from a large scale cross-sectional survey on sports participation in Flanders. Profiles of sports participants were outlined in relation to the organizational setting of sports participation and sports preferences.

It was shown that youngsters in the transition stage of youth cannot be targeted as a single market (Green *et al.*, 2014; Taks and Scheerder, 2006). That is, participation patterns not only differ with regard to sports preferences (Green *et al.*, 2014; Taks and Scheerder, 2006); but also in the way youngsters organize their sporting practice. Whereas 15- to 18-year-old adolescents are more inclined to engage in the traditional club sports system, the transition to adulthood appears to come along with a drop-out from club-organized sport (Balish *et al.*, 2014; Crane and Temple, 2015) and a drop-in to sport light. As the data used in the frame of this study are cross-sectional, however, it is impossible to state whether patterns of drop-out and drop-in are observed in the same person or not. Nevertheless, regarding the general participation rates, it is likely to assume that commonly reported issues of drop-out in adolescence (Balish *et al.*, 2014; Crane and Temple, 2015) should not be perceived as drop-out from sport per se: moving away from sports clubs does not necessarily mean becoming inactive. We therefore suggest future studies on sports participation and drop-out to embrace a more all-encompassing definition of sport and patterns of participation. This means also including non-traditional, informal, self-organized sports activities, as well looking at changes to other contexts and/or activities as a form of drop-out.

Such a change relates to different types of sports activities that are more or less characterized by needs for structural support or facilities (e.g. courts or specific materials), technical or tactical coaching and the presence of other people (solo sports versus team sports). Even though sports-related variables were shown to deliver the largest share of explained variance in the model, it appears that it is also important to take into account underlying motivations, patterns of daily life and other background characteristics that may guide people's choices of activities or participation style. For example, young adults and youngsters with lower SES and youngsters seeking for a healthy lifestyle and/or a positive image of the body (appearance, weight loss) are more likely to enter the sports scene through light settings, whereas adolescents, youngsters with higher SES and people seeking for competitiveness and social interaction are more likely to engage in a sports club.

On the one hand, the advantages of light settings for sports participation are to be highlighted; that is, light ways of organization seem to better suit the needs and sports preferences of (young) adults, resulting in higher participation rates among those groups. Also, the fact that youngsters from lower SES backgrounds are more likely to engage in light settings than in club-organized sport suggests a way in to sport for those young people that have traditionally been found to be inactive and/or out of reach of club-organized sport (Vandermeerschen *et al.*, 2013). On the other hand, light settings could be criticized in terms of the level of intensity they produce. As, on average, club sports participation shows more time-intensive patterns of participation, this is suggested as more effective and efficient in terms of health promotion. This relates to advantages of club sports participation mentioned by previous (longitudinal) research, which reveals that youth club sports participation is more sustainable in light of lifelong sports participation and levels of physical activity (De Montes *et al.*, 2011; Kjønniksen *et al.*, 2009;

Scheerder *et al.*, 2006, 2008; Telama *et al.*, 2005; Wichstrom *et al.*, 2013). For these reasons, it is important for sports providers, such as clubs, to broaden their focus and be aware of current trends and shifts in sports participation to fulfil their role of 'health promoting settings' (Geidne *et al.*, 2013).

This study is not without limitations and makes some suggestions to future research. First, as a subsample of a representative survey on sports participation in 15- to 86-year-old Flemish people, the group of sports active youngsters is relatively small. Particularly when comparing age groups (i.e. adolescents versus young adults), the sample size did not allow for making subdivisions to more specific settings for sports participation, such as after school programmes, activities provided by local sports authorities, in fitness centres and so forth. Due to the sample restrictions, it was impossible to say something about levels of drop-out from (organized) sport that may occur earlier in youth, for example between childhood and adolescence. As mentioned before, the cross-sectional approach of this study does not allow for tracking the evolution of patterns of sports participation over the life-course of a certain person. For future research on drop-out, it is therefore suggested that research investigates not only why and when people drop-out from organized sport (e.g. Balish *et al.*, 2014; Crane and Temple, 2015), but also which activities they subsequently drop-in to from a longitudinal perspective.

Furthermore, the outcomes of this study provide implications to the policy and marketing of traditional sports clubs. According to a study of Jakobsson *et al.* (2012), it seems that club-organized sport is not fully tailored to the demands of all youngsters but appears to select youngsters with specific dispositions and assets in terms of habitus and sports capital to stay in a club during adolescence and later adulthood. To increase their market share, thus to promote lifelong and sustainable sports participation to a wide range of participants, sports clubs are challenged to offer opportunities and market-oriented programmes in a less formal and more flexible atmosphere.

Acknowledgements

This research project was funded by the Flemish Policy Research Centre on Culture, Youth, Sports and Media (supported by the Flemish government).

References

Balish, S.M., McLaren, C., Rainham, D. and Blanchard, C. (2015). Correlates of youth sport attrition: A review and future directions, *Psychology of Sport and Exercise*, *15*, 429–439.

Borgers, J., Thibaut, E., Vandermeerschen, H., Vanreusel, B., Vos, S. and Scheerder, J. (2015). Sports participation styles revisited: A time-trend study in Belgium from the 1970s to the 2000s, *International Review for the Sociology of Sport*, *50*(1), 45–63.

Breedveld, K. and Hoekman, R. (2011). Measuring sports participation in the Netherlands – the need to go beyond guidelines, *European Journal for Sport and Society*, *8*, 117–132.

Breuer, C. and Wicker, P. (2009). Decreasing sports activity with increasing age? Findings from a 20-year longitudinal and cohort sequence analysis, *Research Quarterly for Exercise and Sport*, *80(1)*, 22–31.

Coakley, J. (2008). *Sports in society. Issues and controversies* (10th edition). New York: McGraw-Hill.

Crane, J. and Temple, V. (2015). A systematic review of dropout from organized sport among children and youth, *European Physical Education Review*, DOI: 10.1177/1356336X14555294.

De Montes, L.G., Arruza, J.A., Arribas, S., Irazusta, S. and Telletxea, S. (2011). The role of organized sports participation during adolescence in adults physical activity patterns, *Sport Science Review*, *20 (5/6)*, 37–51.

Downward, P. (2007). Exploring the economic choice to participate in sport. Results from the 2002 general household survey, *International Review of Applied Economy*, *21*(5), 633–653.

Eime, R.M., Sawyer, N., Harvey, J.T., Casey, M.M., Westerbeek, H. and Payne, W.R. (2014). Integrating public health and sport management. Sport participation trends 2001–2010, *Sport Management Review*, available at http://dx.doi.org/10.1016/j.smr.2014.05.004.

Engström, L.-M. (1996). Sweden, in P. De Knop, L-M. Engström, B. Skirstad, M.R. Weiss (eds) *Worldwide trends in youth sport* (pp. 231–243). Champaign, Illinois: Human Kinetics.

Fraser-Thomas, J., Côté, J. and Deakin J. (2005). Youth sport programs: an avenue to foster positive youth development, *Physical Education and Sport Pedagogy*, 10, 19–40.

Geidne, S., Quennerstedt, M., Eriksson, C. (2013). The youth sports club as a health-promoting setting. An integrative review of research, *Scandinavian Journal of Public Health*, 41(3), 269–283.

Gratton, C., Rowe, N. and Veal, A.J. (2011). International comparisons of sports participation in European countries: An update of the COMPASS project, *European Journal for Sport and Society*, 8, 99–116.

Green, K., Thurston, M. and Vaage, O. (2014). Isn't it good, Norwegian wood? Lifestyle and adventure sports participation among Norwegian youth, *Leisure Studies*, DOI: 10.1080/02614367.2014.938771.

Jakobsson, B.T., Lundvall, S., Redelius, K. and Engström, L.-M. (2012). Almost all start but who continue? A longitudinal study of youth participation in Swedish club sports, *Physical Education Review*, 18(1), 3–18.

Kjønniksen, L. Anderssen, N. and Wold, B. (2009). Organized youth sport as a predictor of physical activity in adulthood, *Scandinavian Journal of Medicine and Science in Sports*, 19, 646–54.

Klostermann, C. and Nagel, S. (2014). Changes in German sports participation. Historical trends in individual sports, *International Review for the Sociology of Sport*, 49(5), 609–634.

Kraaykamp, G., Oldenkamp, M. and Breedveld, K. (2013). Starting a sport in the Netherlands. A life-course analysis of the effects of individual, parental and partner characteristics, *International Review for the Sociology of Sport*, 48(2), 153–170.

Mahoney, J.L. and Stattin, H. (2000). Leisure activities and adolescent antisocial behavior: the role of structure and social context, *Journal of Adolescence*, 23, 113–27.

McPherson, B.C., Curtis, J.E. and Loy, J.W. (1989). *The social significance of sport. An introduction to the sociology of sport*. Champaign, Illinois: Human Kinetics.

Meganck, J., Scheerder, J., Thibaut, E. and Seghers, J. (2014). Youth sports clubs' potential as health promoting setting. Profiles, motives and barriers, *Health Education Journal*, early online, art.nr. DOI: 10.1177/0017896914549486.

Nielsen, G., Grønfeldt, V., Toftegaard-Støckel, J. and Andersen, L.B. (2012). Predisposed to participate? The influence of family socio-economic background on children's sports participation and daily amount of physical activity, *Sport in Society: Cultures, Commerce, Media, Politics*, 15(1), 1–27

Pilgaard, M. (2013). Age specific differences in sports participation in Denmark. Is development caused by generation, life phase or time period effects? *European Journal of Sport and Society*, 10(1), 31–52.

Ruseski, J.E., Humphreys, B.R., Hallmann, K. and Breuer, C. (2011). Family structure, time constraints, and sport participation, *European Review of Aging and Physical Activity*, 8(2), 57–66.

Scheerder, J. and Seghers, J. (2011). *Jongeren in beweging. Over bewegingsbeleid, sportparticipatie en fysieke activiteit bij schoolgaande jongeren in Vlaanderen* [Youth sport and physical activity. About sports and physical activity policy, sports participation and physical activity in school-aged youngsters in Flanders]. Leuven: KU Leuven/Afdeling Sociale Kinesiologie en Sportmanagement.

Scheerder, J., Seghers, J., Meganck, J., Vandermeerschen, H. and Vos, S. (2015a). Sportclubs in beeld. Resultaten van het Vlaamse Sportclub Panel 2.0 (VSP2.0) [An image of sports clubs. Results of the Flemish Sports Clubs Survey 2.0]. Leuven: KU Leuven/Onderzoeksgroep Sport- en Bewegingsbeleid.

Scheerder, J., Taks, M. and Lagae, W. (2007). Teenage girls' participation in sports. An intergenerational analysis of socio-cultural predictor variables, *European Journal for Sport and Society*, 4, 133–150.

Scheerder, J., Thomis, M., Vanreusel, B., Lefevre, J., Renson, R., Vanden Eynde, B.and Beunen, G. (2006). Sports participation among females from adolescence to adulthood. A longitudinal study, *International Review for the Sociology of Sport*, 41(3–4), 413–430.

Scheerder, J., Vandermeerschen, H., Meganck, J., Seghers, J. and Vos, S. (2015b). Sports clubs in Belgium, in C. Breuer, R. Hoekman, S. Nagel and H. Van der Werff (eds) *Sport clubs in Europe. A cross-national comparative perspective* (sports Economics, Management & Policy 12) (pp. 47–67). Cham: Springer.

Scheerder, J., Vandermeerschen, H., van Tuyckom, C., Hoekman, R., Breedveld, K. and Vos, S. (2011). *Understanding the game. Sports participation in Europe. Facts, reflections and recommendations*. Leuven: KU Leuven/Policy in Sports and Physical Activity Research Group.

Scheerder, J., Vanreusel, B., Beunen, G., Claessens, A., Renson, R., Vanden Eynde, B. and Lefevre, J. (2008). Lifetime adherence to sport and physical activity as a goal in physical education. In search of evidence from longitudinal data. in J. Seghers and H. Vangrunderbeek (eds). *Physical Education Research. What's the evidence?* (pp. 29–40). Leuven: Acco.

Scheerder, J., Vanreusel, B. and Taks, M. (2005). Leisure-time sport among physical education students: a time-trend analysis of sport participation styles, *European Sport Management Quarterly*, *5(4)*, 415–441.

Scheerder, J. and Vos, S. (2011). Social stratification in adults' sports participation from a time-trend perspective. Results from a 40-year household study, *European Journal for Sport and Society*, *8(1/2)*, 31–44.

Seghers, J., Rutten, C., De Baere, S. and Lefevre, J. (2015). Succesfactoren en redenen van volgehouden lidmaatschap van een club [Success factors and reasons for persistence in club-organised sport], *Tijdschrift voor Lichamelijke Opvoeding*, *2*, 13–18.

Stamm, H. and Lamprecht, M. (2005). Structural and cultural factors influencing physical activity in Switzerland, *Journal of Public Health*, *13*, 203–211.

Taks, M. and Scheerder, J. (2006). Youth sports participation styles and market segmentation profiles: evidence and applications, *European Sport Management Quarterly*, *6(2)*, 85–121.

Telama, R., Yang, X., Viikari, J., Välimäki, I., Wanne, O. and Raitakari, O. (2005). Physical activity from childhood to adulthood. A 21-year tracking study, *American Journal of Preventive Medecine*, *28*, 267–273.

van Bottenburg, M., Rijnen, B. and van Sterkenburg, J. (2005). *Sports participation in the European Union: Trends and differences*. Nieuwegein: W.J.H. Mulier Institute/Arko Sports Media.

Vandermeerschen, H., Vos, S. and Scheerder, J. (2013). Who's joining the club? Participation of socially vulnerable children and adolescents in club-organised sports, *Sport, Education and Society*. DOI: 10.1080/ 13573322.2013.856293.

Vandermeerschen, H., Vos, S. and Scheerder, J. (2014). Towards level playing fields? A time trend analysis of young people's participation in club-organised sports, *International Review for the Sociology of Sport*. DOI: 10.1177/1012690214532450.

Vos, S., Wicker, P., Breuer, C. and Scheerder, J. (2013). Sports policy systems in regulated Rhineland welfare states. Differences in financial structures of sports clubs? *International Journal of Sport Policy and Politics*, 5 *(1)*, 55–71.

Wichstrom, L., von Soest, T. and Kvalem, I.L. (2013). Predictors of growth and decline in leisure time physical activity from adolescence to adulthood, *Health Psychology*, *32*, 775–784.

Wicker, P., Breuer, C. and Pawlowski, T. (2009). Promoting sport for all to age-specific target groups. The impact of sport infrastructure, *European Sport Management Quarterly*, *9(2)*, 103–118.

17

INDOORISING THE OUTDOORS

Tempting young people's interest in lifestyle sports

Lotte Salome and Maarten van Bottenburg

Introduction

Since the late 1980s, there has been a paradoxical development in the sports world that can be best described as the indoorisation of outdoor sports. Typical outdoor sports such as surfing, skiing, snowboarding, mountain climbing and even ski jumping and parachute jumping, which used to be practised exclusively in natural environments, are now being offered by entrepreneurs in controlled indoor centres. Indoor centres such as snow domes and indoor climbing halls offer safe and predictable environments in which these outdoor sports can be consumed without going to a natural environment of mountains, oceans, lakes, rivers and the air (van Bottenburg and Salome, 2010).

Outdoor sports such as surfing and snowboarding are often known as adventure sports, extreme sports, experience sports, alternative sports, and action sports. This collection of terms covers a relatively broad range of sports and physical activities. These range from established and more or less mainstream activities such as snowboarding, through youth sports such as skateboarding, to newly emergent activities like kite-surfing, as well as to high-risk sports such as BASE jumping. In this chapter, the term *lifestyle sports* is used to emphasise the way members of the lifestyle sport cultures describe their activities as lifestyles rather than as sports. The use of this term includes cultures and individual and group identities, as well as the socio-historical context in which the activities emerged, took shape and still exist (Wheaton, 2004). Furthermore, the term is used to emphasise meanings related to personal factors beyond success in competition, and to underline that the activities 'either ideologically or practically provide alternatives to mainstream sports and to mainstream sport values' (Rinehart, 2002, p. 506).

It will be clear from the outset that lifestyle sports are characterised by meanings and properties that do not appear to lend themselves to being practiced in a reconstructed indoor environment. Indeed, these outdoor sports usually take place in wild and desolate natural places, which have not been prepared for sporting activities in advance. The often young practitioners of these sports extol the virtues of being close to nature and being part of natural sceneries. This goes hand-in-hand with a sense of adventure, uncertainty and danger; those who practice these sports wilfully seek out the upper limits and take considered risks (Stranger, 1999). At first sight, this experience of nature and a just-do-it kind of attitude (Wheaton, 2000) is at odds with the artificial and calculated character of the indoor sports centres that have been developed. Whereas those who participate in the outdoor variants of the sports are totally wrapped up in nature, the indoor practitioners must necessarily surrender themselves to technology. While the buzz from outdoor sports comes from adventure, uncertainty and danger, the indoor variants inescapably embrace the elements of control, predictability and calculability.

There is a similar tension with respect to the mutual bond and subculture that has developed among the participants of these sports. Despite the informal ties that are common to the outdoor lifestyle sports, the hard core enthusiasts form various tightly-knit social groups, which outsiders find difficult to penetrate. It takes years of practice and participation – and thus also a major investment in cultural capital – to master the techniques of these sports and to appropriate the shared cultural significance of the sporting styles, clothing, materials, language use and the like (Bourdieu, 1984; Wheaton, 2004). In contrast, gaining access to an indoor sports centre seems to demand no more effort than simply buying a ticket. In comparison to the subcultures that the fervent aficionados of, for example, snowboarding and surfing have built up from the grassroots, visits to the indoor halls are likely to have a fleeting and irregular character from which very few shared meanings can develop. Loynes (1998, p. 35) refers to this as 'recreational capitalism'.

This chapter offers a theoretical exploratory interpretation of the process of indoorisation of outdoor lifestyle sports, or, as Eichberg has called it, the 'artificialisation and interiorisation of the body' (1998, p. 60). From our Dutch perspective, artificial settings such as snow domes and indoor skydive centres provide excellent case studies to investigate this development. Observations, interviews and analyses of textual and visual materials of indoor sports centres were used as sources that provide access to particular accounts of those phenomena, in and through which social reality is constructed (Moisander and Valtonen, 2006).

In particular, we focus on the role of young participants in these indoor lifestyle sports, and the meanings of the artificial sport environments for youth. Following Eichberg, we will argue that natural (to take shelter from bad weather), health or medical and technological explanations do not go far enough. The changes in space are indelibly social, related to broader processes like commercialisation, globalisation and individualisation (Eichberg, 1998).

In the present chapter, the focus will be on the supply side of the market as well as on the demand side. Thus, attention will be devoted to the way in which the rise of this economic market has been embedded in:

1   the structure of the fields in which the new indoor centres in this market are positioned (Bourdieu, 1988);
2   the diverse cultures – in the sense of shared meanings and their representations (Zelizer, 2005) – that have developed in these fields and
3   the broader social processes, which have occurred relatively autonomously from individual action, but have still had a structuring influence on it (Elias, 1977).

The construction of a market

The fact that the indoor centres for outdoor sports have rapidly been able to establish themselves across the globe cannot be seen independently of the acceleration in globalisation, commercial-isation and technological change in the last twenty-five years. The initiatives for these centres were taken by internationally oriented entrepreneurs who can be regarded as outsiders to the mainstream sports world. As far as can be ascertained, the world's first indoor ski centre was opened at the end of the 1980s. At least, that is what SnowDome in Adelaide, South Australia, claimed when it opened its doors in 1988. This idea was also taken up elsewhere, first in Japan, and then later mainly in countries that had poor skiing conditions, but which had nonetheless developed a ski culture partly as a result of their increasing affluence and the rise in popularity of winter sports vacations. Nowadays, one can find these centres all over the world, even in desert regions, such as Bahrain and the indoor snow resort Ski Dubai.

The same process largely applies to the indoor skydiving and indoor surfing centres: a recent, rapid global expansion, fostered by technological innovations and new commercial initiatives. In 1991, the American Thomas Lochtefeld invented the so-called FlowRider, an invention that made a new board sport possible, christened as flowboarding. The FlowRider first came into use in New Braunfels, Texas, in 1991. The FlowRider is now being used across the globe, predominantly in the United States and Europe, but also in Japan, Korea, China, Saudi Arabia and South Africa. Similar and competing developments also took place elsewhere. Vertical wind tunnels for skydiving had originally been developed during the 1950s and 1960s for military purposes and space travel. The first commercial applications of this technology were realised around 1980 and were then replicated worldwide during the 1990s, in Japan and Switzerland, initially. There are now more than twenty commercial indoor skydiving centres in the United States and Europe.

Commercial motives appear to lie behind very many of the innovations in sport facilities of this kind. In this regard, entrepreneurs were not only able to profit from the politics or market deregulation and liberalisation in general, but also the increasing receptiveness of the public, government and sports organisations to commercially run sports facilities in countries where these facilities were traditionally financed and managed by a coalition of national sporting organisations, local sporting clubs and national and local governments. As will be discussed below, the Dutch national government and the NOC*NSF (Dutch Olympic Committee/Dutch Sports Federation) made funding available for the realisation of one of the indoor centres. At the same time, local government agencies adopted a helpful and flexible stance with respect to issuing permits and the sports umbrella organisation and sport federations entered into collaborative relationships with some of the indoor centres with a view to the advancement of elite sport. National borders, national regulatory bodies and national cultural traditions have hardly created any impediment to the global dissemination of these commercial innovations, which have then been given their own local character (Appadurai, 1996; Castells, 1997).

It is self-evident that the developments in new construction, cooling and insulation techniques and the achievement of innovations in water, snow and atmospheric control, which have been enabled by advanced technology, were prerequisites for the indoorisation of outdoor sports. Yet this does not mean that these technological developments should be seen as the driving force behind indoorisation. In so doing, one would run the risk of ignoring the initial idea of using these new technological possibilities to achieve such ends. The development, realisation and response to this idea, and thus the global market of producers and consumers, which has emerged with the indoorisation of outdoor sports, should be viewed as a social construction, in the sense that the use and meaning of these new services had yet to be defined (Collins, 2004).

The idea of offering outdoor sports indoors did not arise from a pre-existing consumer need or interest. 'Consumer demand', argues Randall Collins, 'is not simply an exogenous quantity, but something that is constructed by what is being offered by producers' (Collins, 2004, p. 167). The initiative for the indoorisation of outdoor sports came from entrepreneurs who kept a close eye on each another's activities. Naturally, market research was carried out to be able to underpin and justify the necessary investment. And, without a doubt, just as the prospectus of Dutch Water Dreams reports, this market research discovered that there actually was an interest for such centres among a sizeable group of sports-loving respondents who were, of course, part of the target group. However, this interest is obviously related to the concept that was presented by the producer prior to the realisation of the complex.

This does not mean to say that consumers are merely followers with no will of their own, who do nothing other than consume the products and services on offer along with the meanings that are ascribed to them. Quite the contrary, as Appadurai has noted, 'the production knowledge that is read into a commodity is quite different from the consumption knowledge that is read from the commodity' (Appadurai, 1986, p. 41). Collins contends that in the ongoing flow of social interaction rituals between producers and consumers, the interpretations and meanings that are given to the products and services on one side of the market resonate on the other side, and vice versa (Collins, 2004). Consumers interpret and assess the constructed meanings, which reach them by way of advertisements, internet, stories and so forth, and compare these with their personal experiences and those of others. The meanings of the indoor sports centres are therefore not established in advance. Nor are they determined by the producers or the consumers. Instead there is a constant process of what Erving Goffman has called 'framing' and 'reframing' between the producers and consumers (Goffman, 1974). Both producers and consumers are involved in a continual interactive process, a 'cultural circuit', which not only influences themselves, but also the meanings of the product or service in question (Zelizer, 1988; Lury, 1996; Du Gay *et al.*, 1997; Zukin and Smith Maguire, 2004; Shove and Pantzar, 2005; Sassatelli, 2007). This interaction can have an unintended consequence; namely that, over the course of time, (aspects of) the kinds of sport on offer and their setting can acquire a form, meaning and function that no-one had anticipated and intended in advance (Elias, 1977).

As is generally the case with the development of new markets, the initiative for this interaction lies on the side of the producers. They take the first and most decisive steps 'that begin to pump up material objects into Durkheimian sacred objects, which will in turn generate the biggest profits' (Collins, 2004, p. 168). This principle does not just apply to material products, but also to services. While competing with each other, the producers were the first to give shape to the nature and meaning of the indoor complexes and outdoor sports, which had to be realised according to their visions.

To understand this dream, the meanings that are ascribed to the indoor sports centres should not be understood as intrinsic values that can be derived from the activities themselves. Instead, following Pierre Bourdieu, they should be viewed in relation to the structure of the sports and leisure field, and the various activities that already existed there (Bourdieu, 1988, 1996). When launching and promoting their indoor centres, the entrepreneurs paid particular attention to the meanings surrounding three sub-fields: lifestyle sports, organised competitive sports and elite sport, and the adventure and experience market in the leisure sector.

Meanings in relation to outdoor lifestyle sports

According to Bourdieu, a field effect occurs when it is no longer possible to understand a practice, like the introduction of a new product or service on a market, without knowing the history of this field (Bourdieu, 1980). In this sense, the fact that the producers – when developing and positioning their indoor sports centres – are unable to escape from the dominant meanings of the outdoor lifestyle sports, from which their sport supply partly derives, can be regarded as a field effect.

Research focused on outdoor lifestyle sports has indicated that, on the one hand, commercialisation and commodification processes have sold out lifestyle sports. On the other hand, however, the broader possibilities that these processes offer seem to be beneficial, for example, for sponsorship and professionalisation (Humphreys, 1997). When lifestyle sports became popular with a broad audience in the 1980s, hard core participants tried to protect the exclusiveness and authenticity of their culture. The intrusion of seemingly less committed, less dedicated and thus less authentic participants was not appreciated. Questions of authenticity and the role of 'participants who have been marginalized and ignored by both the core members who are the focus of the research and by the researchers' (Donnelly, 2006, p. 224) have been the subject of discussions in lifestyle sports for years. This complex relationship between lifestyle sports and commercialisation should be re-interpreted against the backdrop of the emergence of artificial sport environments for the experience of these lifestyle sports.

While it is true that the hard core aficionados of the outdoor lifestyle sports do not constitute a large group, the popularity of these sports has grown significantly. The new sport activities were characterised, during the 1960s and 1970s, by their ability to challenge the traditional competitive, rule-bound and male-dominated sport cultures. Also, the sports had things to offer that were difficult to find in other sports, such as the possibility of mastery and perfection in relation to challenging environments (Wheaton, 2004; Breivik, 2010). The popularity of different kinds of these sports expanded since the 1980s, when more and more mostly young people were attracted to the many ways in which the sports represented counter-cultural values (Breivik, 2010). To underscore the young audience of this eclectic collection of risky, individualistic and sensational activities that emphasize freedom and hedonism, the sports were often labelled as 'Gen[eration]-Y sports' (Bennett and Lachowetz, 2004).

In the first stage of their existence, lifestyle sports were predominantly practised by young, white, Western males, often low-income earners or students (Erickson, 2005; Kusz, 2007; Thorpe, 2007c; Robinson, 2008). These committed participants can be considered as real pioneers. With their self-manufactured equipment, they constantly innovated new gear and new activities to create fun and sensational experiences (Thorpe, 2007c).

Artificial settings for lifestyle sports make an explicit connection with the culture of the outdoor lifestyle sports by using slogans and language that appeal to it. For instance, Indoor Skydive Roosendaal advertises that its visitors can experience 'The Ultimate Xperience', implicitly referring to the so-called XSports (extreme sports) and the XGames of the American sports channel ESPN. This indoor centre also claims that its visitors can also get their kicks when it comes to excitement and adventure ('one gets a great adrenaline rush when skydiving').

The experiences that such centres promise attempt to satiate the 'quest for excitement', which, according to Elias and Dunning (1986), characterises modern society. The sporting activities in these centres generate fleeting, pleasant and pleasurable forms of suspense and excitement, which these authors believe are often lacking in the ordinary routines of everyday life. Nonetheless, this suspense and excitement occurs under controlled conditions, thus allowing people the opportunity to experience what Elias has called a 'controlled but enjoyable de-controlling of affects and emotions' (Elias and Dunning, 2008, p. 27).

Needless to say, it is crucial for the indoor centres that the safety of the participants is guaranteed. To minimise the risk of accidents, extensive safety regulations, protocols and procedures are implemented at all indoor centres. However, the emphasis on excitement *and* safety poses a tricky dilemma for the indoor centres. Too great an emphasis on the one (safety) can undermine the very meaning and appeal of the other (excitement). The combination of both desires is the unique selling point: 'At Dutch Water Dreams, you can take part in spectacular white water sports in an environment where safety and comfort take centre stage . . . The advantage of the wild water course compared to a natural wild water setting is that, in the event of a calamity, we are able to turn off the water pumps, and stop the flow of water'. The same applies to indoor skydiving: 'If there is a power failure, then the twelve ventilator fans will carry on turning for a while. This means that you will be able to descend gently and land in a strong net.'

Nonetheless, there is still a danger that an ambiguous meaning will be transmitted: on the one hand, the indoor centres appeal to the hardcore fun sports enthusiast and the adrenaline junkie, yet, on the other, they position themselves in such a way that they also have meaning for rather less courageous daredevils. The dilemma is part and parcel of a broader discrepancy. These enterprises are oriented towards efficiency, predictability, calculability and the control of their service provision. This is a development that George Ritzer has called 'The McDonaldization of Society' (Ritzer, 2008). Yet this rationalisation must not be at the expense of the experience of the sport as a special activity, which can be seen as comparable to experiencing such sports outdoors. The rationalisation thus constantly demands diversification and variation to hold the consumers' interest and keep on surprising them. To achieve this, commercial institutions in the sport, leisure and entertainment industry employ specialists, whom Roberta Sassatelli has characterised as 'motivational professionals' (Sassatelli, 2007). They must guide the consumers to and in their meaningful experience by providing insights into the techniques and experiences with which they can better understand the activities concerned and enjoy them even more.

As Bennett and Lachowetz (2004) argued, lifestyle sports speak to youth culture because of the absence of constraints by teams and rules found in traditional sports. Besides that, for young people, values including creativity, individuality and friendship that are highly prominent in lifestyle sports are seen as predominantly important in sport participation. While the transition from childhood to adulthood is a key risk time for drop-out, lifestyle sports can be seen as activities that are 'independent and conferred a more adult identity upon them' (Coakley and White, 1992). In this regard, lifestyle sports seem to be able to engage young people in the less regulated new sport activities (Tomlinson *et al.*, 2005).

This is in line with figures from a recent Dutch survey about sport participation; in a first attempt to examine the demographic characteristics of Dutch lifestyle sport participants, the survey revealed that in the 16–20 age group, 73 per cent had engaged in a lifestyle sport at least once (Lucassen, Salome and Wisse, 2011). In fact, it is argued that lifestyle sports 'are becoming so central that they are beginning to replace traditional team sports' (Gilchrist and Wheaton, 2011, p. 109). As Taks and Scheerder (2006) conclude from their picture of distinct sport participation profiles and market segments for youth participants, lifestyle sports are new on the scene. There is an increased interest of youngsters in action sports, away from the traditionally organised sports.

Besides the fact that lifestyle sports are of growing interest in the last decade, there are various other trends in these sports. As Breivik (2010) argued, these include the increasing organisation of lifestyle sports – formal regulations, training regimes and safety measures are replacing self-organised, loose and unregulated cultures – and the broadening of the demographic composition of the activities. The expansion in participation in lifestyle sports includes not only young white people, but also participants from various backgrounds, ages and levels of experience, including women, young children and the elderly (e.g. Tomlinson *et al.*, 2005; Wheaton, 2010). While, hitherto, these sports were an almost exclusive area for young, white men, there is nowadays a more varied group of consumers attending the indoor centres for lifestyle sports. Often, these participants are not experienced in lifestyle sports in outdoor environments. Indeed, young people often excel in the indoor versions of lifestyle sports without ever having practiced the sports in a natural environment. Especially in snowboarding and climbing, a complete new participant group has emerged that experiences indoor lifestyle sports without being familiar with the outdoor versions.

All in all, there is no doubt that lifestyle sports in general attract an increasing number of young people. This applies to lifestyle sport participation in controlled indoor settings as well. For young people, these centres offer opportunities to experience new activities in a safe, friendly and accessible environment. Years of time, money and effort to master techniques are not required anymore to feel part of the lifestyle sport culture. Just buying a ticket, no further obligations and little regulations combined with sensation and variation seem to be the keywords. The clear link to the culture of their adventurous outdoor counterparts appears to appeal to them.

Meanings in relation to mainstream sports

The development of competitive sport and elite sport from sporting activities that were initially intended for the leisure market is another example of a field effect in Bourdieu's terms. Competitive sport is the dominant model of sport worldwide – the mainstream sport – with elite sport as the greatest audience puller, and enjoys the non-stop attention of the media.

The rise of the outdoor lifestyle sports can be regarded as a reaction to – or resistance against – these mainstream sports. These sports were not developed by or within the established sports organisations, but came about more-or-less spontaneously from the unregulated activities of young people who, while practicing these sports, began to increasingly align themselves with each other. One of the meanings that they shared was their preference for individual and informal expression in an open and free environment, unhindered by regulations and controls by schools or sports organisations (Wheaton, 2000, 2004). However, the global dissemination and popularisation of these lifestyle sports also went hand-in-hand with a differentiation of performance styles and subcultures within these outdoor sports. The desire and proclivity to continue to distinguish themselves from mainstream sport has continued within certain subgroups. Yet, at the same time, the dominant sport model has been applied to various kinds of sports within the outdoor lifestyle sports. Organised, regulated and standardised disciplines have developed in nearly all lifestyle sports, culminating in competitive and performance-oriented elite sports that are covered by the media. A number of these, such as snowboarding and freestyle skiing, have even been included in the Olympic programme, which can certainly be regarded as *the* symbol of mainstream sport.

Although the commercial indoor sports centres have developed their sports services outside mainstream sport, they cannot escape completely from its sphere of influence. Due to the established balance of power in the field of sport, a relationship with mainstream sport – particularly elite sport – afforded access to funding bodies. In addition to this, a link with mainstream sport – and with elite sport in particular – guarantees free publicity. For example, the SnowWorld ski centre in Landgraaf is used annually for the official FIS European Cup and the Snowboarding World Cup championships, and both receive considerable media attention.

These public flirtations with elite sport are significant for the positioning of the centres. In commercial terms, their function as training centres for elite athletes is subordinate to that of consumer entertainment. The vast majority of the mainly young visitors are not oriented to training for elite sporting performance, but are instead simply looking to have an enjoyable experience. However, the attention on elite sport within these commercial centres prevents too great an emphasis being placed on casual, recreational entertainment.

Just as they must maintain the equilibrium between excitement and safety, the centres also have to keep a watchful eye on the precarious balance between their significance to elite sport and their significance to the broader public. They use the proximity and easy accessibility of their indoor facilities as another unique selling point. Dutch Water Dreams, for example, points out that 'for those who want to go rafting, the Ardennes in Belgium is the closest possibility. Dutch Water Dreams has put an end to this situation.' Their proximity also gives the indoor centres an accessible character to a broader public. Skiing, surfing and parachute jumping can be experienced close-by, at a relatively low cost and can also be tried just the once. The message is that the indoor centres are open to everyone and they lower the threshold: partly due to their proximity, partly due to the limited degree of difficulty and the possibilities to experience an activity without memberships or canteen and cleaning duties.

A successful popularisation ensures a significant growth in visitors. At the same time, an indoor centre can also run the risk of alienating the trendsetting public. Indoor Skydive explicitly calls itself trendsetting. Likewise, the wild water complex Dutch Water Dreams also characterises itself 'as sporty, innovative and rather hip.' They emphasise such meanings by referring to the innovative strength of the sports they offer. They not only created new 'commercial settings' for the practice of these sports (Sassatelli, 2007) but stimulated the development of new sports, with their own rules, meanings and even their own championships. Flowboarding can be seen as a new board sport and is also experienced by the surfers as such. Indeed, the first flowboarding world championships have already taken place, and World Indoor Skydiving Championships are organised annually in the world's largest indoor skydiving wind tunnel, iFly Singapore.

Meanings in relation to leisure experiences

The third field effect, which the indoor centres anticipate, concerns the competition with other providers in the leisure sector. In a commercial struggle to reach the target group in such a way that indoor lifestyle sports become preferable to other fun and exciting activities, the publicity materials produced by the indoor centres do not so much emphasise the sport itself but rather the opportunity to undergo a pleasurable experience (with others). In this regard, Pine and Gilmore (1999) would undoubtedly have used the indoor centres for skiing, surfing and skydiving as typical examples of new enterprises in the 'experience economy'. Following the expansion of the goods economy and then the service economy, according to the authors, the greatest growth that has occurred since the 1990s has been in enterprises that no longer confine themselves to the supply of goods and services but which also provide experiences. It is not so much about the consumer paying for a service but about their buying time to undergo a memorable experience.

Nonetheless, there is an important difference between the meanings that the indoor centres propagate and the ways in which, according to Pine and Gilmore (1999), enterprises in the experience economy operate. Whereas the authors argue in favour of offering an experience to the individual customer ('given that an experience is in itself something personal, no two people can have the same experience', p. 236), the indoor sports centres are focused entirely on groups of (young) consumers. Indeed, they emphasise the social meaning of group visits in fairly elaborate terms. Whether it is for birthdays, wedding parties, business events or school trips, the centres' message is still the same: undergoing the experience together gives pleasure and leads to bonding: 'We can make an unforgettable event not only of your outings with family and friends, but also meetings with, for example, your sports club, student society or another network club . . . From a theme or wedding party to birthdays and anniversaries, Dutch Water Dreams is *the* place to celebrate!' Supply is geared to such meanings. The centres have put together a wide variety of packages with which they cater to the needs of various target groups. They have special rooms for large groups where meetings, office parties and other events can be held. Specific areas can also be fitted out for children's parties and other special groups.

There are two aspects to the meanings that these indoor centres can convey in this regard. First, visits to these centres have a social character: they not only acquire meaning through being an exciting experience of sport, but also because they take place together with other people. As the introduction to this article suggests, in practice, fleeting single visits by individual consumers seldom occur. Nearly all visitors are part of a group. Realising that the experience only acquires a meaning within a social context, Dutch Water Dreams gives every consumer a chip so that a personal film can be downloaded onto his or her cell phone. 'It's fun to show your friends', declares one of the advertisements. Second, the sport is not presented as the primary goal. 'At SnowWorld you can find all the facilities to combine your business meetings with relaxation claims the website of this indoor ski centre', and 'It goes without saying that the meeting rooms can also be booked without making use of the ski pistes . . . If you are not interested in skiing or snowboarding, we have an extensive selection of other activities on offer on our pistes'. All of these alternative activities serve to reinforce the notion that these are leisure centres. In this sense, in their competition with the other providers in the leisure market, the producers have created functions and meanings that transcend the sport itself.

Conclusion

The market for outdoor sports offered indoors was developed under the influence of techno-logical innovations and internationally operating entrepreneurs who have kept a careful eye on their competitors' activities. In so doing, these entrepreneurs have joined the trend towards commodification of sport facilities, which has predominantly taken place outside the system of national sports associations and international sports federations.

During the development of this market, the producers have attempted to ascribe a variety of meanings to the new products and services. Yet these meanings do not stem from the intrinsic values of the products and services themselves. They may be better understood as social constructions, which have emerged not only through the interaction between producers and consumers, in which the initiative was from the producers' side, but also in relation to the structure of the sports and leisure fields and the cultural meanings, which are ascribed to a diverse number of existing activities that take place in these fields.

In light of this structure, when launching and marketing their indoor centres, entrepreneurs must particularly pay heed to the shared meanings around the subfields: the lifestyle sports, organised competitive sports and elite sport, and the experience market of the leisure sector. They define their indoor centres and supply of activities in these centres in competition with, or with reference to the dominant meanings of these subfields. In so doing, they must also determine their position in the field of tension, which emerges between the various layers of meaning, because placing an emphasis on one layer of meaning can have unintended and undesirable consequences for the meanings, which, from another perspective, can be viewed as just as desirable.

The analysis of the construction of the indoorisation of outdoor lifestyle sports and its meanings demonstrates that, as Eichberg (1998) argued, there are more than just natural, health or medical and technological reasons for this development. We have shown that the rise of this economic market is embedded in and influenced by shared understandings and producer and consumer representations in structured fields of outdoor sports, mainstream sports and leisure experience activities.

This chapter is based on van Bottenburg, M. and Salome, L. (2010). The indoorisation of outdoor sports. An exploration of the rise of lifestyle sports in artificial settings. *Leisure Studies*, 29(2), 143–160.

References

Appadurai, A. (1986). *The Social Life of Things. Commodities in Cultural Perspective*. Cambridge: Cambridge University Press.

Appadurai, A. (1996). *Modernity at Large. Cultural Dimensions of Globalization.*Minneapolis: University of Minnesota Press.

Bennett, G. and Lachowetz, T. (2004). Marketing to lifestyles: Action sports and generation Y, *Sport Marketing Quarterly*, *13(4)*, 239–243.

Bourdieu, P. (1980). *Questions de sociologie*. Paris: Editions de Minuit.

Bourdieu, P. (1984). *Distinction. A Social Critique of the Judgement of Taste*. Cambridge: Harvard University Press.

Bourdieu, P. (1988). Program for a sociology of sport. *Sociology of Sport Journal 5(2)*, 153–161.

Bourdieu, P. (1996). Principles of an economic anthropology, in N.J. Smelser and R. Swedberg (eds) *The Handbook of Economic Sociology* (pp. 75–89). New York: Princeton University Press.

Breivik, G. (2010). Trends in adventure sports in a post-modern society, *Sport in Society*, *13(2)*, 260–273.

Castells, M. (1997). *The Power of Identity. The Information Age*. Oxford: Blackwell Publishers.

Coakley, J. and White, A. (1992). Making decisions: gender and sport participation among British adolescents, *Sociology of Sport Journal*, *9*, 20–35.

Collins, R. (2004). *Interaction Ritual Chains*. Princeton/Oxford: Princeton University Press.

Du Gay, P., Hall, S., Janes, L., McKay, H. and Negus, K. (1997). *Doing Cultural Studies. The Story of the Sony Walkman*. Milton Keynes: Open University Press.

Eichberg, H. (1998). *Body Cultures. Essays on Sport, Space and Identity*. London: Routledge.

Elias, N. (1977). *What is Sociology?* New York: Columbia University Press.

Elias, N. and Dunning, E. (1986). *Quest for excitement. Sport and Leisure in the Civilizing Process*. Oxford: Basil Blackwell.

Elias, N. and Dunning, E. (2008). *Quest for excitement. Sport and Leisure in the Civilising process. The Collected Works of Norbert Elias Volume 7*. Dublin: University College Dublin Press.

Erickson, B. (2005). Style matters: Explorations of bodies, whiteness, and identity in rock climbing, *Sociology of Sport Journal*, *22(3)*, 373–396.

Gilchrist, P. and Wheaton, B. (2011). Lifestyle sport, public policy and youth engagement: examining the emergence of parkour, *International Journal of Sport Policy and Politics*, *3(1)*, 109–131.

Goffman, E. (1974). *Frame Analysis. An Essay on the Organization of Experience*. New York: Harper and Row.

Granovetter, M. (1985). Economic action and social structure. The problem of embeddedness, *American Journal of Sociology*, *91(3)*, 481–510.

Humphreys, D. (1997). 'Shredheads go mainstream'? Snowboarding and alternative youth, *International Review for the Sociology of Sport*, *32(2)*, 147–160.

Kusz, K. (2007). Whiteness and extreme sports, in D. Booth and H. Thorpe (eds) *Berkshire Encyclopedia of Extreme Sports* (pp. 357–361). Great Barrington, Massachusetts: Berkshire Publishing Group.

Loynes, C. (1998). Adventure in a bun, *Journal of Experiential Education*, *21(1)*, 35–39.

Lucassen, J., Salome, L. and Wisse, E. (2011). Leefstijlsport, een conceptuele verkenning [A conceptual exploration of lifestyle sports], in J. Lucassen en E. Wisse (eds) *Sporten op de Grens. Studies over Leefstijlsporten [Sports on the Border. Studies on Lifestyle Sports]* (pp. 12–37). Nieuwegein: Arko Sports Media.

Lury, C. (1996). *Consumer Culture*. Cambridge: Polity Press.

Moisander, J. and Valtonen, A. (2006). *Qualitative Marketing Research. A Cultural Approach*. London: Sage Publications.

Pine, B.J. and Gilmore, J.H. (1999). *The Experience Economy. Work is Theatre and Every Business a Stage*. Cambridge: Harvard Business School Press.

Rinehart, R. (2002). Arriving sport: Alternatives to formal sports. In J.J. Coakley and E. Dunning (eds) *Handbook of Sports Studies* (pp. 504–519). London: Sage.

Ritzer, G. (2008). *The McDonaldization of Society* (5th edition). Los Angeles: Pine Forge Press.

Sassatelli, R. (2007). *Consumer Culture. History, Theory and Politics*. London: Sage Publications.

Shove, E. and Pantzar, M. (2005). Consumers, producers and practices. Understanding the invention and reinvention of Nordic walking, *Journal of Consumer Culture*, *5(1)*, 43–64.

Stranger, M. (1999). The aesthetics of risk. A study of surfing, *International Review of Sociology of Sport*, *34(3)*, 265–276.

Taks, M. and Scheerder, J. (2006). Youth sports participation styles and market segmentation profiles: Evidence and applications, *European Sport Management Quarterly*, *6(2)*, 85–121.

Tomlinson, A., Ravenscroft, N., Wheaton, B. and Gilchrist, P. (2005). *Lifestyle Sports and National Sport Policy: An Agenda for Research*. Brighton: University of Brighton.

Tomlinson, J. (2001). *Extreme sports: The Illustrated Guide to Maximum Adrenaline Thrills*. London: Carlton Books.

van Bottenburg, M. and Salome, L. (2010). The indoorisation of outdoor sports. An exploration of the rise of lifestyle sports in artificial settings, *Leisure Studies, 29(2)*, 143–160.

Wheaton, B. (2000). 'Just do it'. Consumption, commitment, and identity in the windsurfing subculture, *Sociology of Sport Journal, 17*, 254–255.

Wheaton, B. (ed.) (2004). *Understanding Lifestyle Sports. Consumption, Identity and Difference*. New York: Routledge.

Wheaton, B. (2010). Introducing the consumption and representation of lifestyle sports, *Sport in Society, 13(7)*, 1057–1081.

Zelizer, V. A. (1988). Beyond the polemics on the market. Establishing a theoretical and empirical agenda. *Sociological Forum, 3(4)*, 614–634.

Zelizer, V. (2005). Culture and consumption, in N. Smelsner and R. Swedberg (eds) *Handbook of Economic Sociology* (pp. 331–354). Princeton: Princeton University Press.

Zukin, S. and Smith Maguire, J. (2004). Consumers and consumption, *Annual Review of Sociology, 30*, 173–197.

18

LIFESTYLE AND ADVENTURE SPORTS AMONG YOUTH

Paul Gilchrist and Belinda Wheaton

Introduction

An important characteristic and intensifying trend in the twenty-first century within Western sporting cultures is an increase in the range and diversity of sports practices, particularly more informal and individualistic activities. A vibrant example of this trend is the emergence and growth of what the academic and popular literature has variously termed extreme, alternative, adventure and lifestyle sports. In this chapter, we consider the growing popularity and significance of these sports, illustrating their impact on the contemporary sporting landscape. We use the term lifestyle sports as an umbrella term to refer to a range of participatory, informal and *stoke[1]*-seeking urban and rural sporting activities, including long-established sports like climbing and surfing through to emergent activities such as snowboarding and parkour. Many of these sports either originated (or, for example surfing, were re-popularised) in North America around the 1960s. With their origins in the counter-cultural social movement of the 1960s and 1970s, many had characteristics that are *different* to traditional rule-bound, competitive and institutionalised sport. They have been characterised by their challenge to the dominant Western 'achievement sport' culture and values (Eichberg, 1998).

First, we explore what lifestyle sports are and the ways in which they have impacted contemporary youth lifestyles, focusing on the UK, where much of our own research has been conducted, and North America, where many of these sports originated and have had most impact on the sportscape. We consider how we can understand and conceptualise the youth (sub)cultures and identities that underpin them, and highlight some of the key trends in their development, including commercialisation. Second, the chapter reviews literature on lifestyle sports as an urban spatial practice and the attendant cultural politics associated with youth lifestyles expressed in urban environments through street sports like skateboarding and parkour/free-running. Third, acknowledging the virtual/real interface at the forefront of youth identities and experiences, we consider the role of digital media in fuelling the popularity, culture and economy of lifestyle sports.

What are lifestyle sports?

A number of characteristics define lifestyle sports (Wheaton, 2013: 28–30). Participants show high commitment in time and/or money and a style of life that develops around the activity.

They have a hedonistic, individualistic ideology that promotes commitment, but often denounces regulation and institutionalisation, and tend to be critical of, or ambivalent to, commercialism and formal person-on-person style competition. They emphasise the aesthetic realm in which one blends with one's environment. Some practitioners refer to their activities as art. The body is used in non-aggressive ways, mostly without bodily contact, yet participants embrace and fetishise notions of risk and danger. Yet while perceptions about risk pervade public debate about adventure sport, the majority of lifestyle sports activities are practiced in controlled ways. Indeed, many activities labelled extreme are actually relatively safe (Booth and Thorpe, 2007: 173) and, according to statistical evidence, cause fewer injuries and deaths than many traditional sports including rugby and boxing (Clemmitt, 2009: 297; James, Barr and LaPrade, this volume). The locations in which these sports are practised are often new or re-appropriated urban and rural spaces, without fixed or delineated boundaries, and lacking regulation and control.

Academics have used a range of labels to characterise these sports including extreme, alternative, lifestyle, whiz, action sports, panic sport, postmodern, post-industrial and new sports. While these labels are used synonymously by some commentators, there are differences that signal distinct emphases or expressions of the activities (Rinehart, 2000; Wheaton, 2013). *Adventure* sports tend to be nature-based, and include more regulated forms of the activities, particularly in education-focused settings. *Action sport* is the term increasingly used by the sports industry, particularly in North America. Initially it described board sports such as skateboarding, snowboarding and surfing. It is now widely used, however, by corporations and media to describe adventure-based and lifestyle activities. Yet, as Jake Burton, the founder of *Burton* snowboards, suggests:

> I think what's a better moniker is maybe that it's a *lifestyle* sport, and a lot of the kids and people that are dong it are just completely living it all the time, and that's what distinguishes snowboarding from a lot of other sports.
>
> *(Burton, 2002; cited in Wheaton 2004: 4; emphasis in the original)*

Unlike some alternative and extreme sports, lifestyle sports are fundamentally about participation, not spectating, either in live or mediated settings. The term lifestyle sport reflects the terminology used by those who participate in these sports, and as discussed below, encapsulates the cultures that surround the activity (Wheaton, 2004; 2013). That is to say, the term *lifestyle* helps encapsulate the ways in which participants, and consumers of the activities, seek out a particular style of life, a way of living that is central to the meaning and experience of participation in the sport, and that gives them a particular and exclusive social identity (Wheaton, 2004). Despite differences in nomenclature, most commentators see such activities as having presented an alternative and potential challenge to traditional ways of seeing, doing and understanding sport (see debate in Rinehart, 2000; Rinehart and Sydnor, 2003; Wheaton, 2004).

Lifestyle sportscapes in the twenty-first century

Lifestyle sports have witnessed unprecedented growth and have drawn participants and followers from increasingly diverse global geographic settings. They continue to develop through a unique historical conjuncture of global communication, corporate sponsorship, and entertainment industries, and recognise the lucrative potential of a global and affluent youth demographic (Thorpe and Wheaton, 2011). A variety of products, services, facilities and events have been created to cater for a growing consumer demand, shaped by consumer trends rooted in changing youth lifestyles and tastes. The self-defined 'worldwide leader' in action sports, ESPN's

X Games (Rinehart, 2008) has played a central role in the global diffusion and expansion of the lifestyle sports industry and culture (Rinehart, 2000). In 1995, the inaugural summer X Games held in Rhode Island (US) featured twenty-seven events in nine categories, ranging from bungee jumping to skateboarding. Following the success of the summer events, ESPN staged the first winter X Games in California in 1997, drawing 38,000 spectators and televised in 198 countries and territories in twenty-one different languages (Pedersen and Kelly, 2000). Blurring the boundaries between music festival and sporting event (Rinehart, 2008), the X Games have been hugely successful in capturing the imagination of the lucrative youth market. The 2002 X Games were watched by 63 million people globally and, in contrast to the ageing Olympic viewership, the average age of these viewers was 20 years (Thorpe and Wheaton, 2011). While in the early years the X Games were all based in North America, they are now also held in Europe, Asia and South America (ESPN.go.com). Audiences have also become increasingly global. The Winter X Games 13, for example, was televised on ESPN's international networks to more than 122 countries (Gorman, 2009).

The outdoor, non-association-based and nomadic nature of these activities makes it hard to accurately measure participation levels. For example, few activities have formal clubs and participants move between different sites. However, from the available sources such as sales of equipment, market research surveys and wide-ranging media commentaries, it is evident that participation in many types of lifestyle and adventure sports continues to grow rapidly, outpacing the expansion of most traditional sports in many Western nations (Tomlinson *et al.*, 2005; Jarvie, 2006; Booth and Thorpe, 2007; Comer, 2010). L'Aoustet and Griffet (2001) claim that in France any observable increase in sports participation can be attributed to non-institutionalised informal sport activities, with surveys showing that 45–60 per cent of the French population now practise informal sports. Sport England's *Active People Survey*s also reveal the increasing popularity of more informal and individualistic sports and lifestyle sports specifically (Gilchrist and Wheaton, 2011). The ever-increasing body of participants and consumers range from the occasional participants who experience a range of alternative and traditional sports; to the 'hard core' committed practitioners who are fully familiarised with the lifestyle, argot, fashion and technical skill of their activity.

Increasing numbers of women and girls participate in many lifestyle sports (Comer, 2010; Thorpe, 2011; Wheaton, 2013), and new consumer markets have developed, including so-called 'tweens' and hen parties. There is some scepticism of the extent to which increasing numbers of female participants challenge the gendered discourses, representations, identities and power relationships in lifestyle sports. As Wheaton enquires, do lifestyle sports 'offer different and potentially more transformatory scripts for male and female physicality, than the hegemonic masculinities and femininities characteristic of traditional sports cultures and identities?' (Wheaton, 2004: 6). Recent research, across a range of sports, suggests that lifestyle sports present *opportunities* for embodied identities that differ from those in traditional sports (Mackay and Dallaire, 2013a; Olive and Phillips, 2013; Thorpe, 2013). In some lifestyle sports, the boundaries of gender identity are expanded but, in most, sporting femininities continue to be 'framed by discourses and practices that perpetuate stereotypes of white heterosexual attractiveness, and masculinities based on normative heterosexuality and whiteness, skill and risk, working within, rather than subverting traditional patterns of gendered and bodily domination in sport' (Wheaton, 2004: 19). This is also the case for many other non-normative lifestyle sporting bodies such as African-American surfers (Wheaton, 2013). Nonetheless, while participants have increasingly broadened to include women, girls and older men, the core market has been middle-class white teenagers and young males, especially among urban activities such as skateboarding.

The ways in which consumers can experience lifestyle sports are also expanding and diversifying. This rapid expansion has led to fragmentation, with enthusiasts engaging in a wide variety of participation styles, supporting new and profitable niche markets (Thorpe and Wheaton, 2011). In surfing, for example, a range of participation styles co-exist including short boards, long boards, paddle-boards and body-boards. Skate-boarding has street and park, ramps and bowl, long-boards and hybrids (Atencio *et al.*, 2009). Mediated sources have also proliferated, from traditional forms like DVDs, films and television shows to internet-based media (see below). There are also those who play video games, buy clothing and accessories, and experience activities through commercial, adventure tourism or education-based adventure-settings. These range from schools to organisations, such as the Scouting movement, to commercial outdoor education operations.

Lifestyle sports, and their associated lifestyles, are significant sites for identity construction and bear some of the central issues and paradoxes of late-modern societies, such as the expression of self-identity becoming increasingly self-reflexive, fluid and fragmented (Wheaton, 2004). In lifestyle sports, consumers are being sold a complete style of life, one that emphasises many of the aspirations of postmodern consumer culture (Wheaton, 2004). Like other 'alternative lifestyle' groupings that have emerged from the counter-culture, lifestyle sports involve 'locally situated identity politics rooted in lifestyle practices' (Hetherington, 1998: 3).

Youth studies and conceptualising lifestyle sports cultures

Sport researchers have adopted a range of concepts and theoretical approaches for examining and conceptualising sporting-based collectivities and their lifestyles and identities. Useful conceptual tools include: subworld (e.g. Crosset, 1995), Bourdieu's ideas of field and distinction (e.g. Kay and Laberge, 2002) and Stebbins' (1992, 2007) serious leisure. Here we focus on subculture, lifestyle and identity as conceptualised within the tradition of youth studies in the UK, which we argue are terms also useful for conceptualising and mapping the cultures of lifestyle sports, and particularly the construction and performance of social identities.

Lifestyle

Despite concerns that as a concept lifestyle lacks theoretical clarity, when used in the sense proposed by Chaney (1996) and Miles (2000), it helps signal that in late capitalism lifestyle is intrinsically linked with patterns of consumption. As King and Church (2013: 68) note:

> Whilst identity is a personal project, lifestyles are a means of personal, social and cultural expression. They capture how social actors understand themselves both as individual entities, and as part of emergent types of networks and groups of social identification inherent of late modernity.

As illustrated above, the participants and consumers of these activities seek out a particular *style of life* that is central to the meaning and experience of participation in the sport and that give them a particular and exclusive social identity (Wheaton, 2004: 4). However while youth in Western societies create identities through consumption, lifestyles are also 'manifestations of the ways young people negotiate with structural constraints in their everyday lives' (Miles, 2000: 35). So, as Miles (2000: 18) argues, we need to conceptualise the concept of lifestyle in a way that 'actively addresses the duality of structure and agency.' It is in this sense that we can start to understand the significance of lifestyle in these sporting cultures. Their consumption is a socially and culturally constructed act, underpinned by determinants of choice such as age, class, gender, sexuality and ethnicity, and which cannot be understood simply in terms of market dynamics, nor in terms of a 'position which seeks to preserve the field of lifestyles and consumption, or at least as a particular aspect of it (such as lifestyle sport), as an autonomous playful space beyond determination' (Featherstone, 1991: 84).

Subculture

Various conceptualisations of subculture have historically been and remain influential in the study of lifestyle sports (e.g. Beal, 1995; Humphreys, 2003; Wheaton, 2007). Since the late 1990s, subcultural scholarship in the context of youth and style has undergone substantial revision, largely in response to criticisms of previous research from or inspired by the University of Birmingham's Centre for Contemporary Cultural Studies (CCCS) (e.g. Muggleton and Weinzierl, 2003a). The body of work (referred to as post-CCCS youth studies), which has (re)conceptualised 'subculture', has received extensive airing in the sociological literature, and is the basis for an extensive discussion in Wheaton (2007). Here, therefore, we highlight key points for understanding lifestyle sport cultures and their identities.

The first point to note is that the term subculture is limited in its applicability to many contemporary youth contexts. It is suggested that more temporary, transient gatherings or 'postmodern tribes' (Featherstone, 1991: 111) characterised by 'fluid boundaries and floating memberships' (Bennett, 1999: 600) have replaced subcultural communities, particularly in style-based contexts. Nonetheless, we can still usefully think about lifestyle sports as subcultures. Many lifestyle sport participants demonstrate more stable, shared and uniform notions of subcultures and forms of status and identity (Kiewa, 2002; Beal and Wilson, 2004; Wheaton, 2003). As Hodkinson's (2002) assessment of the contemporary Goth scene concluded, the 'bounded form' taken by the group did not fit with the postmodern emphasis on cultural fluidity, but could be conceptualised as a re-working of subculture. Hodkinson documented 'group distinctiveness, identity, commitment and autonomy' (2004: 136), terming these aspects as 'cultural substance'.

The second point is that the post-subcultural studies approach has potential for understanding the cultural politics in lifestyle sports (Thorpe and Wheaton, 2013). The approach can help to map, understand and explain the complex and shifting power relations involved in the commercialisation of youth cultures before, during and after the group becomes incorporated into the mainstream. It also brings a greater sensitivity to the multiple voices, subjectivities and experiences *within* the subcultural group – including the marginalised – and can expose the ways in which forms of subcultural capital (economic, physical, embodied, etc.) underpin these power relations and status hierarchies. Post-structuralist conceptions of power at play in post-subcultural theory provoked us to ask questions such as 'who is the subculture resisting, where is the resistance cited, under what circumstances is resistance taking place, and in what forms is it manifest?' (c.f. Barker 2000; in Wheaton, 2007). These questions are important for explorations of how we understand the adaptability of lifestyle sport and youth cultures and to explaining how sport consumers and participants re-work the images and meanings circulated in, and by global consumer culture (e.g. Edwards and Corte, 2010; Rinehart, 2008; Stranger, 2010).

Third, while recognising the importance of (and dominant focus on) micro-political dimensions in analyses of subcultures, there has been a failure to attend to their 'macro political context' (Martin, 2002: 79). Somewhat paradoxically then, at a historic conjuncture when youth protest activities – such as the anti-globalisation and anti-Western movements – have bourgeoned, post-subculturalists have tended to under-politicise youth formations (Muggleton and Weinzierl, 2003b). The emergence of environmental protest groups such as Surfers Against Sewage provide examples of the politicisation of lifestyle sports cultures. Subcultural research, in lifestyle sport as in other spheres, must attend to both the micro-political – the politics of everyday life – and the macro-political, particularly issues of political economy and social stratification (Wheaton, 2013).

Identity

To understand (sub)cultural identity and how it is constructed, contested and (re)made, we have advocated an approach derived from cultural studies and post-CCCS approaches to youth subcultures (Wheaton 2007, 2013). Identity, from this perspective is a dynamic process undergoing constant transformation; about becoming as well as being (Hall, 1990). Drawing on Butler's (1990, 1993) work on gender as a 'performative enactment,' Muggleton (2000: 154) suggests that subcultural identity can usefully be seen as a performance that is never fixed or determinate, but is in a state of flux and change. Central to these identity performances however are the ways in which we perceive others as locating us, and what differentiates us. As the wide-range of empirical research on youth in the cultural studies tradition has demonstrated, claims to authenticity are central to the internal and external status hierarchies in youth subcultures; 'authenticity is something sought, fought over and reinvented' (Brunner, 1989; cited in Rinehart and Sydnor, 2003: 9).

The lifestyle sport participant's group identity is marked by a range of symbolic markers, extending from the specialist equipment used and clothing, to the vehicles driven (such as the long-term status of the VW kombi van in surf culture) and musical taste. There are also less visible aspects that contribute to the social construction, performance and regulation of embodied identity including argot, attitude, forms of physical competence and prowess, and the use of space. As research across a range of different street, mountain and water-based lifestyle sports has demonstrated, although taste and style play an important part in constructing a distinctive sporting identity, members cannot 'buy their way into' the core of the culture (e.g. Wheaton, 2000; Ford and Brown, 2005; Thorpe, 2011). Rather, for core participants, authentic identity tends to be constructed around the embodied performance of the activity, around 'doing it' (Wheaton and Beal, 2003).

The negotiation of space for the expression of community and subcultural identities has long been a thread in youth subcultures (which can be traced back to both the CCCS and Chicago School traditions), essential to how young people define themselves vis-a-vis adults and other young people and how they fashion self-identity. More recently, however, the 'spatial' turn in the social sciences (Warf and Arias, 2009) – particularly through the influence of cultural geography – has alerted youth researchers to the ways in which power inequalities are played out and reproduced through space. As we explore below, the impact of spatiality in lifestyle sporting spaces, exploring the competing uses of social space, and how 'different social groups appropriate and mark out social spaces' (Bennett, 2000: 53), is a growing and productive thread. We consider two spaces considered important to wider processes of developing lifestyles and identities linked to youth leisure activities: lifestyle sport as practised in the urban environment and the impacts of digital media and virtual space in shaping lifestyle sports cultures.

Lifestyle sport in the city

What is increasingly apparent as the twenty-first century lifestyle sportscapes are surveyed is that an alternate spatial configuration is emerging. Sports once practised solely in nature – climbing, surfing, snowboarding, kayaking – can be played in purpose-built, commercialised and controlled artificial settings. Climbing walls, snow domes, white water courses and indoor skydive centres are popular with young people and have put many provincial towns on the sport tourism map (van Bottenburg and Salome, 2010). This trend can be easily dismissed as another sign of the incorporation, commercialisation and commodification of lifestyle sports to the needs of multinational business; or, following George Ritzer's Weberian analysis of the rise of rationalised and calculable products in modernity, an all-to-be expected provision of Disneyfied child-centred and safe environments to satisfy postmodern consumer tastes. Commentators have therefore seen alternative sport as a co-opted sporting movement, increasingly controlled by transnational corporations and media conglomerations in search of a lucrative teenage male consumer audience (Rinehart, 2000). However, as research from the Netherlands has found, the adventure/control, nature/technology, outdoor/indoor binaries present in rigid conceptualisations of lifestyle sports are not helpful as such facilities blur the boundaries between traditional and lifestyle sports. A variety of market segments are catered for and the products offered typically emerge from close interactions between producers and consumers (Salome and van Bottenburg, 2012). We concur with Rinehart and Grenfell (2002: 310) that a continuum is required to understand young people's agency in determining the subcultural meanings and identities that cohere around lifestyle sport space, and which may render sites as inauthentic or authentic.

A grass-roots, do-it-yourself ethic persists in lifestyle sporting cultures around the world. Peripheral places in towns and cities are important to young people in terms of symbolic ownership; a site to hang-out, where adolescents can exercise autonomy and express identities in ways that are important to the making of the self. These areas can be defined, following Bauman's discussion of 'empty spaces', as 'public but not civil', existing on the 'edgelands' of cities in sites surplus to the needs of planners, government and landowners (Bauman, 2000: 94–104). However, users conceptualise these spaces as sites of freedom and possibility outside of commercial and policy interests in the urban landscape (Kociatkiewicz and Kostera, 1999). The emergence of lifestyle sports in 'empty spaces' is well-documented. Improvised sites – skateparks, BMX tracks, parkour training areas – have been constructed throughout towns and cities across the world; a testament to the self-organisation and initiative of children and adolescents to determine their own leisure practices (Edwards and Corte, 2010). In the case of BMX tracks, for instance, Rinehart and Grenfell (2002) note the considerable material and emotional investments made by young people in creating and managing a site and the sense of 'ownership' and accomplishment that accrues. The negotiation of space is habitually achieved not through expensive resources, but body performances and interactions with the environment, so that mere presence of participants and subtle marks etched onto the sporting environment – scuff marks and graffiti tags – stakes a claim to occupation (Saville, 2008; Vivoni, 2009). Informal occupation and territorial marking could be considered as a deliberate spatial tactic, an appropriation of neighbourhood space beyond the surveillance and regulation of adults, sometimes necessitated because access to and ownership of private space is denied to them (Robinson, 2000; Childress, 2004). Thus, 'hanging around, and larking about, on the streets, in parks and in shopping malls, is one form of youth resistance (conscious and unconscious) to adult power' (Valentine *et al.*, 1998: 7).

However, where the histories of lifestyle sports are concerned it is important to remember that 'empty spaces' are not necessarily the 'zone of inattention' identified by Bauman (2000: 103). Proposed builds can create polarised community debate around pro-social and anti-social behaviours expected of participants (Taylor and Marais, 2011). Skate parks in particular have been subjected to negative community reactions around unwelcome externalities – noise pollution, in particular – and associated experimental, illicit or deviant behaviours that could occur – e.g. drinking, drug use, graffiti (Goldenberg and Shooter, 2009). As Steyn explains, 'Skateboarders themselves did little to help this negative image as the subculture developed in the 1980s and the dynamics of their identity became framed by aggressive attitudes, notions of indifference and rebellion, spatially and bodily destruction, and competition' (Steyn, 2004; cited in Drissel, 2013: 115–116). The moral panic over 'unsavoury types' has extended into other forms, styles and scenes within lifestyle sports. Street skaters have come into conflict with police and civic authorities (Vivoni, 2009) and its legal repression is witnessed in many cities around the world. Similarly, the recreational trespassing exercised by urban explorers in London is facing legal challenge on the grounds that participants breach security and cause criminal damage to subterranean and derelict sites that were once part of public infrastructure (Garrett, 2013; Self, 2014).

From the perspective of the young participants involved in lifestyle sports it is often the extra-sporting qualities that are significant. One of the primary drivers behind the creation of spaces for lifestyle sport is a setting for relaxation and social interaction. Young people value them as spaces to socialise outside the home. Champions for the development of skate and parkour parks emphasise their importance to adolescent development. Through managing their own space and leisure time, and relations with other users and authorities, young people can acquire self-confidence, learn new skills and develop peer relations and friendships. For these reasons, public authorities have supported the construction of purpose-built facilities in both suburban and urban locations as they are seen to offer potential resources for positive youth development and active citizenship (Bradley, 2010; Gilchrist and Wheaton, 2011), as well as personal wellbeing and physical health (Dumas and Laforest, 2009). Indeed, there is evidence to suggest that an 'everyday utopianism' (Cooper, 2013) is experienced and expressed in the efforts of teenagers and young adults to establish and evolve their own special sites, in which they articulate hopeful visions of personal transformation and social change (Atkinson, 2009; Gilchrist and Wheaton, 2013).

Encroaching adult intervention has not always been welcome. Over time, the spontaneous and informal nature of lifestyle sports has been seen as under threat, with participants under increasing pressure from both commercial operators and state-funded or sanctioned leisure and education providers to professionalise, institutionalise and regulate. These processes are occurring at both the elite/professional level – to enable the activities to be incorporated in traditional forms of competition such as the Olympic Games, for example – and at grass-roots, where conflicts around the use of space, or concerns about safety, are played-out (Wheaton, 2013).

Under such pressures, divisions are all too common within lifestyle sporting cultures and this can impact on the types of users permitted into the sporting space. Borden (2001) discusses the 'territorialisation of skate parks' in which 'locals' claim a skate park as their own, a process that is underpinned by spatially defined insider (us)/outsider (them) statuses. Divisions are also present among users. Rinehart and Grenfell (2002: 307–308) show how BMX tracks can be captured by a 'middle-class grouping' with the social capital and resources to dominate the planning and management of the site, fashioning it according to their tastes and interests. Participants must also learn about cultural codes and signification. Status hierarchies are present in all lifestyle sports, central to boundaries of inclusion and exclusion and to claims to authenticity and the use of subcultural space (Wheaton and Beal, 2003). Such hierarchies, as Wheaton has shown in her studies of windsurfing culture, emerge from differences in types of activity, equipment, difficulty of manoeuvre to be mastered and executed (requiring most commitment in time) and the most hazardous or risky form of the activity (Wheaton, 2000). As such, lifestyle sport spaces, both informal and formal, improvised and purpose-built, possess complex social relations that can exclude some young people and which orient attitudes and behaviours towards other users of public space (Freeman and Riordan, 2002). There is still a need to consider minority participants' experiences of belonging and exclusion; particularly those that do not fit the 'somatic norm' of the white male. Revealing the gendered and racialised nature of lifestyle sports, and their articulations with sexuality, age and class, is key to understating status and identity in these spaces (Wheaton, 2013).

Further case studies are required of lifestyle sport cultures across a variety of urban settlements too. Not all cities are the same. They carry their own local cultural politics, which defines the nature of sporting participation and opportunity and which colours the social and political significance of the cultures and practices established therein. For example, turning to Northern Ireland, Drissel's (2013) participant observation and interviews with members of the Belfast skateboard scene illustrates how a transnational sport can deconstruct local sectarian divisions through the simple act of staking a subcultural space. He found that unlike the community and sporting spaces used by Protestants and Catholics in Belfast – which have been noted for being heavily segregated by ethno-religious divides – the informal street spaces colonised by young Belfast skaters provide an alternative, a shared space upon which new community relations can be built. Drissel writes: 'Rather than remaining in the fixed ghettoized stasis of Belfast's urban habitus, skateboarders have become *de facto* agents of progressive social change, acting to ameliorate and overcome social constraints through the productive use of space' (2013: 134). The case highlights the importance of analysing the micropolitical – an everyday act of resistance to the bifurcated spatial milieu of youth – alongside the macropolitical, in terms of incremental steps taken by young members of the community toward conflict resolution and peace-building.

As lifestyle sports emerge and take hold in communities, they excite interest, perhaps initial public concern, while over time avenues are explored between young people and external authorities over how the sports can be managed and the ways in which they can be harnessed to fulfil policy agendas for the public good (Gilchrist and Wheaton, 2011). However, there remain problems over the ways in which lifestyle sports have been incorporated into state-sponsored schemes and the (unintended) forms of exclusion and disengagement that accrue (King and Church, 2014). As Daniel Turner's study of skateboarding and sport development in Scotland demonstrates, the needs of policy and community workers and those of the skaters can be at variance, and greater sensitivity is needed to the meanings and personal investments made by young people in the sport. Ostensibly, this is a call to develop shared understandings of the subcultural values and attitudes at play, so that we recognise the impacts the sport development community and its funding models make upon lifestyle sports. For Turner, the 'civilized skater' may well be a product of a bifurcation of participatory cultures. He writes:

> The punk-styled participatory behaviours [of skateboarding] . . . such as aggressive language and mannerisms, territorialism and a lack of interest, or indeed hostility, towards personal health and safety are, in the formal, managed skatepark, removed in order to satisfy other paying customers, insurance requirements and managerial imperatives related to maintaining a high-quality facility
>
> *(Turner, 2013: 1257)*

As other research has found, neoliberal ideologies are increasingly present in both the informal neighbourhood parks and corporate-owned, purpose-built facilites and are rewriting the levels of responsibility and risk to be expected in lifestyle sport spaces and of participants (Howell, 2008). And, as younger participants are attracted to these facilities, we also need to consider the extent to which purpose-built and managed facilities for lifestyle sports fit the requirements of modern family lifestyles, the increasingly structured leisure time exercised by parents on behalf of family members, and the moral duties expected of the good parent. It is not just a relationship between the participant and the (state) authorities that legitimise (or appropriate) the presence of activities within communities that is core to the investigation of youth lifestyles, but those negotiated with the people closest to them.

Lifestyle sport, youth culture and digital media

The mass and niche media are central to lifestyle sporting cultures, fuelling their popularity and transnational cultural influence, as well as being integral to the everyday lives of young people (Gilchrist and Wheaton, 2013). The growth of social media since the 1990s and its social and cultural impacts on adolescence and youth popular culture have been well-documented (Holloway and Valentine, 2003; Miegel and Olsson, 2012; Buckingham, 2013), making it necessary to consider here young people's engagement and the interplay of online and offline practices in the making of sport cultures. The personal and professional uses of new media technologies have had a profound impact on how we view subcultural life, particularly the ways in which it enables interaction and exchange between subcultural groups and participants at a global level. According to Osgerby (2004: 193):

> offering instant communication across the world, new media technologies may have accelerated the dissolution of barriers of time and space, redefining notions of the global and local and offering possibilities for the development of new communities based on affinities of interest, politics or any form of cultural identity.

While we should remain cautious towards the alleged impacts of technologically driven social change, new media technologies play an essential role in the social lives of many young people with websites, blogs and social media tools enabling interaction and social networking between participants as well as being important resources for social support, learning skills, community organisation and the provision of information on participative opportunities and events.

Digital media are seen as an important resource for identity processes of adolescence. They are a mode through which transitions – into developed bodies, adult roles, significant peer relationships, work – can be managed and questions of 'becoming' are pursued (Weber and Mitchell, 2008). By creating their own websites, webpages, blogs, or video channels, young people assemble digital media products, some by way of reflexive consumption of existing media outputs, others from materials available to them, which may be more personal. The result is often a bricolage of influences and ideas that says something about their hopes for the future, belongings and imaginings, as their identities and social relations adapt over time. In this way the internet blurs the relationship between producer and consumer. According to Miles (2003: 230), interactive online media, e.g. video blogs, 'are less about consumption (watching others' content) than exploring models for authorship and production . . . it is the ability to participate as communicative peers that is much more significant and viable for distributed networks than our reconstitution into new consumers'. By making use of digital media young people not only extend user-generated content, they also engage in communities and forge interconnections essential to senses of belonging.

Recent research on lifestyle and action sport cultures has highlighted the creative ways in which internet usage facilitates identity projects for participants and how young adults are engaging in civic, community and political spheres as they pursue their sporting interests in sometimes challenging social and cultural contexts (Gilchrist and Wheaton, 2013). MacKay and Dallaire's (2012, 2013a, b) study of the Montreal-based Skirtboarders, a skateboard crew of young women with an active online presence, reveals the importance of blogs as a form of opposition and resistance to hyper-masculine representations of skateboarding bodies and experiences which circulate within the subculture through traditional sport media and websites in ways that maintain a notion of authenticity among core and elite skateboarders, reinforcing insider–outsider statuses (Wheaton and Beal, 2003; Dupont, 2014). By blogging about a small skateboarding scene involving young women of varied social backgrounds and aspirations, the Skirtboarders create and circulate alternative discourses of the material and ideological meanings of the sport. Their blog profiles female skateboarders only, so promoting the sport among women and girls, with blog entries written by participants expressing a variety of female subject positions in ways that disrupt the normalising disciplinary power of the male-dominated skateboarding culture. Their online presence helps to create an alternative space for young women to articulate more complex poly-gendered identities and subjectivities thereby achieving the self-work and identity-building central to adolescence and young adulthood mentioned above.

Other lifestyle sports are inseparable from a digital environment. Kidder (2012) identifies a real/virtual dialectic at the heart of parkour that explains its transnational development and global cultural ubiquity. The Chicago-based participants studied by Kidder favour online videos downloaded via YouTube and Vimeo to analogue printed coaching manuals and guides. They use social media to make sense of their sport through the sharing of moves, manoeuvres and styles and engage in vibrant discussions on web forums about evolving practices and the deeper philosophical meanings attributed to parkour. User-created videos profile the talent of participants, while web tools and apps like GoogleMaps help to share information on training spots. Websites, blogs and social media are thus important repositories of local scenes and developing customs and cultures. These participant-led discourses, both textual and visual, amount to a dynamic and evolving onscreen pedagogy of the sport that novices must confront to understand its demands (Gilchrist and Wheaton, 2013). For Woermann (2012), in a discussion of freeskiing, the life-world of the freeskier is also partially a screen reality with digital media offering a layer of global comment and interaction that is fundamental to the achievement of bodily actions. In both of these cases, digital media is helping to rewrite how we understand the embodied, athletic and aesthetic demands of lifestyle sports. The digital traces left by lifestyle sports participants reveal the convergences and possibilities of evolving sporting cultures as they borrow from a blend of media, genres, and cultural influences in their evolving scenes and local practices.

Kidder suggests such flows of information and interactions among users online and through offline practices are 'the very essence of Appadurai's global ethnoscapes – ideas and images from around the world become integrated into our aspirations and self-understandings. Even if these objects are incapable of interacting with us; we interact with them. And, we bring them into our other social interactions' (Kidder, 2012: 242). Through this interaction with digital media content, parkour is more than a local phenomenon because participants must negotiate and orient themselves to the global imaginary of the sport. As Kidder states: 'traceurs grapple with fitting their actions and motivations into the virtual parkour canon they access in their lives on-screen' (Kidder, 2012: 244). In this regard, it is less a case of globalisation of a culturally ubiquitous sporting form, and more an example of a truly 'glocalised' sporting culture as participants work with cultural artefacts and resources, making them meaningful to their everyday lives and local conditions (Giulianotti and Robertston, 2004).

Exploring local parkour cultures in the Middle East, Thorpe and Ahmed's (2013) research on traceurs in Gaza has shown how internet videos of parkour became a prime inspiration for young participants. Traceurs in Gaza used social media sites, for example Facebook and YouTube, as a form of informal transnational cultural exchange with other youth to articulate their vibrant local culture and the challenging contexts of participation. The videos and photographs uploaded to the sites relay the everyday risks of participation as bombs fall nearby and gunfire from Israeli forces interrupts training. They communicate the necessity to find spaces at the social margins to practice; the liminal spaces of abandoned pockmarked settlements and unmanned border walls. More importantly, the online presence of the traceurs – PK Gaza – sends a message of hope in a conflict-ridden society. The consumption of the digital media products created by PK Gaza by others in the international parkour community has helped to raise awareness of the problems young people face living in Gaza. Some traceurs have been fortunate enough to be invited to Western Europe to show their skills. These exchanges have helped build alliances within and across the action sport community as participants advocate human rights and social and political justice. As Thorpe and Ahmed (2013: 21) conclude: 'we should not overlook their agency, nor should we assume them to be victims, ideologues or fundamentalists.' The vibrant sporting culture profiled online shows the resilience of young people and their ability to snatch a degree of normality from the jaws of desperation.

Conclusion

In this chapter, we have highlighted a range of lifestyle sports forms, cultures and practices and have critically reflected upon the importance of lifestyle, identity and subculture to understanding their growing popularity and global cultural appeal among young people. Much of the early commentary and research on the institutionalisation and commercialisation of lifestyle sports (reflecting the CCCS approach to youth cultures) focused on the negative effects of incorporation of subcultures as a process that undermined the authentic, oppositional or resistant character of alternative sports (Wheaton and Beal, 2003), typically conceptualising commercialisation as 'a top-down process of corporate exploitation and commodification' (Edwards and Corte, 2010: 1137). Through the limited examples provided here, we have shown the inventiveness and resourcefulness of young people and their ability to fashion their own cultures, identities and experiences in ways that are never fully determined by adults, public authorities, corporate interests or socio-cultural norms. Whether it is the skaters of Belfast, Skirtboarders of Montreal or the traceurs of Gaza, our examples show that lifestyle sports are fundamentally about participation and performance – about *doing it*. The sports are adapted in relation to spatial opportunity, changing cultural tastes, financial pressures, regulatory constraints and the availability of new technologies, but continue to be established worldwide through the agency of young people seeking opportunities for both sport and sociability.

There remain challenging and significant questions to explore in the relationship between youth and lifestyle sports and the social contexts and determinants of participation should be to the fore. In particular, research must attend to the myriad ways in which difference and exclusion is manifest in and through these sport cultures: exposing the complex and contradictory articulations of race, gender, sexuality, class, nationhood, disability/ability in these informal but increasingly globally wide spread spaces and settings in which lifestyle and adventure sports takes place.

Note

1   Stoke is a term used by participants of sports such as surfing to refer to the feeling of enjoyment and thrill they get doing the activity.

References

Atencio, M., Beal, B. and Wilson, C. (2009). The distinction of risk: urban skateboarding, street habitus and the construction of hierarchical gender relations, *Qualitative Research in Sport and Exercise, 1(1)*, 3–20.

Atkinson, M. (2009). Parkour, anarcho-environmentalism and poeisis, *Journal of Sport and Social Issues, 33(2)*, 169–194.

Bauman, Z. (2000). *Liquid Modernity*. Cambridge: Polity.

Beal, B. (1995). Disqualifying the official: An exploration of social resistance through the subculture of skateboarding, *Sociology of Sport Journal, 12(3)*, 252–267.

Beal, B. and Wilson, C. (2004). 'Chicks dig scars': commercialisation and the transformations of skate boarders' identities, in B. Wheaton (ed.) *Understanding Lifestyle Sports: Consumption, Identity and Difference* (pp. 31–54). London: Routledge.

Bennett, A. (1999). Subculture or neo-tribes? Rethinking the relationship between youth, style and musical taste, *Sociology, 33(3)*, 599–617.

Bennett, A. (2000). *Popular Music and Youth Culture: Music, Identity and Place*. Basingstoke: Macmillan.

Booth, D. and Thorpe, H. (2007). *International Encyclopaedia of Extreme Sport*. Great Barrington: Berkshire Reference Works.

Borden, I. (2001). *Skateboarding, Space and the City: Architecture and the Body*. Oxford: Berg.

Bradley, G.L. (2010). Skate parks as a context for adolescent development, *Journal of Adolescent Research, 25(2)*, 288–323.

Buckingham, D. (2013). *Beyond Technology: Children's Learning in the Age of Digital Culture*. Cambridge: Polity Press.

Butler, J. (1990). *Gender Trouble: Feminism and the Subversion of Identity*. London: Routledge.

Butler, J. (1993). *Bodies that Matter: On the Discursive Limits of 'Sex'*. London: Routledge.

Chaney, D. (1996). *Lifestyles*. London and New York: Routledge.

Childress, H. (2004). Teenagers, territory and the appropriation of space, *Childhood, 11(2)*, 195–205.

Clemmitt, M. (2009). Extreme sports: are they too dangerous? *CQ Researcher, 19(13)*, 297–317.

Comer, K. (2010). *Surfer Girls in the New World Order*. Durham, NC, and London: Duke University Press.

Cooper, D. (2013). *Everyday Utopias: The Conceptual Life of Promising Spaces*. Durham, NC: Duke University Press.

Crosset, T. (1995). *Outsiders in the Clubhouse: The World of Women's Professional Golf*. Albany, NY: SUNY Press.

Drissel, D. (2012). Skateboarding spaces of youth in Belfast: negotiating boundaries, transforming identities, *Spaces and Flows: An International Journal of Urban and Extra Urban Studies, 2(4)*, 115–138.

Dumas, A. and Laforest, S. (2009). Skateparks as a health-resource: are they are dangerous as they look? *Leisure Studies, 28(1)*, 19–34.

Dupont, T. (2014). From core to consumer: the informal hierarchy of the skateboard scene, *Journal of Contemporary Ethnography*, 1–26 (online first).

Edwards, B. and Corte, U. (2010). Commercialization and lifestyle sport: lessons from 20 years of freestyle BMX in 'Pro-Town, USA', *Sport in Society, 13(7)*, 1135–1151.

Eichberg, H. (1998). *Body Cultures. Essays on Sport, Space and Identity*. London: Routledge.

Featherstone, M. (1991). *Consumer Culture and Postmodernism* (3rd edition). London, Newbury Park, New Delhi: Sage Publications.

Ford, N. and Brown, D. (2005). *Surfing and Social Theory: Experience, Embodiment and Narrative of the Dream Glide*. London: Routledge.

Freeman, C. and Tamara Riordan, T. (2002). Locating skateparks: the planner's dilemma, *Planning Practice and Research, 17(3)*, 297–316.

Garrett, B.L. (2013). *Explore Everything: Place Hacking the City*. London: Verso.

Gilchrist, P. and Wheaton, B. (2011). Lifestyle sport, public policy and youth engagement: examining the emergence of parkour, *International Journal of Sport Policy and Politics, 3(1)*, 109–131.

Gilchrist, P. and Wheaton, B. (2013). New media technologies in lifestyle sport, in B. Hutchins and D. Rowe (eds) *Digital Media Sport: Technology, Power and Culture in the Network Society* (pp. 169–185). New York: Routledge.

Giulianotti, R. and Robertson. R. (2004). The globalization of football: A study in the glocalization of the 'serious life', *British Journal of Sociology, 55(4)*, 545–568.

Goldenberg, M. and Shooter, W. (2009). Skateboard park participation: a means–end analysis, *Journal of Youth Development*, *4(4)*, 37–48.

Gorman, B. (2009). *ESPN Winter X Games 13 Sets Records Across Platforms*, 2 February. Available at: http://tvbythenumbers.com/2009/02/02/espn-winter-x-games-13-sets-records-across-platforms.

Hall, S. (1990). Culture, identity and diaspora, in J. Rutherford (ed.) *Identity, Community, Culture, Difference* (pp. 224–237). London: Lawrence and Wishart.

Hetherington, K. (1998). *Expressions of Identity: Space, Performance, Politics*. London: Sage.

Hodkinson, P. (2002). *Goth: Identity, Style and Subculture*. Oxford: Berg.

Hodkinson, P. (2004). The Goth scene and (sub) cultural substance, in A. Bennett and K. Kahn-Harris (eds) *After Subculture: Critical Studies in Contemporary Youth Culture* (pp. 353–369). Basingstoke: Palgrave.

Holloway, S. L. and Valentine, G. (2003). *Cyberkids: Children in the Information Age*. London: Falmer Routledge.

Howell, O. (2008). Skatepark as neoliberal playground: urban governance, recreation space, and the cultivation of personal responsibility, *Space and Culture*, *11(4)*, 475–496.

Humphreys, D. (2003). Selling out snowboarding: The alternative response to commercial co-optation, in R. Rinehart and S. Syndor (eds) *To the Extreme: Alternative Sport, Inside and Out* (pp. 407–428). Albany: State University of New York Press.

Jarvie, G. (2006). Sport lifestyles and alternative culture, in G. Jarvie *Sport, Culture and Society: An Introduction* (pp. 267–282). London: Routledge.

Kay, J. and Laberge, S. (2002). The 'new' corporate habitus in adventure racing, *International Review for the Sociology of Sport*, *37(1)*, 17–36.

Kidder, J.L. (2012). Parkour, the affective appropriation of urban space, and the real/virtual dialectic, *City and Community*, 11(3), 229–253.

Kiewa, J. (2002). Traditional climbing: metaphor of resistance or metanarrative of oppression? *Leisure Studies*, *21*, 145–161.

King, K. and Church, A. (2013). 'We don't enjoy nature like that': youth identity and lifestyle in the countryside, *Journal of Rural Studies*, *31*, 67–76.

King, K. and Church, A. (2015). Questioning policy, youth participation and lifestyle sports, *Leisure Studies*, 34(3), 282-302.

Kociatkiewicz, J. and Kostera, M. (1999). The anthropology of empty spaces, *Qualitative Sociology*, *22(1)*, 37–50.

L'Aoustet, O. and Griffet, J. (2001). The experience of teenagers at Marseilles' skate park: emergence and evaluation of an urban sports site, *Cities*, *18(6)*, 413–418.

MacKay, S. and Dallaire, C. (2013a). Skirtboarders.com: skateboarding women and self-formation as ethical subjects, *Sociology of Sport Journal*, *30*, 173–196.

MacKay, S. and Dallaire, C. (2014). Skateboarding women: building collective identity in cyberspace, *Journal of Sport and Social Issues*, 34(6), 548-566.

MacKay, S. and Dallaire, C. (2013b). Skirtboarder net-a-narratives: young women creating their own skateboarding (re)presentations, *International Review for the Sociology of Sport*, *48(2)*, 171–195.

Martin, G. (2002). Conceptualizing cultural politics in subcultural and social movement studies, *Social Movement Studies*, *1(1)*, 73–88.

Miegel, F. and Olsson, T. (2012). A generational thing? The internet and new forms of social intercourse, *Continuum: Journal of Media and Cultural Studies*, 26(3), 487–499.

Miles, S. (2000). *Youth Lifestyles in a Changing World*. Buckingham: Open University Press.

Miles, A. (2003) Softvideography, in M. Eskelinen and R. Koskimaa (eds) *Cybertext Yearbook 2002–2003* (pp. 218–236). Saarijavi: University of Jyvaskyla.

Muggleton, D. (2000). *Inside Subculture: The Postmodern Meaning of Style*. Oxford, UK: Berg.

Muggleton, D. and Weinzierl, R. (eds) (2003a). *The Post-Subcultures Reader*. Oxford: Berg.

Muggleton, D. and Weinzierl, R. (2003b). What is 'post-subcultural studies' anyway?, in D. Muggleton and R. Weinzierl (eds) *The Post-Subcultures Reader* (pp. 3–23). Oxford: Berg.

Olive, R., Louise, M. and Phillips, M. (2015). Women's recreational surfing: a patronising experience, *Sport, Education and Society*, 20(2), 258-276.

Osgerby, B. (2004). *Youth Media*. London: Routledge.

Pedersen, P.M. and Kelly, M.L. (2000). ESPN X games: Commercialised extreme sports for the masses, *Cyber-Journal of Sport Views and Issues 1(1)*. Available at: http://sptmgt.taumu.edu.expnx.htm.

Rinehart, R. and Grenfell, C. (2002). BMX spaces: children's grass roots' courses and corporate-sponsored tracks, *Sociology of Sport Journal*, *19*, 302–314.

Rinehart, R. and Sydnor, S. (eds) (2003). *To the Extreme: Alternative sports, Inside and Out*, Albany: State University of New York Press.

Rinehart, R. (2000). Emerging arriving sport: alternatives to formal sports, in J. Coakley and E. Dunning (eds) *Handbook of Sports Studies* (pp. 504–519). London: Sage.

Rinehart, R. (2008). ESPN's X games, contests of opposition, resistance, co-option, and negotiation, in M. Atkinson and K. Young (eds) *Tribal Play: Subcultural Journeys Through Sport*. Research in the Sociology of Sport, *vol. 4* (pp. 175–195). Bingley, UK: Jai Press.

Robinson, C. (2000). Creating space, creating self: street-frequenting youth in the city and suburbs, *Journal of Youth Studies*, *3*, 429–443.

Salome, L. and van Bottenburg, M. (2012). Are they all daredevils? Introducing a participation typology for the consumption of lifestyle sports in different settings, *European Sport Management Quarterly*, *12(1)*, 19–42.

Saville, S.J. (2008). Playing with fear: Parkour and the mobility of emotion, *Social and Cultural Geography*, *9*, 891–914.

Self, W. (2014). Give the freedom of the city to our urban explorers, *London Evening Standard*, 24 April.

Stebbins, R. (1992). *Amateurs, Professionals and Serious Leisure*. Montreal: McGill Queen's University Press.

Stebbins, R. (2007) *Serious Leisure: A Perspective for Our Time*. London: Transaction Publishers.

Stranger, M. (2010). Surface and substructure: beneath surfing's commodified surface, *Sport in Society*, *13(7)*, 1117–1134.

Taylor, M. and Marais, I. (2011). Not in my back schoolyard: schools and skate-park builds in Western Australia, *Australian Planner*, *48(2)*, 84–95.

Thorpe, H. and Wheaton, B. (2013). Dissecting action sports studies, in D.L. Andrews and B. Carrington (eds) *A Companion to Sport* (pp. 341–358). Oxford: John Wiley and Sons.

Thorpe, H. and Ahmed, N. (2015). Youth, action sports and political agency in the Middle East: lessons from a grassroots parkour group in Gaza, *International Review for the Sociology of Sport*, 50(6), 678-704.

Thorpe, H. and Wheaton, B. (2011). 'Generation X Games', action sports and the Olympic movement: Understanding the cultural politics of incorporation, *Sociology*, *45(5)*, 830–847.

Thorpe, H. (2011). *Snowboarding Bodies in Theory and Practice*. Basingstoke: Palgrave Macmillan.

Tomlinson, A., Ravenscroft, N., Wheaton, B. and Gilchrist, P. (2005). *Lifestyle Sport and National Sport Policy: An Agenda for Research*, Report to Sport England. Accessed from www.sportengland.org/research/ idoc.ashx?docid=a6554a47-29b1-4b02-b3ac-600f3144bf8bandversion=1

Turner, D. (2013). The civilized skateboarder and the sports funding hegemony: a case study of alternative sport, *Sport in Society*, *16(10)*, 1248–1262.

Valentine, G., Skelton, T. and Chambers, D. (1998). Cool places: an introduction to youth and youth cultures, in T. Skelton, and G. Valentine (eds) *Cool Places: Geographies of Youth Cultures* (pp. 1–32). London and New York: Routledge.

van Bottenburg, M. and Salome, L. (2010). The indoorisation of outdoor sports: an exploration of the rise of lifestyle sports in artificial settings, *Leisure Studies*, *29(2)*, 143–160.

Vivoni, F. (2009). Spots of spatial desire: skateparks, skateplazas, and urban politics, *Journal of Sport and Social Issues*, *33(2)*, 130–149.

Warf, B. and Arias, S. (eds) (2009). *The Spatial Turn: Interdisciplinary Perspectives*. London: Routledge.

Weber, S. and Mitchell, C. (2008). Imagining, keyboarding and posting identities: young people and new media technologies, in D. Buckingham (ed.) *Youth, Identity and Digital Media* (pp. 25–48). Cambridge, MA: The MIT Press.

Wheaton, B. and Beal, B. (2003). 'Keeping it real': subcultural media and discourses of authenticity in alternative sport, *International Review for the Sociology of Sport*, *38*, 155–176.

Wheaton, B. (2000) 'New lads?' masculinities and the 'new sport' participant, *Men and Masculinities*, *2*, 434–456.

Wheaton, B. (2003). Lifestyle sports magazines and the discourses of sporting masculinity, in B. Benwell (ed.) *Masculinity and Men's Lifestyle Magazines* (pp. 193–221). *Sociological Review*, Blackwell: Oxford.

Wheaton, B. (ed.) (2004). *Understanding Lifestyle Sports: Consumption, Identity and Difference*. London: Routledge.

Wheaton, B. (2007). Identity, politics, and the beach: environmental activism in 'Surfers Against Sewage', *Leisure Studies*, *26(3)*, 279–302.

Wheaton, B. (2013). *The Cultural Politics of Lifestyle Sports*. London: Routledge.

Woermann, N. (2012). On the slope is on the screen: presumption, social media practices, and scopic systems in the freeskiing subculture, *American Behavioral Scientist*, *56(4)*, 618–640.

SECTION 4

Socialization and youth sport

19

INTRODUCTION

Ken Green

The most significant term in this section of the Handbook and, arguably, the text as a whole is *socialization*. Socialization refers to the processes through which people acquire or are taught (either directly or indirectly, explicit or implicitly, intentionally or unintentionally) and internalize the values, beliefs, expectations, knowledge, skills, habits and practices prevalent in their groups and societies. Put simply, socialization involves the internalization of social norms (shared expectations). It amounts, in other words, to people learning the cultures or ways of life of the groups and wider networks into which they are born and live. Among other things, socialization becomes manifest in what young people take for granted or think of as natural.

The concept of socialization is often criticized in two broad ways. First, socialization is said to be far too static a concept, implying a once and for all occurrence (in the family during infancy and childhood, in particular) rather than a *process*. Conceived as a process, socialization is never total or complete but, rather, ongoing and developmental. Socialization is also criticized for being too deterministic, failing to account for the ways in which (young) people mediate, interpret, adapt and sometimes reject what they learn from their families, schools and peers, for example. Whereas a term such as education implies deliberate guidance, the term socialization is often taken to imply (more or less) conditioned responses to a variety of social influences. It is a gross oversimplification, however, to imagine that the social environment conditions or shapes young people in a deterministic fashion any more than young people are entirely free to shape themselves. Socialization is neither a homogenizing nor all-embracing process (Malcolm, 2008, p. 232). The relationship between young people and socializing agencies such as the family and school is best conceptualized as reciprocal and interactive and one that is, to a greater or lesser extent, contingent upon the former's (more or less conscious) interpretations of the influences of latter (something particularly germane to the socialization of youngsters into youth sport). This is why social scientists talk of negotiation between young people and others in their social networks in an attempt to convey the significance of young people's interpretations of the explicit and implicit messages they receive from the networks they are a part of, such as peers, in general, and friends, in particular. Much research into socialization is, as a consequence, ecological in the sense that it explores socialization processes within the complex networks of relationships that young people inhabit (such as family, friends and school) often at one and the same time. The fact that they do not simply conform to all the norms they are introduced to during primary and secondary socialization is evident in the numerous examples of young people negotiating and compromising on, even rejecting, particular behaviours (for example, playing sport and consuming drugs) as well as embracing them. This is especially apparent when young people begin, more overtly, to construct their own identities from the material of early socialization. Negotiation notwithstanding, it is important to recognize that socialization is inevitable: as young people grow up they cannot help but learn something, '*somewhere* with *somebody*' (Tolonen, 2005: 344; emphases in the original).

The people and groups that (intentionally or unintentionally, directly or directly) pass on particular values, practices and so forth are said to be agents of socialization. Agents of socialization are characteristically subdivided into two categories: primary and secondary. Primary socialization refers to the initial and arguably most influential form of socialization, usually experienced within the family – particularly from parents but also siblings. Secondary socialization, in contrast, refers to those social processes, such as elementary and secondary schooling, and socializing agents, such as PE teachers, peers and friends. Other potentially significant secondary agents of socialization (in terms of time and/or influence) include sports clubs, part-time workplaces and, in particular, the mass media and TV and the internet. Socialization becomes a more or less deliberate and conscious process depending upon the socializing agent(s). Schools, for example, engage consciously (via the formal curriculum) as well as informally (via the so-called hidden or informal curriculum) in the process of (secondary) socialization. The socializing effects of friendship groups, by contrast, tend to be informal via imitation and constraint.

A term commonly associated with socialization is *significant others*; in other words, people who have a significant influence on the thoughts and practices of young people, for example. It is well-established that, among youth especially, decisions regarding participation in sport tend to be tied to encouragement and support from others who are important in their lives (Coakley and White, 1992). Alongside parents and siblings, PE teachers and sports club coaches and officials are often viewed as potentially significant others in youngsters' sporting socialization. In practice, especially 'significant others' for young people are their friends and peers and, through the teenage years especially, these become increasingly significant agents of socialization. This is particularly so with regard to young people's leisure tastes and practices in general and in relation to sport in particular. Thus, secondary socialization from peers can and often does challenge and reinforce primary socialization in the family and secondary socialization in school, evidencing the fact that socialization of young people as they grow older is far from straightforward or unidirectional. For example, much sport tends to be adult led. But as they get older, and start to anticipate adult lives, many youth do not want to be led or organized by adults. The older they get, the more secondary school-aged youngsters tend to favour leisure activities that give them the kinds of independence and autonomy that makes them feel more 'adult-like' (Coakley and White, 1992). It is apparent that young people tend to associate highly structured adult-organized sport with being a child. This is particularly true for girls and young women (Coakley and White, 1992). In this regard, any sports participation must fit in with their preferred self and peer-group identities.

While socialization does not end with adulthood, later stages of the socialization process inevitably build in some way or other upon the foundations laid early on. The significance of early life socialization lies, therefore, in the impact it has on young people's predispositions – what some sociologists refer to as the habitus (Bourdieu, 1977, 1984; Elias, 1994). Habitus can be defined as the durable dispositions that suffuse a person's beliefs, attitudes and behaviours in a particular domain of their lives, such as leisure-sport, or even the whole of their lives – becoming, in effect, what we refer to as second nature or personality (Camic, 1986). On this view, 'the real forces which govern us' (van Krieken, 1998: 47) are our habits or habitus – and it is because we tend not to be aware of the ways in which our seemingly free choices are influenced by deep-seated predispositions (or second nature) that 'the choices involved seem to be made naturally' (Tolonen, 2005: 356). Although a circular and, therefore, problematic concept, habitus has become the default position for sociologists seeking to make sense of the emergence and development of deep-seated and enduring predispositions towards a domain of life such as sport. Young people's sporting habitus are said to be expressed, for instance, when they make sporting and leisure lifestyle choices (albeit often – but not always – within the parameters of their class, gender, ethnic and other socio-cultural conditions). There is, nonetheless, a view that in late- or post-modernity – as their lives have become increasingly individualized – young people can self-socialize by reflexively and consciously choosing groups (such as mountain-bikers, skateboarders and surfers) that will shape them (and their habitus) in ways they wish to be shaped and allow them to develop the kinds of identities they desire.

In keeping with the significance of primary socialization, Section 4: *Socialization and youth sport* opens with two chapters that focus on the significance of childhood and parents for what eventually becomes youths' sporting practices.

In *Parenting and youth sport*, Thomas Quarmby examines the positive and negative influences of parents on enabling their children's sports participation. He portrays the family as not only the first point of socialization but also the key site for childhood socialisation into activities such as sport. Quarmby observes how parents' positive beliefs about activity can lead to the purposeful introduction of sport in the lives of their children through informal play or the purchase of activity-related services. Quarmby highlights the ways in which parents can play a crucial role in relation to several aspects of sports socialization, including not only parental beliefs and values but also specific practices (such as enrolling their children in sports clubs) and strategies (such as the deliberate sampling of a variety of different sports). The things that parents do and say to support and encourage their children's sports participation amount to a combination of active and passive parental practices. In the first instance, parents can provide powerful role models. While role-modelling can be passive and indirect, it is active, direct modelling that appears most influential, especially in the form of joint parent–child participation in sports. Parents also support their children's sports participation by, among other things, paying fees, purchasing sporting equipment, transporting their children to and from activities, and spectating. In doing so, they provide the often crucial emotional as well as practical support. Quarmby observes how the (direct) influence of parents tends to decline with age. He explores this transition (typically during the early secondary years) as youngsters increasingly divide their time between parents, peers and being alone. We are also reminded that the increasingly prominent and influential role of friends should not encourage us to overlook the manner in which the significance of parents persists.

Later on in this section, Holt and Neely point out the manner in which parents continue to play vital roles during the teenage years, not least by providing emotional and tangible support for sport participation. Thus, early parental influences tend to have a profound and lasting effect on sports participation not just during childhood but throughout youth and into adulthood. In this regard, Quarmby cites studies that suggest that youngsters' sporting predispositions and tendencies may even be relatively fixed by age 16. Proficiency gained during childhood is, nevertheless, inevitably dependent upon parental abilities to provide such opportunities during youth which, for some, may be restrained by a variety of factors – a theme picked up in Section 5. In this regard, Quarmby also points up the often gendered nature of parenting practices with mothers tending towards more assistive support in the form of planning and organizing their children's leisure-sport experiences. As Quarmby reminds us, much of the hidden work of sport socialization is carried out by women.

Having explored the significance of primary socialization in the family for youths' sporting experiences, the subsequent chapters in Section 5 draw attention to 'significant others' during secondary socialization, and peer/friendship groups in particular. In *Peer group experiences in youth sport*, Kacey Neely and Nicholas L. Holt note that parents tend to move into the background of teenagers' lives as their daily interactions with peers (whether at school, in sport, or just 'hanging out') become more frequent and important. As they approach and move through the teenage years, young people's leisure is increasingly spent with friends rather than family. According to Neely and Holt, the vast majority of youngsters have what they consider a best friend and many have several good friends. As a consequence, it is likely that young people will be members of several different friendship and peer groups in a variety of settings based, for instance, around school, music and social media, as well as sports. In each and all of these settings, friend and peer group experiences can offer some of the most meaningful aspects of participation by providing, among other things, opportunities to expand social networks, develop friendships and learn a range of social skills. In the process, the dynamism and flexibility of young people's leisure can result in the formation and dissolution, as well as the maintenance, of friendship and peer groups. Neely and Holt suggest that the experiences of youth with their peers need to be understood at a variety of (interrelated) levels – that is, within individuals, within interactions, within relationships and within groups – and explore each of these in depth. As with family socialization, the mechanisms by which friends and peers enable or discourage sports participation involve not merely the transmission of attitudes and values but also 'modelling' of active or inactive pursuits and the provision of psychological support or reinforcement for certain behaviours. It is not just what their friends think about sport and do or do not do in practice that influences young people, however. It is also the opportunities that sport (and, for that matter, any leisure practice) provides for making and sustaining friendships, and the ways in which young people's friendship groups facilitate links with other young people sharing similar interests and situations. Indeed, sport is often a site for the generation of friendships that sport then becomes a means of sustaining. Sports players tend to befriend peers who play their sports (often via those sports) leading to a mutually dependent relationship between young people's friendship and peer-group networks and their involvement in sport. Neely and Holt also point out, however, that as well as enabling and enhancing youth's experiences in sport peers can have detrimental influences. In doing so, they consider the negative consequences of peer group experiences in sport, including tobacco, alcohol and drugs – a relationship explored further by Perreti-Wattel in Section 6 of this Handbook.

In *A personal assets approach to youth sport*, Jean Côté, Jennifer Turnnidge and Matthew Vierimaa examine an increasingly popular model in the field of sports socialization for sports development among youth, namely Positive Youth Development (PYD). In PYD, sport is treated as a vehicle for youths' positive physical, psychological and social development. It focuses upon the so-called 'personal assets' of youth and what the authors refer to as the four Cs: confidence, competence, connection and character. Côté *et al.* link the four Cs to three elements of sport and PYD, namely, activities, relationships, and settings. Côté *et al.* argue that the development of these proximal constructs in young athletes will effectively lead to increased long-term participation, performance and personal development. In doing so, they focus on the three broad ways in which they claim youth are socialized into sports participation: that is, vis-à-vis performance, participation, and personal development. Côté *et al.* suggest that three key elements need to be combined in the design and delivery of quality youth sport programmes:

1   personal engagement in activities
2   quality relationships
3   appropriate settings.

In terms of facilitating and enhancing sports participation, Côté *et al.* point to what they label the Developmental Model of Sport Participation (DMSP). The DMSP has become an especially popular model. The DMSP proposes a common foundation to youth sport programmes focused upon enabling youngsters, with the support of their parents (Quarmby, this volume), to taste a variety of sporting activities during childhood with the emphasis on intrinsic enjoyment (the so-called 'sampling' stage). Thus, the main tenet of the DMSP model is diversity as a precursor to and precondition for the specializing stage in which youngsters commit to one or a few sports and develop the technical and tactical skills in the context of sporting competition. Thereafter, according to the DMSP model, (some) youth enter the investment stage of intensive training and increasingly high-level competition. As we have seen from the earlier chapters in this section, the sampling and investment stages could well pass for a description of what actually happens in practice, in many middle-class families at least. Quarmby shows how parental strategizing typically allows youngsters to experience a range of opportunities prior to selection for recreational and/or performance reasons. Côté *et al.* suggest that the advantage of a diversified foundation in sport during the sampling years resides in the provision of a breadth of experiences that emphasize exploration before commitment to a specific sport activity. Roberts and Brodie (1992) would add that it is also more likely to result in the wide sporting repertoires that often appear a precursor (not to say precondition) to ongoing participation during youth and, ultimately, adulthood.

In their chapter entitled *Understanding take-up, drop-out and drop-off in youth sport*, Jessica Fraser-Thomas, William Falcão and Lauren Wolman examine the reasons youth initially engage in, persist with and/or eventually withdraw from sport. The authors ground their discussion of youth sport take-up within psychological theories of motivation (Competence Motivation Theory, Achievement Goal Theory and Self-Determination Theory) alongside the Expectancy Value and Sports Commitment models. Among other things, Fraser-Thomas *et al.* focus upon drop-out from particular sports (while remaining involved with others) and generalised drop-out (involving withdrawal from all sports). Their observation that youth do not necessarily want to withdraw from sport altogether but can do so because of the intensive nature of their sporting involvement and the lack of other programming options, makes especially interesting reading alongside Borger, Segher and Scheerder's investigation of 'sport light' in Section 3. Fraser-Thomas *et al.* outline models of youth sport withdrawal before focusing upon intrapersonal, interpersonal and contextual factors in youth sport drop-out. Fraser-Thomas *et al.* also explore models of youth sport transitioning and the implications for transitioning out of sport. The authors note that existing research has tended to concentrate on intrapersonal and interpersonal factors in youth sport take-up and withdrawal, thereby overlooking contextual factors at structural, organizational, socio-cultural and policy levels. Each of these themes is addressed in some measure elsewhere in the Handbook. Fraser-Thomas *et al.* conclude that interventions are needed in order to examine all phases of youth sport involvement through the lens of youths' ostensibly basic needs for autonomy, relatedness and competence; in other words, against the backdrop of self-determination theory.

References

Bourdieu, P. (1977). *Outline of a Theory of Practice*. Cambridge: Cambridge University Press.

Bourdieu, P. (1984). *Distinction: A Social Critique of the Judgement of Taste*. (R. Nice, Trans.) Cambridge, MA: Harvard University Press.

Camic, C. (1986). The matter of habit, *American Journal of Sociology*, *91(5)*: 1039–1087.

Coakley, J. and White, A. (1992). Making decisions: Gender and sports participation among British adolescents, *Sociology of Sport Journal*, *9*: 20–35.

Elias, N. (1994). *The Civilizing Process*. Oxford: Blackwell [1939].

Malcolm, D. (2008). *The Sage Dictionary of Sports Studies*. London: Sage Publications.

Roberts, K. and Brodie, D. (1992) *Inner-City Sport: Who Plays and What are the Benefits?* Giordano Bruno: Culemborg.

Tolonen, T. (2005). Locality and gendered capital of working-class youth, *Young, 13(4)*: 343–61.

Van Krieken, R. (1998). *Norbert Elias*. London: Routledge.

20

PARENTING AND YOUTH SPORT

Thomas Quarmby

Introduction

Parents are arguably one of the most important influences on youth sporting practices and their continued engagement. However, a recent article published online in a British newspaper called for parents to be banned from watching their children play sport, arguing that 'parenting hysteria . . . was running riot beyond the white lines' (White, 2014). This raises concern about the immediate influence of parents with regard to youth sport. Against this backdrop, this chapter discusses research concerning parenting and youth sport, examining both the positive and negative influences that parents may have on enabling children's sports participation as well as maintaining or adversely impacting upon their engagement.

Parents as socialising agents

The field of socio-cultural and socio-psychological studies examining the influence of family on youth sports participation is growing. Such studies consistently point to the family as the key social institution and a crucial site for childhood socialisation into activities such as sport (Green, 2010; Rapoport and Rapoport, 1975). Within the family, parents are thought to be the most influential socialising agents for young children's early learning experiences (Kirk, 2005; Shakib and Dunbar, 2004) and the first point of socialisation into sport and other leisure activities. Briefly, socialisation is a process through which children acquire specific values and beliefs that help define their identity and learn the rules and norms for their present and future roles in a particular culture (Kay, 2004). During their initial socialisation into sport, parents have a substantial influence on the extent to which children develop a range of social skills linked to the ideas, attitudes and body movements associated with a given sport (Kirk *et al.*, 1997). Since most children remain in the family environment for many years, this provides repeated and ongoing opportunity for parental socialisation. However, Zeijl *et al.* (2000) argue that the influence of the primary socialising agent declines with age. In their Dutch study of 927 young people, they observed that younger children (aged 10–12) spent a substantial part of their leisure time with their family, parents and siblings in particular. They described children aged thirteen as 'transition children' (Zeijl *et al.*, 2000, p. 297), since they divided their time between parents, peers and being alone, and took an intermediate position between children and adolescents, with adolescents' contact with their peers growing. Despite this tendency, Zeijl *et al.* (2000) concluded that no matter what their age parental influence was still significant, although it was most prominent prior to age thirteen.

Recent studies have suggested that early socialisation in the family, and by parents in particular, can have a profound and lasting effect on sports participation not just during childhood, but over an individual's life course (Birchwood *et al.*, 2008; Haycock and Smith, 2012). A study by Birchwood *et al.* (2008, p. 291) of South Caucasus adults (i.e. from Armenia, Azerbaijan and Georgia) found 'that a distinct and enduring propensity to play sport is acquired during childhood via a culture transmitted by the family'. They observed that family background still made a difference to sports participation when respondents were in their twenties. Birchwood *et al.* (2008) suggested that, as children, individuals acquire a set of deep-rooted predispositions (what Bourdieu would term a habitus) shaped by their social context and transmitted via socialisation in the family. In fact, they argued that these sporting predispositions and tendencies were, irrespective of gender and socio-economic inequalities, relatively fixed by age sixteen (Birchwood *et al.*, 2008). The role of the family and particularly parents as key socialising agents would appear vital, therefore, although the specific mechanisms by which parents influence sporting dispositions was not discussed.

Parental beliefs and values

Parents transmit values to their children and the transmission of parental values, beliefs and practices regarding sport is a vital component of the process of socialisation. A recent study by Wheeler (2011) identified a range of parenting goals, strategies and justifications in the promotion of their children's sports participation. These included the type of personal and social benefits they anticipated their children gaining from sport. For instance, sport provides participants with a myriad of potential physical, social and psychological benefits (Fraser-Thomas *et al.*, 2005) that parents are keen to tap in to. Wheeler's (2011) findings are mirrored in other international literature whereby parents introduced their children to sport due to its purported social and health enhancing benefits. For instance, Shaw and Dawson (2001) indicated that parents were particularly concerned about the health and fitness benefits of their children's leisure sport pursuits, while further Australian work by Macdonald *et al.* (2004) indicated that parent's positive beliefs about activity led to the purposeful introduction of sport in the lives of their children through informal play or the purchase of activity-related services. Wheeler (2011) also found that parents often wanted their children to have experiences that they had not had themselves, and that, by providing opportunities for their children to be involved in a variety of organised sport activities, they could be seen to be meeting the cultural requirements of 'good parenting' (Wheeler and Green, 2012). Moreover, when children play sport, parents feel they are meeting their responsibilities as parents; since youth sports involve enjoyable and valued character building activities believed to help develop and improve their children in particular ways (Coakley, 2009; Vincent and Ball, 2007).

Consistent with previous literature, Wheeler (2011) found that parents also employed a range of strategies to ensure these goals were achieved. First, parents play a significant role in introducing children to sport through, for example, enrolment in sports clubs (Dixon *et al.*, 2008; Gould *et al.*, 2006; Rowley, 1992; Wheeler, 2011). Parents are also responsible for allowing children to sample a variety of different sports, particularly prior to their teenage years (Kirk, 2005). This is key to Côté's (1999) developmental model of sports participation (Côté *et al.*, this volume) in which the sampling years (age 6–13) are viewed as a period when parents develop their children's interest in sport. During these early years, parents are thought to expose children to the sporting domain through a variety of activities that emphasise fun and enjoyment.

Such early experiences in a range of organised sport activities set the foundation for future participation in recreational (MacPhail and Kirk, 2006; MacPhail *et al.*, 2003) and elite sport (Côté, 1999). Furthermore, by allowing the introduction of a wide range of sports, it is argued that the sampling years enable children to become locked in to sport participation (Roberts and Brodie, 1992, p. 60). Becoming locked in to sport during early sport socialisation is, according to Roberts and Brodie (1992), a consequence of the number of different sports that children regularly play and become proficient in during childhood. This, however, is clearly dependent upon parent's abilities to provide such opportunities during youth, which for some, may be restrained by a variety of factors.

Parental practices

The mechanisms and behaviours by which parents influence the sporting engagement of their children can be attributed to a combination of active and passive parental practices (Green, 2010). It is in this area in that most research has been conducted with regard to parenting and youth sport: that is, the things that parents do and say to support sports participation (Wheeler, 2011).

Parental support

Providing support for children's sport activities is one broad example of an active parental practice. Although often used interchangeably, the terms parental support and parental encourage-ment can be distinguished by considering their outcomes (Leff and Hoyle, 1995): parental support can be defined as behaviours that facilitate sports participation (Leff and Hoyle, 1995), while parental encouragement reinforces it (Wheeler, 2011). These terms are not, however, unproblematic in implying that support and encouragement have only positive implications. Studies show that children's sports participation is often dependent on parents' ability to invest the necessary resources of money, time and energy (Coakley, 2009). Elliot and Drummond (2013) suggest that parental support can take the form of investment with regard to the significant financial, logistical and emotional contributions parents make in an effort to provide a positive sporting experience for their children. For example, parents make it possible for their children to participate in sport by paying fees and purchasing (often expensive) sporting equipment (Gould *et al.*, 2008; Kirk *et al.*, 1997; Kay, 2004). In addition, parents provide logistical support by taxiing their children to and from activities. Kirk *et al.* (1997) concluded that parents also make a substantial contribution to their children's sport participation through the commitment of their time and through not only transporting children to venues but also waiting and spectating. It is important to note that for those children regularly engaging in higher levels of sport, these demands can gradually absorb the whole family unit to the point that sport affects the daily, weekly and annual rhythms of family life, with the level of commitment required to provide support having implications for the emotional life of the family (Kay, 2000; Wiersma and Fifer, 2008). Beyond the time demands, parents also make a substantial and vital contribution through providing emotional support (watching activities and discussing them) to both boys and girls (Kirk *et al.*, 1997). It is argued that these types of parental support were significantly related to children's enjoyment and self-esteem (Leff and Hoyle, 1995), while such sources of parental support have also been found to alleviate stress in youth sport (Côté, 1999; Kay, 2004).

However, some parents inappropriately use methods of investment to motivate effort or acquire success (Elliot and Drummond, 2013). This has particular implications, with research indicating that parental rewards can have a negative impact upon children's sports participation by undermining their intrinsic interest (Woolger and Power, 1993). For instance, in their study of the developmental experiences of adolescent swimmers, Fraser-Thomas and Côté (2009) found that some parents financially coerced their children to excel or stay involved in competitive swimming. They reported that parents expected competitive success when they supplied the best resources and regularly reminded their children of the high costs associated with participation (Fraser-Thomas and Côté, 2009). An earlier study by Fraser-Thomas *et al.* (2008) also concluded that the children of parents who offered financial rewards or incentives, for good performances only, were more prone to dropping out of sport.

Parental encouragement

Parental encouragement is closely associated with emotional support since children often turn to their parents for comfort and security. Shakib and Dunbar (2004) suggest that parents share stories about sporting experiences and communicate the importance of sport to their children. In an American study of children aged ten to fourteen years, Duncan *et al.* (2005) found that the most significant type of encouragement or emotional support was parents watching the activity of their children. When children perceived parents to be watching their activity, they reported higher levels of participation (Duncan *et al.*, 2005). It was suggested, therefore, that encouragement of or emotional support for these types was more important than logistical support (Duncan *et al.*, 2005). While positive verbal encouragement can enhance children's enjoyment and satisfaction in sport (Wuerth *et al.*, 2004) so too can excessive encouragement have the opposite effect. Hellstedt (1995) argued for the need to understand parental involvement in children's sport since there is a fine line between positive encouragement and excessive pressure. For instance, it has been reported that some parents lack verbal self-control, offer derogatory remarks and publicly label their children as *pathetic* (Holt *et al.*, 2008). It is also thought that even good-willed comments from parents, such as *good try*, can be misinterpreted by children as an unsuccessful skill attempt and lead to feelings of incompetence, anxiety or embarrassment and thus have negative consequences for their continued engagement (Kanters *et al.*, 2008).

Parental modelling

Family members can be powerful role models in the socialisation process. In fact, the importance of parents as agents of socialisation largely draw from empirical studies that demonstrate relationships between parent and child activity levels (Kay, 2004). Bandura (1986) argues that observational learning occurs when observers (in this case, children) acquire new patterns of behaviour by watching the actions of significant others, namely parents. As such, the modelling of certain actions by parents works to strengthen or weaken children's inhibitions about recently learned behaviours. Since children are frequently exposed to contact with parents, it is perhaps not surprising that parental modelling of sport has received the majority of attention with regard to overall parental influence (Saelens and Kerr, 2008). Parental modelling can be passive and unintentional in the sense that, while not actively promoted or encouraged, attitudes and behaviours can be modelled by parents and imitated by children (Fredericks and Eccles, 2004; Kay, 2004). Indeed, parental attitudes and behaviours can play a significant part in the development of children's sporting dispositions. Parents that transmit values of achievements that depend upon learning and practice, demonstrate work ethic and composure also model non-sport related behaviours that children can transfer to their own sport (Gould *et al.*, 2008). However, the scale of role behaviour in children's sport is further evidenced by parents who display poor conduct and dishonest values. In these cases, such behaviour is likely to be mirrored in children's game play (Elliot and Drummond, 2013).

With regard to children's imitation of specific behaviours, a study by Yang *et al.* (1996) with Finnish children aged nine to fifteen years found that the father's activity was significantly related to their children's activity in present and later life. Yang *et al.* (1996) have argued that fathers exert the most influence on both boys and girls with regard to physical activity and may therefore be a more important socialisation agent. Parents must also be aware that the modelling of sedentary behaviours appears to be even more contagious than sports participation (Green, 2010). While Scheerder *et al.* (2005) suggest that parental sports participation plays a substantial role in children's active involvement in sport they also noted that simple passive modelling of sports participation by parents did not appear to be as effective as active, joint parent-child participation in sports. In Shaw and Dawson's (2001) leisure-based qualitative study with Canadian families, joint family leisure-sport activities were seen to provide parents with time together to 'develop a sense of family and to teach children about values and healthy lifestyles' (Shaw and Dawson, 2001, p. 228). They also suggested that parents engaged in joint participation with their children in a range of sporting activities with some degree of urgency; spending time together before their children got older (Shaw and Dawson, 2001). However, Scheerder *et al.* (2005) suggest that joint participation, while important, may not be as influential as the provision of emotional and even logistical support, particularly as children grow and move towards the teenage years. Arguably, it would appear that children whose parents provide the appropriate levels of support and encouragement are far more likely to participate than children whose parents do not.

Parental roles

As alluded to above, some studies have shown that parents' roles are not necessarily consistent or unproblematic (Kirk *et al.*, 1997). Parents have continued to endorse the gender stereotypical belief that boys are more suited to sports than girls and this continues into middle childhood and adolescence (Fredricks and Eccles, 2004). For many fathers, sport provides a setting in which they feel comfortable and confident as a parent since they draw on past sporting experiences that are consistent with traditionally masculine views of fatherhood (Coakley, 2006). As such, Kay (2009) has argued that sport often features more prominently in fathering than in mothering, though mothers still play a pivotal role in socialising their children into sport, though they do so in different ways. There are, for instance, subtle differences in the types of support that parents provide. A study of parental social support for children's (aged 8–11) outdoor activity suggested that the type of social support afforded by parents differed by gender (Beets *et al.*, 2007). Whereas fathers participated directly with their sons, mothers were found to provide more assistive support and, by planning outdoor activity and play (such as riding bikes, walking or playing in a playground), mothers also positively influenced girls' activity (Beets *et al.*, 2007). This work mirrors previous findings that indicate a tendency for fathers to act as playmates with children, engage in more vigorous 'rough and tumble games' (MacDonald and Parke, 1986, p. 368), while mothers undertake house management responsibilities and engage in less demanding forms of activity with their children (MacDonald and Parke, 1986). A recent study by Haycock and Smith (2012, p. 13) exploring the sporting histories of adults argued that for women, 'it was their mothers who played the major role in planning and organising their early experiences of leisure-sport'. Research by Macdonald *et al.* (2005) and Shaw and Dawson (2001) also revealed that while both parents (male and female) demonstrated equal commitment and responsibility to their children's activities, it was usually mothers who were found to be particularly important in planning and making decisions about their child's activity. In fact, much of the 'hidden' work of sport socialisation (for example, planning, scheduling and organising of leisure) 'falls primarily to women' (Shaw, 2008, p. 699). Arguably, this gendered pattern of parenting may mean that children are likely to be influenced in different ways and at different times. Despite this, the importance of mothers and fathers to the sport socialisation of children cannot be underestimated. Moreover, having two parents who are both supportive and encouraging of sport participation during childhood may help construct sporting biographies that generate greater patterns of participation during young adulthood (Haycock and Smith, 2012).

(Un)Favourable family circumstances

Regardless of their parental beliefs and values, family circumstances may ultimately impact on parents' ability to enact the aforementioned practices. Since parents are significant indicators of social class, it is perhaps not surprising that parents vary in their ability to pass on the kinds of social and cultural capital that is useful for sport (Green, 2010). Evans and Davies (2010) suggest that parents of more middle-class families are better able to invest the significant amounts of time, money, energy and socio-emotional development in their children that provide an important foundation for adulthood participation. Middle-class parents are more likely to possess the material resources (or economic capital) to enable their offspring to engage in sport, but are also more likely to be in a position to transfer their social and cultural capital by virtue of being already actively involved themselves and inclined to pass their love of sport on to their children (Roberts and Brodie, 1992). Haycock and Smith (2012) argue that economic constraints such as the availability of financial resources and transportation clearly influences childhood sport socialisation. However, it is not just class that generates unequal levels of sports participation, but the different family types and structures that are also evident within society (Quarmby and Dagkas, 2010). For instance, the division of labour within families to support participation, particularly where more than one child is involved, is significant, and tends to favour families where parents have a degree of flexibility in their work hours (Kirk, 2005).

Family structure has also been found to have a substantial influence on children's socialisation into sport and the development of sporting dispositions. It has been reported that children from lone parent families tend not to receive the same amount and kinds of support and encouragement for involvement in sport that their two parent, middle-class counterparts do (Dagkas and Stathi, 2007; Macdonald *et al.*, 2004; Quarmby and Dagkas, 2010). Indeed, children from two parent families are far more likely to progress and achieve success in sport (Kay, 2000; Kay *et al.*, 2008). Parents clearly play a key role in introducing and sustaining young children's involvement in sport and are required to meet the financial costs, provide logistical and emotional support as well as adapt family routines to help ensure children can participate and progress in their chosen sport (Kay, 2000; Kay *et al.*, 2008). However, recent changes in family structure may have led 'some sub-groups [to] experience material difficulties' (Kay *et al.*, 2008, p. 8) that ultimately impact on the children's ability to maintain participation in sport.

Implications for youth sport

Notwithstanding class background and family structure, many parents still seek to negotiate these constraints by finding alternative, low cost and localised sporting activities for their children (Shaw, 2008). Parents, as a key part of the central social institution the family, are therefore pivotal in fostering youth participation in sport during the early years, not least because participation usually depends on parental expenditures of time, money and energy (Coakley, 2006). They are highly visible in sport with a range of studies identifying the often unplanned positive and negative influences they exert on children (Frederick and Eccles, 2004). In reality, some parents do have unrealistic expectations and become overly involved in their children's sporting experiences. Unfortunately, it is the stories of parental hysteria that tend to be found disproportionately in media texts, rather than those where parents sacrifice time, money and effort to make children's sporting aspirations a reality.

The evidence would suggest that if parents provide appropriate financial, logistical and emotional support for their children, then a range of positive outcomes such as enjoyment and higher self-esteem can be achieved (Côté, 1999; Leff and Hoyle, 1995). Moreover, such investment may potentially cultivate sporting dispositions that last throughout childhood and beyond. In order to enhance their child's sporting capital, parents should therefore aim to model sporting behaviour, engage in sporting activities with their children wherever possible and encourage children to take part in a range of activities from a young age. Given the increasing pressures on parents however, this may prove difficult. An American study recently indicated that increasing time demands often led to parents limiting their children to one sport (Wiersma and Fifer, 2008). This clearly has implications for their engagement during the sampling years and their chances of becoming locked in to sport. Equally, engaging in practices that counter a child's intrinsic motivation, placing too much pressure on children and holding unrealistic expectations can lead to a range of negative outcomes including heightened anxiety, fear of failure, and disengagement (Fraser-Thomas *et al.*, 2008). However, to better understand sports participation in younger people, the specific parenting practices and family circumstances must be considered and given the disaggregation of family life in the twenty-first century, arguably, no single concept of family or parenting now exists. Hence, fostering sporting dispositions in youth may be mediated by socio-cultural forces that are beyond parental control.

References

Bandura, A. (1986). *Social Foundations of Thought and Action: A Social Cognitive Theory*. Englewood Cliffs, NJ: Prentice-Hall.

Beets, M., Vogel, R., Chapman, S., Pitetti, K. and Cardinal, B. (2007). Parent's social support for children's outdoor physical activity: Do weekdays and weekends matter? *Sex Roles, 56(2)*, 125–131.

Birchwood, D., Roberts, K. and Pollock, G. (2008). Explaining differences in sport participation rates among young adults: Evidence from the South Caucasus, *European Physical Education Review, 14(3)*, 283–298.

Coakley, J. (2009). The good father: Parental expectations and youth sports, in T. Kay (ed.) *Fathering Through Sport and Leisure* (pp. 40–50). Oxford: Routledge.

Côté, J. (1999). The influence of the family in the development of talent in sport, *The Sport Psychologist, 13*, 395–417.

Dagkas, S. and Stathi, A. (2007). Exploring social and environmental factors affecting adolescents' participation in physical activity, *European Physical Education Review, 13(3)*, 369–384.

Dixon, M., Warner, S. and Bruening, J. (2008). More than just letting them play: Parental influence on women's lifetime sport involvement, *Sociology of Sport Journal, 25*, 538–559

Duncan, S., Duncan, T. and Strycker, L. (2005). Sources and types of social support in youth physical activity, *Health Psychology, 24(1)*, 3–10.

Elliott, K. and Drummond, M. (2013). A socio-cultural exploration of parental involvement in junior Australian Rules football, *Asia-Pacific Journal of Health, Sport and Physical Education, 4(1)*, 35–48

Evans, J. and Davies, B. (2010). Family, class and embodiment: Why school physical education makes so little difference to post-school participation patterns in physical activity, *International Journal of Qualitative Studies in Education, 23(7)*, 765–784.

Fraser-Thomas, J. and Côté, J. (2009). Understanding adolescents' positive and negative developmental experiences in sport, *Sport Psychologist, 23(1)*, 3–2

Fraser-Thomas, J., Côté, J. and Deakin, J. (2005). Youth sport programs: An avenue to foster positive youth development, *Physical Education and Sport Pedagogy, 10(1)*, 19–40.

Fraser-Thomas, J., Côté, J. and Deakin, J. (2008). Understanding dropout and prolonged engagement in adolescent competitive sport, *Psychology of Sport and Exercise, 9*, 645–662.

Fredricks, J. and Eccles, J. (2004). Parental influences on youth involvement in sports, in M.R. Weiss (ed.) *Developmental Sport and Exercise Psychology: A Lifespan Perspective* (pp. 144–164). Mornington, WV: Fitness Information Technology.

Gould, D., Lauer, L., Rolo, C., Jannes, C. and Pennisi, N. (2006). Understanding the role parents play in tennis success: A national survey of junior tennis coaches, *British Journal of Sports Medicine*, *40*(7), 632–636.

Gould, D., Lauer, L., Rolo, C., Jannes, C. and Pennisi, N. (2008). The role of parents in tennis success: Focus group interviews with junior coaches, *Sport Psychologist*, *22(1)*, 18–37.

Green, K. (2010). *Key Themes in Youth Sport*. London: Routledge.

Haycock, D. and Smith, A. (2012). A family affair? Exploring the influence of childhood sport socialisation on young adults' leisure-sport careers in north-west England, *Leisure Studies*. DOI: 10.1080/02614367. 2012.715181

Hellstedt, J. (1995). Invisible players: A family system model, in S.M. Murphy (ed.) *Sport Psychology Interventions* (pp. 117–146). Champaign, Illinois: Human Kinetics

Holt, N.L., Tamminen, K., Black, D., Sehn, Z. and Wall, M. (2008). Parental involvement in competitive youth sport settings, *Psychology of Sport and Exercise*, *9(5)*, 663–685.

Kanters, M., Bocarro, J. and Casper, J. (2008). Supported or pressured? An examination of agreement among parents and children on parent's role in youth sports, *Journal of Sport Behaviour*, *31(1)*, 64–80.

Kay, T. (2000). Sporting excellence: A family affair? *European Physical Education Review*, *6(2)*, 151–169.

Kay, T. (2004). The family factor in sport: A review of family factors affecting sports participation, in Sport England (ed.) *Driving up Participation: The Challenge for Sport* (pp. 39–60). London: Sport England.

Kay, T., Armour, K., Cushion, C., Thorpe, R. and Pielichaty, H. (2008). *Are We Missing the Coach for 2012?*. Loughborough University: Institute of Youth Sport.

Kay, T. (2009). Introduction: Fathering through sport and leisure, in T. Kay (ed.) *Fathering Through Sport and Leisure* (pp. 1–6). London: Routledge.

Kirk, D. (2005). Physical education, youth sport and lifelong participation: the importance of early learning experiences, *European Physical Education Review*, *11(3)*, 239–255.

Kirk, D., O'Connor, A., Carlson, T., Burke, P., Davis, K. and Glover, S. (1997). Time commitments in junior sport: Social consequences for participants and their families, *Physical Education and Sport Pedagogy*, *2(1)*, 51–73.

Leff, S. and Hoyle, R. (1995). Young athletes' perceptions of parental support and pressure, *Journal of Youth and Adolescence*, *24(2)*, 187–203

Macdonald, D., Rodger, S., Ziviani, J., Jenkins, D., Batch, J. and Jones, J. (2004). Physical activity as a dimension of family life for lower primary school children, *Sport, Education and Society*, *9(3)*, 307–325.

Macdonald, D., Rodger, S., Abbott, R., Ziviani, J. and Jones, J. (2005). 'I could do with a pair of wings': Perspectives on physical activity, bodies and health from young Australian children, *Sport, Education and Society*, *10(2)*, 195–209.

MacDonald, K. and Parke, R. (1986). Parent–child physical play: The effects of sex and age of children and parents, *Sex Roles*, *15(7)*, 367–378.

MacPhail, A. and Kirk, D. (2006). Young people's socialisation into sport: Experiencing the specialising phase, *Leisure Studies*, *25(1)*, 57–74.

MacPhail, A., Gorely, T. and Kirk, D. (2003). Young people's socialisation into sport: A case study of an athletics club, *Sport, Education and Society*, *8(2)*, 251–267.

Quarmby, T. and Dagkas, S. (2010). Children's engagement in leisure time physical activity: exploring family structure as a determinant, *Leisure Studies*, *29(1)*, 53–66.

Rapoport, R. and Rapoport, R. (1975). *Leisure and the Family Lifecycle*. London: Routledge.

Roberts, K. and Brodie, D. (1992). *Inner-city Sport: Who Plays, and What are the Benefits?* Culemborg: Giordano Bruno.

Rowley, S. (1992). *TOYA (Training of Young Athletes Study): Identification of Talent*. London: The Sports Council.

Saelens, B. and Kerr, J. (2008). The family, in A. Smith and S. Biddle. (ed.) *Youth Physical Activity and Sedentary Behaviour* (pp. 267–294). Leeds: Human Kinetics.

Scheerder, J., Vanreusel, B., Taks, M. and Renson, R. (2005). Social stratification patterns in adolescents' active sports participation behaviour: a time trend analysis 1969–1999, *European Physical Education Review*, *11(1)*, 5–27.

Shakib, S. and Dunbar, M. (2004). How high school athletes talk about maternal and paternal sporting experiences, *International Review for the Sociology of Sport*, *39(3)*, 275–299.

Shaw, S. (2008). Family leisure and changing ideologies of parenthood, *Sociology Compass*, *2(2)*, 688–703.

Shaw, S. and Dawson, D. (2001). Purposive leisure: Examining parental discourse on family activities, *Leisure Sciences*, *23(4)*, 217–231.

Vincent, C. and Ball, S. (2007). 'Making up' the middle-class child: Families, activities and class dispositions, *Sociology*, *41(6)*, 1061–1077.

Wiersma, L. and Fifer, A. (2008). 'The schedule has been tough but we think it's worth it': The joys, challenges and recommendations of youth sport parents, *Journal of Leisure Research*, *40(4)*, 505–530.

Wheeler, S. (2011). The significance of family culture for sport participation, *International Review for the Sociology of Sport*, *47(2)*, 235–252.

Wheeler, S. and Green, K. (2012). Parenting in relation to children's sports participation: generational changes and potential implications, *Leisure Studies*. DOI: 10.1080/02614367.2012.707227

White, J. (2014). The time has come to ban parents watching their offspring play school sport. *The Telegraph* [Online], 10 January 2014. Available from: www.telegraph.co.uk/sport/columnists/jimwhite/10564509/The-time-has-come-to-ban-parents-watching-their-offspring-play-school-sport.html [Accessed 11 January 2014].

Woolger, C. and Power, T. (1993). Parent and sport socialisation: Views from the achievement literature, *Journal of Sport Behaviour*, *16(3)*, 312–318.

Wuerth, S., Lee, M. and Alfermann, D. (2004). Parental involvement and athletes' career in youth sport, *Psychology of Sport and Exercise*, *5(1)*, 21–33.

Yang, X., Telema, R. and Laakso, L. (1996). Parents physical activity, socioeconomic status and education as predictors of physical activity and sport among children and youths – A twelve year follow up study, *International Review for the Sociology of Sport*, *31(3)*, 274–289.

Zeijl, E., Poel, Y., Bois-Reymond, M., Ravesloot, J. and Meulman, J. (2000). The role of parents and peers in the leisure activities of young adolescents, *Journal of Leisure Research*, *32(3)*, 281–302.

21

PEER GROUP EXPERIENCES IN YOUTH SPORT

Kacey Neely and Nicholas Holt

Introduction

Peer group experiences can provide youth with opportunities to acquire a range of skills, attitudes, and behaviours that influence their development (Rubin *et al.*, 1998; 2006). Good peer relationships during the teenage years are a marker of social competence (Morison and Masten, 1991) and predictive of healthy development in adulthood (Parker and Asher, 1987). Peer group experiences may also represent some of the most meaningful aspects of participation in youth sport. For instance, youth sport provides individuals with opportunities to expand their social networks, develop friendships and learn a range of social skills, such as how to work with other people (e.g. Holt *et al.*, 2009; Holt *et al.*, 2008). Given the achievement demands often associated with sport, combined with the unique public nature of performances and the prominent roles played by parents and coaches, youth sport provides a particularly interesting social context in which to study peer group experiences (cf. Weiss and Stuntz, 2004).

Compared to coach and parental influence, peer group experiences in youth sport remain relatively unexplored. Indeed, as Smith (2003) suggested, 'it is puzzling the degree to which research on peers has paled in comparison [to research on coaches and parents] given the relevance of these social agents and the vast array of research questions that could be pursued, (p. 26). Fortunately, however, a body of research has emerged examining various aspects of peer group experiences in youth sport. Detailed and thorough reviews of peer group experiences in sport have been published elsewhere (e.g. Smith, 2007; Smith and McDonough, 2008; Weiss and Stuntz, 2004). In order to build on and complement these existing reviews, this chapter discusses the peer group experiences in youth sport literature using a framework of social complexity (Rubin *et al.*, 1998; 2006).

The importance of peer group experiences during the adolescent period

During their adolescence, individuals essentially transition from being children to becoming adult members of society (Petersen, 1988). Youth is therefore characterised by numerous social, emotional, cognitive and physical transitions. From a social perspective, most youth go through a process of becoming less reliant on their parents as they gain an increasing level of independence. Simultaneously, peers (i.e. individuals of equal standing; Smith, 2007) begin to fulfill a more important role in their lives (Lerner *et al.*, 2005). This is not to say that parents are no longer important. In fact, research in youth sport shows parents continue to play vital roles during the teenage years by providing emotional and tangible support for sport participation (e.g. Côté, 1999). Nonetheless, in general terms, parents tend to move into the background of teenagers' lives as their daily interactions with peers (whether at school, in sport or just hanging out) become more frequent and important.

Peer group structures

About 80 per cent of youth report they have a 'best friend' and five or more 'good friends' (Hartup and Overhauser, 1991). Youth typically participate in a range of different peer groups in various settings (e.g. school, sport teams or hanging out with friends). There is a fluidity to these social networks, in that the composition may change, even over a period of a few weeks, as some peers leave the network while other peers join (Cairns *et al.*, 1995). In the context of sport, while a team may remain together for the duration of a season, some players leave and new players arrive at the start of every new season. Peer groups are important to boys and girls, but girls typically report more intimate social relationships than boys (Urberg *et al.*, 1995).

The social complexity of peer group experiences

Several theoretical frameworks are relevant to the study of peer group experiences in sport, including Sullivan's (1953) interpersonal theory of psychiatry, Bandura's (1986) social cognitive theory and Harter's (1978; 1981; 1987) competence motivation theory (see Smith, 2007; Smith and McDonough, 2008; Weiss and Stuntz, 2004 for reviews). In this chapter, we have used another approach, Rubin *et al.*'s (1998; 2006) framework of social complexity, to conceptualise and organise the peer group experiences in sport literature.

Rubin *et al.* (1998) claimed that the experiences of youth with their peers 'can best be understood by referring to several levels of social complexity: within individuals, within interactions, within relationships, and within groups' (p. 623). Rubin and colleagues proposed a 'nested' framework of peer group experiences, which means events and processes within each level (i.e. within individuals, interactions, relationships and groups) are constrained and influenced by events and processes within other levels. Hence, a series of interdependent and reciprocal relationships depict peer group experiences at different levels of social complexity.

In the following sections, we describe each level of social complexity and briefly provide examples of youth sport research pertinent to each of these levels. We then go on to discuss the interdependent and reciprocal nature of these levels of social complexity and provide some examples of youth sport studies that have examined factors across different levels.

Within individuals

The Rubin *et al.* (1998; 2006) framework begins with the individual. Although individuals are not considered as a level of social complexity per se, they influence subsequent levels of peer group experience. In other words, peer group experiences originate from the individuals who form the group. From a social complexity perspective, individual characteristics are relatively stable (that is, factors at other levels of social complexity are more dynamic and less stable). In sport, for example, athletes' psychological characteristics have been associated with leadership ability and status. In a study of girls' high school soccer teams, Glenn and Horn (1993) found teammates rated a player favourably on leadership ability if she was:

1 a skilled player;
2 confident in her soccer skills;
3 displayed instrumental and expressive behaviours.

As Weiss and Stuntz (2004) observed, these findings suggested that being a leader on a team is based on a combination of personal, physical and psychological characteristics.

Within interactions

Interactions are short-term social exchanges that stem from individuals' behaviours. Interactions are usually dyadic (i.e. between pairs) and change in response to fluctuating circumstances of the social situation. Interactions are related to individuals' own goals in a social situation, and their understanding of their partners' thoughts, as well as demands of the context. During interactions youth may cooperate, compete, fight or attempt to resolve conflict.

Interactions represent one of the most difficult levels of social complexity to study because of the methodological challenges posed by the need to look at fluctuating behaviours and interactions in a particular context. Using a qualitative approach that combined interviews and ethnographic observations with female soccer players (*M* age = 13.0 years; *SD* = 1.2) from two teams, Holt *et al.* (2008) found short-term interactions involved individuals integrating new teammates into the team after try-outs and learning to engage with different types of peers. Furthermore, players decided to resolve conflicts with teammates for the good of the team.

Within relationships

Interactions are shaped by longer-term relationships (a higher order level of social complexity). Relationships are defined by the characteristics of individuals, the types of interactions that take place and individuals' history of earlier relationships. Friendships are an example of the within relationships level. Peer friendships research centres around three issues:

1 whether or not an individual has friends;
2 who those friends are; and
3 the quality of the friendships.

(Hartup, 1999; Weiss and Smith, 1999)

Weiss, Smith and Theeboom (1996) interviewed thirty-eight youth athletes from the United States (aged 8–16 years) about their 'best sport friendships'. Positive and negative dimensions of sport friendship were identified through content analysis. In a follow-up study, Weiss and Smith (1999) used these positive and negative dimensions as the basis for the development and validation of a questionnaire to assess friendship quality in sport (The Sport Friendship Quality Scale or SFQS). The SFQS has twenty-two items representing the following six factors: self-esteem enhancement and supportiveness, loyalty and intimacy, things in common, companionship and pleasant play, conflict resolution and conflict. The creation of the SFQS stimulated a body of research examining associations between friendship quality and various psychosocial and behavioural variables (Carr and Fitzpatrick, 2011). In a study with youth tennis players, for example, Weiss and Smith (2002) found higher perceptions of companionship and pleasant play, things in common, and conflict resolution were associated with tennis enjoyment and commitment.

Within groups

Relationships are further embedded in and influenced by groups (the highest level of social complexity), which are networks of relationships within relatively clearly defined boundaries (Rubin *et al.*, 1998; 2006). Groups are more than an aggregate of individuals, interactions and relationships. Rather, groups have features that are not necessarily found at lower levels of social complexity, such as shared norms, processes such as task and social cohesion, and hierarchical organisation. Groups help define the type and range of interactions and relationships that occur within them. For instance, youth sport teams may have different group features than cliques of friends at school.

Several studies in youth sport have examined peer acceptance (or popularity), which is a group level construct that can be defined as how a group views an individual and determines her or his status (Weiss and Stuntz, 2004). For instance, when youth have been asked to choose factors that would make them popular or well-liked among their classmates, boys consistently report being good at sport, whereas factors such as being pretty and getting good grades are more highly valued social acceptance criteria for girls (e.g. Adler *et al.*, 1992; Chase and Drummer, 1992). The gender-appropriateness of sports has also been linked with higher social acceptance. Girls who play traditionally feminine sports such as volleyball and gymnastics and boys who play traditionally masculine sports such as football and baseball typically have high social acceptance among their peers (Holland and Andre, 1994). Peer group acceptance has also been studied in relation to a range of other constructs at different levels of social complexity.

Research examining factors at different levels of social complexity

We have described factors at different levels of social complexity that can be used to understand peer experiences in sport. Rubin *et al.* (1998; 2006) acknowledged that the multifaceted nature of their framework is a challenge to researchers seeking to study peer group experiences. Nonetheless, several studies in youth sport have examined associations between factors at different levels of social complexity.

Using the SFQS (Weiss and Smith, 1999), researchers have examined associations between peer friendship and peer acceptance. Applying the Rubin *et al.* (1998; 2006) framework, peer friendships would be an example of a within relationship level construct and peer acceptance an example of a within group level construct. For example, Smith (1999) found higher perceptions of peer acceptance and friendship influenced physical self-worth and effect which, in turn, influenced higher motivation for physical activity among youth.

Researchers have also examined associations between perceived competence (which can be construed as an individual level factor) and peer acceptance (a group level construct). For instance, Weiss and Duncan (1992) examined physical competence and peer acceptance in sport using children's self-report (to assess perceived competence and perceived peer group acceptance) and teachers' ratings (to assess actual competence and peer group acceptance). Higher perceived and actual peer acceptance was associated with higher perceived and actual physical competence. Peer acceptance was also positively associated with motivational variables of perceived success, future expectations for success, and stability and personal control attributions for success. Furthermore, Moran and Weiss (2006) showed that for female high school athletes, peer acceptance and friendship quality, along with perceived competence, and instrumental and expressive behaviours, predicted self-ratings of leadership. Smith (2007) observed that these findings, together with other research on the benefits of friendship quality, suggest a meaningful association exists between peer group experiences and individuals' self-perceptions. This reflects the 'nested' features of levels of social complexity and ways in which factors at one level influence factors at another level.

Parents' influence on peer group experiences

Despite the fact that teenagers are gaining increasing independence, parents still exert influence over peer group experiences in general and friendships more specifically. In one study (not in a sporting context), Ducharme, Doyle and Markiewicz (2002) found teenagers who were securely attached to their fathers had fewer conflicts with their peers compared to teenagers with less secure attachment to their fathers. In a follow-up to an earlier study (Ullrich-French and Smith, 2006), Ullrich-French and Smith (2009) examined how multiple social constructs (including peer acceptance, friendship and parent–child relationships) influenced motivation to continue in sport one year later among soccer players (aged 10–14 years). Positive perceptions of multiple social relationships predicted higher enjoyment and perceived competence. More specifically, greater perceived competence, more positive friendship quality, and the combination of mother relationship quality and peer relationships predicted continued involvement on the same team. These studies show that the quality of relationships between youths and their parents can influence youths' peer group experiences and motivation for sport participation.

Coaches' influences on peer group experiences

A particularly interesting feature of peer group experiences in sport is that they occur in a context that includes other highly involved adults, namely, coaches. Looking at the influence of coaches on peer group experiences, Ommundsen, Roberts, Lemyre and Miller (2005) found a perceived mastery-oriented motivational climate (i.e. emphasising effort, personal improvement and skill development) positively predicted perceptions of friendship quality with a nominated best friend in soccer. In contrast, a perceived performance-oriented environment (i.e. emphasising normative comparison and public evaluation) negatively predicted friendship quality. These findings suggest coaches play an important role in structuring peer group experiences in sport settings.

Negative consequences of peer group experiences in sport

The majority of the research we have reviewed above has focused on some of the more positive features of peer group experiences in sport. Indeed, there may be a popular view that sport participation is associated with a range of healthy behaviours, but this is not *consistently* supported by empirical evidence. For example, four systematic reviews have examined the association between sport participation (defined as participation in organised high school and collegiate sports) and health behaviours related to alcohol, tobacco and illicit drug use (Diehl *et al.*, 2012; Kwan *et al. and* Cairney, 2013; Lisha and Sussman, 2010; Martens *et al.*, 2006). Overall, findings from these reviews can be summarised as follows: Sport participation is associated with a lower use of tobacco (cigarettes) and illicit drugs, but increased use of alcohol during youth and emerging adulthood, particularly among young males. The use of alcohol among youth who play sport may be due to some of the social norms and peer group interactions that occur in particular sporting contexts. Holt and Jones (2008) described how, in certain sport settings, such as amateur rugby in the UK, there may be social norms and a culture that actually encourages the consumption of alcohol.

It is imperative to gain better understandings of the reasons why athletes are at greater risk for certain negative behaviours compared to youth who are not engaged in sport (Kwan *et al.*, 2013). The study of peer group experiences provides one way of examining this issue. Recently, Bruner *et al.* (2014) sought to understand how membership of a sport team may influence behaviours using the concept of social identity. Social identity is based on three peer-related concepts: the importance of being a group member (cognitive centrality), positive feelings associated with group membership (in-group affect), and perceptions of similarity, bonding, and belongingness with other group members (in-group ties) (Cameron, 2004). Bruner *et al.* had 329 male and female athletes (*M* age = 15.88 years; *SD* = 1.25) complete questionnaires assessing social identity, task and social cohesion, and pro-social and antisocial behaviours before, during and after their sport seasons. Findings revealed that in-group affect was positively related to pro-social behaviours towards teammates (e.g. providing constructive feedback) but not to anti-social behaviours towards opponents (e.g. deliberately fouling opponents). In-group ties had no significant relation to pro-social behaviours toward opponents, but did have a negative effect on antisocial behaviours toward teammates and opponents. Task cohesion mediated a positive effect for in-group ties on pro-social behaviours towards teammates, and a negative effect for in-group ties and in-group affect on antisocial behaviours toward teammates and opponents. Social cohesion mediated a positive effect for in-group ties on antisocial behaviour toward opponents.

These findings suggest that strong perceptions of in-group affect and task cohesion are beneficial for promoting more pro-social behaviour toward teammates and less antisocial behaviours toward teammates and opponents, but strong in-group ties and social cohesion may actually increase the likelihood of youth displaying anti-social behaviours toward teammates and opponents. Understanding the nature of peer group experiences within sport teams over time may be a critical factor in learning more about associations between sport participation and positive and negative health behaviours. Furthermore, as some aspects of peer group experiences can be influenced by parents (Ullrich-French and Smith, 2009) and coaches (Ommundsen *et al.*, 2005), there may be several potentially modifiable factors that can be targeted by interventions seeking to promote positive health behaviours and developmental outcomes through sport.

Advancing peer relationships research in youth sport

We have been able to organise much of the sport peer group experiences literature around the framework proposed by Rubin *et al.* (1998, 2006). We must emphasise, however, that this framework has rarely been used in individual studies, although several studies have considered aspects of peer group experiences at different levels of social complexity. We suspect that the sport peer group experiences literature may be advanced by the more explicit use of the Rubin *et al.* framework in order to examine associations between factors at different levels of social complexity to provide more complete accounts of peer experiences in sport. For instance, Holt *et al.* (2008) were able to examine factors at interaction, relationship and group levels in their qualitative study of female soccer players, which provided in-depth insights into the fluctuating nature of peer group experiences over a season. Though it may not be necessary, or even possible, for all levels of social complexity to be included in a single study, the Rubin *et al.* framework is a valuable tool that can assist in the design of studies (e.g. examining associations between constructs at different levels of social complexity) and the planning of programmes of research (such as a series of studies for a PhD thesis).

Methodological considerations

Research is often driven by the availability of valid measurement instruments. In the youth sport peer group experiences literature, the availability and use of the SQFS (Weiss and Smith, 1999) has led to the creation of a strong body of research examining associations between friendship quality and a range of psychosocial and behavioural outcomes. Similarly, qualitative interviews and ethnographic observations have been used to examine various dimensions of peer group experiences (e.g. Holt *et al.*, 2008). However, Murphy-Mills *et al.* (2011) suggested a reliance on the use of self-report questionnaires and qualitative interviews may 'limit the nature of the information collected on influence of peers within the sport context by restricting the ability of researchers to conduct studies that fully examine the complex, reciprocal, and dynamic nature of peer interactions in youth sport' (p. 161).

Murphy-Mills *et al.* (2011) proposed the use of an innovative approach called the state space grid (Lewis *et al.*, 1999) within a dynamic systems perspective to study athlete dyad *interactions*. The state space grid is created from observational data that represents all of the possible behavioural states within a system and graphically shows the reciprocal nature of these interactions over time, thus allowing youth sport researchers to examine the content and structure of peer interactions.

Given that a dynamic system is comprised of reciprocal interactions between two individuals who influence and are influenced by each other (Lewis, 2000), two athletes within a team would act as the components within a system. Murphy-Mills *et al.* (2011) explained that using the state space grid would enable researchers to examine patterns of interactions, and how they emerge and change over time (e.g. during the course of a season). Since the within interaction level represents a major measurement challenge for assessing peer group experiences, the state space grid may offer a new methodological approach that could be used in conjunction with questionnaires, interviews and/or ethnographic observations to examine different elements of social complexity that characterise peer group experiences in sport.

Conclusion and future directions

Through their interactions with peers, youth can acquire a range of skills and attributes that are important for development. As we have shown, a strong body of evidence is accumulating. Nevertheless, we agree with Smith (2007) that the research base on peer group experiences in sport 'remains thin and many questions remain unanswered. This leaves tremendous opportunities for sport psychology researchers' (p. 51).

In advancing the literature, Rubin *et al.*'s (1998; 2006) framework of social complexity can be used to understand the nested levels of social relationships that characterise peer group experiences. Although the complexity of this framework creates measurement challenges, the use of multiple data collection techniques and new methodological approaches may help advance the knowledge base in this area (Murphy-Mills *et al.*, 2011). It is also important to consider that peer groups (and the individuals, interactions, relationships and group processes therein) are fluid and change over time, which necessitates longitudinal research designs. Finally, peer group experiences in sport are also influenced by other social agents, such as parents (Ullrich-French and Smith, 2009) and coaches (Ommundsen *et al.*, 2005). By understanding more about the complexity of peer group experiences, we may be able to establish more sophisticated explanations of how and why sport participation is associated with both positive and negative health behaviours. Hence, peer group experiences remain a particularly salient topic for youth sport researchers and an area ripe for further study.

References

Adler, P.A., Kless, S.J. and Adler, P. (1992). Socialization to gender roles: Popularity among elementary school boys and girls, *Sociology of Education*, *65*, 169–187.

Bandura, A. (1986). *Social foundations of thought and action: A social cognitive theory*. Englewood Cliffs, NJ: Prentice-Hall.

Bruner, M.W., Boardley, I.D. and Côté, J. (2014). Social identity and prosocial and antisocial in youth sport, *Psychology of Sport and Exercise, 15*, 56–64. DOI: 10.1016/j.bbr.2011.03.031

Cairns, R.B., Leung, M., Buchanan, L. and Cairns, B.D. (1995). Friendships and social networks in childhood and adolescence: Fluidity, reliability, and interrelations, *Child Development, 66*, 1330–1345.

Cameron, J.E. (2004). A three-factor model of social identity, *Self and Identity, 3*, 239–262. DOI: 10.1080/13576500444000047

Carr, S. and Fitzpatrick, N. (2011). Experiences of dyadic sport friendships as a function of self and partner attachment characteristics, *Psychology of Sport and Exercise, 12*, 383–391. DOI: 10.1016/j.psychsport.2011.03.003.

Chase, M. A. and Drummer, G.M. (1992). The role of sport as a social status determinant for children, *Research Quarterly for Exercise and Sport, 63*, 418–424.

Côté, J. (1999). The influence of the family in the development of talent in sport, *The Sport Psychologist, 13*, 395–417.

Diehl, K., Thiel, A., Zipfel, S., Mayer, J., Litaker, D.G. and Schneider, S. (2012). How healthy is the behavior of young athletes? A systematic literature review and meta-analyses, *Journal of Sports Science and Medicine, 11*, 201–220.

Ducharme, J., Doyle, A.D. and Markiewicz, D. (2002). Attachment security with mother and father: Associations with adolescents' reports of interpersonal behaviour with parents and peers, *Journal of Social and Personal Relationships, 19*, 203–231.

Glenn, S.D. and Horn, T.S. (1993). Psychological and personal predictors of leadership behaviour in female soccer athletes, *Journal of Applied Sport Psychology, 5*, 17–34. DOI: 10.1080/10413209308411302

Harter, S. (1978). Effectance motivation reconsidered: Toward a developmental model, *Human Development, 21*, 34–64. DOI: 10.1159/000271574

Harter, S. (1981). A model of intrinsic mastery motivation in children: Individual differences and developmental change, in W.A. Collins (ed.) *Minnesota Symposium on Child Psychiatry*, vol. 14 (pp. 215–255). Hillsdale, NJ: Erlbaum.

Harter, S. (1987). The determinants and mediational role of global self-worth in children, in N. Eisenberg (ed.) *Contemporary topics in developmental psychology* (pp. 219–242). New York: Wiley.

Hartup, W.W. (1999). Constraints on peer socialization: Let me count the ways, *Merrill-Palmer Quarterly, 45*, 172–183.

Hartup, W.W. and Overhauser, S.M. (1991). Friendships, in R.M. Lerner, A.C. Petersen, and J. Brooks-Gunn (eds) *Encyclopedia of adolescence*, vol. 1 (pp. 378–384). New York: Garland.

Holland, A. and Andre, T. (1994). Athletic participation and the social status of adolescent males and females, *Youth and Society, 25*, 388–407. DOI: 10.1177/0044118X94025003005

Holt, N.L. and Jones, M.I. (2008). Future directions for positive youth development and sport research, in N.L. Holt (ed.) *Positive youth development through sport* (pp. 122–132). London: Routledge.

Holt, N.L., Black, D.E., Tamminen, K.A., Mandigo, J.L. and Fox, K.R. (2008). Levels of social complexity and dimensions of peer experience in youth sport, *Journal of Sport & Exercise Psychology, 30*, 411–431.

Holt, N.L., Tamminen, K.A., Tink, L.N. and Black, D.E. (2009). An interpretive analysis of life skills associated with sport participation, *Qualitative Research in Sport and Exercise, 1*, 160–175. DOI: 10.1080/19398440902909017

Holt, N.L., Tink, L.N., Mandigo, J.L. and Fox, K.R. (2008). Do youth learn life skills through their involvement in high school sport? *Canadian Journal of Education, 31*, 281–304.

Kwan, M., Bobko, S., Faulkner, G., Donnelly, P. and Cairney, J. (2013). Sport participation and alcohol and illicit drug use in adolescents and young adults: A systematic review of longitudinal studies, *Addiction, 39*, 497–506. DOI: 10.1016/j.addbeh.2013.11.006

Lerner, R.M., Brown, J.D. and Kier, C. (2005). *Adolescence: Development, diversity, and context* (Canadian edition.). Toronto: Pearson.

Lewis, M. D., Lamey, A.V. and Douglas, L. (1999). A new dynamic system method for the analysis of early socioemotional development, *Developmental Science, 2*, 457–475. DOI: 10.1111/1467-7687.00090

Lewis, M.D. (2000). The promise of dynamic systems approaches for an integrated account of human development, *Child Development, 71*, 36–43. Champaign. DOI: 10.1111/1467-8624.00116

Lisha, N.E. and Sussman, S. (2010). Relationship of high school and college sports participation with alcohol, tobacco, and illicit drug use: A review, *Addictive Behaviours, 35*, 399–407. DOI: 10.1016/j.addbeh.2009.12.032

Martens, M.P., Dams–O'Connor, K. and Beck, N.C. (2006). A systematic review of college student–athlete drinking: Prevalence rates, sport-related factors, and interventions, *Journal of Substance Abuse Treatment*, *31*, 305–316.

Moran, M.M. and Weiss, M.R. (2006). Peer leadership in sport: Links with friendship, peer acceptance, psychological characteristics, and athletic ability, *Journal of Applied Sport Psychology*, *18*, 97–113. DOI: 10.1080/10413200600653501

Morison, P. and Masten, A.S. (1991). Peer reputation in middle childhood as a predictor of adaptation in adolescence: A seven-year follow-up, *Child Development*, *62*, 911–1007.

Murphy-Mills, J., Bruner, M. W., Erickson, K. and Côté, J. (2011). The utility of the state space grid method for studying peer interactions in youth sport, *Journal of Applied Sport Psychology*, *24*, 159–174. DOI: 10.1080/10413200.2010.545101

Ommundsen, Y., Roberts, G.C., Lemyre, P. –N. and Miller, B.W. (2005). Peer relationships in adolescent competitive soccer: Associations to perceived motivational climate, achievement goals, and perfectionism, *Journal of Sports Sciences*, *23*, 977–989. DOI: 10.1016/j.psychsport.2008.06.007

Parker, J.G. and Asher, S.R. (1987). Peer relations and later personal adjustment: Are low-accepted children at risk? *Psychological Bulletin*, *102*, 357–389.

Petersen, A.C. (1988). Adolescent development, in M.R. Rosenzweig (ed.) *Annual review of psychology*, vol. 39 (pp. 583–607). Palo Alto, CA: Annual Reviews.

Rubin, K.H., Bukowski, W.M. and Parker, J.G. (1998). Peer interactions, relationships, and groups, in W. Damon (series ed.) and N. Eisenberg (vol. ed.) *Handbook of child psychology: vol. 3 Social, emotional, and personality development* (5th edition) (pp. 619–700). New York: Wiley.

Rubin, K.H., Bukowski, W.M. and Parker, J.G. (2006). Peer interactions, relationships, and groups, in W. Damon, R.M. Lerner, and N. Eisenberg (eds), *Handbook of child psychology: vol. 3 Social, emotional, and personality development* (6th edition) (pp. 571–645). New York: Wiley.

Smith, A.L. (1999). Perceptions of peer relationships and physical activity participation in early adolescence, *Journal of Sport & Exercise Psychology*, *21*, 329–350.

Smith, A.L. (2003). Peer relationships in physical activity contexts: A road less travelled in youth sport and exercise psychology research, *Psychology of Sport and Exercise*, *4*, 25–39. DOI: 10.1016/S1469-0292 (02)00015-8

Smith, A. L. (2007). Youth peer relationships in sport, in S. Jowett (ed.) *Social psychology in sport* (pp. 41–54). Champaign, Illinois: Human Kinetics.

Smith, A.L. and McDonough, M.H. (2008). Peers, in A. L. Smith and S.J.H. Biddle (eds) *Youth physical activity and sedentary behavior: Challenges and solutions* (pp. 295–320). Champaign, Illinois: Human Kinetics.

Sullivan, H.S. (1953). *The interpersonal theory of psychiatry*. New York: Norton.

Ullrich-French, S. and Smith, A.L. (2006). Perceptions of relationships with parents and peers in youth sport: Independent and combined prediction of motivational outcomes, *Psychology of Sport and Exercise*, *7*, 193–214. DOI: 10.1016/j.psychsport.2005.08.006.

Ullrich-French, S. and Smith, A.L. (2009). Social and motivational predictors of continued youth sport participation, *Psychology of Sport and Exercise*, *10*, 87–95. DOI: 10.1016/j.psychsport.2008.06.007.

Urberg, K.A., Degirmencioglu, S.M., Tolson, J.M. and Halliday-Scher, K. (1995). The structure of adolescent peer networks, *Developmental Psychology*, *31*, 540–547.

Weiss, M.R. and Duncan, S.C. (1992). The relationship between physical competence and peer acceptance in the context of children's sports participation, *Journal of Sport and Exercise Psychology*, *14*, 177–191.

Weiss, M.R. and Smith, A.L. (1999). Quality of youth sport friendships: Measurement development and validation, *Journal of Sport & Exercise Psychology*, *21*, 145–166.

Weiss, M. R. and Smith, A. L. (2002). Friendship quality in youth sport: Relationship to age, gender, and motivational variables, *Journal of Sport and Exercise Psychology*, *24*, 420–437.

Weiss, M.R., Smith, A.L. and Theeboom, M. (1996). 'That's what friends are for': Children's and teenagers' perceptions of peer relationships in the sport domain, *Journal of Sport & Exercise Psychology*, *18*, 347–379.

Weiss, M.R. and Stuntz, C.P. (2004). A little friendly competition: Peer relationships and psychosocial development in youth sport and physical activity contexts, in M.R.Weiss (ed.) *Developmental sport and exercise psychology: A lifespan perspective* (pp. 165–196). Morgantown, WV: Fitness Information Technology.

22

UNDERSTANDING TAKE-UP, DROP-OUT AND DROP-OFF IN YOUTH SPORT

Jessica Fraser-Thomas, William Falcão and Lauren Wolman

Sport has been proposed as a context for youths' positive physical, psychological and social development (Fraser-Thomas *et al.*, 2005), encouraging extensive research examining factors associated with participation, and fuelling concern regarding withdrawal (e.g. Gould *et al.*, 1982). Current research suggests 50–70 per cent of youth in western nations participate in sport programmes (e.g. Clark, 2008; Physical Activity Council, 2014), while 20–50 per cent of participants typically leave sport programmes each year (Delorme *et al.*, 2011; Pelletier *et al.*, 2001; Ullrich-French and Smith, 2009), with a 35 per cent withdrawal rate commonly cited in the literature (e.g. Gould, 1987). The reasons youth initially engage in, persist with and/or eventually withdraw from sport are extensive and interrelated, yet the study of withdrawal presents various methodological and practical challenges. Given these complexities, we begin the chapter by providing definitions of youth sport take-up, drop-out and drop-off, and providing an overview of the chapter.

We root our discussion of youth sport take-up within five theories of motivation widely adopted in sport psychology to explain youths' sport engagement:

1 Competence Motivation Theory (Harter, 1978, 1981)
2 Achievement Goal Theory (Nicholls, 1979, 1984)
3 Value Expectancy Theory (Eccles, 1984; Eccles and Harold, 1991)
4 Self-Determination Theory (Deci and Ryan, 1987; Ryan and Deci, 2000)
5 Sport Commitment Model (Carpenter *et al.*, 1993; Scanlan *et al.*, 1993).

Motivation, conceptualized as the reasons that we do what we do (Reeve, 2014), drives the theoretical foundation of the first section. This is followed by an applied discussion of research utilizing motivation frameworks to examine intrapersonal, interpersonal, and contextual factors that dynamically interact to influence youths' reasons for taking up sport (Weiss and Williams, 2004).

Next, we discuss drop-out and drop-off, and are reminded that 'youth sport drop-outs cannot be considered as a single entity' (Butcher *et al.*, 2002, p. 160). Butcher and colleagues exemplified sport scientists' challenges in defining drop-out, while providing a rationale for including a discussion of drop-off in the current review. They used a retrospective design to examine ten-year sport participation profiles of 1,387 high school students, finding that 94 per cent withdrew from a sport over the ten-year period. Of those, 71 per cent continued participation in at least one sport following withdrawal from another, 55 per cent began a new sport within one year of withdrawal and 11 per cent re-joined the same sport after one to six years. Their findings re-emphasize the distinction between two important concepts that have persisted throughout the literature: *activity-specific drop-out*, whereby individuals discontinue a specific sport activity while continuing others, and *domain-general drop-out*, whereby individuals permanently withdrawal from all sport activities (Gould, 1987). In this chapter, we consider all types of youth discontinuation from sport, whether permanent or temporary, from one or all sport activities. Specifically, we outline key models of sport withdrawal and transition, and discuss current research in the context of motivation theories. We conclude the chapter with suggestions for further examination, exploration and critical reflection, as the field continues to move forward.

Youth sport take-up

In their review entitled *The why of youth sport involvement*, Weiss and Williams (2004) suggest the most common reasons youth engage in sport are:

- physical competence (e.g. learning skills, being accomplished, showing improvement);
- social acceptance (e.g. being with friends, belonging, gaining approval from significant others);
- enjoyment (e.g. excitement, interest, fun).

Below, five prominent theories of motivation provide diverse lenses to understand and examine youth sport take-up; they collectively highlight the importance of competence, social approval and enjoyment as reasons motivating youth to engage in sport.

Theoretical models of motivation

Competence Motivation Theory (CMT; Harter, 1978, 1981) proposes that individuals are motivated by their inherent curiosity and desire to feel competent. Specifically, CMT suggests individuals seek to achieve mastery and experience reinforcing outcomes in different domains (e.g. cognitive, social, physical). CMT also emphasizes the necessity of optimal challenge levels in mastery attempts, to foster intrinsic motivation and feelings of competence. Social agents (e.g. parents, coaches) play an important role in creating mastery opportunities, providing reinforcement, encouraging independent mastery attempts, and serving as behaviour models (Wheeler, Quarmby in this section). When children receive positive reinforcement for independent mastery attempts, they internalize self-rewards and are encouraged to seek their own goals, complete tasks without the help of adults and evaluate themselves positively. Conversely, children who do not receive encouragement or approval for independent mastery attempts, may internalize dependency, develop externally defined goals and engage in 'self-punishing systems' (Harter, 1978, p. 54). Essentially, children's feelings of competence are driven by a motivation cycle of mastery attempts and self-evaluations, which can lead to positive outcomes (e.g. self-esteem, internal control) and motivation, or negative outcomes (e.g. anxiety, lack of control) and decreased motivation.

Achievement-Goal Theory (AGT; Nicholls, 1979, 1984) assumes individuals engage in activities to achieve competence in a personally or socially valued goal. Specifically, AGT focuses on understanding *why* individuals try to achieve a goal, for task- and/or ego-orientated reasons. Task-oriented individuals use internal, personal and self-referenced criteria to assess their achievements; they perceive competence as the mastery of a skill, learn through moderately challenging tasks, apply high effort and experience mastery as an 'end in itself' (Nicholls, 1984, p. 331). In contrast, ego-oriented individuals assess achievements using external and social comparisons; they perceive competence as success relative to others, choose tasks to easily show ability, apply only sufficient effort to out-perform others and experience mastery as a 'means to an end' (Nicholls, 1984, p. 330). AGT is among the most widely utilized theories in examining youth sport involvement, with task and ego goal orientations offering clear conceptual measures of young people's competence beliefs.

Expectancy-Value Model (EVM; Eccles, 1984; Eccles and Harold, 1991) suggests individuals' choices, persistence and effort in an activity are influenced by their expectations of success (i.e. how they think they will do) and subjective task value (i.e. importance they attribute to being successful). Expectations of success and subjective task value are influenced by individual, social and cultural factors, including individuals' goals, ability perceptions, affective memories and interpretations of experiences. Essentially, these factors can lead youth to have positive expectations of success and high value of an activity, increasing their likelihood of choosing, persisting, and showing effort within the activity. On the other hand, negative outcomes emerge in the case of low expectations of success and task value, and decrease motivation.

Self-Determination Theory (SDT; Deci and Ryan, 1985, Ryan and Deci, 2000) suggests motivation varies on a self-determination continuum from intrinsic motivation, to extrinsic motivation and amotivation, which is mediated by feelings of competence, relatedness and autonomy. The most self-determined form of motivation is intrinsic, as individuals partake in behaviours for their own sake, to gain knowledge, accomplish and experience stimulation. Individuals are more likely to find activities interesting, satisfying and enjoyable if their competence, relatedness and autonomy needs are met. Extrinsic motivation leads to engagement in activities for more instrumental reasons, with four subtypes conceptualized according to self-determination levels:

- integrated (i.e. most self-determined; congruent with one's values and needs),
- identified (i.e. in line with personal goals),
- introjected (i.e. to demonstrate ability/feelings of worth) and
- externally regulated (i.e. least self-determined; controlled by external demands/rewards).

Finally, amotivation occurs when individuals engage in an activity without intent as they fail to see a connection between actions and outcomes, often due to decreased fulfillment of autonomy, competence and relatedness needs.

Sport Commitment Model (SCM; Carpenter *et al.*, 1993; Scanlan *et al.*, 1993) offers a sport-specific model of commitment, providing insight into individuals' desires to continue participation in sport. SCM suggests that enjoyment (i.e. fun, pleasure), personal investment (i.e. time, effort), social constraints (i.e. social expectations, obligation to the activity) and involvement opportunities (i.e. perceived or actual benefits) positively influence commitment, while involvement alternatives (i.e. other activities) can diminish individuals' commitment to an activity. Weiss, Kimmel and Smith (2001) highlighted enjoyment as the strongest predictor of commitment, proposing it mediates the relationship between all variables and sport commitment, thus having central importance in youths' sport participation.

Intrapersonal, interpersonal and contextual factors in youth sport take-up

The five theoretical models above offer unique lenses through which to interpret youth sport take-up. While the models collectively highlight competence, social acceptance and enjoyment as critical within the motivational process, these motives are primarily intrapersonal in nature. Individuals' motives do not exist in isolation; they are significantly influenced by interpersonal and contextual factors. This section focuses on interacting influences contributing to youths' motives through three primary pathways:

- providing opportunities and experiences
- offering feedback
- modelling behaviours and values.

First, social agents' provision of sport opportunities plays a critical role in youths' motivation. In a systematic review of parental correlates of child physical activity, parental modelling and support were found to impact children's task value (Gustafson and Rhodes, 2006), with other studies emphasizing similar influences of peers (Sallis, *et al.*, 2000). According to EVM, social agents (e.g. parents, coaches, peers, siblings) can facilitate children's early positive memories of sport, which subsequently influence task selection and persistence (Eccles, 1984; Eccles and Harold, 1991). In line with CMT, social agents can also provide challenging activities through optimally facilitated goals, activities and competitions, fostering interest, effort, success, positive experiences, pleasure and intrinsic motivation (Keegan *et al.*, 2009; Papaioannou *et al.*, 2008). Further, numerous studies have supported AGT and SDT, finding task-involved coaching climates increase athletes' perceptions of competence, relatedness and autonomy, resulting in higher intrinsic motivation (e.g. Sarrazin *et al.*, 2002; Stein *et al.*, 2012).

Social agents also play important roles in offering feedback to youth, and modelling values and behaviours. Recent advances to seminal works highlight that encouraging, constructive feedback, where coaches also demonstrate belief in their athletes, can increase intrinsic motivation, participation and performance (Bray *et al.*, 2014; Smith *et al.*, 1979; Vallerand and Reid, 1988). Additionally, consistent with CMT and EVM, researchers have found children's goals, evaluation systems, performance expectations and commitment are influenced by adult modelling and expectations (Carpenter *et al.*, 1993; Papaioannou *et al.*, 2008; Scanlan *et al.*, 1993).

Finally, it is important to acknowledge socio-cultural contextual factors, influencing youths' sport engagement, leading to under-representation of numerous groups. For example females, new immigrants, children in single parent families, children in families of lower socio-economic status, as well as children living in large cities and rural areas experience numerous barriers to participation related to financial cost and practical accessibility (Clark, 2008; Holt *et al.*, 2011; Vella *et al.*, 2014). Although intervention research aimed to address socio-cultural disparities is challenging, one study found that youth with specialized school physical education teachers and opportunities to attend sporting events are more likely to engage in sport programmes, offering promising policy considerations (Vella *et al.*, 2014).

Youth sport drop-out

Research in sport drop-out has more exploratory roots than the theory-driven study of take-up. Orlick's (1974) study among sixty drop-out youth athletes was among the first to highlight withdrawal concerns:

For many children, competitive sport operates as a kind of failure factory which not only effectively eliminates the 'bad ones' but also 'turns off' many of the 'good ones'. The programmes, by their present structure and emphasis and the agents of these programmes (i.e. the coaches), often appear to work together in a kind of conspiracy to eliminate children, particularly if they are of less skill levels (p. 25) . . . Programmes and their agents seem so caught up in the winning ethic that the drop out appears to be part of the price that is being paid . . . in a short sighted quest for 'victory'.

(Orlick, 1974, p. 25 and p. 27)

Orlick's early research spurred a large body of work in the decades that followed, leading to diminished concerns. Extensive questionnaire-based studies concluded that 'conflicts of interest' and 'other things to do' were consistently among top reasons for withdrawal. However, a lack of fun, coach conflicts, perceived low abilities, too much pressure and poor team atmosphere remained prominent reasons, with differences determined by gender, age, level of experience, level of competition, sport type and culture (e.g. Gould *et al.*, 1982; Klint and Weiss, 1986; Molinero *et al.*, 2006; Rottensteiner *et al.*, 2013). A key limitation of early drop-out research was that it examined primarily superficial reasons for withdrawal (e.g. lack of fun), and failed to uncover sources of these issues (e.g. why sport was not perceived as fun) (Burton, 1988). Two models emerged from early attrition research, expanding initial conceptualizations of drop-out:

1   Gould's (1987) Model of Youth Sport Withdrawal (MYSW);
2   Lindner *et al.*'s (1991) Model of Voluntary Youth Sport Withdrawal (MVYSW).

Youth sport withdrawal models

The first component of Gould's (1987) MYSW addresses the issue of definition (discussed in the introduction), suggesting drop-out be distinguished as activity-specific (i.e. discontinuation from a specific sport activity) or domain-general (i.e. permanent withdrawal from all sport activities). The second component speaks to child-controlled withdrawal (i.e. child makes withdrawal decision) versus externally-controlled (i.e. child withdraws for reasons out of their control – injuries, being cut, programme cost). The third component draws upon elements of the social exchange theory (Thibaut and Kelley, 1959), focusing on children's cost-benefit analysis of sport engagement. Finally, the fourth component acknowledges surface level reasons for withdrawal of a personal (e.g. not having fun) and/or situational (e.g. programme too serious) nature, while drawing attention to the underlying theoretical motives for these reasons (e.g. AGT, CMT).

Lindner and colleagues' (1991) MVYSW focuses on voluntary (i.e. child-controlled) withdrawal, highlighting the interaction between environmental, developmental and sport-related factors. Environmental factors include youths' attraction to other leisure activities and social opportunities, as well work, school and/or family responsibilities. Developmental factors include youths' growing desire for autonomy and independence, and changing physical bodies and psychosocial needs. Finally, sport-related factors include motivation, burnout, cost, time investment, coaches and injury.

Both models reflect comprehensive and innovative frameworks for their time, but as Lindner *et al.* (1991) outlined, their model is 'complex', 'awkward' and 'cumbersome' (p. 6 and 8), and empirical testing in its entirety is 'nearly impossible' (p. 12). Consequentially, little research has used these models. In their systematic review, Balish and colleagues (2014) conclude the majority of attrition research has been conducted at intrapersonal (i.e. psychological) and interpersonal (i.e. social-environmental) levels, with much less considering biological, institutional, community and policy factors. As such, we next discuss intrapersonal and interpersonal factors influencing withdrawal, driven by the five theoretical motivation models previously outlined; we then explore broader contextual factors at structural, organizational, socio-cultural and policy levels.

Intrapersonal, interpersonal and contextual factors in youth sport drop-out

Intrapersonal factors

Intrapersonal factors are the most prominently examined correlates of youth sport drop-out, often through SDT (Balish *et al.*, 2014). For example, two large prospective studies conducted in Canada and France found drop-out was associated with lower intrinsic motivation (for stimulation, knowledge and accomplishment), and higher extrinsic motivation and amotivation; drop-out athletes also experienced lower competence, autonomy and relatedness than persistent athletes (Pelletier *et al.*, 2001; Sarrazin *et al.*, 2002). Similarly, Ryska, Hohensee, Cooley and Jones (2002) found drop-out athletes participated primarily for extrinsic reasons (e.g. social recognition) rather than intrinsic reasons (e.g. challenge). Weiss and Weiss (2003) also used SDT, with SCM, to examine profiles of high-level gymnasts that might be at risk of drop-out. Participants were clustered into commitment profiles according to the constructs of SCM. Entrapped athletes (i.e. low on enjoyment and benefits; high on costs, attractive alternatives and investments) and vulnerable athletes (i.e. moderate on enjoyment, benefits, costs and attractive alternatives; high on investments) scored significantly lower on intrinsic motivation and higher on amotivation than attracted athletes (i.e. high on enjoyment, benefits, investments; low on costs and attractive alternatives). Entrapped and vulnerable athletes also scored lower on effort and persistence in training. Profiles suggested attracted athletes were 'enthusiastic', vulnerable athletes appeared 'obligated' and entrapped athletes seemed 'malcontented' (pp. 242–244).

CMT has also guided prospective studies of withdrawal. For example, Ommundsen and Vaglum's (1997) investigation of Norwegian soccer players found low perceived competence was associated with drop-out, yet this relationship was unaffected by the importance athletes afforded to soccer competence. Authors proposed athletes' withdrawal might serve as a coping strategy to diminish the importance of their sport when their competence is low, thus preserving their self-esteem. Further, several studies have shown intrapersonal differences dependent on gender, age and sport experience. Typically, females and/or less experienced athletes are more likely to withdraw due to lower perceived competence, poorer social engagement, less enjoyment and more emotional challenges (Butcher *et al.*, 2002; Keathley *et al.*, 2013; Molinero *et al.*, 2006; Rottensteiner *et al.*, 2013).

Interpersonal factors

Given the bi-directional influences of intrapersonal and interpersonal factors, SDT, coupled with AGT, again frame much of the withdrawal research on interpersonal factors. Numerous recent longitudinal studies using structural equation modelling highlight important roles of coaches, parents, and peers/teammates in creating task-oriented motivation climates (i.e. emphasizing learning, effort, self-improvement and mastery over time), subsequently fulfilling athletes' needs for competence, autonomy and relatedness, in turn contributing to youths' task-orientation and intrinsic motivation, and consequentially facilitating persistence rather than withdrawal (e.g.

Cervelló *et al.*, 2007; Jõesaar *et al.*, 2011; Le Bars *et al.*, 2009; Quested *et al.*, 2013; Sarrazin *et al.*, 2002). Studies also suggest facilitation of an ego-oriented climate (i.e. outcome emphasis, success defined as winning/outperforming one's opponent) increases athletes' likelihood of withdrawal (Cervelló *et al.*, 2007; Jõesaar *et al.*, 2011). However, these models do not explain all the variance in youths' drop-out, thus other theories need also be considered (Jõesaar *et al.*, 2011). Guillet, Sarrazin, Carpenter, Trouilloud and Cury (2002) drew upon components of SCM, SDT and Social Exchange Theory (Thibaut and Kelley, 1959) finding sport commitment accounted for 44 per cent of the variance in adolescent handballers' withdrawal. Lower commitment was associated with higher social constraints (pressure), lower perceived benefits (competence, autonomy, relatedness, progress, coach support, playing time) and more alternative opportunities.

While very few intervention studies have examined withdrawal, Barnett *et al.* (1992) conducted a study among eighteen youth sport coaches; eight engaged in a two-and-a-half-hour Coach Effectiveness Training session (Smith *et al.*, 1979), while ten made up the control group. Despite equal win-loss records, drop-out rate in trained coaches' teams was 5 per cent, compared to untrained coaches' teams at 26 per cent, re-emphasizing the substantive role of significant others in influencing youths' withdrawal. Coaches may have the greatest influence on youths' withdrawal, followed by teammates and friends (Armentrout and Kamphoff, 2011; Rottensteiner *et al.*, 2013). In a study of adolescent swimmers who had all considered withdrawal at some point, only engaged athletes emphasized the critical role of coaches' open communication during difficult times; drop-out athletes recounted no similar experiences (Fraser-Thomas *et al.*, 2008b). Other studies suggest lack of a solid peer group and/or 'best friend' (Fraser-Thomas *et al.*, 2008a, 2008b; Ullrich-French and Smith, 2009), and negative peer experiences such as teasing, bullying and unhealthy peer competition (Armentrout and Kamphoff, 2011; Patrick *et al.*, 1999) also contribute to withdrawal. Evidence again suggests differences according to gender, with girls being more likely to withdraw due to interpersonal conflicts and perceived pressure from coaches, parents or peers (Butcher *et al.*, 2002, Gould *et al.*, 1982; Keathley *et al.*, 2013; Molinero *et al.*, 2006; Rottensteiner *et al.*, 2013).

Contextual factors

Recent research in the field highlights the importance of studying structural, organizational, socio-cultural, and policy factors in youth withdrawal. While Balish and colleagues' (2014) review found minimal evidence supporting these correlates, they highlight the value of further investigations. We identify three key areas of interest:

1 programme structure
2 relative age effects
3 community size.

Programme structure

In Fraser-Thomas and colleagues' (2008a) examination of the developmental pathways of drop-out and engaged adolescent swimmers, drop-outs demonstrated a clear trend of early specialization. Namely, while both groups spent equal time in training and competition, drop-outs spent less time in extracurricular activities and unstructured playful sport, more time in sport-specific training from a younger age (i.e. deliberate practice; Ericsson *et al.*, 1993), had their first training camp at an earlier age, and more often considered themselves the youngest in their training group. Prior research among Canadian hockey players, Russian swimmers and Swedish tennis players indicates a similar pattern – youth who engaged in earlier intensive training withdrew from their sport at earlier ages (Barynina and Vaitsekhovskii, 1992; Carlson, 1988; Wall and Côté, 2007). Another recent study highlighted the mean age of withdrawal across an American state hockey organization was only ten years – much lower than traditionally reflected in the literature (Armentrout and Kamphoff, 2011). Some researchers have cautioned that early systematized training may be a significant risk to children's healthy development and lead to burnout (e.g. Donnelly, 1993; Smith, 1986). Others have emphasized that more opportunities for play-based sport can offer a solid foundation for intrinsic motivation, skill development and subsequent competence (Côté *et al.*, 2009). Our review suggests more longitudinal research is needed to better understand long-term effects of early specialization (Baker *et al.*, 2009).

Closely tied to early specialization is the issue of time, consistently cited as a reason for withdrawal (e.g. Butcher *et al.*, 2002; Gould *et al.*, 1982; Molinero *et al.*, 2006). Armetrout and Kamphoff's (2011) study with parents of withdrawn athletes re-emphasizes the tremendous practical, emotional and financial tolls of sport on families, with one parent stating, 'I told him we can't afford it and we didn't have the time' (p. 128). While financial and practical barriers related to time are well recognized as influencing youths' initial sport participation among families of low socio-economic status (e.g. Clarke, 2008; Vella *et al.*, 2014), little research has examined these barriers among those already invested. As policies aimed to address these issues, such as Canada's Children's Fitness Tax Credit, remain largely unsuccessful (Spence *et al.*, 2010), it appears barriers should be further studied in relation to continued participation (Vella *et al.*, 2014), even among those of relatively high socio-economic status (Armetrout and Kamphoff, 2011).

The issues of early specialization coupled with time, practical and financial investment speak collectively to issues of programme structure. It appears youth do not necessarily want to engage in domain-general withdrawal (i.e. from all sport activities), but they do so because of the intensive structure of their programme, and the lack of other programming options available (e.g. Fraser-Thomas *et al.*, 2008b; Rottensteiner *et al.*, 2013). As one parent outlined, 'the competition level is pushed too far at too young of an age' (Armentrout and Kamphoff, 2011, p. 128). Burton, O'Connell, Gillham and Hammermeister's (2011) recent intervention study offers considerations for alternative competitive programming approaches. Their empirically-based 'competitively engineered' programme aimed to maximize enjoyment through high action and scoring, enhanced personal involvement, close scores and positive social relationships, leading to a 50 per cent decrease in attrition rates in a children's flag football team. Collectively, these findings suggest further investigation and consideration of programme structure, particularly through intervention research, is necessary to better understand and reduce withdrawal.

Relative age effects (RAE)

A second contextual factor of interest in withdrawal involves RAE, which emerged from youth sports' registration cut off dates by chronological age. Originally intended to equalize competition, RAE appear to have accentuated some disparities (Cobley *et al.*, 2009). Barnsley *et al.* (1985) were among the first to outline RAE in sport, finding Canadian hockey players who made it to professional levels were approximately four times more likely to be born in the first than the last quarter of the calendar year. Despite extensive work examining RAE in relation to participation and performance over the past three decades, studies have only recently examined RAE in drop-out. Three large scale investigations among French basketball players (N=44,498) (Delorme *et al.*, 2011), Canadian hockey players (N=14,325) (Lemez *et al.*, 2014) and Belgian soccer players (N=1,745) (Helsen *et al.*, 1998) suggest robust RAE for drop-out, meaning drop-out is over-represented among youth born later in the sport calendar year, and under-represented among those born earlier.

Few studies have examined underlying roots of RAE; however, Lemez and colleagues (2014) found young hockey players who withdrew had more often experienced a lack of progression within their sport. Relatively younger players may experience a significant size disadvantage and lower sense of competence, given that talent identification is often based on physical attributes, and relatively older children are typically more physically developed (Barnsley *et al.*, 1992; Cobley *et al.*, 2009; Helsen *et al.*, 1998). Balish *et al.* (2014) had insufficient evidence to suggest height, weight, and body mass index were associated with withdrawal, but two studies indicate drop-out athletes may be significantly shorter and at earlier stages of puberty than their teammates (Figueiredo *et al.*, 2009; Fraser-Thomas, *et al.*, 2008a). There are also likely cyclical elements to RAE, whereby relatively older players receive more attention, better coaching, more playing time and more rewards for their investment (Barnsley *et al.*, 1992; Cobley *et al.*, 2009; Helsen *et al.*, 1998). As such, there are growing calls for policy modifications to minimize the disparities created through RAE (Cobley *et al.*, 2009; Delorme *et al.*, 2011; Lemez *et al.*, 2014).

Community size

A final line of contextual research in youth sport drop-out focuses on community size. The seminal work of Curtis and Birch (1987) on 'birthplace effect' showed that youth born (and presumably engaging in sports) in smaller communities are over-represented in elite sport (Côté *et al.*, 2006; Turnnidge *et al.*, 2014). Recent examinations of hockey players (N=15,565; Imitiaz *et al.*, 2014) and swimmers (N=181; Fraser-Thomas *et al.*, 2010) found youth in cities greater than 500,000 were 2.9 and 4.7 times more likely to withdraw, respectively. Authors proposed several hypotheses to explain this disparity. For example, programmes in larger cities may be more institutionalized, placing a greater focus on winning (i.e. ego-oriented climate), while smaller communities may offer options for involvement at diverse levels with lower levels of investment. Smaller communities may also have more accessible open spaces and recreational facilities for children to engage in unstructured and organized sport, in turn providing more opportunities to develop skills and competence. Marsh (1987) also proposed the 'big fish small pond' effect, whereby youths' social comparison in smaller communities may lead to a greater sense of competence for more children. Finally, Fraser-Thomas *et al.* (2010) found that youth in smaller communities experienced more supportive relationships (i.e. from parents, coaches, peers). Smaller teams, lower coach-athlete ratios and more one-on-one coaching may be fundamental to youths' positive sport experiences (e.g. Fraser-Thomas *et al.*, 2008a, 2008b; Hellison, 2003).

In sum, significant research advances have furthered understanding of youth sport drop-out over the past four decades, particularly regarding interpersonal and intrapersonal factors. Our review of programme structure, RAE and community size widens the lens through which we comprehend drop-out, yet examination of broader contextual factors (i.e. structural, organizational, socio-cultural and policy) remains in its infancy. As such, future research must continue to unpack interacting contextual factors contributing to withdrawal, while intervention research and subsequent policies should be built upon evidence-based foundations.

Drop-off: transitioning out of youth sport

Unlike drop-out, the term drop-off is not commonly cited in the literature; however, we argue the concepts are closely related. Specifically, drop-off may be better suited to capture the natural progressions of youths' involvement in sports throughout development such as withdrawal from one sport and continuation in another, which is currently conceptualized within drop-out definitions (Gould, 1987; Lindner *et al.*, 1991). In this section, we outline two sport development models focused on youths' trajectories, stages and transitions through sport:

1   Developmental Model of Sport Participation (DMSP; Côté and Fraser-Thomas, 2011).
2   Developmental Perspective on Transitions Faced by Athletes (DPTFA; Wylleman and Lavallee, 2004).

Models of youth sport transitioning

The DMSP (Côté, 1999; Côté and Fraser-Thomas, 2011; see also Côté in this section) proposes youth engage in three key sport trajectories:

1   recreational participation through sampling
2   elite performance through sampling
3   elite performance through early specialization.

Each trajectory entails different types and frequencies of training, and varying involvement in other activities, which impact performance, health and psychosocial outcomes. With regards to drop-off, the DMSP proposes the transition between trajectories is possible at any time. For example, an athlete on a path to high performance sport may choose to reduce their involvement to a recreational level. Further, individuals on any trajectory may choose to drop-out permanently, resulting in more probable negative outcomes; early specialization is proposed as the path most likely to lead to drop-out.

The DPTFA (Wylleman and Lavallee, 2004) provides an overview of factors influencing individuals' stages and transitions throughout sport at athletic, psychological, psychosocial and academic/vocational levels. At the athletic level, sport participants may pass through four stages (although not all individuals pass through each stage):

1   initiation (into organized sport)
2   development (involving increased training and competition)
3   mastery (into high performance sport)
4   discontinuation.

At the psychological and psychosocial levels, children are initially influenced primarily by parents and siblings, and increasingly by peers and coaches during adolescence and young adulthood. At the academic/vocational level, influences include transitions of primary school, secondary school, higher education and/or vocational training/professional occupation. The DPTFA also highlights the interactive and interdependent normative and non-normative factors influencing young people's sport development. Normative transitions are predictable and anticipated events, generally associated with age (e.g. moving junior to senior competition level). In contrast, non-normative transitions are unexpected and involuntary events (e.g. de-selection or injury).

Intrapersonal, interpersonal and contextual factors in youth sport transitions

In contrast to models of take-up and drop-out, models of drop-off focus on the role of several contextual factors, such as athletes' sport trajectories, development and programme availability.

With regard to sport trajectories, the DMSP and DPTFA suggest children and adolescents' common pattern of taking up and dropping out of different sports (Butcher *et al.*, 2002; Gould *et al.*, 1982) may reflect normative transitions, as children 'try different sports in the same way they might try on different coats, sampling preferences until they find the one they like best (Burton, 1988, p. 245). Long-term outcomes of different sport trajectories have only recently been studied, with conflicting results. Namely, two large-scale longitudinal studies in Belgium and Canada found youths' involvement in recreational and school-based sport were associated with prolonged sport participation into adulthood (Curtis *et al.*, 1999; Vanreusel *et al.*, 1997); however, youths' earlier higher-frequency sport involvement has also been associated with more positive long-term physically active behaviours (Kjønniksen *et al.*, 2009; Tammelin *et al.*, 2003).

From a developmental perspective, graduation from primary and/or secondary school presents a normative transition that often threatens youths' continued sport participation, due to competing priorities (e.g. academics, jobs) or lack of programming (Lim *et al.*, 2011; Wyllemann and Lavallee, 2004; Zick *et al.*, 2007). This may be particularly true for youth in team sports, as school and community team programmes are generally less available during adulthood (Zick *et al.*, 2007). These studies re-affirm the importance of continued study of contextual factors in relation to drop-off, to in turn build stronger collaborations between sport agencies, and increase availability of organized community sport programming for youth transitioning into adulthood (Collins and Buller, 2000; Eime and Payne, 2009; Lim *et al.*, 2011).

Interpersonal and interpersonal factors also influence youths' drop-off from sport. DMSP and DPTFA highlight the role of parents, peers and coaches in athletes' sport development and transitions, with coaches' facilitation of enjoyment and focus on athletes' personal and social development playing a fundamental role in athletes' long-term involvement (Côté and Fraser-Thomas, 2011 Wylleman and Lavallee, 2004). Youth sport participants often intend to return to sport following an adjustment period, but attempts are often met with frustration (Lim *et al.*, 2011; Lunn, 2010; Zick *et al.*, 2007). While some successfully navigate their way to a new team (e.g. varsity), many often discontinue shortly thereafter, faced with challenges of adjusting to new teammates, coaches and expectations, leading to stress, feelings of inadequacy and disorientation (Green, 2005). Retirement can be accompanied by a further sense of identity loss and physiological changes (e.g. Warriner and Lavallee, 2008). One positive adaption to the drop-off process involves transitioning to lifestyles sports (e.g. golf and running) and personal fitness (Chapter 17), which can help former participants re-integrate sport and physical activity into their life (Lunn, 2010). Evidently, continued sport participation during both normative and non-normative transitions is greatly influenced by social support and personal needs (e.g. interests, competence, attitudes) (Hirvensalo and Lithvnen, 2011; Lim *et al.*, 2011 Lunn, 2010).

Future research

As interest and concern surrounding youth sport take-up, drop-out and drop-off remain paramount, more advanced research designs will be necessary to advance knowledge. In particular, longitudinal designs would allow more comprehension of youths' sport development over time and crucial transitions, given reasons and rates of participation and withdrawal change with age (Balish *et al.*, 2014; Butcher *et al.*, 2002; Weiss and Williams, 2004; Wylleman and Lavallee, 2004). Benefits and potential risks of certain sport trajectories (e.g. early specialization) will only be fully understood with rigorous longitudinal designs examining training and competition demands, and adaptations to these demands at each stage of development according to sport, gender, etc. (Baker *et al.*, 2009). While many researchers have shifted in this direction over the past decade (e.g. Butcher *et al.*, 2002; Fraser-Thomas *et al.*, 2008a; Le Bars *et al.*, 2009; Pelletier *et al.*, 2001; Sarrazin *et al.*, 2002), their designs have been somewhat limited by retrospective recall or over-simplification of drop-out as failure to re-register. Rather than nearly exclusive reliance on self-report questionnaires, longitudinal research should draw upon additional innovative approaches including observation, case studies, journaling and photo-elicitation (Balish *et al.*, 2014 Quested *et al.*, 2013).

There is also tremendous potential to advance knowledge through intervention research. While theoretical understanding of youth sport involvement is abundant, further work must draw upon motivation, withdrawal and transition models to develop effective interventions. Researchers may also consider implementing gender-specific interventions, given consistent evidence of differences in psychosocial constructs such as coach and peer relationships, and values related to sport participation (Butcher *et al.*, 2002; Keathley *et al.*, 2013; Rottensteiner *et al.*, 2013). Further, intervention research offers an optimal platform for examining contextual factors. For example, interventions designed around RAE could focus on coach education, modifying age groupings (i.e. one-year versus two- and three-year groupings), implementing quotas of age distributions on each team and/or shifting the competitive focus to later stages of development (Barnsley *et al.*, 1992; Delorme *et al.*, 2011; Helsen *et al.*, 1998).

Finally, we propose the re-consideration of definitions and conceptual models of youth sport involvement. Gould's 1987 suggestion that 'the lack of appropriate operational definitions has plagued previous research' (p. 79) appears to remain true. Despite typologies and classification systems for drop-out (e.g. Gould, 1987; Lindner *et al.*, 1991), the logistical complexities of applying these frameworks seem to have discouraged rather than encouraged further research. Additionally, typologies often suggest withdrawal represents a healthy sampling and transitioning process of multiple sports throughout youth (Balish *et al.*, 2014; Butcher *et al.*, 2002; Côté and Fraser-Thomas, 2011; Gould, 1987), in contrast to original reasons for studying drop-out – that it is negative for children's development (e.g. Burton, 1988; Gould, 1987).

In moving research forward, it may be more fruitful to re-define drop-out as *only* permanent withdrawal from all sports (i.e. a more concerning type); all other forms of withdrawal, attrition, discontinuation and transfer could be considered within bodies of youth sport development research. The current trend of deciphering drop-outs' extensive characteristics (e.g. age, sport type, investment, abilities, competition levels) in order to appropriately classify their drop-out type prior to study could be abandoned. Instead, conceptual and theoretical models of sport development and transition could integrate such characteristics, essentially absorbing important factors of current drop-out classification systems. We believe this re-definition of drop-out would allow for less muddied waters in the study of drop-out, while also facilitating increased efforts towards a growing body of rich research on youth sport profiles, trajectories, stages and transitions, which is gradually contributing to important policy (e.g. Canada's Long Term Athlete Development Model, Canadian Sport for Life, 2014; Australia's Foundation Talent Elite Mastery Framework, Australian Sports Commission, 2014).

Conclusion

In sum, critical to advancing knowledge are more multi-level models that consider contextual factors in addition to intrapersonal and interpersonal factors, drawing upon multiple theoretical concepts, and recognizing interacting effects (Balish *et al.*, 2014; Weiss and Williams, 2004). While there is a wealth of theory driving current work, Gould (1987) suggested, 'quite possibly these theories are not comprised of independent psychological constructs, and may at times discuss the same constructs under the guise of different labels' (p. 78). Tremendous knowledge has advanced our understanding of youths' take-up, drop-out and drop-off in sport over the past several decades, but researchers must continue to work closely with programmers, coaches and policy makers to assure optimal opportunities for all youths' engagement and development in sport.

References

Armentrout, S.M. and Kamphoff, C.S. (2011). Organizational barriers and factors that contribute to youth hockey attrition, *Journal of Sport Behaviour, 34(2),* 121–136.

Australian Sports Commission (2014). Foundations, talent, elite, and mastery, retrieved from the Australian Sports Commission website: www.ausport.gov.au/ais/pathways.

Baker, J., Cobley, S. and Fraser-Thomas, J. (2009). What do we know about early sport specialization? Not much! *High Ability Studies,* 20(1), 77–89.

Balish, S.M., McLaren, C., Rainham, D. and Blanchard, C. (2014). Correlates of youth sport attrition: A review and future directions, *Psychology of Sport and Exercise, 15,* 429–439.

Barnett, N.P., Smoll, F.L. and Smith, R.E. (1992). Effects of enhancing coach–athlete relationships on youth sport attrition, *The Sport Psychologist, 6,* 111–127.

Barnsley, R.H., Thompson, A.H. and Barnsley, P.E. (1985). Hockey success and birthdate: The relative age effect, *Canadian Association of Health, Physical Education, and Recreation, 51,* 23–28.

Barnsley, R.H., Thompson, A.H. and Legault, P. (1992). Family planning: Football style. The relative age effect in football, *International Review of Sport Sociology, 27,* 77–87.

Barynina, I.I. and Vaitsekhovskii, S.M. (1992). The aftermath of early sports specialization for highly qualified swimmers, *Fitness and Sport Review International, 27(4),* 132–133.

Bray, S.R., Martin Ginis, K.A., Cairney, J., Marinoff-Shupe, D. and Pettit, A. (2014). '*They believe I can do it . . . Maybe I Can!' The effects of interpersonal feedback on relation-inferred self-efficacy, self-efficacy, and intrinsic motivation in children's sport.* Paper presented at the annual Sport Participation Research Initiative Conference. Ottawa: Canada.

Burton (1988). The drop-out dilemma in youth sports: Documenting the problem and identifying solutions, in R.M. Malina (ed), *Young athletes: Biological, psychological, and education perspectives* (pp. 245–266). Champaign, Illinois: Human Kinetics.

Burton, D., O'Connell, K., Gillham, A.D. and Hammermeister, J. (2011). More cheers and fewer tears: Examining the impact of competitive engineering on scoring and attrition in youth flag football, *International Journal of Sports Science and Coaching, 6(2),* 219–228.

Butcher, J., Lindner, K. and Johns, D.P. (2002). Withdrawal from competitive youth sport: a retrospective ten-year study, *Journal of Sport Behaviour, 25(2),* 145–163.

Canadian Sport For Life (2014). *Long term athlete development model stages.* Retrieved from Canadian Sport for Life website: http://canadiansportforlife.ca/learn-about-canadian-sport-life/ltad-stages.

Carlson, R. (1988). The socialization of elite tennis players in Sweden: An analysis of players' backgrounds and development, *Sociology of Sport Journal, 5,* 241–256.

Carpenter, P.J., Scanlan, T.K., Simons, J.P. and Lobel, M. (1993). A test of the Sport Commitment Model using structural equation modelling, *Journal of Sport and Exercise Psychology, 15(2),* 119–133.

Cervelló, E.M., Escartí, A. and Guzmán, J.F. (2007). Youth sport drop-out from the achievement goal theory. *Psicothema, 19(1),* 65–71.

Clark, W. (2008). Kids' sports. *Canadian Social Trends.* (Catalogue no. 11–0008-X). Ottawa, ON: Statistics Canada.

Cobley, S., Baker, J., Wattie, N. and McKenna, J. (2009). Annual age-grouping and athlete development: A meta-analytical review of relative age effects in sport, *Sports Medicine, 39,* 235–256.

Collins, M.F. and Buller, J.R. (2000). Bridging the post-school institutional gap in sport: evaluating champion coaching in Nottinghamshire, *Managing Leisure, 5(4),* 200–221.

Côté, J. (1999). The influence of the family in the development of talent in sport, *The Sport Psychologist, 13,* 395–417.

Côté, J., Lidor, R. and Hackfort, D. (2009). ISSP position stand: To sample or to specialize? Seven postulates about youth sport activities that lead to continued participation and elite performance, *International Journal of Sport and Exercise Psychology, 7(1),* 7–17.

Côté, J. and Fraser-Thomas, J. (2011). Youth involvement and positive development in sport, in P.R.E. Crocker (ed.) *Sport psychology: A Canadian Perspective* (2nd edition) (pp. 226–255). Toronto: Pearson Prentice Hall.

Côté, J., Macdonald, D.J., Baker, J. and Abernethy, B. (2006). When 'where' is more important than 'when': Birthplace and birthdate effects on the achievement of sporting expertise, *Journal of Sport Sciences*, *24*, 1065–1073.

Curtis, J.E. and Birch, J.S. (1987). Size of community of origin and recruitment to professional and Olympic hockey in North America, *Sociology of Sport Journal*, *4*, 229–244.

Curtis, J., McTeer, W. and White, P. (1999). Exploring effects of school sport experiences on sport participation later in life, *Sociology of Sport Journal*, *16*, 348–365.

Deci, E.L. and Ryan R.M. (1987). The support of autonomy and the control of behaviour, *Journal of Personality and Social Psychology*, *53*(6), 1024–1037.

Delorme, N., Chalabaev, A. and Raspaud, M. (2011). Relative age is associated with sport drop-out: Evidence from youth categories of French basketball, *Scandinavian Journal of Medicine and Science in Sports*, *21*, 120–128.

Donnelly, P. (1993). Problems associated with youth involvement in high-performance sport, in B.R. Cahill and A.J. Pearl (eds) *Intensive participation in children's sport* (pp. 95–126). Champaign, Illinois: Human Kinetics.

Eccles, J.C. (1984). Sex differences in achievement patterns, in T. Sonderegger (ed.) *Nebraska symposium of motivation* (pp. 97–132). Lincoln, NE: University of Nebraska Press.

Eccles, J.C. and Harold, R.D. (1991). Gender differences in sport involvement: Applying the Eccles' expectancy-value model, *Journal of Applied Sport Psychology*, *3*, 7–35.

Eime, R.M. and Payne, W.R. (2009). Linking participants in school-based sports programs to community clubs, *Journal of Science and Medicine in Sport*, *12*(2), 293–299.

Ericsson, K.A., Krampe, R.T. and Tesch-Römer, C. (1993). The role of deliberate practice in the acquisition of expert performance, *Psychological Review*, *100*, 363–406.

Falcão, W.R., Bloom, G.A. and Gilbert, W.D. (2012). Coaches' perceptions of a coach training program designed to promote youth developmental outcomes, *Journal of Applied Sport Psychology*, *24*(4), 429–444.

Figueiredo, A., Gonçalves, Coelho-e-Silva, M. and Malina, R. (2009). Characteristics of youth soccer players who drop out, persist or move up, *Journal of Sports Sciences*, *27*(9), 883–891.

Fraser-Thomas, J.L., Côté, J. and Deakin, J. (2005). Youth sport programmes: An avenue to foster positive youth development, *Physical Education and Sport Pedagogy*, *10*, 19–40.

Fraser-Thomas, J., Côté, J. and Deakin, J. (2008a). Examining adolescent sport drop-out and prolonged engagement from a developmental perspective, *Journal of Applied Sport Psychology*, *20*, 318–333.

Fraser-Thomas, J., Côté, J. and Deakin, J. (2008b). Understanding drop-out and prolonged engagement in adolescent competitive sport, *Psychology of Sport and Exercise*, *9*(5), 645–662.

Fraser-Thomas, J., Côté, J. and Macdonald, D.J. (2010). Community size in youth sport settings: Examining developmental assets and sport withdrawal, *PHENex Journal*, *2(2)*, 1–9.

Goodger, K., Gorely, T., Lavallee, D. and Harwood, C. (2007). Burnout in sport: A systematic review, *The Sport Psychologist*, *21*: 127–151.

Gould, D. (1987). Understanding attrition in children's sport, in D. Gould and M.R. Weiss *Behavioural issues* (vol. 2) (pp. 61–85). Champaign, Illinois: Human Kinetics.

Gould, D., Feltz, D., Horn, T. and Weiss, M.R. (1982). Reasons for discontinuing involvement in competitive youth swimming, *Journal of Sport Behaviour*, *5*, 155–165.

Green, B.C. (2005). Building sport programmes to optimize athlete recruitment, retention, and transition: toward a normative theory of sport development, *Journal of Sport Management*, *19*(3), 233–253.

Guillet, E., Sarrazin, P., Carpenter, P.J., Trouilloud, D. and Cury, F. (2002). Predicting persistence or withdrawal in female handballers with social exchange theory, *International Journal of Psychology*, *37*(2), 92–104.

Gustafson, S.L. and Rhodes, R.E. (2006). Parental correlates of physical activity in children and early adolescents, *Sports Medicine*, *36*, 79–97.

Harter, S. (1978). Effectance motivation reconsidered: Toward a developmental model, *Human Development*, *21*, 34–64.

Harter, S. (1981). A model of intrinsic mastery motivation in children: Individual differences and developmental change, in A. Collins (ed), *Minnesota symposium on child psychology* (vol. 14) (pp. 215–255). Hillsdale, NJ: Erlbaum.

Hellison, D. (2003). *Teaching responsibility through physical activity* (2nd edition). Champaign, Illinois: Human Kinetics.

Helsen, W.F., Starkes, J.L. and Van Winckel, J. (1998). The influence of relative age on success and drop-out in male soccer players, *American Journal of Human Biology*, *10*, 791–798.

Hirvensalo, M. and Lintunen, T. (2011). Life-course perspective for physical activity and sports participation, *European Review of Aging and Physical Activity*, *8(1)*, 13–22.

Hollembeak, J. and Amorose, A.J. (2005). Perceived coaching behaviours and college athletes' intrinsic motivation: a test of self-determination theory, *Journal of Applied Sport Psychology*, *17(1)*, 20–36.

Holt, N.L., Kingsley, B.C., Tink, L.N. and Scherer, J. (2011). Benefits and challenges associated with sport participation by children and parents from low-income families, *Psychology of Sport and Exercise*, *12(5)*, 490–499.

Imitiaz, F., Hancock, D.J., Vierimaa, M. and Côté, J. (2014). Place of development and drop-out in youth ice hockey, *International Journal of Sport and Exercise Psychology*, *12(3)*, 234–244.

Jõesaar, H., Hein, V. and Hagger, M.S. (2011). Peer influence on young athletes' need satisfaction, intrinsic motivation and persistence in sport: A twelve-month prospective study, *Psychology of Sport and Exercise*, *12*: 500–508.

Keathley, K., Himelein, M.J. and Srigley, G. (2013). Youth soccer participation and withdrawal: Gender similarities and differences, *Journal of Sport Behaviour*, *36(2)*, 171–188.

Keegan, R.J., Harwood, C.G., Spray, C.M. and Lavallee, D.E. (2009). A qualitative investigation exploring the motivational climate in early career sports participants: Coach, parent and peer influences on sport motivation, *Psychology of Sport and Exercise*, *10*, 361–372.

Kjønniksen, L. Anderssen, N. and Wold, B. (2009). Organized youth sport as a predictor of physical activity in adulthood, *Scandinavian Journal of Medicine and Science in Sports*, *19(5)*, 646–654.

Klint, K.A. and Weiss, M.R. (1986). Dropping in and dropping out: Participation motives of current and former youth gymnasts, *Canadian Journal of Applied Sport Sciences*, *11*, 106–114.

Le Bars, H., Gernigon, C. and Ninot, G. (2009). Personal and contextual determinants of elite young athletes' persistence or dropping out over time, *Scandinavian Journal of Medicine and Sport Science*, *19*, 274–285.

Lemez, S., Baker, J., Horton, S., Wattie, N. and Weir, P. (2014). Examining the relationship between relative age, competition level, and drop-out rates in male youth ice-hockey players, *Scandinavian Journal of Medicine and Science in Sports*, *24(6)*, 935–942.

Lim, S.Y., Warner, S., Dixon, M., Berg, B., Kim, C. and Newhouse-Bailey, M. (2011). Sport participation across national contexts: a multilevel investigation of individual and systemic influences on adult sport participation, *European Sport Management Quarterly*, *11(3)*, 197–224.

Lindner, J.K., Johns, D.P. and Butcher, J. (1991). Factors in withdrawal from youth sport: A proposed model, *Journal of Sport Behaviour*, *14*, 3–18.

Lunn, P.D. (2010). The sports and exercise life-course: a survival analysis of recall data from Ireland, *Social Science and Medicine*, *70(5)*, 711–719.

Marsh, H.W. (1987). The big fish, little pond effect on academic self-concept, *Journal of Educational Psychology*, *79*, 280–295.

Molinero, O., Salguero, A., Tuero, C., Alvarez, E. and Márquez, A. (2006). Drop-out reasons in young Spanish athletes: Relationship to gender, type of sport and level of competition, *Journal of Sport Behaviour*, *29(3)*, 255–269.

Nicholls, J.G. (1979). Quality and equality in intellectual development: The role of motivation in education, *American Psychologist*, *34*, 1071–1084.

Nicholls, J.G. (1984). Achievement motivation: Conceptions of ability, subjective experience, task choice, and performance, *Psychological Review*, *91*, 328–346.

Ommundsen, Y. and Vaglum, P. (1997). Competence, perceived importance of competence and drop-out from soccer: A study of young players, *Scandinavian Journal of Medicine and Science in Sports*, *7*, 373–383.

Orlick, T. (1974). The athletic drop-out: A high price for inefficiency, *CAPHERD Journal (November–December Volume)*, 21–27.

Papaioannou, A.G., Ampatzoglou, G., Kalogiannis, P. and Sagovits, A. (2008). Social agents, achievement goals, satisfaction and academic achievement in youth sport, *Psychology of Sport and Exercise*, *9*, 122–141.

Patrick, H., Ryan, A.M., Alfeld-Liro, C., Fredricks, J.A., Hruda, L.Z. and Eccles, J.S. (1999). Adolescents' commitment to developing talent: The role of peers in continuing motivation for sports and the arts, *Journal of Youth and Adolescence*, *28*, 741–763.

Pelletier, L.G., Fortier, M.S., Vallerand, R.J. and Brière, N.M. (2001). Associations among perceived autonomy support, forms of self-regulations, and persistence: A prospective study, *Motivation and Emotion*, *25*, 279–306.

Physical Activity Council (2014). *2014 participation report*. Retrieved from Physical Activity Council website: www.physicalactivitycouncil.com/PDFs/current.pdf.

Quested, E., Ntoumanis, N., Viladrich, C., Haug, E., Ommundsen, Y., Van Hoye, A., Mercé, J., Hall, H.K., Zourbanos, N. and Duda, J.L. (2013). Intentions to drop-out of youth soccer: A test of the basic needs theory among European youth from five countries, *International Journal of Sport and Exercise Psychology, 11(4)*, 395–407.

Reeve, J.M. (2014). *Understanding motivation and emotion* (6th edition). Hoboken, NJ: Wiley and Sons.

Rottensteiner, C., Laakso, L., Pihlaja, T. and Konttinen, N. (2013). Personal reasons for withdrawal from team sports and the influence of significant others among youth athletes, *International Journal of Sports Science and Coaching, 8(1)*, 19–32.

Ryan, R.M. and Deci, E.L. (2000). Self-determination theory and the facilitation of intrinsic motivation, social development, and well-being, *American Psychologist, 55(1)*, 68–78.

Ryska, T.A., Hohensee, D., Cooley, D. and Jones, C. (2002). Participation motives in predicting sport drop-out among Australian youth gymnasts, *North American Journal of Psychology, 4(2)*, 199–210.

Sallis, J.F., Prochaska, J.J. and Taylor, W.C. (2000). A review of correlates of physical activity of children and youth, *Medicine and Science in Sports and Exercise, 42*, 963–975.

Sarrazin, P., Vallerand, R., Guillet, E., Pelletier, L. and Cury, F. (2002). Motivation and drop-out in female handballers: a 21-month prospective study, *European Journal of Social Psychology, 32(3)*, 395–418.

Scanlan, T.K., Carpenter, P.J., Schmidt, G.W., Simons, J.P. and Keeler, B. (1993). An introduction to the sport commitment model, *Journal of Sport and Exercise Psychology, 15(1)*, 1–15.

Smith, R.E. (1986). Towards a cognitive-affective model of athletic burnout, *Journal of Sport Psychology, 8*, 36–50.

Smith, R.E., Smoll, F.L. and Curtis, B. (1979). Coach effectiveness training: A cognitive behavioural approach to enhancing relationship skills in youth sport coaches, *Journal of Sport Psychology, 1*, 59–75.

Spence, J.C., Holt, N.L., Dutove, J.K. and Carson, V. (2010). Uptake and effectiveness of the Children's Fitness Tax Credit in Canada: The rich get richer, *BMC Public Health, 10*, 356–361.

Stein, J., Bloom, G.A. and Sabiston, C.M. (2012). Influence of perceived and preferred coach feedback on youth athletes' perceptions of team motivational climate, *Psychology of Sport and Exercise, 13*, 484–490.

Tammelin, T., Näyhä,, S. Hills, A.P. and Järvelin, M-R. (2003). Adolescent participation in sports and adult physical activity, *American Journal of Preventive Medicine, 24(1)*, 22–28.

Thibaut, J.W. and Kelley, H.H. (1959). *The Social Psychology of Groups*. Oxford, England: John Wiley.

Turnnidge, J. Hancock, D.J. and Côté, J. (2014). The influence of birth date and place of development on youth sport participation, *Scandinavian Journal of Medicine and Science in Sports, 24*, 461–468.

Ullrich-French, S. and Smith, A. (2009). Social and motivational predictors of continued youth sport participation, *Psychology of Sport and Exercise, 10*, 87–95.

Vallerand, R.J. and Reid, G. (1988). On the relative effects of positive and negative verbal feedback on males' and females' intrinsic motivation, *Canadian Journal of Behavioural Science, 20*, 23 –250.

Vanreusel, B., Renson, R., Beunen, G., Claessens, A.L., Lefevre, J., Lysens, R., Vanden Eynde B. and Leuven, K.U. (1997). A longitudinal study of youth sport participation and adherence to sport in adulthood, *International Review for the Sociology of Sport, 32(4)*, 373–387.

Vella, S.A., Cliff, D.P. and Okely, A.D. (2014). Socio-ecological predictors of participation and drop-out in organised sports during childhood, *International Journal of Behavioural Nutrition and Physical Activity, 11*, 62–71.

Wall, M. and Côté, J. (2007). Developmental activities that lead to drop-out and investment in sport, *Physical Education and Sport Pedagogy, 12(1)*, 77–87.

Warriner, K. and Lavallee, D. (2008). The retirement experiences of elite female gymnasts: self-identity and the physical self, *Journal of Applied Sport Psychology, 20(3)*, 301–317.

Weiss, M.R., Kimmel, L.A. and Smith, A.L. (2001). Determinants of sport commitment among junior tennis players: Enjoyment as a mediating variable, *Pediatric Exercise Science, 13:* 131–144.

Weiss, W.M. and Weiss, M.R. (2003). Attraction- and entrapment-based commitment among competitive female gymnasts, *Journal of Sport and Exercise Psychology, 25*, 229–247.

Weiss, M.R. and Williams, L. (2004). The why of youth sport involvement: A developmental perspective on motivational processes, in M.R. Weiss (ed.) *Developmental sport and exercise psychology: A lifespan perspective* (pp. 223–268). Morgantown, WV: Fitness Information Technology.

Wylleman, P. and Lavallee, D. (2004). A developmental perspective on transitions faced by athletes, *Developmental sport and exercise psychology: A lifespan perspective* (pp. 507–527). West Virginia: Fitness Information Technology.

Zick, C.D., Smith, K.R., Brown, B.B., Fan, J.X. and Kowaleski-Jones, L. (2007). Physical activity during the transition from adolescence to adulthood, *Journal of Physical Activity and Health, 4(2)*, 125–137.

23

A PERSONAL ASSETS APPROACH TO YOUTH SPORT

Jean Côté, Jennifer Turnnidge and Matthew Vierimaa

A personal assets approach to youth sport

The personal and social development of young people in sport is a rhetoric that is used globally by sport organizations, coaches and parents to promote sport among youth. However, questions surrounding *What constitutes development?* and *How does development occur in sport?* are issues that coaches, parents and policy makers struggle to agree upon. These fundamental questions have created several debates among researchers and policy makers in terms of how youth sport programmes should be structured. For example, a number of researchers see youth sport as the initial step in talent development programmes aimed at developing the *performance* of elite level athletes (e.g. Ford *et al.*, 2009). Several sport programmes are designed with this primary objective and therefore focus on the development of fundamental movement patterns and sport performance skills. Such programmes are characterized by the long-term goal of achieving elite performance. Unfortunately, this is often at the cost of short-term gratification and enjoyment (Côté and Abernethy, 2012). Other researchers advocate that youth sport programmes should maximize time spent in physical activity as a way to diminish issues related to lack of exercise among youth (e.g. Janssen and LeBlanc, 2010). Accordingly, several youth sport programmes have been developed with the goal of increasing physical activity *participation* through sport and diminishing the impact of diseases related to inactivity and obesity. Finally, numerous researchers propose that sport is an ideal activity to teach and transmit positive life values to young people (e.g. Danish, Petitpas and Hale, 1993). Several sport programmes, such as Sports United to Promote Education and Recreation (SUPER; Danish, 2002), Play it Smart (Petitpas *et al.*, 2004), The First Tee (The First Tee, 2005), Going for the Goal (Danish *et al.*, 1993) and Teaching Personal and Social Responsibility (TPSR; Hellison, 2003) are specifically designed to achieve this objective of facilitating personal development through sport.

Although youth sport has the potential to promote a number of important outcomes in young people's development, including performance, participation and personal development (i.e. the 3 Ps; Côté *et al.*, 2008), when programmes focus on a sole objective, it limits their potential contribution to the overall development of youth. Furthermore, specific youth sport programmes that focus on one of the Ps will often use specifically trained personnel and intervention programmes that can be costly and potentially difficult to sustain (Turnnidge *et al.*, 2012). Instead of focusing on one outcome, in this chapter we will present a global vision for youth sport through a new framework that accounts for the mechanisms necessary for a developmentally sound approach to youth sport involvement and that can be incorporated in the different trajectories of the Developmental Model of Sport Participation (DMSP; see Côté and Abernethy, 2012 for a review).

The DMSP provides a common foundation to youth sport programmes that focuses on the idea of trying out various forms of sporting activities during childhood and getting involved in activities that are inherently enjoyable such as deliberate play. The DMSP, however, does not clearly incorporate the dynamic elements and processes that interact to explain and predict the achievement of Performance, Participation and Personal Development. A Positive Youth Development (PYD) approach to youth sport programming will be used next to start building a framework for sport that focuses on the personal assets of youth. First we will use the PYD concepts of the Cs system (confidence, competence, connection and character) to reframe sport as an activity that should prioritize personal assets among youth. Second we will link three dynamic elements of sport and PYD – *activities*, *relationships* and *settings* – to the Cs and the Ps, and present these elements as the integrated mechanisms that constitute youth sport.

The 4 Cs: confidence, competence, connection and character

The PYD approach has been developed using an asset-building perspective on youth development, which views youth in a positive light and focuses on building personal assets (Benson, 2003). One of the predominant frameworks that originated from this asset-building approach to youth development is Lerner *et al.*'s (2005) 5 Cs. Lerner and colleagues (2005) suggest that PYD occurs as youth acquire the five latent variables that make up the 5 Cs: competence, confidence, connection, character and caring/compassion. An extensive body of research has been conducted using this framework in extra-curricular activities which lends support to this conceptualization of PYD. While PYD research began in developmental psychology, it has rapidly gained in popularity among youth sport researchers (see Holt, 2008; Holt and Neely, 2011 for a review).

In reviewing the extant sport literature, Côté and colleagues (2010) proposed a collapsed 4 Cs framework for studying PYD in a youth sport context. This revised framework integrates caring and compassion with character, due to the similarity and overlap among these constructs within the sport literature. Using the 4 Cs framework, Vierimaa and colleagues (2012) have since proposed a measurement approach to assess competence, confidence, connection and character using existing sport specific instruments and techniques. While the validation of this approach is ongoing, this line of research represents the re-alignment of the 5 Cs framework to more accurately reflect the unique aspects of the youth sport context.

The first construct comprising the 4 Cs is competence, which is defined as individuals' perception of their ability in a given area (e.g. sport; Weiss and Ebbeck, 1996). The broad general definition of competence includes multiple domain specific-areas (e.g. social, cognitive, academic and vocational). However, in discussing the 4 Cs in relation to the youth sport context, it is preferable to limit our conceptualization of competence to the sport domain. Second, just as sport competence reflects an individual's actual ability or performance in sport, confidence is indicative of the degree to which one believes that he/she can be successful in sport (Vealey, 1986). More specifically, confidence within the 4 Cs framework represents a narrowing of confidence from one's global self-worth (Jeličić *et al.*, 2007) to domain-specific beliefs regarding one's ability to be successful in a given sport (Feltz and Chase, 1998). Third, the construct of connection comprises the quality of an athlete's relationships with all individuals involved in sport, and the nature and degree of interactions that make up these relationships (e.g. Jowett and Poczwardowski, 2007; Smith, 2007). The multiple types of relationships that exist in youth sport have the potential to positively affect the personal growth of young athletes. Character is the final construct in the 4 Cs framework, and includes the concepts of sportspersonship and moral development (Shields and Bredemeier, 1995). Thus, character can be defined as a sense of responsibility, integrity, empathy and respect (Côté and Gilbert, 2009).

Collectively, the 4 Cs represent a parsimonious framework whereby the development of these proximal constructs in young athletes will effectively lead to increased long-term participation, performance and personal development in sport. Lerner, Dowling and Anderson (2003) have described contribution as the ultimate outcome of a focus on the 4 Cs in extra-curricular activities; in other words, through the development of the 4 Cs, youth are more likely to give back and contribute to their self, family, community and society. Thus, just as each of the 4 Cs is uniquely linked to aspects of sport performance and participation, they jointly facilitate healthy personal development and civic engagement. Based on the evidence reviewed in this section, it becomes apparent that if the 4 Cs are the central focus of sport programmes, the ultimate outcomes of performance, participation and personal development (3 Ps) are more likely to emerge from sport involvement.

Three dynamic elements of development

By focusing on the personal, social and physical setting features of different activities (e.g. play, practice, sampling, specialization), the DMSP infers that the positive outcomes of sport result from the personal engagement, social relationships and settings that comprise a play or practice activity in sport (Côté *et al.*, 2008). These dynamic elements of sport involvement within the DMSP are consistent with the nested system approach of Bronfenbrenner's ecological systems theory (1995) and the vast amount of youth sport research that is focused on youth development (see Holt, 2008; Holt and Neely, 2011 for a review). When combining the features of the DMSP, previous youth sport research and ecological systems theory, we can suggest a set of key elements that should be combined to design and deliver quality youth sport programmes. These three elements are:

1   personal engagement in activities
2   quality relationships
3   appropriate settings.

1 Personal engagement in activities

Bronfenbrenner (1995) suggested that proximal processes are a critical catalyst for human development, acting as mechanisms of organism–environment interaction. In accordance with the DMSP, we suggest that 'personal engagement in activities' acts as proximal process to promote the development of the 4 Cs in sport. In the DMSP, 'personal engagement' is more probable to occur when diversity in sport precedes specialization and when a mixture of play and practice activities are integrated in youths' sport experiences.

First, the main tenet of the DMSP is that diversity should precede specialization in sport (Côté and Abernethy, 2012). Diversity during childhood sport allows young athletes to experience a range of opportunities and then select (or be selected to) a specific path during adolescence, entering either the recreational or specializing years. The advantage of a diversified foundation in sport during the sampling years is that it provides young athletes with a breadth of experiences that emphasize exploration before commitment to a specific sport activity. Empirical evidence (e.g. Busseri *et al.*, 2006; Fredericks and Eccles, 2006) shows that a breadth of experiences in early development is an indicator of continued involvement in more intense activities later in life and of successful development of personal assets such as the 4 Cs. The most important aspect of diversity during the sampling years is that it reduces the intensity of involvement in one sport during childhood. Furthermore, youth sport programmes built around the concepts of diversity have a protective effect against negative outcomes such as burnout, dropout and injuries (Fraser-Thomas *et al.*, 2008a; Fraser-Thomas *et al.*, 2008b; Law *et al.*, 2005).

Second, a mixture of play and practice activities with more play during childhood and increasing practice time during adolescence is a central feature of the DMSP. Côté *et al.* (2013) recently reviewed the literature on youth sport activities and provided a taxonomy of activities that could be generally categorized as either practice or play. The fundamental difference between practice and play resides in the general goal that the activity aims to achieve in a specific sporting situation. The goal of practice activities is to improve performance, whereas the goal of play activities is to have fun. The various practice and play activities that constitute sport fulfill different needs in youth and ultimately affect their current and future sport involvement. The intrinsically-motivating and self-directed nature of primarily play-oriented activities contrasts with the outcome-oriented and often adult-driven nature of mainly practice-oriented activities.

Most youth sport programmes are designed from an adult perspective around the activities of structured practice. For example, organized youth sport programmes are adapting models of development that focus on long-term athlete development, skill acquisition and institutional-ization instead of focusing on the inherent enjoyment of participating in various forms of sporting activities (Côté *et al.*, 2011). To achieve its full potential in terms of the development of the Cs and achieving the full range of the Ps, sport programmes should offer youth diverse sporting experiences during childhood, including youth-led activities (Coakley, 1983; Côté *et al.*, 2013). Through exposure to adult-led and youth-led activities, youth will be able to extract unique developmental benefits that would otherwise be difficult to attain if they were exposed to only one type of activity (Imtiaz *et al.*, 2014; Larson *et al.*, 2005). The incorporation of both adult-led activities and peer-led activities into the sport experience of youth requires adults (e.g. coaches and parents) to diminish their direct involvement in sport and sometimes, to change their relationships with the youth sport participants.

This section suggests that personal engagement in activities will have a positive impact on the personal assets of youth involved in sport and the long-term objectives of performance, participation and personal development. Youth sport programmes should be designed to enhance the engagement of youth in the various activities of sport by focusing on the personal and social motives that drive youth to participate in sport. The adult-led and peer-led activities that constitute sport are the proximal processes that structure the experiences and personal engagement of youth in sport.

2 Quality relationships

A central issue within the PYD and sport literature has been the exploration of the social and contextual factors that can foster positive developmental outcomes. Previous research consistently highlights that one of the most influential components of the sport environment is the social interactions that occur within the sport context (e.g. Petitpas *et al.*, 2005). Consistent with this perspective, studies suggest that the manner in which social agents, such as coaches, parents, peers and siblings, interact with young athletes can have important implications for the outcomes that youth derive from their sport participation (e.g. Jowett and Poczwardowski, 2007; Keegan *et al.* and Lavallee, 2009; Ullrich-French and Smith, 2006). For instance, in an exploration of a model sport programme for athletes with disabilities, Turnnidge, Vierimaa and Côté (2012) found that social factors, including coach–athlete relationships, peer interactions and the creation of a supportive team environment, were the central processes contributing to positive developmental outcomes. The facilitation of the 4 Cs and ultimately, the 3 Ps in sport may therefore depend not only on youths' engagement in appropriate sporting activities, but also on the quality of the social interactions that occur within each of these unique contexts.

Coaches

It is well documented that coaches play an integral role in shaping youths' performance, participation and personal development (Smith and Smoll, 2007; Vella *et al.*, 2011). For example, studies indicate that coaches can influence athletes' performance by adopting positive interpersonal styles, such as transformational leadership behaviours or autonomy-supportive behaviours (Charbonneau, Barling and Kelloway, 2001; Gillet *et al.*, 2010). A number of studies also suggest that coaches can affect youths' decisions to participate in sport. More specifically, findings indicate that coaches can influence a number of outcomes related to participation, including sport enjoyment, self-determined motivation and sport persistence (e.g. Álvarez *et al.*, 2009; Pelletier *et al.*, 2001). Finally, there is an emerging body of research exploring coaches' contributions to youths' personal development (e.g. Côté *et al.*, 2010; Vella *et al.*, 2011). Indeed, Côté and Gilbert (2009) proposed that a critical component of coaching effectiveness is improving athletes' competence, confidence, connection and character (i.e. the 4 Cs). Previous research indicates that positive coach–athlete relationships can be characterized by coaches who include their athletes in decision-making processes, display care and concern for their athletes, evaluate their athletes' performance based on self-referenced improvements and effort, acknowledge their athletes' feelings and input, promote interactive discussions and behave in a clear and consistent manner (e.g. Becker, 2013; Erickson *et al.*, 2011, Mageau and Vallerand, 2003; Pelletier *et al.*, 2001). Collectively, these studies illustrate the important role that coaches may play in promoting personal assets in youth sport and achieving the outcomes of performance, participation and personal development.

Parents

Parent–athlete relationships represent another critical element of the youth sport experience. Not only are parents often the primary socializing agents for youths' initial experiences with sport (Wuerth *et al.*, 2004), but they also serve as significant role models for youths' attitudes and behaviours within the sport context (Fredricks and Eccles, 2004). Positive perceptions of parental relationships are linked with a myriad of athlete outcomes, including enjoyment, perceived competence and continued sport participation (e.g. Ullrich-French and Smith, 2006). Building upon the qualitative works of Bloom (1985) and Côté (1999) with elite athletes, numerous studies have illustrated the pivotal role that parents play in the process of athlete development, including providing emotional, informational, tangible and companionship or network support. Through these forms of support, parents can have an important influence on an athlete's acquisition of the 4 Cs and the 3 Ps. For example, evidence suggests that parents can model critical life skills for athletes, such as displaying respect, maintaining control of one's emotions and demonstrating a strong work ethic (e.g. Fraser-Thomas and Côté, 2009; Knight *et al.*, 2011). In doing so, parents can help young athletes acquire these important personal development outcomes. Previous research also demonstrates how parents' roles evolve throughout development, ranging from a leadership role during childhood to a more supporting role during adolescence (Côté, 1999; Fraser-Thomas *et al.*, 2013).

Peers

Although the sport literature has predominantly focused on how adult socializing agents, such as coaches, can shape youth development, there is growing recognition that peer interactions represent an important vehicle through which to accrue positive developmental outcomes (Rubin *et al.*, 2006). As youth progress through their athletic trajectories, peer relationships can become an increasingly salient social context. This is highlighted by the fact that as youth develop, they tend to rely less on their parents and more on their peers as a source of competence information (Horn, 2004). Serving as both friends and competitors, peers can also encourage youth to improve their athletic skills (Bloom, 1985).

Peer relationships can also have significant implications for participation-related outcomes. Previous research indicates that sport-related friendships can enhance youths' enjoyment of and commitment to sport (e.g. Weiss and Smith, 2002), as well as their perceived competence and self-determined motivation (Ullrich-French and Smith, 2006). Collectively, these findings indicate that peers are important sources of motivation for young athletes. Athletes can also acquire key personal development outcomes through their interactions with peers. For example, Holt and colleagues (Holt *et al.*, 2008; Holt *et al.*, 2009) found that athletes' social skill development was facilitated through their peer interactions, rather than through direct teaching by the coach. While further research in this area is needed, evidence exists to suggest that peers can positively contribute to youth's development, both as athletes and as well-rounded individuals.

Siblings

Another potentially important social factor is the quality of an athlete's sibling relationships (Bloom, 1985; Côté, 1999). Wold and Anderssen (1992) suggest that youth whose siblings participate in sporting activities are more likely to be involved in sport themselves. Previous research also indicates that siblings can have a positive influence on youth's development of physical, emotional and psychological skills (Fraser-Thomas *et al.*, 2013). However, there is also evidence to suggest that sibling relationships may be linked to some negative outcomes, such as feeling jealous, isolated, resentful or frustrated (Bloom, 1985, Côté, 1999; Fraser-Thomas *et al.*, 2008b; Harwood and Knight, 2009). These conflicting findings illustrate the need for further research on the sibling-athlete relationship and its influence on youths' acquisition of the 4 Cs and 3 Ps.

Other relationships

It is important to note that there are several other potentially important relationships within the sport environment. These may include, but are not limited to, athletes' relationships with coaches, officials, volunteers and sport administrators. In addition, it is essential to recognize that all of the relationships discussed in this section do not occur in isolation from one another and the interactions between the different relationships may have a significant influence on the quality of youths' sport experiences. For example, the athlete's relationship with their coach may shape their perceptions of the peer relationships occurring within the team. In addition, there may be instances where adults serve as both a parent and coach for young athletes or when youth are both siblings and teammates. The complex intricacies of such relationships and their influences on youth development are certainly a worthy area of future study.

It is evident from the literature reviewed in this section that quality relationships are part of the dynamic elements in sport that affect the development of personal assets (i.e. the 4 Cs), and ultimately, the acquisition of the 3 Ps. At a practical level, sport programmes that work at fostering quality relationships in youth sport, as well as enhancing youth's personal engagement in activities and the appropriate features of sport settings, will have a positive effect on the personal assets of youth, helping to facilitate the long-term objectives of increasing performance, participation and personal development.

3 Appropriate settings

A physical sport context that is in line with youths' need to play, develop skills and have fun is the third and final element of the dynamical structure that impact the 4 Cs and the 3 Ps in youth sport. Recent studies have focused on the physical environment of successful sport organizations or communities to identify features that distinguish positive sport environments (e.g. Balish and Côté, 2013; Côté *et al.*, 2006; Henriksen *et al.*, 2010a; Henriksen *et al.*, 2010b; Henriksen *et al.*, 2011). These studies demonstrate that the physical setting of the sport environment is a factor that affects the acquisition of personal assets (4 Cs) and the long-term outcomes of performance, participation and personal development.

Henriksen and colleagues (2010a; 2010b; 2011) studied three Scandinavian sport organizations in kayak, sailing, and track and field that consistently produced elite level athletes. These studies showed that sport environments that are accessible and provide opportunities for diversification, while supporting quality relationship and proximal role models, facilitate the development of talent in sport. Further, these findings are consistent with studies that examined the birthplace of professional athletes in various countries and in different sports showing a strong tendency for elite level athletes to be born in smaller cities rather than in big urban centres (MacDonald and Baker, 2013). The community features of successful clubs and small cities appear to create an integrated physical space that have a very powerful influence on athletic success and long-term performance in sport (Balish and Côté, 2013).

In terms of continued participation, two recent studies of young Canadian ice hockey players over a period of six years showed an association between place of development and long-term participation (Imtiaz *et al.*, in press; Turnnidge *et al.*, 2012;). These studies suggest that larger cities are associated with decreased sport participation and higher dropout rates, while smaller cities are associated with increased sport participation and prolonged engagement in youth ice hockey. These findings suggest that sport programmes in smaller cities are more conducive towards promoting prolonged participation in sport.

Fraser-Thomas *et al.* (2010) explored the relationships between city size and personal development in a sample of swimmers. Their findings indicated that swimmers who were part of clubs in smaller cities (less than 500,000) scored significantly higher on indicators of personal development such as commitment to learning, positive identity, empowerment and support, than swimmers who trained in bigger cities (greater than 500,000). These findings suggest that city size may not only influence performance and participation, but also personal development. Athletes in smaller cities appear to gain more positive assets from participating in sport than athletes in bigger cities.

Barker's (1968) behaviour setting theory offers theoretical anchors that shed light on how the physical setting may influence participation, performance and personal development in sport. Barker defined a behaviour setting as a unit of the environment in which physical and social elements interact to influence individual behaviours. More specifically, a behaviour setting has two distinct properties: (a) a specific set of time, place and objects, and (b) a specific set of behaviour patterns (Scott, 2005). In the context of our developing framework, *Appropriate settings* refers to the first property (a specific set of time, place and objects) of Barker's behaviour setting while the second property (a specific set of behaviour patterns) focuses on the quality relationships and personal engagement in activities. Although the basic unit of analysis of a *behaviour setting* requires both the physical and social properties, studies of different sport contexts allow us to propose some features of physical settings that are most likely to lead to positive outcomes.

The sport studies reviewed in this section are consistent with the principles of positive youth development and the eight setting features identified by the National Research Council and Institute of Medicine (NRCIM, 2002). Four of these features relate to the physical environment:

1   a safe environment in which youth develop,
2   an appropriate structure in which children experience a stable environment,
3   the availability of opportunities for skill building and
4   the integration of family, school and community efforts.

Furthermore, findings of studies of successful clubs and communities allow us to add two additional features of appropriate settings that are more specific to sport:

1   accessibility to different sport contexts is more important than the quality of the sport facilities and equipment;
2   sport contexts with fewer people increase youth personal effort and involvement in different roles and positions.

Studies reviewed in this section show that appropriate settings promote the personal assets of youth in sport and affect youth's long-term performance, participation and personal development. Understanding the links between the physical environment and patterns of behaviours in sport can help design sport systems that nurture the development of the 4 Cs and ultimately have a positive impact on the 3 Ps. The features of successful sport communities (i.e. appropriate settings) provide the final dynamic element of our framework that interacts with personal engagement in activities and the quality relationships to promote successful development in sport.

A personal assets framework to sport

The consideration of personal factors (i.e. personal engagement in activities), interpersonal factors (i.e. quality relationships) and physical contexts (i.e. appropriate settings) is necessary to fully understand the processes through which development in sport and through sport occurs. The integration and interaction of these three dynamic elements help us to understand the process in sport by which changes in the individual's personal assets take place (e.g. confidence, competence, connection and character) and eventually, influence the long-term outcomes of sport in terms of participation, performance and personal development. Figure 23.1 outlines the components of the Personal Assets Framework to Sport that creates conditions over time for positive experiences and optimal development in sport. The figure presents an ecological approach

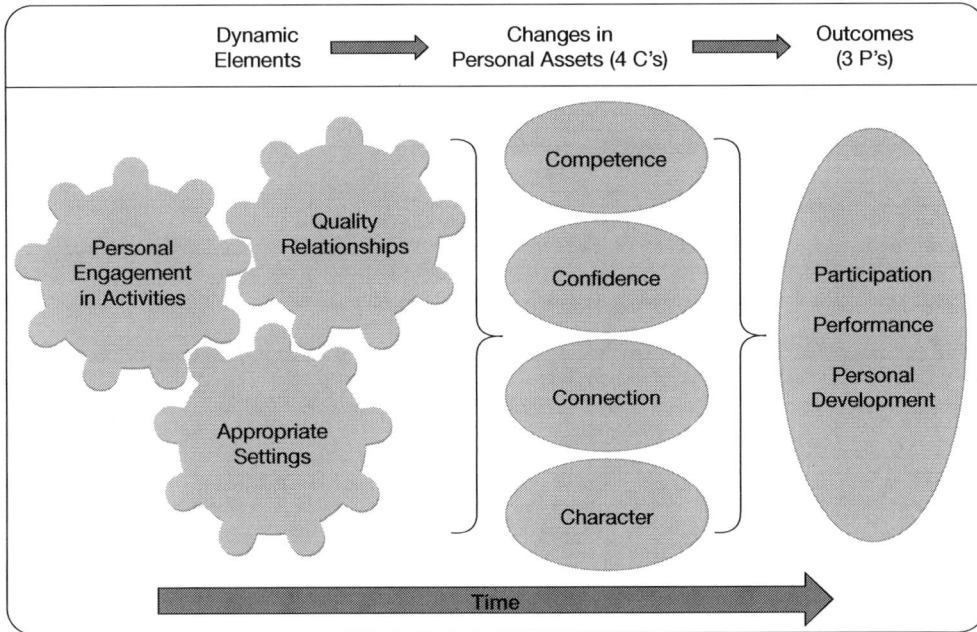

Figure 23.1 The Personal Assets Framework for Sport

to sport that can be integrated in the different pathways of the DMSP to better understand the mechanisms that constitute healthy development in sport.

Derived from ecological systems approaches (e.g. Barker, 1968; Bronfenbrenner, 1995), the framework in Figure 23.1 suggests that three conditions are necessary for fostering optimal development in sport. First, the dynamic elements of personal engagement in activities, quality relationships and appropriate settings constitute a system that should be integrative and complementary to help propel youth towards positive experiences in sport. Second, there should be an alignment between the dynamic elements (activities, relationships and settings) and the personal assets of competence, confidence, connection and character (4 Cs) so that the 3 Ps (participation, performance and personal development) evolve from this process. Third, the overemphasis on one outcome during the early years of involvement in sport will diminish the contribution that sport can make to the total development of a person.

In conclusion, two questions were posed at the beginning of this chapter: *What constitutes development?* and *How does development occur in sport?* The Personal Assets Framework to Sport (Figure 23.1) provides a dynamical structure that identifies the variables in sport that constitute development and the process by which personal assets and outcomes are acquired. The Personal Assets Framework to Sport serves to highlight the dynamic elements and personal assets that should be combined and aligned to design and deliver youth sport programmes that promote performance, participation and personal development within the different pathways of the DMSP. This chapter helps to demonstrate that the ultimate objectives of sport (3 Ps) are not mutually exclusive and that effectively designed sport programmes can contribute to the development of youth in sport and as a person.

References

Álvarez, M. S., Balaguer, I., Castillo, I. and Duda, J. L. (2009). Coach autonomy support and quality of sport engagement in young soccer players. *The Spanish Journal of Psychology*, *12*: 138–148.

Balish, S. and Côté, J. (2013). The influence of community on athletic development: An integrated case study. *Qualitative Research in Sport, Exercise, and Health*. DOI: 10.1080/2159676X.2013.766815.

Barker, R. G. (1968). *Ecological Psychology: Concepts and Methods for Studying the Environment of Human Behaviour*. Stanford, CA: Stanford University Press.

Becker, A. (2013). Quality coaching behaviours. In P. Potrac, W. Gilbert and J. Denision (eds), *Routledge Handbook of Sports Coaching* (pp. 184–195). New York: Routledge.

Benson, P. L. (2003). Developmental assets and asset-building communities: Conceptual and empirical foundations. In R. Lerner and P. L. Benson (eds) *Developmental Assets and Asset Building Communities: Implications for Research, Policy and Practice* (pp. 19–43). New York: Kluwer.

Bloom, B. S. (1985). *Developing Talent in Young People*. New York: Ballantine.

Bronfenbrenner, U. (1995). Development ecology through space and time: A future perspective. In P. Moen, G. H. Elder, and K. Luscher (eds), *Examining Lives in Context: Perspectives on the Ecology of Human Development* (pp. 619–647). Washington, DC: American Psychological Association.

Busseri, M. A., Rose-Krasnor, L., Willoughby, T. and Chalmers, H. (2006). A longitudinal examination of breadth and intensity of youth activity involvement and successful development. *Developmental Psychology*, *42*(6): 1313–1326.

Charbonneau, D., Barling, J. and Kelloway, E. K. (2001). Transformational leadership and sports performance: The mediating role of intrinsic motivation. *Journal of Applied Social Psychology*, *31*: 1521–1534.

Coakley, J. J. (1983). Leaving competitive sport: retirement or rebirth? *Quest*, *35*(1): 1–11.

Côté, J. (1999). The influence of the family in the development of talent in sport. *The Sport Psychologist*, *13*: 395–417.

Côté, J. and Abernethy, B. (2012). A developmental approach to sport expertise. In S. Murphy (ed), *The Oxford Handbook of Sport and Performance Psychology* (pp. 435–447). New York: Oxford University Press.

Côté, J., Coakley, C. and Bruner, M. W. (2011). Children's talent development in sport: Effectiveness or efficiency? In S. Dagkas, and K. Armour (eds), *Inclusion and Exclusion Through Youth Sport* (pp. 172–185). London, UK: Routledge.

Côté, J., Ericsson, K. A. and Law, M. P. (2005). Tracing the development of athletes using retrospective interview methods: A proposed interview and validation procedure for reported information. *Journal of Applied Sport Psychology*, *17*: 1–19.

Côté, J., Erickson, K. and Abernethy, B. (2013). Practice and play in sport development. In J. Côté and R. Lidor (eds), *Conditions of Children's Talent Development in Sport* (pp. 9–20). Morgantown, WV: Fitness Information Technology.

Côté, J. and Gilbert, W. (2009). An integrative definition of coaching effectiveness and expertise. *International Journal of Sport Science and Coaching*, *4*: 307–323.

Côté, J., MacDonald, D., Baker, J. and Abernethy, B. (2006). When 'where' is more important than 'when': Birthplace and birthdate effects on the achievement of sporting expertise. *Journal of Sport Sciences*, *24*: 1065–1073.

Côté, J., Strachan, L. and Fraser-Thomas, J. (2008). Participation, personal development, and performance through sport. In N. L. Holt (ed), *Positive Youth Development Through Sport* (pp. 34–45). London: Routledge.

Danish, S. (2002). *SUPER (Sports United to Promote Education and Recreation) Programme Leader Manual*. (3rd edition). Richmond, VA: Life Skills Center, Virginia Commonwealth University.

Danish, S. J., Petitpas, A. L. and Hale, B. D. (1993). Life development intervention for athletes: Life skills through sports. *The Counselling Psychologist*, *21*: 352–385.

Erickson, K., Côté, J., Hollenstein, T. and Deakin, J. (2011). Examining coach–athlete interactions using state space grids: An observational analysis in competitive youth sport. *Psychology of Sport and Exercise*, *12*: 645–654.

Feltz, D. L. and Chase, M. A. (1998). The measurement of self-efficacy and confidence in sport. In J. Duda (ed), *Advancements in Sport and Exercise Psychology Measurement* (pp. 63–78). Morgantown, WV: Fitness Information Technologies.

The First Tee. (2005). *Longitudinal effects of The First Tee Life Skills Education Programmes on Positive Youth Development*. University of Virginia: M. Weiss.

Ford, P.R., Ward, P, Hodges, N.J. and Williams, A.M. (2009). The role of deliberate practice and play in career progression in sport: The early engagement hypothesis. *High Ability Studies*, 20: 67–75.

Fraser-Thomas, J., Côté, J. and Deakin, J. (2008a). Understanding dropout and prolonged engagement in adolescent competitive sport. *Psychology of Sport and Exercise*, 9: 645–662.

Fraser-Thomas, J., Côté, J. and Deakin, J. (2008b). Examining adolescent sport dropout and prolonged engagement from a developmental perspective. *Journal of Applied Sport Psychology*, 20: 318–333.

Fraser-Thomas, J., Côté, J. and MacDonald, D. (2010). Community size in youth sport settings: Examining developmental assets and sport withdrawal. *Physical and Health Education Academic Journal, North America*, 2, July. 2010. Available at: http://ojs.acadiau.ca/index.php/phenex/article/view/6/1162. Date accessed: 05 Jul. 2010.

Fraser-Thomas, J., Strachan, L. and Jeffery-Tosoni, S. (2013). Family influence on children's involvement in sport. In J. Côté and R. Lidor (eds), *Conditions of Children's Talent Development in Sport* (pp. 179–196). Morgantown, WV: Fitness Information Technology.

Fredricks, J. A. and Eccles, J. S. (2004). Parental influences on youth involvement in sports. In M.R. Weiss (ed), *Developmental Sport and Exercise Psychology: A Lifespan Perspective* (pp. 145–164). Morgantown, WV: Fitness Information Technology.

Fredricks, J. A. and Eccles, J. S. (2006). Is extracurricular participation associated with beneficial outcomes? Concurrent and longitudinal relations. *Developmental Psychology*, 42(4): 698–713.

Gillet, N., Vallerand, R. J., Amoura, S. and Baldes, B. (2010). Influence of coaches' autonomy support on athletes' motivation and sport performance: A test of the hierarchical model of intrinsic and extrinsic motivation. *Psychology of Sport and Exercise*, 11: 155–161.

Harwood, C. and Knight, C. (2009). Understanding parental stressors: An investigation of British tennis-parents. *Journal of Sport Sciences*, 27(4): 339–351.

Hellison, D. (2003) *Teaching Responsibility Through Physical Activity* (2nd edition). Champaign, Illinois: Human Kinetics.

Henriksen, K., Stambulova, N. and Roessler, K.K. (2010a). A holistic approach to athletic talent development environments: A successful sailing milieu. *Psychology of Sport and Exercise*, 11: 212–222.

Henriksen, K., Stambulova, N. and Roessler, K. K. (2010b). Successful talent development in track and field: considering the role of environment. *Scandinavian Journal of Medicine and Science in Sports*, 20: 122–132.

Henriksen, K., Stambulova, N. and Roessler, K. K. (2011). Riding the wave of an expert: A successful talent development environment in kayaking. *The Sport Psychologist*, 25: 341–362.

Holt, N. L. (2008). *Positive Youth Development Through Sport*. London: Routledge.

Holt, N.L., Black, D.E., Tamminen, K.A., Fox, K.R. and Mandigo, J.L. (2008). Levels of social complexity and dimensions of peer experiences in youth sport. *Journal of Sport and Exercise Psychology*, 30: 411–431.

Holt, N. L. and Neely, K. C. (2011). Positive youth development through sport: a review. *Revista iberoamericana de psicología del ejercicio y el deporte*, 6(2): 299–316.

Holt, N. L., Tamminen, K. A., Tink, L. N. and Black, D. E. (2009). An interpretive analysis of life skills associated with sport participation. *Qualitative Research in Sport and Exercise*, 1: 160–175.

Horn, T. S. (2004). Developmental perspectives on self-perceptions in children and adolescents. In M. R. Weiss (ed), *Developmental Sport and Exercise Psychology: A Lifespan Perspective* (pp. 165–196). Morgantown, WV: Fitness Information Technology.

Imtiaz, F. Hancock, D. J. and Côté, J. (2014). Examining the experiences of athletes in adult-led and peer-led youth sport. Manuscript submitted for review.

Imtiaz, F., Hancock, D. J., Vierimaa, M. and Côté, J. (in press). Place of development and dropout in youth ice hockey. *International Journal of Sport and Exercise Psychology*.

Janssen, I. and LeBlanc, A. G. (2010). Review Systematic review of the health benefits of physical activity and fitness in school-aged children and youth. *International Journal of Behavioural Nutrition and Physical Activity*, 7: 1–16.

Jeličić, H., Bobek, D., Phelps, E., Bobek, D., Lerner, J. V. and Lerner, R. M. (2007). Using positive youth development to predict contribution and risk behaviours in early adolescence: Findings from the first two waves of the 4-H study of positive youth development. *International Journal of Behavioural Development*, 31(3): 263–273.

Jowett, S. and Poczwardowski, A. (2007). Understanding the coach-athlete relationship. In S. Jowett and D. Lavallee (eds), *Social Psychology in Sport* (pp. 3–14). Champaign, Illinois: Human Kinetics.

Keegan, R., Harwood, C., Spray, C. and Lavallee, D. (2009). A qualitative investigation exploring the motivational climate in early career sports participants: Coach, parent and peer influences on sport motivation. *Psychology of Sport and Exercise*, 10: 361–372.

Knight, C. J., Neely, K. C. and Holt, N. L. (2011). Parental behaviours in team sports: How do female athletes want parents to behave? *Journal of Applied Sport Psychology, 23*: 76–92.

Larson, R., Walker, K. and Pearce, N. (2005). A comparison of youth-driven and adult-driven youth programmes: Balancing inputs from youth and adults. *Journal of Community Psychology, 33*: 57–74.

Law, M., Côté, J. and Ericsson, K. A. (2007). Characteristics of expert development in rhythmic gymnastics: A retrospective study. *International Journal of Sport and Exercise Psychology, 5*: 82–103.

Lerner, R. M., Dowling, E. M. and Anderson, P. M. (2003). Positive youth development: Thriving as the basis of personhood and civil society. *Applied Developmental Science, 7*(3): 172–180.

Lerner, R. M., Lerner, J. V., Almerigi, J. B., Theokas, C., Naudeau, S., Gestsdottir, S., Naudeau, S., Jeličić, H., Alberts, A., Ma, L., Smith, L. M., Bobek, D. L., Richman-Raphael, D., Simpson, I., DiDenti Christiansen, E. and von Eye, A. (2005). Positive youth development, participation in community youth development programmes, and community contributions of fifth grade adolescents: Findings from the first wave of the 4-H Study of Positive Youth Development. *Journal of Early Adolescence, 25*: 17–71.

MacDonald, D. J. and Baker, J. (2013). Circumstantial development: Birthdate and birthplace effects on athlete development. In J. Côté and R. Lidor (eds), *Conditions of Children's Talent Development in Sport* (pp. 197–208). Morgantown, WV: Fitness Information Technology.

Mageau, G. and Vallerand, R. (2003). The coach-athlete relationship: A motivational model. *Journal of Sport Sciences, 21*: 883–904.

National Research Council and Institute of Medicine (2002). *Community Programmes to Promote Positive Youth Development*. Washington, DC: National Academy Press.

Pelletier, L. G., Fortier, M. S., Vallerand, R. J. and Brière, N M. (2001). Associations among perceived autonomy support, forms of self-regulation, and persistence: A prospective study. *Motivation and Emotion, 25*: 279–306.

Petitpas, A. J., Cornelius, A. E., Van Raalte, J. L. and Jones, T. (2005). A framework for planning youth sport programmes that foster psychosocial development. *The Sport Psychologist, 19*: 63–80.

Petitpas, A. J., Van Raalte, J. L., Cornelius, A. and Presbrey, J. (2004). A life skills development programme for high school student-athletes. *The Journal of Primary Prevention, 24*: 325–334.

Phelps, E., Zimmerman, S., Warren, A. E. A., Jeličić, H., von Eye, A. and Lerner, R. M. (2009). The structure and developmental course of positive youth development (PYD) in early adolescence: Implications for theory and practice. *Journal of Applied Developmental Psychology, 30*(5): 571–584.

Rubin, K. H., Bukowski, W. and Parker, J. (2006). Peer interactions, relationships, and groups. In N. Eisenberg (ed), *Handbook of Child Psychology: Social, Emotional, and Personality Development* (6th edition, pp. 571–645). New York: Wiley.

Scott, M. M. (2005). A powerful theory and a paradox: Ecological psychologists after Barker. *Environment and Behaviour, 37*(3): 295–329.

Shields, D. L. L. and Bredemeier, B. J. L. (1995). *Character Development and Physical Activity*. Champaign, Illinois: Human Kinetics.

Smith, A. L. (2007). Youth peer relationships in sport. In S. Jowett, and D. Lavallee (eds), *Social Psychology in Sport* (pp. 41–54). Champaign, Illinois: Human Kinetics.

Smith, R. E. and Smoll, F. L. (2007). Social-cognitive approach to coaching behaviours. In S. Jowett, and D. Lavallee (eds). *Social Psychology in Sport* (pp. 75–90). Champaign Illinois: Human Kinetics.

Turnnidge, J., Hancock, D. J. and Côté, J. (2012). An investigation of contextual factors and sport participation in Ontario minor ice hockey. *Scandinavian Journal of Medicine and Science in Sports*. DOI: 10.1111/sms.12002

Turnnidge, J., Vierimaa, M. and Côté, J. (2012). An in-depth investigation of a model sport programme for athletes with disabilities. *Psychology, 3*: 1131–1141.

Ullrich-French, S. and Smith, A. L. (2006). Perceptions of relationships with parents and peers in youth sport: Independent and combined prediction of motivational outcomes. *Psychology of Sport and Exercise, 7*: 193–214.

Vierimaa, M., Erickson, K., Côté, J. and Gilbert, W. (2012). Positive youth development: A measurement framework for sport. *International Journal of Sports Science and Coaching, 7*: 601–614.

Vealey, R. (1986). Conceptualization of sport-confidence and competitive orientation: Preliminary investigation and instrument development. *Journal of Sport Psychology, 8*: 221–246.

Vella, S., Oades, L. G. and Crowe, T. P. (2011). The role of the coach in facilitating positive youth development: Moving from theory to practice. *Journal of Applied Sport Psychology, 23*: 33–48.

Weiss M.R. and Ebbeck, V. (1996). Self-esteem and perceptions of competence in youth sport: Theory, research, and enhancement strategies. In O. Bar-Or (ed), *The Encyclopaedia of Sports Medicine: Vol. 5. The Child and Adolescent Athlete* (pp. 364–382). Oxford: Blackwell Science.

Weiss, M. R. and Smith, A. L. (2002). Friendship quality in youth sport: Relationship to age, gender, and motivational variables. *Journal of Sport and Exercise Psychology, 24:* 420–437.

Wold, B and Anderssen, N. (1992). Health promotion aspects of family and peer influences on sport participation. *International Journal of Sport Psychology, 23:* 343–359.

Wuerth, S., Lee, M. J. and Alfermann, D. (2004). Parental involvement and athletes' career in youth sport. *Psychology of Sport and Exercise, 5:* 21–33.

SECTION 5

Social divisions and youth sport

24

INTRODUCTION

Ken Green

Sport does not create social divisions but it is affected by them. In addition, sport can deepen or diminish existing divisions, as well as throw them into sharp relief. Youth sport, and developments therein, are almost inevitably dependent upon the impact of such social divisions as class, gender, ethnicity and disability, as well as the intersections between them. Not only is the momentum behind particular developments in youth sport rooted in particular sections of youth (white, middle-class males' propagation of particular lifestyle sports, for instance), developments in youth sport are unlikely to affect all youths to the same extent or even in similar ways. Consequently, in Section 5 of the Handbook, the various contributors examine the key social divisions in youth sport, as well as the interrelations between them.

In their opening chapter, *Playing an unequal game? Youth sport and social class*, Jeroen Scheerder and Hanne Vandermeerschen explore the significance of social class for youth sport. They remind us that the link between social class and sports participation has become one of the most frequently analyzed issues in sports participation, both empirically and theoretically. It will remain so if, as appears likely, economic inequalities between the *haves* and the *have nots* continue to widen. Scheerder and Vandermeerschen focus upon the consequences of an unequal distribution of socio-economic (money and education, especially) as well as social and cultural resources (such as sporting family members and club memberships) for the general recreational and sporting opportunities of youth and their resultant sporting capital (assets in the form of tastes, knowledge and social relationships). Scheerder and Vandermeerschen point out the manner in which social class not only affects general sports participation but also preferences for particular sports. Many working-class youths, for instance, lack the diversity of experiences and, therefore, interests found among middle-class youth. Scheerder and Vandermeerschen note how the emphasis on social class as *an*, even *the*, explanatory factor in relation to sports participation has been increasingly challenged by those who argue that in post-modern societies social stratification along traditional lines has faded and youth (sub)cultures have been de-coupled from social class. Along with most analyses of class patterns in sports participation, however, they conclude that on the basis of empirical findings, youths' leisure and sporting choices continue to be circumscribed by structural factors and particularly class differentials or gradients.

The gendered character of sport – in terms of participation (rates, frequency, forms and venues) and experiences (meanings and motivations, for example) – has been amply demonstrated over the last half a century or more. The historical gendering of sports participation notwithstanding, there have been some marked changes in females' relationships with sport in recent decades,

259

alongside the undoubted continuities. Sport is no longer a male preserve. It has become a normal part of many girls' and women's everyday lives. Females in the developed world are now playing far more sport than previous generations and have been closing the gap on males. Nevertheless, despite a narrowing of sex differences in sports participation over recent decades, gendered patterns persist and boys and men continue to do more. In *Sexuality, gender and youth sport*, Jan Wright reflects upon the continuities and changes in relation to gender-based inequalities and the (re)production of gender norms. In the process, Wright reflects upon girls' limited access to and differing experiences of sports as well as the ways various sporting practices celebrate particular forms of (hegemonic) masculinity. At the same time, she points out the actual and potential use of youth sport as a tool for empowering rather than merely inhibiting, restricting or delimiting girls' and young women's experiences. Among other things, Wright explores the socially constructed nature of the ostensible lack of interest and sporting abilities among girls (and some boys), noting that the majority of young girls *do* like sport and would like to do more. Amid widespread recognition that gender differences are best explained in terms of the construction of masculinities and femininities, Wright highlights the persistence of a kind of 'soft essentialism' – an implicit underlying tendency to explain any remaining differences in sports participation between males and females in terms of fundamental natural differences. Against this backdrop, Wright argues that changes in gender norms have not been as profound as might have been hoped or, for that matter, anticipated. In schools and the wider communities, sport still remains a site where boys and young men are socialized into and feel free (even encouraged) to express the beliefs and behaviours associated with hegemonic masculinities. One consequence is that sport remains, at best, an awkward experience for male youth who do not measure up to the requirements, be they physical or socio-psychological. Nor, she adds, have lifestyle sports been the utopian site of resistance to normative gender relations that they were initially viewed as. Although the expression of masculinity may differ from that associated with traditional team sports, lifestyle sports have also become sites for masculine identity production, 'where heterosexuality is for the most part the unspoken norm'. Finally, Wright signposts arenas for future research noting that very little is known about 'how young lesbians, gay men or transgender young people negotiate the discourses and practices of youth sports'.

In *Youth sport, race and ethnicity*, Scott Fleming provides a brief overview of the background to current understandings of how experiences of youth sport are shaped by race, racism and ethnicity. After seeking to bring some 'operational clarity' to key concepts such as race, Fleming provides an account of the neglect of youth sport in studies of race/ethnicity alongside a policy overview illustrating the absence of careful and considered approaches to sport development and educational policy for minority ethnic groups, before summarizing what is known about particular contemporary themes and issues.

It is fair to say that our understandings of race/ethnic issues in the broad arena of sport appear substantially different in the second decade of the twenty-first century than they did half a century ago. Among other things, the Human Genome Project (mapping human genetic diversity) has demonstrated that the concept of race has no scientific validity based, as it is, upon superficial, morphological (visible physical traits) differences, such as skin colour. It seems, therefore, that racial theories represent an ideological *ex-post facto* rationalization of preferred views of the (sporting) world and preferred (sporting) practices; put simply, convenient justifications for the subjugation of peoples. Discussion of race/ethnicity and sport has been further complicated by the fact that the ethnic map continues to change as newer immigrant minorities (from East Asia, Latin America, the Middle-east, North Africa and Eastern Europe, for example) are increasingly dispersed around the globe (Roberts, 2009). While the white–black axis remains influential in sport (and in elite sport, in particular), in terms of engagement with sport generally and youth sport in particular, South Asian Muslim groups are probably the group most researched nowadays, not least because of the seeming significance of religion and religiosity to sports participation. As Fleming indicates, these factors go part way to explaining the contemporary preference for the term ethnicity with its emphasis upon culture (or way of life), including religion (and religiosity, in particular; see Walseth, this book), language, country of origin, cultural norms, family and identity.

When studying youth sport and ethnicity, it is important to keep in mind that, globalizing tendencies notwithstanding, nearly everything that youth do in the name of sport and physical recreation has ethnic connotations, not least as the product of one or another culture or cultures: cricket in England, petanque in France, baseball in the United States, Aussie rules in Australia, bandy in Norway and so forth. Thus, ethnicity is not a minority issue in youth sport, even though it is usually treated as one – it is a facet of all sport. In addition, while there are variations in ethnic participation in sport – that is, between ethnic groups; between males and females within and between ethnic groups; and between sports (e.g. cricket, skiing, kabbadi, basketball and badminton) – there are few examples of substantial and exclusive involvement in any activity among only one ethnic group. Nevertheless, as Walseth (this volume) notes, Muslim youth are significantly underrepresented in sport in Europe. This is partly explained by potentially competing priorities. Some aspects of Islam – for example, the Islamic ideal of gender-segregation and particular gendered items of clothing (such as the hijab [the headscarf] worn by Muslim females) – serve to hinder sports participation among Muslim youth, and girls in particular. In addition, the significance of so-called 'host' sporting cultures should not be under-estimated. Frelier and Breedveld (2009: 112), for example, have revealed how in the Netherlands, as in many countries, sports clubs in particular can 'breathe a very "Dutch" atmosphere' and 'that . . . makes people from ethnic minorities shy away from what is quite often typically Dutch'. Walseth and Strandbu (2014) have made a similar point regarding Norwegian sporting culture. It is also worth bearing in mind that, as Birchwood *et al.* (2008) have observed, there may well be a dearth of genuine interest in Western sports not only in Muslim countries but among Muslim groups in Western societies, where cultural, non-material barriers to sport participation can prove highly resilient irrespective of the existence of suitable preconditions for sports participation.

Where religion does not have a substantial impact upon the (sporting) way of life of particular majority ethnic groups (in the the United States, Australasia and Western world, for example), this tends to be because religiosity – the degree to which people regard themselves as religious – is relatively weak and/or the religion itself (Christianity, for example) does not strongly circumscribe many aspects of people's lifestyles, including leisure and sport. While there may be room for manouevre and accommodation between culture and religion, this appears less likely in the case of Muslims – for whom there is usually little or no separation of religious and secular activities. In such cases, religion and religiosity impacts upon whole swathes of everyday life. In her chapter entitled *Sport, youth and religion*, Kristin Walseth focuses on the religions most studied by those interested in the relationship between youth, sport and religion – the religions that are also shaping up to be the global ideological schism of the twenty-first century, namely Christianity and Islam. After unpicking the fluctuating relationship between religions of one kind or another and sport, Walseth identifies the values that enable particular religions, such as Christianity and Islam, to potentially coalesce reasonably amicably with sport. Both Christian and Muslim youth can, she observes, find support for their participation in sports in their religious texts. Both, for example, encourage youth to take care of their bodies and their health. Nonetheless, the culture in Islam is one of physical activity rather than sports per se. In Islam, Walseth observes, physical activity is perceived as important first and foremost because exercising is interpreted as a way of taking care of the body and the body is perceived as a gift from Allah (God). Moreover, physical activity is considered important because of the recreational dimension to Islam. One might reasonably conclude, therefore, that Muslims would be involved in sports and physical activity. Despite this seemingly favourable position from which to cultivate sport and physical recreation among Muslim youth, Walseth notes that they tend to be significantly underrepresented in sports in Europe. This seeming contradiction is, Walseth suggests, explained in part by potentially competing priorities: physical activity and even sport may be encouraged in Islam as long as it does not take precedence over faith. Hence, sports participation is far from straightforward among Muslims. Indeed, some aspects of Islam serve to hinder sports participation among Muslim youth, and girls in particular. The Islamic ideal of gender segregation and particular gendered items of clothing are instances of such barriers. Among other facets of the interrelationships between religion and youth sport, Walseth reflects upon areas of actual as well as potential conflict between the teachings and requirements of both Christianity and Islam, in principle, and the actions required in many competitive sports, in practice.

In *Youth sport and dis/ability*, Donna Goodwin takes as her starting point the fact that youth experiencing disability tend to be significantly less active than their non-disabled peers. Goodwin reminds the reader of the domain assumptions underpinning the two dominant perspectives on disability, namely the so-called medical and social models. The increasingly successful application of science, in general, and medicine, in particular, in combating illness and disease over the past two centuries has resulted in the dominance of scientific models of health and illness. The corresponding privileging of what became known as the medical model of disability meant that those medical and educational experts (such as doctors and educational psychologists) charged with the diagnosis of, and prescription for, disability tended to focus upon young people's particular mental or physical impairments in the medical terms associated with dis/functionality. Consequently, the term disability has come to be used to refer to biomedical conditions that limit a person's ability to perform specific tasks with the result that those with disabilities are often viewed in terms of their level of functional ability to perform physical and sporting tasks. In response to the individualistic and de-contextualized – and, correspondingly, partial – views of individuals with disability manifest in medical models, an alternative social model emerged in the latter decades of the twentieth-century to challenge the 'personal tragedy view of disability' (Fitzgerald, 2006: 756). From this perspective, disability (like other social dynamics such as race and gender) was conceptualized as a social construct rather than a biological or medical category. Thus, it is now generally accepted that medicalized diagnoses ignore wider social processes (of stigmatization, for example) and the general socially constructed physical (for example, sports facilities without disabled access) and cultural (such as sports and games that, in unmodified form, are inaccessible to youngsters with disabilities) barriers to participation in wider, supposedly able-bodied, societies. In this manner, social models or explanations express a view of people with disabilities as constrained by situations that, in their effects, disable (and, as a consequence, oppress) them – not as an unavoidable consequence of their disability, as such, but rather because of the ways in which people and institutions respond or, more often, do not respond to them and their needs. In practice, their engagement with various institutions (such as education and sport) is mediated by a wide variety of socially constructed restrictions – which often go hand-in-hand with impoverishment and multiple disadvantages – such as a lack of private transport and equipment and inaccessible school and sports buildings as well as discriminatory attitudes. Goodwin observes that the medical model remains the default or common-sense model of sports participation (and not merely among youth). In confronting a range of issues, Goodwin utilises the 'Paralympic paradox' to illustrate the tensions and inadequacies of representing Paralympian (and, for that matter, any disabled sportsperson) as an impaired athlete.

In their chapter *Unpacking gender/sexuality/race/disability/class to understand the embodied experiences of young people in contemporary physical culture* (what might be termed intersectionality), Laura Azzarito and Doune Macdonald highlight the ways in which sport impacts young people's experiences – specifically in terms of 'the complex articulation of gender/sex, race/ethnicity, social class, and disability'. Azzarito and Macdonald explore how youth perform, practice and express their multidimensional identities in plural and fluid ways in specific physical culture contexts. They argue that an examination of the contradictions and fluidity of gender/sex relations at the intersection of race, disability and social class allows for new and fresh insights into youths' subjective experiences in sport and wider physical cultures. Among other things, Azzarito and Macdonald pinpoint the ways in which sport can reproduce racialized, heteronormative, able-bodied masculinities as well as the transformative possibilities associated with the potential for sport to 'bridge differences and potentially enable and encourage young women and men to experience their bodies and construct their identities in positive, confident, and affirmative ways'. The concept of intersectionality, they conclude, enables a more adequate understanding of the complex relations between of sport, identity and opportunity. It allows, for example, a better appreciation of the ways in which the social dynamics of gender, sexuality, race and class intersect to 'other' and exclude many young people from sport.

Rounding off Section 5 of the Handbook, Karin Redelius and Håkan Larsson report on a growing area of research: youth sports in relation to human rights. Human rights are social inventions; they are, in other words, socially constructed. As such they may be granted or rejected. In the world of sport, they are often contested. To become real and meaningful, rights need to be agreed upon and then protected by transnational institutions and countries (as well as their own institutions). Nowhere perhaps, is this more apparent than with children and young people. Redelius and Larsson 'discuss the possibilities for children and young people to have something to say about their participation in sport', specifically in relation to the intentions indicated in the *United Nations' Convention on the Rights of the Child*. Redelius and Larsson take sport, and club sport in particular, as their focus and, more specifically, the significance of training, competition and ranking for the rights of young people in sport. In doing so, the authors tease out the potentially unintended consequences of (club) sport for youngsters' perceptions of enjoyment and development as well as their likely adherence to sport.

Studies of youth sport and sporting lives are inevitably drawn back time and time again to the significance of social divisions of one kind or another – either in isolation or, increasingly, in conjunction; in other words, whether the old predictors of youth's lives (social class and gender, in particular) have become less significant for sports participation than for previous generations and, if not, the extent to which youths are able to take personal charge of their sporting biographies. Notwithstanding compelling evidence (from studies of youth more generally) that, since the 1970s, youth cultures have fragmented and no longer map neatly onto the various social divisions (Roberts, 2008), it is clear that all of the contributors to this section subscribe to the view that class, gender and ethnicity and dis/ability retain their significance, albeit to a greater or lesser extent.

References

Birchwood, D., Roberts, K. and Pollock, G. (2008) Explaining differences in sport participation rates among young adults: Evidence from the South Caucasus, *European Physical Education Review*, 14(3): 283–300.

Fitzgerald, H. (2006). Disability and physical education, in D. Kirk, D. Macdonald and M. O'Sullivan (eds) *The Handbook of Physical Education*. (pp. 752–66). London: Sage.

Frelier, M. and Breedveld, M. (2009) Participation of ethnic minorities in Dutch sports clubs, in ISSA (International Sociology of Sport Association) (2009) (eds) *Sport: Passion, Practice and Profit*. World Congress of Sociology of Sport, 2009. Utrecht, 15–18 July: 111–112.

Roberts, K. (2008). *Youth in Transition. In Eastern Europe and the West*. Basingstoke: Palgrave Macmillan.

Walseth, K. and Strandbu, Å. (2014). Young Norwegian-Pakistani women and sport: How does culture and religiosity matter? 20(4): 489–507.

25

PLAYING AN UNEQUAL GAME?

Youth sport and social class

Jeroen Scheerder and Hanne Vandermeerschen

Introduction

The social stratification of sports participation is a recurring topic in the academic literature on sports. The link between social class and sports participation has been frequently analysed, both theoretically and empirically. The insights of the French sociologist Pierre Bourdieu (1930–2002) concerning the relationship between social position and lifestyle have been both inspiring and influential for this field of study (e.g. Bourdieu, 1978, 1988; Ohl, 2000; Stempel, 2005). Since research on social stratification has mostly focused on adults, the relation between youth sport and social class seems to be somewhat underestimated (Scheerder *et al.*, 2005a; Scheerder *et al.*, 2005c). Yet, perhaps more than ever, the topics of social difference in general, and social inequality in particular, are worthy of investigation.

In the first part of this chapter, we argue why the relation between youth sport and social class is an issue of concern. The chapter then proceeds with a brief overview of some recent international research findings. This informs us about the present situation, reporting to what extent youth sports participation is currently linked to social class. In order to have a more detailed view, a case study based on youth sport in Flanders (Belgium) is presented in the third section. The case study makes it possible to study youth sport and its social stratification over a broader time frame, since the Flemish data allow depiction of the development of sports participation over a time span of several decades. Yet, as argued by Dagkas and Stathi (2007), it is one thing to identify social groups participating less; understanding *why* they participate less is even more important. Therefore, in a fourth section, explanations of the relationship between youth sport and social class are explored, both based on theoretical understandings as well as empirical findings from the literature. We conclude the chapter by considering opportunities for the future and a potential way forward.

Social class, and its relation with youth sport, constitute the central theme of this chapter. However, the term social class is not without polemic. A multitude of definitions and operationalisations exist in the literature, and it has repeatedly been questioned whether the idea of a social class remains relevant to our current society (e.g. Beck, 1992; Waters, 1994). We have chosen not to dwell on this debate here. Rather, it is important for the reader to know that, when using the term social class in this chapter, we mean a person's socio-economic position in general.

When using the term social stratification, we mean a system of social classification in which entire categories of people are ranked in a social hierarchy. Based upon an unequal distribution of valued resources – such as money, education, occupation, housing, an affluent and attractive lifestyle, and interesting and enjoyable recreational opportunities – people are assigned to different social classes and acquire distinct social statuses. In this way, people with a higher class standing are more likely to consume more of the things that society values, compared to persons in lower social groups. Moreover, these distinct patterns of social ranking seem to persist across generations. Studies on sports participation generally refute the idea that sport has become more democratic and egalitarian in social class terms. In fact, since the 1950s, empirical research has continuingly shown that participation in sports activities is characterised by social differences, reflecting the social stratification patterns that exist in society (e.g. Bourdieu, 1978; Lüschen, 1963; 1969; Moens and Scheerder, 2004; Renson, 1976; Scheerder *et al.*, 2002; Scheerder *et al.*, 2005b; Scheerder and Vos, 2011; von Euler, 1953; Wilson, 2002).

Youth sport and social class: why it matters

There are at least two fundamental arguments regarding why the relation between youth sport and social class is an important academic and societal issue. The first argument relates to efficiency (i.e. *utilitarian legitimation*), whereas the second argument involves social justice (i.e. *moral legitimation*) (Elling and Claringbould, 2005). However, before discussing these two core arguments, it is necessary to consider how sport is currently viewed in society.

Youth sports participation is generally considered as positive leisure, mainly because sports participation is said to be linked to a large number of benefits as well as being used as an instrument to reach broader objectives. Traditionally, elements such as character building, discipline, fair play or teamwork have been mentioned as positive effects of practicing sport for young people. More recently, sport has been said to contribute to 'positive youth development' (Danish *et al.*, 2004; Fraser-Thomas *et al.*, 2005; Holt, 2008; see also Côté *et al.*, this volume). Sport is also believed to help develop social capital (Nicholson and Hoye, 2008), to engender social inclusion (Bailey, 2008) and to foster empowerment (Lawson, 2005). Apart from benefits within the educational, psychological and/or social realm, more general references to well-being and public health are often made. The alleged benefits of sports are not only mentioned in the academic literature, they also abound in political discourses, and correspond to commonly-held beliefs. From a policy perspective, it is important to observe that the claimed benefits go well beyond the individual level. Sport is believed to contribute to the wider community and/or to society as a whole (Bailey, 2008; Jarvie, 2003).

Yet, this optimistic view of sport and its positive effects has been heavily criticized (e.g. Coakley, 2011; Coalter, 2007). A major criticism is that many of the claims lack empirical evidence. Second, sport can also entail negative consequences (Waddington, 2000). Examples involve bullying (Donnelly and Coakley, 2002), discrimination (Elling and Knoppers, 2005) or the risk of sport-related injuries. Thus, the downsides of sports tend to be minimised. Third, potential positive effects often are dependent upon the context and conditions of the sports practice, which are easily overlooked (Bloyce and Smith, 2010; Coakley, 2011; Waddington, 2000).

Nevertheless, it is plausible to suggest that sport can be expected to bring some benefits to young people (Bailey, 2008). Youngsters can only take advantage of any potential benefits, however, if they are participating effectively (Bailey, 2008; Vandermeerschen, Vos and Scheerder, 2013). This leads us to the first, utilitarian argument regarding why it is desirable to study and be aware of the relation between youth sport and social class: it is important in terms of (policy) *efficiency*. If sports can contribute to (public) health, to social inclusion and so forth – factors that benefit broader society – it is in the interest of all to make sure that as many young people as possible find their way into sports, regardless of their social background.

At the same time, in order to fully grasp what is at stake when referring to youth sport and social class, one should also take the second, moral argument into account, that is, the idea of *social justice*. If sports participation leads to positive effects in other areas of life, in the interests of social justice it is necessary to ensure that these benefits are accessible to all. And there is more. Depending on the definition of 'need' (Dean, 2013; Veal, 2002), sports may be considered as a right. For example, the right to practice sports has been acknowledged in the *European Sport for All Charter* (COE, 1975; 1980), as well as in the United Nations' *International Charter of Physical Education and Sport* (UN/UNESCO, 1978). If we accept the idea of sports as a right, guaranteeing the possibility to do sports is imperative regardless of the potential benefits. In practice, however, this has not always been self-evident.

Whereas the efficiency argument has to do with participation (as many youngsters as possible), the social justice argument mainly relates to *opportunities* for participation (opportunities for all). A similar focus on opportunities can be found in the capability approach as proposed by Sen (2009). In his work on social justice, Sen argues that what matters is that an individual has the capability to do the things 'he or she has reason to value' (Sen, 2009: 231). In other words, a person has a *real* opportunity to do things. Put differently, according to this approach, the focus is not so much on what a person ends up doing, but rather on what a person is able to do, whether or not he or she makes use of that opportunity (Sen, 2009: 235). In our context, this implies that every individual should have the real opportunity to take part in sports, regardless of his or her social background.

If we accept the idea of sports as a social right – and, therefore, the idea that sports should be available to all, at least in theory – it is necessary to monitor the extent to which there is non take-up of provisions, and whether this potential non take-up is socially stratified. Since public money is spent on sport provisions, it is important to know whether all societal groups benefit from it. In order to answer this question, in the next section, empirical findings with regard to youth sports participation and social class will be presented, based on the available academic literature.

International evidence

Providing a brief overview of research findings with regard to youth sport and social class is not an easy task, since comparison between research findings is made difficult by the many differences in definitions and conceptualisations of both sport and social class. In addition, the notion of physical activity is often used in studies, rather than sport. The latter can lead to some confusion, since physical activity can cover different meanings. In what follows, some key findings are presented without being exhaustive. The focus lies on youth sport and aspects related to socio-economic status. However, physical activity is also considered, at least when it refers to leisure-time physical activity. Physical education, on the other hand, is not taken into consideration, since we focus solely on sports in a voluntary and, therefore, extra-curricular context.

Findings with regard to the relation between youth sport and social class vary across studies. In some studies, no evidence for a link between sports participation and socio-economic status is found. This is the case, for example, in the research of Nàdori and Szilasi (1976), who investigated a potential link between the sports participation of Hungarian boys and girls on the one hand, and the socio-professional status of their fathers (intellectual versus working class) on the other. Nor did Jakobsson *et al.* (2012) find significant differences between young people's participation in club-organised sports and their parents' educational level and economic capital. Nevertheless, the majority of studies do report significant differences in sports participation according to socio-economic background: a higher socio-economic status generally being associated with a higher likelihood of sports participation (e.g. Grunden, 1970; Hasbrook, 1986; Laakso and Telama, 1981; Renson *et al.*, 1978; Schafer, 1969; Scheerder *et al.*, 2005a; 2005c; Sisjord, 1994; Taks *et al.*, 1993). Toftegaard-Støckel *et al.* (2011), for instance, found sports participation to be associated with parents' employment status; adolescents with at least one unemployed parent being less likely to participate in sports. La Torre *et al.* (2006) studied both parents' educational levels and work activities and the relationship with extra-curricular physical activity. They observed a positive relationship between physical activity and both educational level and occupation of the parents. Fernandes *et al.* (2012) found higher levels of sports practice during leisure time for adolescents from the highest socio-economic status. Studying participation in club-organised sport, Vandermeerschen *et al.* (2013, 2014) found that parental education and income poverty continue to influence the likelihood of participation.

Research findings also suggest, however, that the social stratification of participation depends partially on the organisational context. Indeed, Santos *et al.* (2004) found that adolescents from the higher social strata chose significantly more organised physical activities. Socio-economic status is more strongly related to organised physical activities compared to non-organised physical activities. Based on a survey among Finnish youngsters, Laakso *et al.* (2008) stated that organised youth sport is regulated by the socio-economic status of the parents, whereas this is not the case for unorganised leisure-time physical activity. The analyses of Telama *et al.* (2009), on the same data, revealed that there is an increase in the social inequality in participation in organised physical activity.

Finally, though less frequently investigated among youngsters, social class not only affects general sports participation; it also influences the preference for particular sports. Studying the issue from a life-course perspective, Kraaykamp *et al.* (2012) found that the socio-economic status of the parents influenced the chance of starting a sport, especially a high status sport. In other words, parents stimulate the enrolment in highbrow sport activities. Kraaykamp *et al.* (2012) concluded from their study that intergenerational transmission (from parents to their off-spring) of sporting preferences tends to be lifelong.

In summary, the international evidence suggests that sports participation is still socially stratified, youngsters from higher social strata being more likely to participate in sports, especially in an organised context. In addition, the choice of specific sports also tends to be linked to social class. These findings are in line with conclusions from the broader field of youth studies. For example, Sletten (2010) has found that families' financial situations have a significant effect on participation in social leisure-time activities, with participation in structured leisure-time activities being particularly affected. Overall, research indicates that leisure practices are closely related to material and social circumstances (Shildrick and MacDonald, 2006).

Case-study: social stratification patterns in sports participation in Flanders

In order to examine whether changes have occurred in the relationships between youth sports participation and social class, we need empirical data that allow for a time-trend analysis. In Flanders (Belgium), among other countries such as Denmark, England, the Netherlands, Spain, Sweden and Switzerland (for an overview, see Scheerder *et al.*, 2011), such long-term sports participation data are available over a timespan of several decades. In Flanders, youth sports participation data have been collected since the late 1960s for boys and since the late 1970s for girls (Scheerder *et al.*, 2005a, 2005c). The so-called *Study on Movement Activities in Flanders* (SMAF) consists of a large repeated cross-sectional survey among high school adolescents aged 13–18. Participation in (club-organised) sports is measured every ten years. To ensure an accurate comparison between both sexes, we will focus here on the results from 1989, 1999 and 2009. The multivariate analysis is carried out with club-organised sports participation as the dependent variable. Pupils were considered to be club participants if they practised at least one sport in a club-organised context during the twelve months prior to the investigation, regardless of the frequency, the intensity or the level of their sports practice. As a consequence both competitive as well as recreational forms of club-organised sports participation were included. The background variables were sex, age and the socio-economic status (SES) of the family. The SES variable was based on the highest educational achievement of both the father and the mother, as well as their socio-professional status. For further details about the SMAF survey, we refer to Scheerder and Vos (2011) and Vandermeerschen *et al.* (2013, 2014).

A multilevel model, performed by Vandermeerschen *et al.* (2014), revealed that sports participation among youth, aged 13–18 years, continued to be socially stratified during the preceding three decades (Table 25.1). More precisely, the findings indicate that, during the past decades, sex and parental SES remained important predictors for sports participation in a club-organised context. Yet, their effect and interconnection changed. Whereas the inequality between boys and girls decreased, social inequality persisted when it came to active participation in a sports club. Albeit to a somewhat lesser degree, age also influenced the likelihood of club-organised sports participation. Younger adolescents were more likely to be actively involved in club-organised sports. This effect remained almost the same throughout the whole period of observation – a finding confirmed by a pooled model, including interactions with *year of observation* (table not shown). Thus, the results indicated that social stratification of club-organised sports participation still exists. Sex, SES and age continue to determine the likelihood of club participation by Flemish youth. Moreover, as again confirmed by the pooled model mentioned above, for boys the impact of SES increased in recent decades.

Table 25.1 Multilevel regression results for participation in club-organised sports among school-aged adolescents in Flanders, 1989-2009, in odds ratios (standard error)

	1989		*1999*		*2009*	
Constant	1.270★	(0.142)	1.564★★★	(0.147)	1.234★	(0.105)
Age (centred at 16)	0.945★	(0.027)	0.891★★★	(0.026)	0.897★★★	(0.028)
Sex						
Male (ref.)						
Female	0.463★★★	(0.051)	0.610★★★	(0.066)	0.707★★	(0.082)
SES of the parents	1.015	(0.081)	1.275★	(0.125)	1.519★★★	(0.166)
Interaction female★SES	1.610★★★	(0.206)	1.349★	(0.176)	1.003	(0.149)
Variance components						
School level	0.391★★★	(0.083)	0.238★★★	(0.073)	0.073	(0.138)
Intraclass correlation coefficient	0.044		0.017		0.002	
Log likelihood	-1350.03		-1188.14		-951.60	

★ $p < 0.05$, ★★ $p < 0.01$, ★★★ $p < 0.001$

In search of explanations

Observing the social stratification of sports participation leads us to wonder to what extent this is a matter of differences in preference, social exclusion, or both (Liu, 2009). There is no definite answer to this question (Liu, 2009). More research is needed to fully comprehend the relationships between youth sport and social class. Qualitative research can be particularly insightful for understanding the choices of young people. Though some notable studies have been conducted on this topic (e.g. Humbert, 2006; Wright *et al.*, 2003), there is still a need for more information concerning the experiences and meanings of less privileged youngsters with regard to leisure-time sports and physical activity. Nonetheless, the current literature already offers important insights that might enable us to better understand the relationships between youth sport and socio-economic background, and research has indicated there is more at stake than merely different preferences. While it is not possible to be exhaustive, in what follows, some key insights are highlighted.

An important line of theory and findings is linked to culture. Though certainly not without criticisms, the work of Bourdieu remains essential for understanding the demand for sport and how different interests are created and to a certain extent inter-generationally transmitted (Bourdieu, 1984, 1990). Bourdieu's cultural reproduction theory, his insights with regard to (i) the social desire among people to distinguish themselves from others and (ii) people's relationships with their bodies (and, by extension, the concept of symbolic violence) have proved of great value in recognising the social and structural component in what might otherwise mistakenly be perceived as a purely individual matter (Bourdieu, 1984, 1990; Bourdieu and Passeron, 1970). In their research on young people and sports, Coakley and White (1992) found that youngsters from lower social strata tended to avoid participation in 'middle class sports' to shun ridicule or rejection from significant others. More recently, studying sports participation in the South Caucasus, Birchwood *et al.* (2008) have found that the propensity to practice sports is transmitted via the family culture. This implies that it is not just education leading to sports practice, but that the family culture influences both the propensity to do sports as well as the likelihood of a high educational achievement (Birchwood *et al.*, 2008).

To fully understand the relationships between youth sport and social class – or the social stratification of sports participation more generally – it is necessary to remember that sports participation is not a separate experience in young people's lives. Rather, it is dependent upon the way they view themselves, and their position in the broader social world (Coakley and White, 1992; McCulloch *et al.*, 2006). Similarly, as explained by Sen (2009: 282–283), people will tend to adjust their desires and expectations to what seems feasible to them, given their own circumstances. As a consequence, the social stratification of youth sports participation is affected by the presence or absence of a social gap in society in general. If a society is strongly stratified, larger inequalities in sports participation will be observed, whereas in more equal societies, also in sports participation, social differences will tend to be smaller (Coalter, 2013; Green *et al.*, 2013).

As mentioned earlier, the emphasis on social class has been challenged. For example, the individualisation thesis (e.g. Bauman, 2000; Beck, 1992; Giddens, 1991; 1994) claims that social stratification along traditional lines has faded. According to individualisation theory, identity would be less predetermined than several decades ago, but continuously shaped by youths' own, individual choices. Also with regard to youth culture, it has been argued that youth (sub)cultures have gained independence from social class (Shildrick and MacDonald, 2006). Yet, on the basis of empirical findings, while one can possibly challenge the notion of class, it cannot be denied that social structural inequalities continue to influence the leisure-related 'choices' of youth

(McCulloch *et al.*, 2006; Shildrick and MacDonald, 2006). In other words, cultural preferences are partially determined by structural conditions. Young people of all social strata may well have to face an increasing amount of choices, but these choices are still directed and, to some extent, circumscribed by structural factors (McCulloch *et al.*, 2006).

In addition, the organisational culture of sports can impede young people from participating, even in those many cases where there is no question of formal exclusion (Elling and Claringbould, 2005). Doherty and Chelladurai (1999) argue that in terms of organisational culture, a distinction should be made between a culture of similarity versus a culture of diversity. In organisations with a culture of similarity, people are expected to fit in and to follow the value system and perspectives of the homogeneous dominant group (Doherty and Chelladurai, 1999: 288). In organisations with a culture of diversity, on the other hand, there is an underlying respect for differences, and bringing one's own and unique values and attitudes into an organisation, while sharing the organisational goals, is accepted (even valued) (Doherty and Chelladurai, 1999: 288). Doherty and Chelladurai observe that most sports organisations present a culture of similarity. As a consequence, marginalised groups are often expected to take over the hegemonic traditions, standards and norms from the dominant group, which are erroneously perceived as neutral or objective (Elling and Claringbould, 2005). This can cause young people to withdraw, or retain from participating. In sum, discrimination can be institutionalised and covert (Elling and Claringbould, 2005). This also indicates that social power relations continue to govern the field of sports (Elling, 2002; Elling and Claringbould, 2005; Sugden and Tomlinson, 2002).

Finally, on a more practical level, there can be many barriers to sports participation for young people as well. First, the availability and accessibility of sporting facilities can be a major obstacle (Elling and Claringbould, 2005). Facilities can be limited in certain areas, or can be too expensive to realistically access. The research of Dollman and Lewis (2010) demonstrates that access to facilities for organised sports is more limited for young people from underprivileged neighbourhoods. In the qualitative research of Humbert *et al.* (2006), youngsters from a low socio-economic background stressed the importance of environmental factors in enabling them to do sports. They stated that safe, accessible, affordable, high quality facilities were essential for their participation (Humbert *et al.*, 2006: 478). This was less to the fore among young people from higher social strata. In addition to suitable facilities, time constraints should also be mentioned. Time constraints can prevent young people participating in sport, regardless of their social background. However, the study of Humbert *et al.* (2006) revealed that whereas youngsters from a higher socio-economic background experience time constraints because of other scheduled commitments (such as music lessons), young people from a low socio-economic background were more likely to mention family responsibilities, such as the care for a younger sibling. Finally, parental support plays a role as well. Dollman and Lewis (2010) have found that girls from lower social strata in particular receive less parental support, both instrumental (buying equipment, providing transport, for instance) and affective (such as permission and encourage-ment). Instrumental support is linked to material resources more generally. Clearly, though not the only determinant, a lack of resources is still an important explanatory factor, holding back less privileged young people from partaking of sports (Jehoel-Gijsbers, 2009).

Identifying the way forward

In this chapter, we have tried to show that youth sports participation remains socially stratified. So far, Sport for All policies – implemented with variable efforts, depending on the region or country, as well as the political and economic climate – have generally not been able to adequately deal with this issue. Social inequality in youth sports seems to be deeply rooted. Given the complexity of the problem and its link with social inequality in society in general, as demonstrated in this chapter, it is unlikely that the problem will disappear soon. Nevertheless, it is important to continue – or, rather, to intensify – the struggle for real sports opportunities for all young people, as a matter of social justice.

While certainly not pretending to have any miracle solution at hand, we would like to conclude this chapter by mentioning three considerations that might offer some guidance in effectively enhancing social equality in youth sport. A first point is the necessity to take the needs of disadvantaged young people into account and work on a demand-oriented basis. If we are to enhance sports opportunities, it is important to listen to the voices of *all* young people (MacPhail *et al.*, 2003), and to adjust to it where and when necessary. Awareness of the presence of a dominant culture in the current sporting provision, being ready to question *what* is usually done, and *how* it is normally done, are all necessary in order to open up sport to people from all social strata. Second, but closely related to the first point, is the requirement to encourage participation in its broadest sense. People from all social strata should be involved in all levels of sports organisations, including the level of decision-making (Bailey, 2008; Long *et al.*, 2002). Within the framework of sports clubs, for example, it is important to ensure (or at least actively strive for it) that social diversity is reflected in the board and among the trainers. In other words, it is not sufficient to attract new members as consumers, ownership also needs to be shared. This is the only way to make structural progress towards a more inclusive sports sector. Third, social inequality in youth sports is linked to broader social cleavages in contemporary society. Therefore, though it affects the core of sports, the sports sector can hardly deal with this issue alone. Rather, it seems that partnerships will be necessary, with youth workers, for example, and the social sector more generally. Crossing traditional boundaries between sectors, and sharing knowledge and expertise, might demand additional efforts, since exploring new pathways is not always easy. However, it is likely to prove rewarding.

References

Bailey, R. (2008). Youth sport and social inclusion. In: N.L. Holt (ed). *Positive Youth Development Through Sport*. (pp. 85–98). London: Routledge.

Bauman, Z. (2000). *Liquid Modernity*. Cambridge: Polity.

Beck, U. (1992). *Risk Society. Towards a New Modernity*. London: Sage.

Birchwood, D., Roberts, K. and Pollock, G. (2008). Explaining differences in sports participation rates among young adults. Evidence from the South Caucasus, *European Physical Education Review, 14*(3), 283–298.

Bloyce, D. and Smith, A. (2010). *Sport Policy and Development. An Introduction*. London: Routledge.

Bourdieu, P. (1978). Sport and social class. *Social Science Information, 17*(6), 819–840.

Bourdieu, P. (1984). *Distinction. A Social Critique of the Judgement of Taste*. Cambridge, MA: Harvard University Press.

Bourdieu, P. (1988). Program for a sociology of sport, *Sociology of Sport Journal, 5*(2), 153–161.

Bourdieu, P. (1990). *In Other Words. Essays Towards a Reflexive Sociology*. Cambridge: Polity.

Bourdieu, P. and Passeron, J.C. (1970). *La Reproduction. Eléments Pour une Theorie du Système D'enseignement*. Paris: Minuit.

Coakley, J. (2011). Youth sports. What counts as 'positive development'? *Journal of Sport and Social Issues, 35*(3), 306–324.

Coakley, J. and White, A. (1992). Making decisions. Gender and sports participation among British adolescents, *Sociology of Sport Journal, 9*, 20–35.

Coalter, F. (2007). *A Wider Social Role for Sport. Who's Keeping the Score?* London: Routledge.

Coalter, F. (2013). Game plan and the spirit level. The class ceiling and the limits of sports policy? *International Journal of Sport Policy and Politics, 5*(1), 3–19.

COE (1975). *The European Sport for All Charter*. Strasbourg: Council of Europe.

COE/CDS (1980). *The European Sport for All Charter. Text and background.* 2nd edition. Strasbourg: Council of Europe/Committee for the Development of Sport.

Dagkas, S. and Stathi, A. (2007). Exploring social and environmental factors affecting adolescents' participation in physical activity, *European Physical Education Review, 13*(3), 369–384.

Danish, S., Forneris, T., Hodge, K. and Heke, I. (2004). Enhancing youth development through sport, *World Leisure, 46*(3), 38–49.

Dean, H. (2013). The translation of needs into rights. Reconceptualising social citizenship as a global phenomenon, *International Journal of Social Welfare, 22,* S32-S49.

Doherty, A.J. and Chelladurai, P. (1999). Managing cultural diversity in sport organizations. A theoretical perspective, *Journal of Sport Management, 13,* 280–297.

Dollman, J. and Lewis, N.R. (2010). The impact of socioeconomic position on sports participation among South Australian youth, *Journal of Science and Medicine in Sport, 13,* 318–322.

Donnelly, P. and Coakley, J. (2002). *The Role of Recreation in Promoting Social Inclusion* (Perspectives on Social Inclusion Working Paper Series). Toronto: Laidlaw Foundation.

Elling, A. (2002). *Ze Zijn er (niet) Voor Gebouwd. In- en Uitsluiting in de Sport naar Sekse en Etniciteit [They are (not) Made for it. Inclusion and Exclusion in Sport by Sex and Ethnicity].* Nieuwegein: Arko Sports Media.

Elling, A. and Claringbould, I. (2005). Mechanisms of inclusion and exclusion in the Dutch sports landscape. Who can and wants to belong? *Sociology of Sport Journal, 22,* 498–515.

Elling, A. and Knoppers, A. (2005). Sport, gender and ethnicity. Practices of symbolic inclusion/exclusion, *Journal of Youth and Adolescence, 34(4)* 257–268.

Fernandes, R.A., Reichert, F.F., Monteiro, H.L., Freitas Júnior, I.F., Cardoso, J.R., Ronque, E.R.V. and De Oliveira, A.R. (2012). Characteristics of family nucleus as correlates of regular participation in sports among adolescents, *International Journal of Public Health, 57*(2), 431–435.

Fraser-Thomas, J.L., Côté, J. and Deakin, J. (2005). Youth sport programs. An avenue to foster positive youth development, *Physical Education and Sport Pedagogy, 10*(1), 19–40.

Giddens, A. (1991). *Modernity and Self-identity. Self and Society in the Late Modern Age.* Cambridge: Polity.

Giddens, A. (1994). Living in a post-traditional society. In: U. Beck, A. Giddens and S. Lash (eds). *Reflexive Modernisation. Politics, Tradition and Aesthetics in the Modern Social Order.* (pp. 56–109). Cambridge: Polity.

Green, K., Thurston, M., Vaage, O. and Roberts, K. (2013). '[We're on the right track, baby,] we were born this way'! Exploring sports participation in Norway, *Sport, Education and Society,* DOI: 10.1080/13573322.2013.769947.

Grunden, C. (1970). Sport and social background. A study of 13- and 15-year-old children, *Bulletin of Physical Education, 8,* 36–40.

Hasbrook, C.A. (1986). The sport participation–social class relationship. Some recent youth sport participation data, *Sociology of Sport Journal, 3*(2), 154–159.

Holt, N.L. (2008). Introduction. Positive youth development through sport. In: N.L. Holt (ed). *Positive Youth Development Through Sport.* (pp. 1–8). London: Routledge.

Humbert, M.L., Chad, K.E., Spink, K.S., Muhajarine, N., Anderson, K.D., Bruner, M.W., Girolami, T.M., Odnokon, P. and Gryba, C.R. (2006). Factors that influence physical activity participation among high- and low-SES youth, *Qualitative Health Research, 16*(4), 467–483.

Jakobsson, B.T., Lundvall, S., Redelius, K. and Engström, L.-M. (2012). Almost all start but who continue? A longitudinal study of youth participation in Swedish club sports, *European Physical Education Review, 18(1),* 3–18.

Jarvie, G. (2003). Communitarianism, sport and social capital. Neighbourhood insights in Scottish Sport, *International Review for the Sociology of Sport, 38*(2), 139–153.

Jehoel-Gijbers, G. (2009). *Kunnen alle kinderen meedoen? Onderzoek naar de maatschappelijke participatie van arme kinderen [Can all Children Participate? A Research on the Societal Participation of Poor Children].* The Hague: Netherlands Institute for Social Research.

Kraaykamp, G., Oldenkamp, M. and Breedveld, K. (2012). Starting a sport in the Netherlands. A life-course analysis of the effects of individual, parental and partner characteristics. *International Review for the Sociology of Sport, 48*(2), 153–170.

La Torre, G., Masala, D., De Vito, E., Langiano, E., Capelli, G. and Ricciardi, W. (2006). Extra-curricular physical activity and socioeconomic status in Italian adolescents, *BMC Public Health, 6(22),* DOI: 10.1186/1471–2458–6-22.

Laakso, L. and Telama, R. (1981). Sport participation of Finnish youth as a function of age and schooling, *Sportwissenschaft, 11,* 28–45.

Laakso, L., Telama, R., Nupponen, H., Rimpela, A. and Pere, L. (2008). Trends in leisure time physical activity among young people in Finland, 1977–2007, *European Physical Education Review*, *14*(2), 139–155.

Lawson, H.A. (2005). Empowering people, facilitating community development, and contributing to sustainable development. The social work of sport, exercise, and physical education programs, *Sport, Education and Society*, *10*(1), 135–160.

Liu, D.-L. (2009). Sport and social inclusion. Evidence from the performance of public leisure facilities, *Social Indicators Research*, *90*, 325–337.

Long, J., Welsh, M., Bramham, P., Butterfield, J., Hylton, K. and Lloyd, E. (2002). *Count me in. The Dimensions of Social Inclusion through Culture and Sport*. London: Department of Culture, Media and Sport.

Lüschen, G. (1963). Soziale schichtung und soziale mobilität bei jungen sportlern, *Kölner Zeitschrift für Soziologie and Sozial Psychologie*, *15*, 74–93.

Lüschen, G. (1969). Social stratification and social mobility among young sportsmen. In: J.W. Loy and G. Kenyon (eds). *Sport, Culture and Society*. (pp. 258–276). New York: MacMillan.

McCulloch, K., Stewart, A. and Lovegreen, N. (2006). 'We just hang out together'. Youth cultures and social class, *Journal of Youth Studies*, *9*(5), 539–556.

MacPhail, A., Kirk, D. and Eley, D. (2003). Listening to young people's voices. Youth sports leaders' advice on facilitating participation in sport, *European Physical Education Review*, *9*(1), 57–73.

Moens, M. and Scheerder, J. (2004). Social determinants of sports participation revisited. The role of socialization and symbolic trajectories. *European Journal for Sport and Society*, *1*(1), 35–49.

Nàdori, L. and Szilasi, G. (1976). The influence exerted by the local social milieu on extra-mural physical and sport activity of school youth, *International Review of Sport Sociology*, *11*(1), 49–64.

Nicholson, M. and Hoye, R. (2008) (eds). *Sport and Social Capital*. Oxford: Elsevier.

Ohl, F. (2000). Are social classes still relevant to analyse sports groupings in 'postmodern' society? An analysis referring to P. Bourdieu's theory (Review article), *Scandinavian Journal of Medicine and Science in Sports* 10: 146–55.

Renson, R. (1976). Social status symbolism of sports stratification, *Hermes*, *10*, 433–443.

Renson, R., Beunen, G., De Witte, L., Ostyn, M., Simons, J. and Van Gerven, D. (1978). The social spectrum of the physical fitness of 12 to 19-year-old boys. In: M. Ostyn, G. Beunen and J. Simons (eds). *Kinanthropometry II*. (pp. 104–118). Baltimore, MD: University Park Press.

Santos, M.P., Esculcas C. and Mota, J. (2004). The relationship between socioeconomic status and adolescents' organised and non–organised physical activities, *Pediatric Exercise Science*, *16*, 210– 218.

Schafer, W.E. (1969). Some sources and consequences of interscholastic athletics. In: G.S. Kenyon (ed.) *Aspects of Contemporary Sport Sociology* (Proceedings of the C.I.C. Symposium on the Sociology of Sport; University of Wisconsin, November 1968). (pp. 41–42). Chicago, Illinois: Athletic Institute.

Scheerder, J., Taks, M., Vanreusel, B. and Renson, R. (2005a). Social changes in youth sports participation styles 1969–1999. The case of Flanders (Belgium), *Sport, Education and Society*, *10*(3), 321–341.

Scheerder, J., Vanreusel, B., Taks, M. and Renson, R. (2002). Social sports stratification in Flanders 1969–1999. Intergenerational reproduction of social inequalities? *International Review for the Sociology of Sport*, *37*(2), 219–245.

Scheerder, J., Vanreusel, B. and Taks, M. (2005b). Stratification patterns of active sport involvement among adults. Social change and persistence, *International Review for the Sociology of Sport*, *40*(2), 139–162.

Scheerder, J., Vanreusel, B., Taks, M. and Renson, R. (2005c). Social stratification patterns in adolescents' active sports participation behaviour. A time trend analysis 1969–1999, *European Physical Education Review*, *11*(1), 5–27.

Scheerder, J., Vandermeerschen, H., van Tuyckom, C., Hoekman, R., Breedveld, K. and Vos, S. (2011). *Understanding the Game: Sport Participation in Europe. Facts, Reflections and Recommendations* (Sport Policy and Management 10). Leuven: University of Leuven/Research Unit of Social Kinesiology and Sport Management.

Scheerder, J. and Vos, S. (2011). Social stratification in adults' sports participation from a time-trend perspective. Results from a 40-year household study, *European Journal for Sport and Society*, *8*(1+2), 31–44.

Sen, A. (2009). *The Idea of Justice*. London: Penguin

Shildrick, T. and MacDonald, R. (2006). In defence of subculture. Young people, leisure and social divisions, *Journal of Youth Studies*, *9*(2), 125–140.

Sisjord, M.-K. (1994). *Youth, Sport and Social Stratification* (Paper presented at the 12th Symposium of the International Sociology of Sport Association; Bielefeld; 1994).

Sletten, M.A. (2010). Social costs of poverty. Leisure time socializing and the subjective experience of social isolation among 13–16-year-old Norwegians, *Journal of Youth Studies*, *13*(3), 291–315.

Stempel, C. (2005). Adult participation sports as cultural capital. A test of Bourdieu's theory of the field of sports, *International Review for the Sociology of Sport*, *40*(4), 411–432.

Sugden, J. and Tomlinson, A. (2002). *Power Games. A Critical Sociology of Sport*. London: Routledge.

Taks, M., Renson, R., Vanreusel, B., Beunen, G., Claessens, A., Colla, M., Lefevre, J., Ostyn, M., Schueremans, C., Simons, J. and Van Gerven, D. (1993). Sociocultural determinants of sport participation among 13- to 18-year-old Flemish girls, 1979–1989'. In: W. Duquet, P. De Knop and L. Bollaert (eds). *Youth Sport: A Social Approach*. (pp. 50–58). Brussels: VUBPress.

Telama, R., Laakso, L., Nupponen, H., Rimpelä, A. and Pere, L. (2009). Secular trends in youth physical activity and parents' socioeconomic status from 1977 to 2005, *Pediatric Exercise Science*, *21*, 462–474.

Toftegaard-Støckel, J., Nielsen, G., Ibsen, B. and Andersen, L.B. (2011). Parental, socio and cultural factors associated with adolescents' sports participation in four Danish municipalities, *Scandinavian Journal of Medicine and Science in Sports*, *21*(4), 606–611.

UN/UNESCO (1978). *International Charter of Physical Education and Sport*. New York: United Nations Educational, Scientific and Cultural Organization.

Vandermeerschen, H., Vos, S. and Scheerder, J. (2013). Who's joining the club? Participation of socially vulnerable children and adolescents in club-organised sports, *Sport, Education and Society*. DOI: 10.1080/13573322.2013.856293

Vandermeerschen, H., Vos, S. and Scheerder, J. (2014). Towards level playing fields? A time trend analysis of young people's participation in club-organised sports, *International Review for the Sociology of Sport*. DOI: 10.1177/1012690214532450

Veal, A. (2002). *Leisure and Tourism Policy Planning*. 2nd edition. Oxon: CAB International.

von Euler, R. (1953). Idrottsrörelsen av i dag. En sociologisk studie. In: Sveriges Riksidrottsförbund (ed). *Svensk Idrott. En Ekonomisk, Historisk och Sociologisk Undersökning*. (pp. 16–19). Malmö: Allhem.

Waddington, I. (2000). *Sport, Health and Drugs. A Critical Sociological Perspective*. London: E. and F.N. Spon.

Waters, M. (1994). Succession in the stratification system. A contribution to the 'death of class' debate, *International Sociology*, *9*(3), 295–312.

Wilson, T.C. (2002). The paradox of social class and sports involvement. The roles of cultural and economic capital, *International Review for the Sociology of Sport*, *37*(1), 5–16.

Wright, J., MacDonald, D. and Groom, L. (2003). Physical activity and young people. Beyond participation, *Sport, Education and Society*, *8*(1), 17–33.

26

SEXUALITY, GENDER AND YOUTH SPORT

Jan Wright

Why is sexuality and gender an issue in youth sport?

There are two main themes underpinning most research and writing on gender, sexuality and youth sports: a concern with social inequalities based on gender and sexuality, and a concern with sport as a site where limiting gender norms are (re)produced for boys, girls, young women and men. The two themes are not distinct but are often intertwined in discussions of gender and sexuality in relation to youth sports. For example, girls' limited access to and different experience of sports, such as the different codes of football, are not only about fewer resources or opportunities but about the ways the practices associated with football as a traditional male sport celebrate and train boys and young men for particular forms of (hegemonic) masculinity, thereby putting at risk the claim to being appropriately female of those girls and women who might want to play. In addition, such practices also work to exclude and put at risk those boys who do not demonstrate socially valued forms of masculinity in their performance of the game, or who choose not to play the game. These themes have been explored in relation to school sports, community and club youth sports, contemporary and action sports and from the perspectives of sociology of sport and cultural studies.

An additional theme also requires some attention. More recently, and less well covered in academic literature, is the use of youth sport as a tool for empowering girls and challenging gender relations in local communities. Although the idea of empowering girls through sport is not new and indeed has been part of the argument for encouraging girls' participation since the nineteenth century (Scraton, 1992) and for minority communities in developed countries (Cooky, 2009), more recently this has become a global endeavor targeting girls in disadvantaged communities, in the context of sport for development and peace (Hayhurst, 2013; Right to Play International, 2012).

Approaching the topic

Approaching the topic of gender, sexuality and youth sports is made complex through a history of different theoretical positions and different motivations prompting research in the area. The other difficulty in approaching the topic is not because of any dearth of research on gender, sexuality and sport, but because there is so little research that clearly identifies itself as focusing on youth sport. Much of the research, for example on gender, sexuality and contemporary sports (e.g. skateboarding and youth subcultures), is clearly about young people. Since it is mostly teenagers and young adults who participate, however, participants are not identified necessarily by age. Classic works such as Messner's (2009, 2011) study of gender production in youth sports through his examination of adult volunteers in sport and Ian Wellard's (2007) collection, *Rethinking Gender and Youth Sports*, are more targeted. However, to only focus on these would ignore a wealth of other research. The approach taken then has been an inclusive one, using edited collections on sociology of sport, database searches of journals such as, *Sociology of Sport, Sport Education and Society, Journal of Sport and Social Issues*, following up on references in articles, relying on my own and colleagues knowledge of writers in the field and chasing up their most recent work through Google searches. I have tried to cover literature from North America, UK, Australia and New Zealand and to a lesser extent Europe. I feel remiss in not referencing more work from Asia, Africa and South America. One of the challenges has been the proliferation of research in the fields of sociology of sport and cultural studies exploring sporting youth subcultures from a multitude of perspectives. In this writing, race and ethnicity are difficult to tease out from gender and sexuality, for example, Atencio, Beal and Yochim's (2013) study of the reproduction of *Skurban* masculinities in media and marketing productions associated with skateboarding. I have therefore tried to pull out those themes related specifically to gender and sexuality; the intersection of race, ethnicity, social class and gender are covered in other chapters in this Handbook.

Gender inequalities

The home page for the 2013 conference of International Working Group on Women in Sport (IWG) epitomizes the liberal feminist approach that prompted the first arguments and research on girls' unequal access and opportunities in sport. The page includes a summary of the UK report from the Women's Sport and Fitness Foundation (WSFF) headed, 'Startling gender gap between UK school-aged girls and boys' (IWG, 2013). The report points to schools as holding the key to addressing the alleged gap in participation levels. The findings of this report are not new, nor is the advice to schools, which is in itself disturbing. However, what the report points to is the endurance of concerns (and solutions) from similar reports in the 1970s and 1980s when liberal feminist approaches to gender inequalities were at their height.

The theme of gender inequalities in sport has arguably been historically the earliest and most persistent in the literature on gender and youth sports. This literature has focused on the unfair exclusion, for the most part of girls and young women, from sports that have been dominated in numbers, attention and resources by boys and young men. With a more nuanced attention to privilege within groups of girls and boys, notions of exclusion have more recently been extended to specific groups of girls and, to a lesser extent, boys (e.g., Wellard, 2002, 2012). The literature on gender inequalities, for the most part, seems to respond to the idea that the absence of particular groups of children and young people from sport, mostly girls and young women, limits their access to important social and personal experiences that are valuable for themselves, their health and for society – the *goods* of sport, which have been seen to benefit boys and young men.

The majority of the literature, from a sociological perspective, attributes girls' and some boys' lack of interest to the social structures and practices associated with sports themselves or to competing interests in young people's lives. Research that involves interviews with teachers, coaches and organisers, those who set up the conditions for young people's participation, suggest that gender differences in interest and ability are taken for granted and indeed are actively, if unintentionally, constructed by the practices (Cooky, 2009; Flintoff, 2008; Messner, 2009). For example, many of the sports organization, council and sporting personnel Cooky (2009) interviewed (regarding reasons for girls' lower participation in community sports) explained this in terms of girls' lack of interest and ability in sports – characteristics that her respondents saw as inherent in being female. In this ethnographic study contrasting the approaches of local councils and their support for girls' sport, Cooky also demonstrated how this lack of interest, as manifest in their non-attendance, was socially constructed in the many different and subtle ways in which the sports were presented.

As research consistently reports, the majority of young girls *do* like sport and would like to do more (Bailey *et al.*, 2011). They are excluded from sport for 'a variety of often competing and complex factors' (Wellard, 2011, p. 46), such as the influence of friends and family, a perceived lack of skill and knowledge for the sports on offer, negative experiences of sport and physical education (PE) at school, competing interests and priorities, costs and transport. A study by Eime and colleagues (2008), for example, demonstrated how the decisions of the young rural women (sixteen to seventeen years) were contingent on other priorities associated with transitions during adolescence. While the girls in their study enjoyed their involvement in community sports, their desire to succeed educationally was a critical factor in decisions to move from structured club sport to more flexible individual activities.

In response to the many reports on girls, *and it is always girls*, low participation in both school and community sport, over the past 45 years numerous programmes and initiatives have been instituted, some of which have targeted women's participation and have had flow on effects for girls, such as Title IX in the United States, and others that have specifically targeted girls. These have been supported by local and national governments, and by philanthropic and corporate sponsorship. The latter include, most recently, programmes such as the Canadian Women's Sports Foundation (WSF) community project, GoGirlGo! (WSF, 2011), which describes itself as an 'award winning curriculum and sports education programmes, which works to improve the health of sedentary girls and keeps girls involved in physical activity by supporting programmes and organizations that work with girls', and the UK School Sports Partnership Programme (SSPP), where girls and young women were one group targeted to improve participation. Flintoff (2008) investigated how gender equity issues were taken up by teachers involved in the SSPP. She concludes that there was little evidence of improved 'inclusivity' and explains this in terms of: the prevalence of essentialist masculinist discourses associated with competitive sport practices; and the positioning of the teachers within an equality of access or difference discourse, which assumed categorical differences between girls' and boys' interests and capabilities. Like others working in this area (e.g., Wellard 2011), Flintoff (2008, p. 395) asks, 'How could gender equity permeate practices associated with youth sport in ways that would ensure all boys and girls have a quality experience?' This seems to remain a perennial question to which there is, as yet, no definitive answers.

Although those writing about PE might pose questions that include boys as well as girls, in the literature on community sports less attention is paid to boys' experiences of exclusion. The few exceptions attend specifically to boys in non-traditional male sports (Chimot and Louveau, 2010; Wellard, 2002). There seems to have been little attention to the experiences of boys who 'dropout' of sports, nor is there any strong discourse about gender inequalities as they relate to boys and young men in this literature. A notable exception to the latter is the work of Messner on gender, families and youth sports, *It's All for the Kids* (Messner, 2009). While the study reported in the book primarily focused on the adults involved with youth sports, Messner concludes from his observations that youth sports coaches' views of children are explained by an ascendant gender ideology he calls 'soft essentialism': 'a shared belief in natural differences between girls and boys that exists alongside more relativized and non-categorical views of girls and boys as flexible choosers in social life, and still largely categorical views of men and women' (Messner, 2011, p. 166). Messner argues that this ideology (in the context of the middle class practices of team sports) is harder on boys than it is on girls.

> Rather than being a focus of gender revolution, . . . youth sports has become an ideal site for the construction of adult narratives that appropriate the liberal feminist language of 'choice' for girls, but not for boys, in ways that help to recreate and naturalize the continuing gender inequalities in professional class work and family life.
>
> *(Messner, 2011, p. 154)*

The research reported in this section points to the complexities of researching and theorizing inequalities in youth sport, and the different discourses that have come into play over time and within different social and cultural contexts. It is clear that gender equality cannot be examined without attention to the specificities of context and the diverse identifications of the girls and boys, young men and women involved in the any study.

Constructing masculinities and femininities

With the influence of social constructionist theories and particularly poststructuralist feminism, queer theory and masculinities theory, attention has turned to sport and associated cultural sites as spaces where discourses and practices (re)produce hierarchies of gender norms for boys and girls, young women and men. This is proposed as happening not only through the practices associated with sport itself, but through the images of sport produced in and through media coverage of sport events, commentary on sports and athletes and the marketing of sports and non-sports related products. These texts serve as discursive resources for how young people come to understand gender and sexuality and how they constitute their own gender and sexual identities, both in relation to sport and in their lives more broadly. Research and writing from these perspectives include the analysis of images and written texts such as those produced by the media, advertising, marketing and textbooks (e.g., Atencio *et al.*, 2013; Cooky, 2011; Grahn, 2012; Rinehart, 2005). Research informed by a social constructivist perspective also includes work that examines the ways interactions and practices in sporting contexts shape gender identities and attitudes to sport and physical activity, and how participants negotiate gender relations in differing sporting contexts (Atencio *et al.*, 2009; Chimot and Louveau, 2010; Garrett, 2004; Kivel and Kleiber, 2000; MacPhail *et al.*, 2009; Wilson *et al.*, 2001).

While there have obviously been shifts in what constitutes socially valued forms of masculinity and femininity, the research on the construction of gender suggests that the changes in gender norms have not been as profound as one might like. Sport continues to be valued in schools and communities as a space where boys and young men learn and express the attributes of hegemonic masculinity (Connell, 2008). As such, sport becomes a dangerous place for those boys who do not *measure up*; boys, who are not *good* at sport, who are small, develop at a slower rate, or who choose not to participate, face violence, ridicule and humiliation (Wellard, 2012). Sport is a place where bodies are displayed and, in school contexts, where participation is more difficult to avoid. For example, research demonstrates how change rooms and practices such as playing teams with shirts off/on leave boys vulnerable to bullying and victimization (Drummond, 2011). Such practices also confirm the masculine identities of these boys as lower in value than the forms of masculinity expressed by those other boys who are successful in sports. Those boys who dare to participate in a *feminine* sports, such as rhythmic gymnastics or dance (Chimot and Louveau, 2010; Gard 2008), are also confronted with considerable challenges. Chimot and

Louveau (2010), for example, describe the different strategies the boys in their study, who participated in rhythmic gymnastics, had to implement to deal with the pressure from family and peers to discontinue their participation, and to negotiate between the negative masculine identity ascribed to them by others and the one they defined for themselves. As Messner (2011) suggests, for some boys, particularly in comparison to middle class girls, there seem still to be fewer choices, and more rigid lines around what constitutes socially valued forms of masculinity in sporting contexts.

In contrast to the relatively small amount of research on the experiences of boys in sport, there is considerably more research on the ways women and girls negotiate the terrain of sport as a male domain. Some of this research, which will be explored further under the topic of 'subculture research', documents the ways in which girls and young women are excluded by forms of symbolic violence (homophobia), which challenge their femaleness, particularly when they attempt to participate in traditional male sports and sports that demand strong physical bodies and aggressive play. In this context when culturally valued forms of femininity clash with the forms of physicality required of their sport, they are required to negotiate conflicting expectations. Much of this research, however, also seeks to explore the opportunities in and through sport for resistance and challenging gender norms.

As will become evident below (under youth sport subcultures) and, as researchers such as Cooky (2011), Azzarito (2011) and Heywood (2007) argue, while there may appear to have been more changes in what constitutes female physicality, the underpinning *flows* of power have changed little. These researchers all acknowledge that Title IX has made a substantial difference in the numbers of girls and young women participating in sport. As Cooky (2011, p. 210) points out, 'sport is no longer reserved for an elite group of highly skilled girls and women, but appears as a normal part of girls' and women's everyday lives' (Heywood and Dworkin, 2003). She points particularly to the success of the U.S. soccer team in the 1999 Women's World Cup 'as an emotionally riveting spectacle of girls' and women's empowerment in sport . . . part of the cultural imagery of Girl Power!' (Cooky, 2011, p. 211). With the very public successes of athletes such as the Williams sisters, and various iconic female athletes across Australia, UK, Canada and the United States, it looked like feminism had been successful and equality had finally been achieved in sport and that, in a post-feminist world, girls could do anything.

However, as Cooky (2011, p. 211) and others (Azzarito, 2011; Heywood, 2007) argue, the successes of elite athletes and teams did not translate into 'increased participation, increased opportunities, or broader shifts in the *structural* landscape of sport'. While elite female tennis players might command the same prize money and earn equal pay, these achievements rarely trickled down to the average female athlete (Cooky, 2011). While media images of athletes promoted new forms of female physicality, 'the power chick' who was strong and competitive was also, like the Williams sisters, Sharapova and others, 'heterosexy and feminine' (p. 219). In the late 2000s, Cooky argues, the marketing of female athletes has become even more sexualized and associated with what she calls 'strip culture', with athleticism downplayed as athletes, such as Sharapova, pose in underwear. She argues that

> the lack of popular cultural texts [compared to those associated with Girl Power in the late 1990s] today addressing girls as sport participants, spectators and consumers suggests that Girl Power! served primarily as a marketing discourse, rather than a sustained and ongoing instrument of political change in girls' lives.
>
> *(Cooky, 2011, p. 223)*

In the neoliberal landscape of the 2000s, feminist social researchers, (e.g., Azzarito 2011; Cooky, 2011; Heywood, 2007), argue that female athletes and those who look up to them, are encouraged to become entrepreneurial individualists, rather than recognize the structural inequalities still facing girls every day and in sport. Heywood (2007), for example, argues that programmes such as WSF GoGirlGo, through their marketing, encourage girls and young women to emulate the 'future [post-feminist] girl' who is celebrated for her 'desire, determination and confidence to take charge of her life, seize chances, and achieve her goals' (Harris 2004; quoted in Heywood 2007, p. 103). In her analysis of GoGirlGo, Heywood demonstrates how in the marketing of the programmes,

> the female athlete and female athleticism and strength are literal embodiments of Girl Power, the subject who is, through her accomplishment and good lessons she learns in sport, supposed to develop her strength, health and self-confidence and apply these to her career goals.
>
> *(Heywood, 2007, p. 115)*

Such post-feminist messages, Cooky (2011, p. 217) argues, obscure 'the structural inequalities girls face every day' and promote 'individualism and individual empowerment over collective empowerment'. The hierarchies of femininity promoted in and through sport thus (re)produce social values promoted in contemporary western neoliberal societies, such as an emphasis on individual responsibility for achievement and self-development. These are values, Cooky and Heywood argue, that continue to privilege those young women who are able to make their own way – girls and young women who have the economic, social and cultural capital to succeed.

Gender, sexuality and youth sport sub-cultures

One prominent area of scholarship in the sociology of sport is the exploration of the ways in which, what have been called variously contemporary sports/action sports/'new' youth sports/lifestyle sports, (re)produce or offer sites of resistance for normative gender relations. Most of these sports, such as skateboarding, windsurfing, surfing and snowboarding, are characterized by 'creative, aesthetic, and performative expressions of their activities' (Wheaton, 2004, p. 298). Participants, according to Wheaton look for pleasure in the buzz, the ecstasy of speed, being at one with the environment, the standing still of time; they engage in 'playful practices' (Midol and Broyer, 1995, quoted in Wheaton, 2004, p. 298) and often take risks. For some, part of the excitement is the subversive challenge to mainstream culture. In the early writing on these alternative sports, great hopes were expressed that, in their challenges to mainstream culture, these sports would provide spaces that encouraged 'femininity and masculinity to be embodied in a variety of shapes and ways that allow power to be embodied in ways not tied to domination or gender, (Whitson, 1994, p. 368).

This hope has become a theme in much of the research on subcultures in relation to gender. For example, Rinehart (2005, p. 232) asks whether 'the much-vaunted alternative ethos of action sports lead to a concomitant paradigm shift in fundamental attitudes towards race, class, gender differences within these sports forms?' The answer seems quite complex, however. In general it seems that the power to define relations and identities in lifestyle sports still rests with the boys and men in the sports. These sports are still sites of hegemonic masculine identity production, although the expression of that masculinity might be differ from that valued in traditional team sports. In her study of 'competing masculinities in the windsurfing culture', Wheaton (2004), for example, demonstrates how, 'despite windsurfing's counter cultural heritage and the *feminized* appearance of some male windsurfers . . . traditional *hegemonic* masculinity predominates at the *core* of the subculture' (Wheaton, 2004, p. 136). In another example, Waitt (2007, p. 107) remarks of the youth surfing subculture that he was studying: 'I was struck by how surfing remains an initiation into a normative expression of European manhood'. As the quote from Atencio and colleagues (Atencio *et al.*, 2009) below suggests, gendered hierarchies still operate in skateboarding, particularly in its street or free versions.

> Masculine habituses were most closely associated with risk-taking behaviours and technical prowess; they became significantly rewarded with social and cultural capital. Conversely, women's habituses were considered as lacking in skill and aversive to risk-taking. Women thus came to be positioned as inauthentic participants in the street skateboarding social field and were largely excluded from accessing symbolic capital.
>
> *(Atencio* et al.*, 2009, p. 3)*

It would seem that the practices of male participants in these new sports still exclude girls and young women because of their assumed feminine qualities, which either make their participation unsuitable or less valued. This is not to say that there are not exceptions both within and between sports. In skateboarding, for example, in the paper cited above, Atencio *et al.* (2009) describe corporately organized 'All Girl' events and niche media that supported the female skateboarders in their study. Thorpe (2005), in her study of women in snowboarding, describes how women, in the sport from the very early days, benefited from the commercialization of the sport, and were able to command high salaries and compete on an equal level to men in the Olympics. She describes how women worked collaboratively to form women's companies and were involved in marketing and brand development, including clothing and women's boards: 'The increasingly active and significant role of the female snowboarder suggests that the gender relations in snowboarding are dynamic, rather than fixed, and contested, rather than agreed.' (Thorpe, 2005, p. 81) However, Thorpe goes on to argue that 'much of the evidence of positive progress is superficial' (p. 83). In a way similar to the shifts in female athleticism described above by Cooky, competition both in sport and in the marketplace also encouraged individualism with women snowboarders becoming less supportive of each other. Thorpe concludes that 'the snowboarding industry employs a variety of overt and covert strategies to reinforce female 'otherness' and male superiority'. In ways that resonate with Waitt's (2007) discussion of surfing, she writes:

> The masculinity of snowboarding appears common sense through the emphasis on male physicality and power with a focus on war, violence, injury and risk taking. The prominence of the male physicality in snowboarding is a 'subtle form of symbolic domination rather than overt physical control, which contributes to the reproduction and reinforcement of power relations inherent in the existing gender order' (Gillett and White 1992: 363).
>
> *(Thorpe, 2005, p. 87)*

Sexuality and youth sport

The social construction of masculinities and femininities in and through sport clearly points to gendered or sexual hierarchies where heterosexuality is for the most part the unspoken norm (Wellard, 2012). What this means is that issues of sexuality per se seem to be rarely addressed in relation to youth sports – for example, we know very little about how young lesbians, gay men or transgender young people negotiate the discourses and practices of youth sports. What little research there is focuses primarily on school sport and PE and the symbolic and real violence of homophobia and its effects on, mostly young men's, participation. If youth sports mimic sports more generally then as a site where 'hegemonic masculinities are made and remade' (Wellard 2012, p. 104) they are unlikely to be a welcoming environment for sexual minorities. Wellard suggests that in environments highly regulated by adults within and outside the school context, gay and lesbian young people have fewer options than when they are adults.

At the same time, some sports serve as spaces where women whose bodies do not conform to normative heterosexual forms of femininity can enjoy themselves and find like-minded young women. The young lesbian women in Kivel and Klieber's (2000) study, for example, chose their sports in high school for their potential to provide opportunities for meeting other women like themselves. Some sports provided a safe place in which to express their sexuality. On the other hand, the gay boys in the same study tended to avoid sports, preferring not to be in or around the kind of 'male atmosphere', the macho attitude and violence in sports 'where they separated the males from the females' (p. 224). Others lesbian and gay youth in this study distanced themselves from sports that might have led to their identification as gay or lesbian.

While there has been a rise in organized sporting events and specific competitions or teams for those identifining as gay and lesbian, there is little research on how these impact young people. Does the public nature of the gay games, for example, open up possibilities for a more public expression of identity? Do young people seek out such opportunities? How inclusive are competitive contexts such as the gay games for all bodies and capabilities? In general, research on the experiences of young gay, lesbian, transgender and transsexuals is an area in community and club sports is an area missing from the youth sport research.

Sport for development: empowering girls through sport

A recent area of prominence in relation to gender and youth sport, which has received only limited academic attention, is the sport and development programmes focused specifically on 'empowering' young women and girls. Many of these programmes are motivated by the UN millennium Development Goal – 'promoting gender equality and the empowering of women' (United Nations, 2013). This call has been taken up and supported through funding, resources and personnel by non-government organisations (NGOs), sport federations, transnational corporations (TNCs) and UN agencies in developing countries and communities throughout the world (Hayhurst, 2013). On the International Platform on Sport and Development (2013a) website, Sport and Development 'refers to the use of sport as a tool for development and peace'. While there are initiatives reported on the website that address children and youth development more broadly, gender is targeted as an area of specific interest. The website argues that, 'In recent years, there has been a significant shift from advocating for 'gender equity in sport' towards using 'sport for gender equity and personal development' (2013b). Sport thus becomes a tool for enhancing 'girls' sense of agency, self-empowerment and personal freedom, in promoting their social inclusion and social integration in their communities, in challenging oppressive gender norms and lastly in offering girls opportunities for leadership and achievement'. The website describes a number of case studies, such as the Kenyan Moving the Goal Posts Project, to illustrate how sports programmes in developing countries have achieved this. Other projects (such as the Nike Girls Effect campaign) go further to imagine girls as 'agents of development . . . capable of bringing about "unparalleled social and economic change to their families, communities and countries" (Girl Effect 2001)' (Hayhurst, 2013, para.1.1).

Despite the proliferation of these projects, there has been little research into their effects. Two notable exceptions are Brady's (2005) analysis of the outcomes of a large scale mixed-sex

NGO supported programme in the slums of Nairobi and an experimental pilot project in traditional Upper Egyptian villages and Hayhurst's (2013) study of girls' experiences of a corporate funded gender and development martial arts programme. Brady found that the girls' involvement in sport, though very different in each programme, helped to build their 'social assets' through assisting the girls build social networks and by bringing them into 'the public sphere', thereby beginning 'to transform gender norms' (p. 36).

Hayhurst (2013, p. 1) also argues that the programme she studied achieved many of its stated goals: 'the . . . programme increased the young women's confidence, challenged gender norms, augmented their social networks, improved their physical fitness and was useful in providing employment opportunities'. She points to the complex and subtle forms of agency and opposition, 'subversive agency', that the girls exerted in challenging traditional gender norms in the face of opposition and verbal and physical abuse from their communities. Like Cooky, Azzarito and Heywood, however, Hayhurst, also argues that Girl Effect programmes place the onus on the girls and young women as agents of change, often in the face of considerable community resistance, and without structural support 'in their quest to challenge gender norms' (para.8.4). Hayhurst argues that at this point in time, 'there seems to be a lack of understanding as to how the intentions of these programmes . . . are actually *translated in practice* – particularly into their wider communities and through their interactions with family members' (para.8.6, italics in the original).

Identifying ways forward for the future

Although the area of gender and sport has been one of the perennial areas of sport research, there are still important areas, particularly in relation to youth sport, that have yet to be explored. Clearly from the research discussed above, despite changes in the nature of sport and greater social acceptance of a diverse range of femininities and masculinities, sport remains one of the more (perhaps one of the most) conservative sites for the acceptance of difference and the (re)production of narrow and limiting gender norms. Are youth sports, as Messner (2011, p. 166) suggests, 'largely a homosocial realm run by men' or are there new configurations that provide viable alternatives? This is a fruitful space for further research; research, for example, into organizations such as *i9 Sport* (Anderson, 2012), an American corporate franchise which claims to offer a different experience for children and youth, including one that is 'gender-integrated'.

While there has been a shift towards research on masculinities in sport, there is still a considerable gap in the literature on the experiences of boys and young men in (or not in) youth sport, particularly in relation to the experiences of young men who identify as gay. More research is needed into the experiences of young gay, lesbian transsexual and transgender participants in youth sports in general and in sports that are specifically designated as gay and lesbian sports.

In relation to youth subculture sport, Wheaton (2007, p. 296) suggests that studies need to be 'more attentive to poststructuralist, postmodernist and postcolonial debates around difference', with greater attention to girls' and young women's involvement in subcultures and to 'how different, contradictory, and competing femininities and masculinities are constructed and exhibited in various lifestyle sport subcultural settings'. The same could be said of all aspects of youth sport, in its various manifestations in schools, communities and clubs, and in relation to young people in western and non-western countries, including the impact of neoliberalism and globalization on the ways in which gender plays out in youth sports.

References

Anderson, E. (2012). i9 and the transformation of youth sport. *Journal of Sport and Social Issues, 37*(1): 97–111.

Atencio, M., Beal, B. and Wilson, C. (2009). Distinction of risk: Urban skateboarding, street habitus, and the construction of hierarchical gender relations. *Qualitative Research in Sport and Exercise, 1*(1): 3–20.

Atencio, M., Beal, B. and Yochim, E. C. (2013). 'It ain't just black kids and white kids': The representation and reproduction of authentic 'skurban' masculinities. *Sociology of Sport Journal, 30*: 153–172.

Azzarito, L. (2010). Future Girls, transcendent femininities and new pedagogies: toward girls' hybrid bodies? *Sport Education and Society, 15*(3), 261–275.

Bailey, R., Wellard, I. and Dismore, H. (2005). Girls and physical activities: A summary review. *Education and Health, 23*(1): 3–5.

Brady, M. (2005). Creating safe spaces and building social assets for young women in the developing world: A new role for sports. *Women's Studies Quarterly, 33*(1/2): 35–49.

Chimot, C. and Louveau, C. (2010). Becoming a man while playing a female sport: The construction of masculine identity in boys doing rhythmic gymnastics. *International Review for the Sociology of Sport, 45*(4): 436–456.

Connell, R. (2008) Maculinity construction and sports in boys' education: a framework for thinking about the issue. *Sport Education and Society, 13*(2):131–145.

Cooky, C. (2009). 'Girls just aren't interested': The social construction of interest in girls' sport. *Sociological Perspectives, 52*(2): 259–284.

Cooky, C. (2011). Do girls rule? Understanding popular culture images of girl power and sport. In S. S. Prettyman and B. Lampman (eds), *Learning Culture through Sports: Perspectives on Society and Organized Sports* (pp. 210–226). Lanham: Rowman and Littlefield.

Drummond, M. (2011). Sport, the body and boys' constructions of masculinity. In S. Georgakis and K. Russell (eds), *Youth Sport in Australia* (pp. 85–96). Sydney: University of Sydney Press.

Eime, R. M., Payne, W. R., Casey, M. M. and Harvey, J. T. (2010). Transition in participation in sport and unstructured physical activity for rural living adolescent girls. *Health Education Research, 25*(2): 282–293.

Flintoff, A. (2008). Targeting Mr Average: Participation, gender equity and school sport partnerships. *Sport Education and Society, 13*(4): 393–411.

Garrett, R. (2004). Gendered bodies and physical identities. In J. Evans, B. Davies, and J. Wright (eds), *Body Knowledge and Control: Studies in the Sociology of Physical Education and Sport* (pp. 140–156). London and New York: Routledge.

Gillett, J. and White, P. (1992). Male bodybuilding and the reassertion of hegemonic masculinity: A critical feminist perspective, *Play and Culture, 5*(4): 358–369.

Girl Effect (2011). The Girl Effect, Retrieved from www.girleffect.org 26/12/2013.

Grahn, K. (2014). Youth athletes, bodies and gender: gender constructions in textbooks used in coaching education in Sweden. *Sport Education and Society, 19*(6): 735–75.

Harris, A. (2004). *Future Girl: Young Women in the 21st Century.* New York: Routledge.

Hayhurst, L. M. C. (2013). Girls as the 'new' agents of social change? Exploring the 'girl effect' thought sport, gender and development programmes in Uganda. *Sociological Research Online, 18*(2): 8. Retrieved from www.socresonline.org.uk/18/2/8.html.

Heywood L. and Dworkin, S. L. (2003) *Built to Win: The Female Athlete as Cultural Icon.* Minneapolis: University of Minnesota Press.

Heywood, L. (2007). Producing girls: Empire, sport and the neoliberal body. In J. Hargreaves and P. Vertinsky (eds), *Physical Culture, Power and the Body* (pp. 101–120). London and New York: Routledge.

International Platform on Sport and Development (2013a). *Learn More.* Retrieved from www.sportanddev. org/en/learnmore/ 26/12/2013.

International Platform on Sport and Development (2013b) *Sport and Gender.* Retrieved from www. sportanddev.org/en/learnmore/sport_and_gender/ 26/12/2013.

IWG (2013). *Catalyst eNewsletter: Report shows startling gender gap in physical activity between UK school-aged girls and boys.* Retrieved from www.iwg-gti.org/catalyst/may-2012/report-shows-startling-gender-ga/

Kivel, B. D. and Kleiber, D. (2000). Leisure in the identity formation of lesbian/gay youth: Personal, but not social. *Leisure Studies, 22*(4): 215–232.

MacPhail, A., Collier, C. and O'Sullivan, M. (2009). Lifestyles and gendered patterns of leisure and sporting interests among Irish adolescents. *Sport Education and Society, 14*(3): 281–299.

Messner, M. A. (2009). *It's All for the Kids: Gender, Families and Youth Sports.* Berkeley: University of California Press.

Messner, M. A. (2011). Gender ideologies, youth sports and the production of soft essentialism. *Sociology of Sport Journal, 28*(2), 151–170.

Midol, N. and Broyer, G. (1995). Towards an anthropological analysis of new sport cultures: The case of whiz sports in France. *Sociology of Sport Journal, 12,* 204–212.

Right to Play International (2012). Chapter 4: Sport and gender: Empowering girls and women. Retrieved from www.righttoplay.com/International/our…/Final_Report_Chapter_4.pdf 26/12/2013

Rinehart, R. (2005). 'Babes' and boards: Opportunities in new millenium sport. *Journal of Sport and Social Issues, 29:* 232–255.

Scraton, S. (1992) *Shaping Up to Womanhood: Gender and Girls' Physical Education.* Milton Keynes: Open University Press.

Thorpe, H. (2005). Jibbing the gender order: females in the snowboarding culture. *Sport and Society: Cultures, Commerce, Media, Politics, 8*(1): 76–100.

United Nations (2013) *Goal 3: Promote gender equality and empower women.* Retrieved from www.un.org/millenniumgoals/gender.shtml 26/12/2013.

Waitt, G. (2007). (Hetero)sexy waves: surfing, space, gender and sexuality. In I. Wellard (ed), *Rethinking Gender and Youth Sport* (pp. 99–126). London and New York: Routledge.

Wellard, I. (2002). Men, sport, body performance and the maintenance of 'exclusive masculinity'. *Leisure Studies, 21:* 235–247.

Wellard, I. (2007). Introduction: Young people, gender, physical activity and sport. In I. Wellard (ed), *Rethinking Gender and Youth sport* (pp. 1–11). London: Routledge.

Wellard, I. (2011). Girls and physical activities: An update. *Education and Health, 29*(3): 46–50.

Wellard, I. (2012). Sexuality and youth sport. In S. Dagkas and K. Armour (eds), *Inclusion and Exclusion through Youth Sport* (pp. 100–112). London and New York: Routledge.

Wheaton, B. (2004). 'New lads'? Competing masculinities in the windsurfing culture. In B. Wheaton (ed), *Understanding Lifestyle Sports. Consumption, Identity and Difference* (pp. 131–153). London and New York: Routledge.

Wheaton, B. (2007). After sport culture: Rethinking sport and post-subcultural theory. *Journal of Sport and Social Issues, 31*(3): 283–307.

Whitson, D. (2002). The embodiment of gender: Discipline, domination and empowerment. In S. Scraton and A. Flintoff (eds), *Gender and Sport: A Reader* (pp. 227–240). London: Routledge.

Wilson, B., White, P. and Fisher, K. (2001). Multiple identities in a marginalized culture: female youth in an 'inner-city' recreation/drop-in center. *Journal of Sport and Social Issues, 25*(3): 301–323.

WSF (2011). GoGirlsGo! Retrieved from www.womenssportsfoundation.org/en/home/programmes/gogirlgo

27

YOUTH SPORT, RACE AND ETHNICITY

Scott Fleming

Introduction

The *Routledge Adolescence and Society Series* includes an edited collection entitled *Young People's Involvement in Sport* (Kremer *et al.*, 1997). On its cover is a photograph of six young lads wearing soccer kit in what looks as though it might be a training session (but probably isn't). One of the lads is white; the others are from minority ethnic groups. The rest of the book has 269 pages of text, yet there is barely a mention of race, racism(s), ethnicity or specific ethnic groups. The paradox is not merely a matter of choosing an appropriate image for marketing a book; it is a reflection of the neglect of race and ethnicity in the discourses around youth sport more generally. For though there have been some important contributions to the sports studies literature linked to ethnicity before and since, this element of the topic of youth sport remains relatively under-researched and therefore insufficiently understood.

In this chapter, I provide a brief overview of the background to the current understanding of how experiences of youth sport are shaped by race, racism and ethnicity. It reflects my own research interests in this area that go back almost thirty years, and my commitment to anti-racism informed by aspects of critical race theory (Hylton, 2010; Hylton and Long, 2005). Following an attempt to bring some operational clarity to key concepts, the chapter has three further sections: an account of landmark edited collections that highlight the neglect of youth sport in studies of ethnicity and racism; a policy overview again illustrating the absence of careful and considered approaches to sport development and educational policy for minority ethnic groups; and, a summary of what is known about particular contemporary themes and issues.

A conceptual platform

There are some important premises upon which this chapter is predicated. First, the term race has been used in different ways – as classification (Banton, 2004), as signifier (Cashmore, 2004) and as synonym (van den Berghe, 2004). It remains contested and problematic. On an operational level, as Saeed and Kilvington (2011: p. 603) suggest, 'arguably, "race" in contemporary society is defined by skin colour as this is the most obvious method of distinction between "races"'. However, they go on to explain that such distinctions are without scientific basis in biology. In brief, the term race was applied to the appearance of human beings as a taxonomic classification of sub-species (Tobias, 1972 [1961]), but without clear distinctions. Differences within a so-called race are much greater than the differences between races, and for this reason as well as others the concept has no analytical purchase (Fleming, 2001). This fundamental concern is not new. First published in 1964, UNESCO (1972: p. 68) was unambiguous, 'Pure races – in the sense of genetically homogeneous populations – do not exist in the human species'. That race continues to be used in many current discourses by, for example, politicians, broadcast media, and even some academic writers, tells us something about the (mistaken) resilience of the concept.

Second, a much more useful conceptual point of departure for discussions about race and youth sport is ethnicity – and this is a distinction that does not originate in the semantics of vocabulary (see also Stein, 2004). Ethnicity may be thought of as the shared cultural identity of the members of a particular group that make it distinct from other groups. Linked to collective history and tradition, it is often concerned with the expression of cultural difference. For those interested in cricket, the historical accounts linked to that sport in the Caribbean and the Indian sub-continent illustrate the point (Bose 2002; James 2013 [1963]), especially in the rivalries of opposition.

Third, whether or not it is widely recognised that there are conceptual flaws in accounts of race, there exists what Saeed and Kilvington (2011: p. 603) have referred to as 'race thinking' which, they argue, is prevalent in western culture. Specifically, a commitment to the idea of race and the linked attitudes and beliefs about the characteristics of so-called racial groups provides a basis for racism – especially when associated with assumptions about superiority and inferiority. Also a contested concept, racism is manifest in the behaviour of individuals and groups as well in organisations, institutions and even societies. Importantly, it is clear that racism has multiple origins and methods of expression and has been experienced in a variety of ways – for example, by different groups and during different historical periods. Hence, it has become customary for some scholars to refer to 'racisms' (Long and Spracklen, 2011b).

Fourth, youth sport in Britain needs to be set within a wider demographic and cultural context. The 2011 census showed that over the preceding two decades, England and Wales became more ethnically diverse (ONS, 2012). Moreover, population projections indicate that the ethnic composition of Britain will continue to change, with slow growth among Black Caribbean groups but with an increasing proportion of South Asian groups, Chinese and 'other' ethnic groups (Rees *et al.*, 2012). The centres of population density among minority ethnic groups are the major urban cities, and there are key linkages between ethnicity and class that help to frame youth sport. Indeed, sports participation remains stubbornly and positively related to household income (Farrell and Sands, 2002). All of this is set a prevailing climate of a return to old political debates about immigration and the evident appeal of some anti-immigration sentiment, as well as fears about terrorism and Islamophobia (Bi, 2011).

Fifth, there has been a tendency in some aspects of sports policy discourse to assume homogeneity among minority ethnic groups in Britain and this has operated on (at least) three levels (Fleming, 2007 [1994]): treating all minority ethnic groups as though they are the same; treating all members of a broadly defined group as though they are the same (e.g. South Asians); treating all members of more narrowly defined groups as though they are the same (e.g. Muslims). It is important, therefore, that the heterogeneity of minority ethnic groups is not neglected in any careful consideration of the youth sport.

Sixth, this chapter addresses themes around ethnicity linked to youth sport. To do so it has been necessary isolate ethnicity from the other demographic characteristics of young people – in particular, class, gender and dis/ability, which are relevant and important. Yet it is clear that a properly nuanced consideration of multi-dimensional young people in Britain requires recognition of the intersectionality of these and other variables (Azzarito and Macdonald, this volume; Watson and Scraton, 2013).

Mapping the terrain

Notwithstanding the failure to address explicitly the linkages between ethnicity and youth sport, it is, of course, possible to infer a lot about youth sport from various sources from the sociology and social psychology of sport, more generally, and from some accounts of sporting lives (Holland, 1997; Ismond, 2003; King, 2004). Since the early 1980s, there has been a series of landmark volumes that have charted the development of the body of knowledge. The first was Ernest Cashmore's *Black Sportsmen* (1982). Republished in 2013, it was concerned primarily with the experiences of elite male athletes from a variety of sports including athletics, boxing and soccer. It was not without critics, notably Bruce Carrington (1986) who noted the atypicality of the respondents whose narratives were featured ('not every black youth gets involved in sport', p. 5), the retrospective nature of the narrative accounts and inherent problems of the accuracy of recall, the narrowness of the range of sports considered and the inferences drawn from them, and the failure to address class relations. All of these comments were reasonable (if together they seemed a little churlish), but they should not detract from the profound influence of Cashmore's work on sport and youth studies more widely around that time (Cashmore, 2012 [1987]; Cashmore and Troyna, 1981; 2013 [1982]). In *Black Sportsmen* there were analytical points that still resonate over thirty years later (which presumably helps to explain the decision to republish). They include:

1   the prospect of blackness for kids;
2   all or nothing from families;
3   expectations of failure among teachers;
4   twice as hard for blacks.

Each tells its own tale around themes of identity, the perception of limited prospects for upward social mobility, the consequences of stereotypes and the impact of racism.

Almost a decade later, the second landmark volume was Grant Jarvie's (1991) edited collection *Sport, Racism and Ethnicity*. Wider in scope and variable in quality, it included chapters on the influence of racism on South Asian male youth (Fleming, 1991) and on young African-Caribbean and South Asian women (Lovell, 1991). Both were based on ethnographic studies, each within an educational context. The former was a typology of the experiences of racisms in a north London secondary school (Fleming, 1995); the latter was based at a community college in Coventry and was notable for also being one of the first feminist contributions to address in an empirical study the leisure lives of women from minority ethnic groups in Britain. From these, however, an understanding of youth sport *per se* can only be inferred (at best).

The remaining two landmark volumes were also edited collections. Published in 2001, the first, *'Race', Sport and British Society*, was edited by Ben Carrington and Ian McDonald. The second, *Sport and Challenges to Racism*, was edited by Jonathan Long and Karl Spracklen and published in 2011. These two volumes emanate from two of the British Universities at the vanguard of a sustained commitment to the sociology of 'ethnic relations' in sport and leisure – the University of Brighton (see, especially, Burdsey, 2007; 2011) and Leeds Metropolitan/ Beckett University (see, especially, Hylton, 2009; Spracklen, 2013). Coincidentally, with the three collections separated by ten-year gaps, each provides a snapshot of the emphases and priorities for researchers at the particular time, and helps to chart the progress and sophistication of the understanding of the complex issues that were addressed.

Chapters by Carrington and McDonald (2001b) on sub-elite cricket and by Johal (2001) on the engagement of South Asian males in soccer shed light on the experiences of youth sport for members of minority ethnic groups, but these were secondary to the main themes of racism and social exclusion. Extending the reach of the exposition of racism in sport internationally, Long and Spracklen's (2011a) volume confirmed its continued prevalence at elite and grass-roots levels. In the conclusion they note that sport should become a site of resistance and might include: 'demanding changes in sporting structures and procedures' and 'demanding representation in sports governance to try and pull the levers of power' (Long and Spracklen 2011c, p. 250). Rather than elaborating on this in relation to the infrastructure of British sport (which would inevitably embrace youth sport), however, they set out a manifesto for anti-racism through legislation, campaigning, education and action.

In summary then, it is clear that the links between ethnicity and youth sport have not been a major focal point for researchers other than in the sense that youth sport has been and remains a site for racism – and why wouldn't it be?

The policy domain

A review of sport policy since the early 1980s and of some of the evidence that has helped to inform it provides a further context for the consideration of ethnicity in relation to youth sport. As part of the Sport for All campaign, the then Sports Council (1982) launched a major policy document, *Sport in the Community . . . The Next Ten Years*. In order to increase participation target groups were identified, and these included ethnic minorities. Based on an assimilationist model of ethnic relations, schemes were devised and implemented often based on a limited and/or stereotypical appreciation of the groups for whom provision was intended – for instance, attempts were made to attract under-represented minority groups to: 'existing facilities for sports of *direct interest*' (Sports Council, 1982, p. 36; emphasis added).

The rationale for the choice of ethnic minorities as a target group was not argued or evidenced persuasively, at least not publicly; and the schemes seemed to be based on assumptions about stereotypes (Fleming, 2007 [1994]). At a time when, as Cashmore (2013 [1982]) demonstrated, some young African-Caribbean men were experiencing elite level success in working class sports, the absence of high profile South Asian sports performers seemed to be cause for concern and policy intervention. In short, and with the benefit of hindsight, this was all rather simplistic.

A policy update, *Sport in the Community – Into the 90's* (sic), was published by the Sports Council in 1988. By that time there was better evidence about patterns of actual participation, and it had become clear that South Asians were, indeed, under-represented. There was also an acknowledgement that: 'a lack of understanding [remained] about the needs of different ethnic minority groups, and in many areas service delivery is inadequate' (p. 30). An appetite for empirical work of wider scope and greater quality had been established and a study by Verma *et al.* (1991) was commissioned. Later published as *Winners and losers: Ethnic minorities in sport and recreation* (Verma and Darby, 1994), it addressed the intersections of ethnicity and gender among different minority ethnic groups. Its conclusions identified a set of factors that influenced involvement in sport and physical activity including the cultural traditions of minority ethnic groups, as well as the combination of racism and sexism from providers of sporting and recreational facilities and within society at large. Interestingly, it also noted the factors that affect *all* sports participants (e.g. age, class, gender, social skills and self-confidence) and challenged the suggestion that minority ethnic groups in general show less interest, enthusiasm and aptitude for sport and physical recreation than their white peers.

By 2000, Sport England had conducted an extensive survey of over 3,000 adults (the youngest of whom were sixteen), and consistent with findings of the General Household Survey in 1996, the data showed that minority ethnic groups were disproportionately under-represented (Rowe and Champion, 2000). As if to make the point about the dangers of treating all minority ethnic groups as a single lumpen mass, the data also revealed (among other things) that black African men and black other men and women were over-represented, while men and women who classified themselves as black Caribbean or Bangladeshi participated less than the averages for all men and all women. There were also some interesting data about patterns of participation in specific sports, but the analyses did not incorporate age as a factor. Importantly too, a sizeable minority (8 per cent) of all participants indicated that they had had a 'negative experience of sport due to ethnicity'.

The health benefits derived from physical activity are well established (Hardman and Stensel, 2009), and it was inevitable that different levels of engagement in sport would be linked to public health among children and young people (Maguire and Collins, 1998). Policy and media rhetoric associated with childhood obesity in particular has sometimes been reactionary and even sensational, but rigorous epidemiological reviews have shown trends linked to ethnicity. Specifically, having noted some methodological caveats, Fischbacher *et al.* (2004) concluded that low levels of physical activity among minority ethnic groups of South Asian origin may contribute to increased risk of diabetes and coronary heart disease. Drawing upon the *Health Survey for England (1999–2004)*, Williams *et al.* (2011) confirmed that even though South Asians born in the UK reported higher levels of physical activity than those born elsewhere, overall physical activity levels were very low among all South Asians.

In view of this, it is surprising that there were only fleeting mentions of ethnicity as a major consideration in *Driving up participation: The challenge for sport*, a collection of academic papers commissioned by Sport England (2004) to address priorities from the UK Government's strategy for sport and physical activity *Game Plan* (DCMS/Strategy Unit, 2002). For example, Rowe, Adams and Beasley (2004) re-stated the evidence of participation patterns from Sport England's (2000) survey, and Rowe *et al.* (2004) commented on the overall demographic profile of England with an acknowledgement of the importance of sensitivity to the barriers that impact on minority ethnic groups and: 'to provide the *types of activities that appeal to them* within environments that are accessible and welcoming' (p. 11; emphasis added). In contrast to the similar aspiration from over twenty years earlier (Sports Council, 1982 – above), however, this ambition was at least founded on the evidence of extensive surveys that explored not only participation patterns but preferences too (Rowe and Champion, 2000). There were also mentions of the influence of ethnicity in Long's (2004) exposition of the demographics of a greying society and a plea for recognition of the heterogeneity of older people, and in Kay's (2004) overview of the role of the family as a socialising agency into sport and variability in family structure linked to cultural factors. Overall, though, full and careful consideration of ethnicity is conspicuous by its absence and in particular in its relation to youth sport.

Even the excellent systematic review of literature on ethnicity, sport and physical recreation by Long *et al.* (2009, p. 28) pays only scant attention specifically to youth sport, noting that the Sports Equity Index (Sport England, 2005a) drew on the 2002 *Young People and Sport Survey* to demonstrate that, like their adult counterparts, young people (aged 6–16) from (Black and Minority Ethnic) communities had below average levels of participation for taking part in both casual (at least once a month) and regular (at least once a week) sport (excluding walking). Of particular concern is evidence from Broderson *et al.* (2007) and Woodfield *et al.* (2002) that these discrepancies are already well established by age 11. All in all, it is clear that the linkages between ethnicity and youth sport have been largely neglected by academic researchers.

In parallel with sport development policy, an important context for the engagement of young people in sport was (and continues to be) through schooling. During the 1980s, the physical education (PE) profession in Britain was slow to respond to the challenges posed by a culturally diverse society. Initially, curricula and pedagogy adopted a colour–blind approach (Bayliss, 1989), and the implication was clear: 'treating all children the same [meant] treating them all like white children and probably like white middle class children' (Williams, 1989, p. 163). There followed a problems approach to PE for minority ethnic groups where black and South Asian children and young people were seen as the problem rather than inappropriate curricula and teaching methods (Bayliss, 1983, 1989).

As part of an overall policy and practice imperative, multicultural PE was designed to cultivate empathy among children and young people, to help them to question prejudice and to develop their open-mindedness (National Curriculum Council, 1990). Predictably, it was the subject of scathing critique. Based on a continuation of a commitment to an assimilationist stance, there was an implicit notion of cultural superiority (Mullard, 1985) and of the introduction of a mechanism for coercion and control. More specifically, Cole (1986: p. 124) drew attention to the preoccupation with 'safe cultural sites' – of which PE was one (alongside art, dance, drama, music and domestic science) – and the tokenism which was caricatured as 'let's dress up and eat Chinese food' (Katz, 1982: p. 13) and 'saris, samosas and steel bands' (Troyna and Carrington, 1990). There were questionable assumptions about the potential of multicultural PE for enhancing the self-esteem of black and South Asian youth (Cole, 1986), as well as the possibility that cultural distinctiveness was reinforced unintended ways, racist stereotypes were consolidated, and ethnic antagonism exacerbated (Fleming, 1992). Most important of all, a multicultural approach to PE failed to acknowledge and address the centrality of racism in the experiences of young people from minority groups.

Later, in the aftermath of the death of Stephen Lawrence, the publication of the Macpherson Report (Home Office, 1999) was a pivotal moment in criminal justice as well as the politics of ethnic relations in Britain. It recommended amendments to the National Curriculum in order to value cultural diversity and prevent racism (Benn, 2000), but in spite of case study evidence (e.g. Benn *et al.*, 2011), the effects of any such changes are yet to be evidenced unequivocally. The challenge for the education sector was set out by Benn:

> The dilemma of moving towards greater valuing of cultural diversity is related to what Bullivant (1981) called the 'pluralist dilemma' in Western societies which results from the juxtaposition of different, but unequal, cultures within a democratic and liberal society.

If it is true that the National Curriculum in England and Wales homogenises the educational experiences of children and young people, then the same fundamental questions about multicultural education apply: what is the anchor for the homogeneity? In other words, the same as what/whom and based on what criteria?

Throughout, the effects of stereotyping continue to haunt the perceptions of many in the PE profession. They may not be as crass as some reported by Bayliss (1983, pp. 6–7) over thirty years ago, for instance: 'blacks will never make good swimmers because their bones are heavier'; 'blacks run faster because they have wider nostrils and can breathe in more oxygen'; and 'blacks have an extra muscle at the top of their legs which helps them run faster'. Yet anecdotally at least they have remained resilient to the contradictory empirical evidence (Fleming, 2001).

Ethnicity and youth sport – key themes and issues

Despite the neglect of ethnicity in considerations of youth sport for minority ethnic groups in Britain, there are some over-arching points to make. First, sport continues to act as a vehicle for the expression of ethnic identity and pride as well as a site of racism. Both shape the un/willingness of young people from minority ethnic groups to engage in sport and physical activity. Second, the history of sport development policy initiatives serve as a reminder that minority ethnic groups do not necessarily perceive and express their sporting preferences in the same way as providers anticipate, or as each other (Bi, 2011) – and there exists evidence of 'frustrated demand' (Rowe and Champion, 2000, p. 4). Third, there is something very familiar about many of the attempts to summarise the links between sports participation and ethnicity (and this chapter is no different). Yet there are still relatively unexplored areas of enquiry that add texture to appreciation the complexity of the young lives of members of minority ethnic groups – some of them from within the UK (Long et al., 2009), others with a valuable international dimension (e.g., Bandyopadhyay, 2011; Benn et al., 2011; Long and Spracklen, 2011). Fourth, there is a clear public health imperative related to sport and physical activity – particularly for young people and especially from groups who are under-represented. Some of the inability and/or unwillingness to take part is a matter of personal circumstances and individual choice. Yet when trends of non-participation among specific minority ethnic groups are evident, these transcend personal troubles and become public issues (Mills, 2000 [1959]). Fifth, a variety of campaigns and campaigning organisations have been launched that are committed to positive action, these can be found in an annotated appendix prepared by sportscotland (2001). Among the thirty-five initiatives listed, many are aimed at women (and presumably girls, in some instances at least) and have a local focus (e.g. Blackburn Asian Women's Project, Sandwell Asian Women's Exercise and Recreation Activities). Others are country-wide programmes (e.g. Sporting Equals, Scottish Asian Sports Association Competition), and others still have a focus on a specific sport (e.g. Tackle Racism in Rugby League, Basketball Rejects Racism).

Looking ahead, recommendations for sports policy linked to minority ethnic groups and sport have been synthesised by Long et al. (2009, pp. 62–64) – many are as important now as they were when published first. There are some that apply in particular to youth sport. Edited for brevity, they include:

- sport administrators should ensure that mainstream equality policies are integrated into sport;
- national governing bodies and other sport organisations/providers should promote racial equality and ensure a wider understanding of racisms that is fit for purpose;
- sports councils should be willing to take risks and innovate around sport and physical recreation to make gains;
- training is needed to offer those working in sport an understanding of the needs of minority ethnic communities;
- dialogue should be promoted with Black and minority ethnic communities and efforts made to empower members of local communities;
- good practice ideas and successes should be regularly disseminated.

Acknowledgements

I am extremely grateful to Ken Green and Andy Smith for their patience and forbearance during the preparation of this chapter.

References

Azzarito, L. and Macdonald, D. (2016). Unpacking gender/sexuality/disability/social class to understand the embodied experiences of young people in contemporary physical culture. In K. Green and A. Smith (eds) *The Routledge Handbook of Youth Sport*. London: Routledge.

Bandyopadhyay, K. (2010). Ed. *Why Minorities Play or Don't Play Soccer*. London: Routledge.

Banton, M. (2004). Race: as classification. In E. Cashmore (ed.) *Encyclopedia of Race and Ethnic Studies* (pp. 333–333). London: Routledge.

Bayliss, T. (1983). *Physical education in a multiethnic society*. London: Inner London Education Authority.

Bayliss, T. (1989). PE and racism: making changes, *Multicultural Teaching*, 7 (2), 18–22.

Benn, T. (2000). Valuing cultural diversity: the challenge for physical education. In S. Capel and S. Piotrowski (eds) *Issues in Physical Education* (pp. 64–77). London: Routledge.

Benn, T., Pfister, G. and Jawad, H. (2011) Eds. *Muslim Women and Sport*. London: Routledge.

Bi, S. (2011). Sporting equality for BME communities, *Journal of Policy Research in Tourism, Leisure and Events*, 3 (2), 204–208.

Bose, M. (2002). *History of Indian cricket*. Revised edition. London: Andre Deutsch.

Burdsey, D. (2007). *British Asians and Football: Culture, Identity, Exclusion*. London: Routledge.

Burdsey, D. (2011). *Race, Ethnicity and Football: Persisting Debates and Emergent Issues*. London: Routledge.

Carrington, B. and McDonald, I. (2001a). Eds. *'Race', Sport and British Society*. London: Routledge.

Carrington, B. and McDonald, I. (2001b). Whose game is it anyway? Racism in local league cricket. In B. Carrington and I. McDonald (eds) *'Race', Sport and British Society* (pp. 49–69). London: Routledge.

Carrington, B. (1986). Social mobility, ethnicity and sport, *British Journal of Sociology of Education*, 7 (1), 3–18.

Cashmore, E. (2004). Race: as signifier. In E. Cashmore (ed.) *Encyclopedia of Race and Ethnic Studies* (pp. 334–336). London: Routledge.

Cashmore, E. (2012 [1987]). *The Logic of Racism*. London: Routledge Revivals.

Cashmore, E. (2013 [1982]). *Black Sportsmen*. London: Routledge Revivals.

Cashmore, E. and Troyna, B. (1981). Just for white boys? Elitism, racism and research, *Multiracial Education*, 10 (1), 43–48.

Cashmore, E. and Troyna, B. (2013 [1982]). Eds. *Black Youth in Crisis*. London: Routledge Revivals.

Cole, M. (1986). Multicultural education and the politics of racism in Britain, *Multicultural Teaching*, 5 (1), 20–24.

Department for Culture Media and Sport/Strategy Unit. (2002). *Game Plan: a strategy for delivering Government's sport and physical activity objectives*. London: DCMS/Strategy Unit.

Farrell, L. and Sands, M.A. (2002). Investigating the economic and demographic determinants of sporting participation in England, *Journal of the Royal Statistical Society: Series A (Statistics in Society)*, 165 (2), 335–348.

Fischbacher, C.M., Hunt, S. and Alexander, L. (2004). How physically active are South Asians in the United Kingdom? A literature review, *Journal of Public Health*, 26 (3), 250–258.

Fleming, S. (1991). Sport, schooling and South Asian male youth culture. In G. Jarvie (ed.) *Sport, Racism and Ethnicity* (pp. 30–57). London: Falmer.

Fleming, S. (1992). Multiculturalism in the physical education curriculum: the case of South Asian male youth, dance and South Asian dance, *Multicultural Teaching* 11 (1), 35–38.

Fleming, S. (1995). *'Home and Away': Sport and South Asian Male Youth*. Aldershot: Avebury.

Fleming, S. (2001). 'Racial' science and black and South Asian physicality. In B. Carrington and I. McDonald (eds) *Race, Sport and British Society* (pp. 105–120). London: Routledge.

Fleming, S. (2007 [1994]). Sport and South Asian youth: the perils of false universalism and stereotyping. In A. Tomlinson (ed.) *The Sport Studies Reader* (pp. 289–297). London: Routledge.

Hardman, A.E. and Stensel, D.J. (2009). *Physical Activity and Health – The Evidence Explained*. 2nd edition. Abingdon: Routledge.

Holland, B.L. (1997). Surviving leisure time racism: the burden of racial harassment on Britain's black footballers, *Leisure Studies*, 16 (4), 261–277.

Home Office (1999). The Stephen Lawrence Inquiry: Report of an Inquiry by Sir William Macpherson of Cluny, Cm 4262–I. London: Home Office.

Hylton, K. (2009). *Race and Sport: Critical Race Theory*. London: Routledge.

Hylton, K. (2010). How a turn to critical race theory can contribute to our understanding of race, racism and anti-racism in sport, *International Review for the Sociology of Sport*, 45 (3), 335–354.

Hylton, K. and Long, J. (2005). Race, sport and leisure: lessons from critical race theory, *Leisure Studies*, 24 (1), 81–98.

Ismond, P. (2003). *Black and Asian Athletes in British Sport and Society – A Sporting Chance?* Basingstoke: Palgrave Macmillan.

James, C.L.R. (2013 [1963]). *Beyond a Boundary*. 50th Anniversary edition. Durham, NC: Duke University Press.

Jarvie, G. (1991). ed. *Sport, Racism and Ethnicity*. London: Falmer.

Johal, S. (2001). Playing their own game: the South Asian football experience. In J. Long and K. Spracklen (eds) *Sport and Challenges to Racism* (pp. 153–169). Basingstoke, Hampshire: Palgrave Macmillan.

Katz, J.H. (1982). Multicultural education: games educators play, *Multiracial Education*, 10 (2), 11–18.

Kay, T. (2004). The family factor in sport: a review of family factors affecting sports participation. In *Driving up Participation: The Challenge for Sport* (pp. 39–60). London: Sport England.

King, C. (2004). *Offside Racism – Playing the White Man*. Oxford: Berg.

Kremer, J., Trew, K. and Ogle, S. (1997). Eds. *Young People's Involvement in Sports*. London: Routledge.

Long, J. (2004). Sport and the ageing population: do older people have a place in driving up participation in sport? In *Driving up Participation: The Challenge for Sport* (pp. 28–38). London: Sport England.

Long, J., Hylton, K., Spracklen, K., Ratna, A. and Bailey, S. (2009). *Sysematic Review of Literature on Black and Minority Ethnic Communities in Sport and Physical Recreation*. London: Sport England.

Long, J. and Spracklen, K. (2011a). Eds. *Sport and Challenges to Racism*. Basingstoke, Hampshire: Palgrave Macmillan

Long, J. and Spracklen, K. (2011b). Positioning anti-racism in sport and sport in anti-racism. In J. Long and K. Spracklen (eds) *Sport and Challenges to Racism* (pp. 3–18). Basingstoke, Hampshire: Palgrave Macmillan

Long, J. and Spracklen, K. (2011c). So what has changed (and what has to change)? In J. Long and K. Spracklen (eds) *Sport and Challenges to Racism* (pp. 247–256). Basingstoke, Hampshire: Palgrave Macmillan

Lovell, T. (1991). Sport, racism and young women. In G. Jarvie (ed.) *Sport, Racism and Ethnicity* (pp. 58–73). London: Falmer.

McGuire, B. and Collins, D. (1998). Sport, ethnicity and racism: the experience of Asian heritage boys, *Sport, Education and Society*, 3 (1), 79–88.

Mills, C.W. (2000 [1959]). *The Sociological Imagination*. Oxford: Oxford University Press.

National Curriculum Council (1990). *The Whole Curriculum*. London: NCC.

Office for National Statistics (2012). *Ethnicity and National Identity in England and Wales 2011*. London: ONS.

Rees, P., Wohland, P., Norman, P. and Boden, P. (2012). Ethnic population projections for the UK, 2001–2051, *Journal of Population Research*, 29 (1), 45–89.

Rowe, N., Adams, R. and Beasley, N. (2004). Driving up participation in sport: the social context, the trends, the prospects and the challenges. In *Driving up Participation: The Challenge for Sport* (pp. 6–13). London: Sport England.

Rowe, N., Beasley, N. and Adams, R. (2004). Sport, physical activity and health: future prospects for improving the health of the nation. In *Driving up Participation: The Challenge for Sport* (pp. 14–26). London: Sport England.

Rowe, N. and Champion, R. (2000). *Sports Participation and Ethnicity in England*. London: Sport England.

Saeed, A. and Kilvington, D. (2011). British-Asians and racism within contemporary English football, *Soccer and Society*, 12 (5), 602–612.

Sports Council (1982). *Sport in the Community . . . The Next Ten Years*. London: Sports Council.

Sports Council (1988). *Into the 90's*. London: Sports Council.

Sport England (2004). *Driving up Participation: The Challenge for Sport*. London: Sport England.

sportscotland (2001). *Sport and Ethnic Minority Communities: Aiming at Social Inclusion*. Edinburgh: sportscotland.

Spracklen, K. (2013). *Whiteness and Leisure*. Basingstoke: Palgrave Macmillan.

Tobias, P.V. (1972 [1961]). The meaning of race. In P. Baxter and B. Sansom (eds) Race and Social Difference (pp. 19–43). Harmondsworth: Penguin.

Troyna, B. and Carrington, B. (1990). *Education, Racism and Reform*. London: Routledge.

UNESCO (1972 [1964]). Proposals on the biological aspects of race. In P. Baxter and B. Sansom (eds) *Race and Social Difference* (pp. 68–73). Harmondsworth: Penguin.

Van Den Berghe, P.L. (2004). Race: as synonym. In E. Cashmore (ed.) *Encyclopedia of Race and Ethnic Studies* (pp. 336–337). London: Routledge.

Verma, G.K. and Darby, D.S. (1994). *Winners and Losers*. London: Falmer.

Verma, G.K., MacDonald, A., Darby, D. and Carroll, R. (1991). *Sport and Recreation with Special Reference to Ethnic Minorities*. Manchester: Manchester University Press.

Watson, B. and Scraton, S. (2013). Intersectionality and Leisure Studies. *Leisure Studies*, 32 (1), 35–47.

Williams, A. (1989). Physical education in a multicultural context. In A. Williams (ed.) *Issues in Physical Education for the Primary Years* (pp. 160–172). Lewes: Falmer.

Williams, E.D., Stamatakis, E., Chandola, T. and Hamer, M. (2011). Assessment of physical activity levels in South Asians in the UK: findings from the Health Survey for England, *Journal of Epidemiology and Community Health*, 65 (6), 517–521.

28

SPORT, YOUTH AND RELIGION

Kristin Walseth

A chapter such as this cannot cover all religions and their attitudes to sports. Neither is it possible to cover all the national examples of religious organizations offering sports to youth. Because it is impossible to be representative of all of them, I have chosen to focus on Christianity and Islam because these are the religions most studied by scholars linking youth, sport and religion. Because most of the research focusing on sports is from western countries (Europe, North America, Oceania), there is a clear bias in the chapter. The chapter will be structured around a focus on Christianity and sport followed by Islam and sport. These sections will focus on the understanding of physical activity and sports in the two religions, followed by a description of Christian and Muslim organizations offering sports to youth and, finally, on how Christian and Muslim athletes manage their religious identity within the sport context. A distinction is drawn between Christianity and Islam as religions (official Christianity/Islam) and belief in Christianity/Islam as a manifestation of religiosity (unofficial Christianity/Islam) (Kamrava, 2006).

Christianity

Understandings of sports in Christianity

The relationship between organized religion and sports has not always been congenial. Within a Christian context, medieval preachers often denounced those festive gatherings and sporting contests because they were invariably occasions for drunkenness and often associated with riots and bloodshed. The issue of whether sports should be played on Sundays was an important source of friction between sport and religion in the eighteenth and nineteenth centuries. A shift in the search for sporting respectability came in the mid-nineteenth century, as the ideology of Muscular Christianity became widely adopted in English public schools. Athletes and the religious became allied in the promotion of health and fitness of mind and body, along with the quest for self-improvement and the moral elevation of the soul (Magdalinski and Chandler, 2002). In both Britain and the United States, the Muscular Christianity movement began not as a passion for competitive games but rather as a concern for healthy diet, fresh air, and firm muscles. Good health seemed especially scarce in England's industrial cities. Health crusaders considered the body as a sacred temple of god, requiring regular attention and cleansing (Baker, 2007: 38).

Such an alliance also paved the way for the later development of athletic missionaries, as well as the YMCA. According to Baker (2007), the ideological pioneers of Muscular Christianity came from highly privileged backgrounds, were trained in the classics at private boys' schools, and received degrees from universities. What these men pronounced from their elite position, the YMCA implemented at the grassroots. The YMCA was not an easy convert to the gospel of sport, however. It was born of Protestant piety, not playfulness. In England, the land of the association's birth, it initially barely endorsed physical exercise programmes. The goal of the YMCA at this time was to 'improve the spiritual, mental and social condition of young men and to promote evangelical religion among young men' (Baker, 2007: 48). The Church's suspicious and ambivalent attitude toward play, pleasure and sport is underlined by Johnston (1983).

It should be noted that the YMCA shared a pronounced gender bias with Muscular Christianity, which represented a reaction against the feminization of American middle-class culture that occurred during the first half of the nineteenth century. It was assumed that both men and women could benefit from proper diets, healthy walks and gymnastic exercises, but competitive sports were not perceived as the proper sphere for women. The stronger the emphasis on competitive sports, the greater the identification of Muscular Christianity with manliness (Baker, 2007). This observation has parallels in Messner's (1992) work on sport and masculinities. Messner shows how the development of modern sports in the United States in the nineteenth century was concerned with socializing boys into a certain kind of manliness and building character.

In Dahl's (2008) study of the comprehension of body, movement and sport in Christianity, Islam and Buddhism, she identifies such Christian Protestant values as asceticism, rationality, individuality, determination and work ethic. She concluded that these values fit well with the values of competitive sports. However, leading scholars today argue that while the quest for excellence in any human endeavor is a positive goal, success, enhanced performance and winning in sports are certainly not the central messages of the Christian gospel (Baker and Parker, 2013; Brock, 2012). Leading Catholic voices, such as Novak (1994), point to the Protestant work ethic and Marxist ideology as the major forces that transformed sport into a soulless utilitarian endeavor.

Christian organizations offering sports to youth

This brief historical overview linking sport and Christianity explains the relationship that exists today between sport and Christianity in the United States, as well as the large numbers of organizations mixing sports and evangelism. Christian religious symbols and discourses are more common and present in everyday life in the United States than in Europe. This is particularly true for sports. However, in recent decades similar developments have occurred in Europe. U.S. groups such as Fellowship of Christian Athletes and Athletes in Action (AIA) now have sister organizations in Europe such as Christians in Sport in Britain and Christian Sports Contact (KRIK) in Norway and Sweden. The common goal of these organizations seems to be evangelism, and sport has become a central way of reaching out to athletes. The Norwegian organization KRIK stands out as a particular interesting organization since it is run for and by youth. KRIK is the fastest-growing religious organization in Norway and arranges youth camps with thousands of participants and hundreds of youth volunteering as leaders. Even though the goal of KRIK is evangelism, the youth who participate in the organization seem to seek KRIK out because of the social aspect of the activities, and because the sporting activities offered are less concerned with performance and competition than sport activities within ordinary sport clubs (Storli, 2011; Trysnes, 2010).

Schroeder and Scribner's (2006) study of an evangelical Christian college in the United States shows that Christianity played a significant role in athletic department's cultures by constraining its membership, influencing its pedagogy and guiding department decisions. The morals taught in the department – hard work, discipline, perseverance, humility and graciousness – were connected to the Christian faith by coaches who believed in these assumptions and incorporated prayer into the athletic experience. Faith influenced how athletes were dealt with. Coaches were concerned with their athletes spiritually, emotionally, socially and academically. Coaches were expected to be role models. Outwardly, winning was not valued as much for the outcome as for the process. However, there were other indications that winning was of primary importance to the culture. The clearest evidence of winning's importance was the dismissal of a coach that many participants praised for improving the moral quality of his players. His contract was not renewed after a season where his team had poor athletic results (Schroeder and Scribner, 2006: 50). Another study from Canada reported on a local church-sponsored hockey league, which was successful when they collectively decided to play hockey in a manner that reflected Christian values. Fair play was a stated goal in the league and body contact, fights, swearing on the ice and drinking beer in the locker room were prohibited (Dunn and Stevenson, 1998). The mere existence of this hockey league indicates that there are aspects of competitive sports, such as ice hockey, which are difficult to handle for Christian athletes. Thus, we shall now turn to the experiences of Christian athletes in sports.

Religiosity among Christian athletes

Hoffman (1992) argues that there might be conflict between Christianity and the actions required in many competitive sports. Studies of elite athletes associated with AIA indicated that some of the elite athletes avoided moral conflict by clearly separating their religious beliefs from sports participation. They asked no questions and played as everyone else did (Stevenson, 1991, 1997). Such an approach – that accepts unethical and violent behavior on the field of play but not off it – is what Walsh and Guilianotti (2007) aptly term 'white line fever', whereby sporting arenas are special spheres where the rules of life do not apply. Nonetheless, most of the elite Christian athletes in Stevenson's studies were troubled by conflicts between their religious beliefs and what their actions as athletes. In practice, these athletes sometimes found it impossible to give full expression to their Christian faith. Despite their strong commitment to their faith, some admitted to compromising their Christian identity because they needed to be accepted by the team or in their sport. Examples of dilemmas mentioned included parties and drinking or from violations of the accepted rules of a sport, such as holding an opponent's shirt, pushing an opponent when the referee was not aware, injuring opponents (Stevenson, 1991, 1997).

Even though research illustrates the dilemmas experienced by some Christian athletes, as well as the fact that athletes drop out of sport due to these dilemmas (Neale, 1969; Stevenson, 1991, 1997), anecdotal evidence suggests that most elite athletes who identify themselves as Christians do not play sports differently to others (Coakley, 2007). Some stories indicate that they merge their religious beliefs and sport participation by emphasizing the ascetic aspects of sport. Asceticism refers to discipline, self-denial, and avoiding bodily pleasures. Embracing this philosophy helps athletes give moral meaning to their actions in sports (Coakley, 2007).

The studies referred to above are few and focus on young men involved in religious organizations (AIA, an evangelical Christian college, and a Christian hockey league). According to Coakley (2007), there have been no studies of Christian athletes who are not members of similar organizations. This is underlined by Watson and Parker (2013) who argue that there is a distinct lack of interview-based research that explores how modern-day Christian athletes reconcile their religious beliefs with modern sporting culture. Moreover, the experiences of Christian female athletes seems to be completely absent. As we will see, this stands in marked contrast to the growing literature on Muslim girls' experience in sports.

Islam

Understandings of sports in Islam

In Islam, physical activity is perceived as important first and foremost because exercising is interpreted as a way of taking care of the body and the body is perceived as a gift from Allah. It is, therefore, important for Muslims to take care and not damage their bodies – through drugs and alcohol, for example (Walseth and Fasting, 2003). Islam encourages Muslims to be strong and to seek the means of strength (Amara, 2008). Moreover, physical activity is important in Islam due to the recreational aspect of Islam. The Islamic literature, particular the hadiths (reports of the sayings or actions of the Prophet and his companions), are full of stories about the Prophet and how he encouraged people to be involved in physical activities. Al-Qaradawy (1992) interpreted one such hadith to mean that the lives of Muslims should consist of both seriousness and play, and that all ought to have some leisure time. The Islamic literature also tells us that the second caliph, Umar Ibn Khattab, stated: 'Teach your children swimming and archery, and tell them to jump on the horse's back' (Qaradawy, 1992: 296). There is, in addition, another strong hadith that tells the story of the Prophet who raced with his wife Aisha in order to please her, to enjoy himself and to set an example for his companions. Aisha said: 'I raced with the Prophet and beat him in the race. Later, when I had put on some weight, we raced again and he won.' Then he said, referring to the previous occasion: 'this cancels that [a draw]' (Qaradawy, 1992: 293). This last example seems to be especially important for Muslim women because it explicitly shows that Muhammad requested women to run.

Due to the Islamic texts' positive attitudes toward physical activity and sport, one might expect all Muslims to be very physically active and involved in sports. Muslim youth are, however, significantly underrepresented in sports in Europe (Benn *et al.*, 2011; Strandbu and Bakken, 2007; Walseth and Fasting, 2004). One reason for this is that other aspects of Islam seem to function as practical barriers to youths' sports participation (particularly for girls). Of particular importance here is the Islamic ideal of gender segregation and the use of the hijab (the headscarf worn by Muslim women).

In Amara's (2008) *Introduction to the study of sport in the Muslim world*, he included the Fatwa (a ruling on a matter of Islamic law, issued by a recognized religious authority) on the question of sport (www.islamonline.net). The Islam Online website has a strong link with the European Council of Fatwa and Research. The Fatwa has included some tips for Muslim practising sports:

1   A Muslim should not occupy himself with sports to the extent that leads to neglecting religious and other duties.
2   A Muslim is not permitted to give himself loose rein in practicing sports in a way that involves inflicting harm on others. Practicing sports in crowded streets, for example, thus causing traffic jam is not an Islamic way of example.
3   Blind fanaticism in favor or against a team has nothing to do with Islam, for this really contradicts the Islamic teachings calling for unity and love.
4   While practicing sports there should be no room for foul words, bad behavior and slandering.

5   Islam does not allow matches or games that involve both sexes, in a way that opens channels for seduction, temptation and corruption.

6   Islam rejects also all games and sports that stir sexual urge or encourage moral perversion such as women practicing dancing and being watched by the public.

(Amara, 2008: 538)

The argument that sport is encouraged in Islam, providing it does not take precedence over faith, is also underlined by Jawad, Al-Sinani and Benn (2011). Similarly, the argument that sport should not be too *exciting* for the male audience is underlined in Abdelrahman's (1992) interview of religious leaders in Egypt.

Muslim organizations offering sport to youth

While Christian organizations offering sporting activities to their members has been a common phenomena for decades, Muslim organizations are new actors in this arena. In Britain, Amara and Henry (2010) show that Muslim organizations offering sports activities to their members have become a common phenomenon, particularly in cities with substantial Muslim populations such as London, Leicester and Birmingham. Muslim organizations in these cities offer a range of sports activities from karate and badminton to fitness, swimming as well as recreational activities for the elderly.

Amara and Henry's (2011) study reveals that the religious criteria for the selection and organization of sports activities are constructed around *Shari'a* guidance (the moral code and religious law of Islam). The general (minimum) rules that are adopted first and foremost concern the non-mixing of sexes. Other important parameters involve the dress code in a public domain (e.g. in a sports hall), general Islamic rules of *halal* (permitted) and *haram* (forbidden), and a code of conduct which, among other things, regulates relations between the Muslim community and other communities, including the laws of the state. Amara and Henry's (2011) study indicates that practicing sports is seen as a religious obligation. Nonetheless, the us and them dichotomy, the prejudice against Muslim communities, and the subsequent lack of funding opportunities are limiting the sports activities offered by Muslim communities in Britain (Amara and Henry, 2010).

In Norway, a similar development has taken place, though on a much smaller scale than in Britain. Walseth (2015) shows that Muslim organizations in Norway offer sports as a way of gathering Muslim youth together. The sports offered are influenced by Islamic theology. The findings indicate that the general Islamic rules that are adopted first and foremost concern the non-mixing of the sexes something that is particularly evident in the context of swimming. Other theologically influenced frames mentioned were sport during Ramadan and attitudes towards violent sports activities. When asked about the religious criteria for the selection and organization of sporting activities, Muslim sports organizations in Norway responded that they chose sports activities that appeared to be particularly popular among youth and did not offer sports activities mentioned in Islamic literature such as riding horses, wrestling or archery. This is similar to findings in Amara and Henry's (201) British study, in which the selection of sports activities tends to be dictated by the availability of sports facilities and not necessarily by the literal interpretation of the Islamic texts.

The participants in the Norwegian study had different attitudes toward *violent* sports such as boxing. Some of the participants stressed that they were not willing to support sports that were violent because this was seen as being in conflict with the Islamic ethos. Their argument is in accordance with a Fatwa on the question of boxing (Amara, 2008), which argues that boxing should not be permitted, although others accepted the practice of all sports being officially recognized by the sports federations.

Mosques in the Norwegian study offered some sex-segregated sporting activities for women only (mostly swimming, but also some badminton and volleyball). These activities were arranged by each women's committee within the mosque, though none of the mosques has female teams competing in the national leagues. The study revealed that, within Muslim organizations, sports activities for boys and men were more common than for girls and women. Some mosques have established their own cricket and football teams for boys. The goal behind the initiatives appeared to be to support Muslim (male) youth in their identity work. The organizations wanted their youth to develop identities as Norwegian Muslims, indicating that the ultimate goal is to be well-integrated (having education, jobs) as well as proud of one's identity as Muslims (Walseth, 2015).

Religiosity among Muslim athletes

There has been a substantial growth in research on Muslim youth and sport over the last ten to twenty years, within which two different approaches can be discerned. The first focus has been on sport in Muslim societies including, for example, sporting heroines in the Muslim world (Hargreaves, 2000) and the opportunities and barriers girls and young women in Muslim countries face in relation to sports participation (Benn *et al.*, 2011; Pfister, 2000, Sehlikoglu, 2013; Tlili, 2010; Walseth and Fasting, 2003). The second and most common focus has been on religiosity among Muslims living in Diasporas and, more specifically, how this affects their involvement in physical activity and sports (Ahmad, 2011; Benn *et al.*, 2011; Farooq and Parker, 2009; Palmer, 2009; Ratna, 2011; Strandbu, 2005; Walseth, 2006).

The main source of research on Muslim youth and sport in Muslim countries is a collection edited by Benn *et al.* (2011), entitled *Muslim Women and Sport*. Among other things, the various contributors highlight the challenges and explore the opportunities for Muslim women in sports in the Muslim countries of Bahrain, Iran, Oman, Syria, Turkey, Palestine, Arab Emirates, Bosnia, Morocco and Iraq. The book illustrates the diversity of barriers women encounters in sports. This variety is, of course, due to the great diversity of political and national contexts. As an example, Koca and Hacisoftaoglu (2011) reveal how one female Muslim elite athlete in Turkey fought for the right to wear Islamic dress in competition, while Muslim sportswomen in other Muslim countries adopted Western dress and demanded acceptance of their decision by their families and peers. Most of the authors in this collection concluded that women's sports tend to be less valued than men's sports, though it should be stressed that this seems to be more of a cultural than a religious issue. Another common issue in the book is the focus on body culture and Islamic concern for modesty.

Muslim women's participation in elite sports witnessed a breakthrough in the 1984 Olympics when Nawel Moutawakel from Morocco became the first Muslim woman to win a goal medal. Another factor influencing Muslim women's sporting options around that time was the first staging of the Islamic Women Games in 1993. The Games involved only female athletes and the competitions were barred to male attendees and the media. The objective of the games was to create suitable conditions for the participation of women in sporting activities in compliance with Islamic codes. The games have been controversial among some western feminists. Some argue that Muslim women instead should fight for the opportunity to participate in the Olympics. The *Atlanta plus* project run by a French feminist argued for the exclusion of Muslim countries from the Olympics if they did not allow participation of female athletes from their countries (Amara, 2008). The perspective has been influential. At the London Olympics in 2012, after considerable pressure from the International Olympic Committee, every national delegation had at least one female athlete representing.

A study of young Egyptian Muslim women's involvement in sports (Walseth and Fasting, 2003) found that the women interpreted Islam in a way that encouraged participation in sports. All the informants noted, however, that Islam preferred Muslim women to wear the hijab. Some of the informants thought this was a barrier for their sporting participation because they wore a kind of veil (krimar and nikab) which, in addition to covering the hair, also covered the chest. It was, according to these informants, almost impossible to practice their sport while wearing this veil. As a result, these women had to exercise at home or in sex-segregated training studios. The informants thought that participation in sports was almost impossible because of the way sport was organized in Egypt at that time. Since there were very few sex-segregated sporting arenas, these women could not participate in competitive sports. However, the women stressed that it was not the requirements concerning veils and sex segregation that limited their participation in sports. Rather, according to these women, it was the Egyptian society's secular organization of sport that limited them.

In the Muslim Diaspora, some of the same experiences recurred. Recent research underscores the struggle young Muslim women continue to face when they try to combine their right to religious expression with physical activity and participation in sports in Europe, North America and Australia (Ahmad, 2011; Jiwani and Rail, 2010; Manal and Oliver, 2012; Palmer, 2009; Ratna, 2011). The studies by Ratna (2010) and Ahmad (2011) reveal that British Asian girls choose to fight for the right to play football (soccer) while maintaining their religious identity. The British Asian female footballers in Ratna's study negotiated their entrance into sports using various techniques. Some made reference to the Koran to empower themselves and justify their participation in football. Some engaged in the establishment of Muslim sports organizations to ensure that they could play football within an Islamic framework, while others preferred to oppose sexism and racism by focusing on becoming highly skilled female footballers.

One of the especially significant issues identified by researchers is the lack of gender-segregated sports facilities and the lack of recognition of the hijab as part of sporting gear in Western countries (Ahmad, 2011; Benn *et al.*, 2011a; Dagkas et.al., 2011; Guerin *et al.*, 2003; Jiwani and Rail, 2010; Wray, 2002). Ahmad's (2011) research illustrated how the hijab was a barrier to sport participation in Britain where football organizations discriminated against Muslim women, as evidenced in the FIFA hijab ban in 2007.[1] The veiled Muslim women in her study challenged traditional cultural ideals by competing in football at the Women's Islamic Games in Iran. The games became a safety zone where religious identities were not threatened, and where the hijab did not present a barrier. The women not only negotiated their values by rejecting cultural ideals of femininities while holding onto their Muslim identity, but also negotiated these values within British football and found a space for themselves representing Britain in the Women's Islamic Games. Nonetheless, the wearing of the hijab remains a contested issue in Western countries. Pfister (2011) writes that there has been a dramatic increase in the number of Muslim girls wearing the hijab in Denmark in recent years. 'Doing Islam has become a widespread habit, in some cases almost a fashion', according to Pfister (2011: 61). The wearing of the hijab is often perceived by non-Muslims as a sign of subordination and discrimination. However, Muslim girls claim various reasons for wearing it. For some, it is a reflexive choice and sign of resistance while, for others, wearing the hijab is an embodiment of faith, an expression of the belief that covering their bodies is the right way to be in the world (Pfister, 2011).

Studies by Benn *et al.* (2011a), Strandbu (2005; 2012) and Wray (2002) show how young Muslim women's faith is embodied and how sports challenge women's right to embody their faith. Strandbu's studies of Norway concluded that some of the Muslim girls actually preferred gender-segregated physical activity. Their reasons cannot be attributed to strict parents that deny their daughters' participation in any physical activity whatsoever. Instead, the girls had internalized cultural ideas and values. That explains, moreover, why participating in gender-integrated sports embarrassed the girls. The girls opted out of gender-integrated physical activity because they did not see it as a natural thing to do.

The blurring of culture and religion in these stories is not new; it can be seen in older research (Sfeir, 1985; Zaman, 1997). The inter-relationship between religion and culture is also described in Benn *et al.*'s (2011b) book, *Muslim Women and Sport*. Despite the increased focus on Islam as *embodied*, there does also seem to be a recent tendency among young European Muslims to separate culture from religion (Ramadan, 2004). This has consequences for sport participation in the sense that culture seems to inhibit Muslim girls' involvement in sports insofar as traditional gender roles give girls responsibility for younger siblings and traditional female household chores. In separating culture from religiosity, Muslim girls give themselves an opportunity to concentrate exclusively on the religious sources of prescriptions concerning sports, while previous research was shown to encourage Muslim women to participate in sports (Amara, 2008; Jawad *et al.*, 2011; Walseth and Fasting, 2003). These arguments corroborate the findings of Ratna (2011) and Walseth (2006): By separating religion and culture, Muslims can argue that Islam supports women's involvement in sporting activities.

The great diversity within a group of young Muslim women is also stressed in Palmer's (2009) study from South Australia. The study explored the ways in which a group of young Muslim refugee women experienced playing on a football team. The study focused on how these women articulated their social identities through the traditions of Islam and the resources of Western popular culture, and how this was expressed on the football pitch.

Because Muslim women are less likely than men to be involved in sports in both Muslim countries and Europe (Benn *et al.*, 2011b), the focus of research has mainly been one the reasons for this divergence. As such, the research on Muslims and sports has focused on women and not men. Some new research has focused on Muslim athletes and their experiences of combining religiosity with sport participation.

Burdsey's (2010) study of religiosity in English first-class cricket reveals how Islam plays a major part in players' lives, but does not necessarily influence their cricket careers *per se*. Religion seems to be the driving force behind the players' identity construction, with sport serves as a mere tool to assist that process. Farooq and Parker's (2009) study of sports and physical education in independent Muslim schools in Britain placed a similar emphasis on sports and illustrated how young Muslim males used sport and religion as tools in their reflexive identity work. Sports were perceived as strategic sites for the development of Muslim masculine identities.

Current status and future research

Based on the above, it seems evident that Christian and Muslim youth can find religious support for their participation in sports. Both Islam and Christianity encourage youth to take care of their bodies and their health. In Christianity, these arguments have historical origins in *Muscular Christianity*. In Islam, the basis is the hadiths about the Prophet encouraging Muslims to be involved in physical activities. Despite such encouragement, sport participation can create problems for athletes due to the culture of modern sports. As an example, to hurt one's opponent is controversial in Islamic as well as Christian theology. Despite these dilemmas, on the field Christian and Muslim athletes do not appear to play sports differently than others. In Islam, however, the differences between boys' and girls' approaches to sports are greater than among

Christians. One evident reason for this is Islam's prescriptions for sex segregation. A survey conducted in Norway on youth participation in sports underlines this point. The survey found that youth (both boys and girls) who identified themselves as Christians were more likely to participate in sport clubs than either youth who belonged to other religions or youth identifying with no religion. In contrast, the survey showed that being a Muslim made it less likely that a girl would participate in sport clubs (Strandbu and Bakken, 2007).

The encouragement to practice sports in the religion's ethos is embraced and incorporated by religious organizations. While Christian organizations have been offering sports to youth for decades, Muslim organizations are only just beginning. Both seem to have evangelism as a goal, though Muslim organizations seem to have a broader focus which includes integration work. From a political perspective, Christian evangelism through sports seems to be perceived as less controversial than Islamic evangelism. This can be seen in the problems that Muslim organizations encounter in obtaining political and financial support for their sports activities and in the open critique of these activities as segregated activities that prevent integration (Amara and Henry, 2010). There is a lack of research on these organizations. Because the Muslim organizations are new agents in this field, it is important to follow their development. At present, we only have research on this from a British and Norwegian perspective. It would be interesting to discover whether this is a development taking place in other Western countries as well. In particular, we need knowledge about the purposes of such organizations.

The experiences of Muslim youth in sports in the Diaspora have been a central focus of research in the past decade. Here we find a wealth of studies mainly focusing on Muslim girls. In contrast, few studies have focused on how Muslim male athletes manage their religiosity in sports. Even more evident is the almost total lack of studies that have focused on how religiosity is dealt with by Christian youth athletes. An obvious reason for this unequal and biased focus is that Muslim girls have been less involved in sports than their male counterparts and Christian youth. As such, the natural focus of research has been on exploring the reason for this absence, and collecting knowledge on how sports can be adapted to Muslim girls' needs. However, it can also be argued that the continued focus is a result of Orientalism and a Western research obsession with 'the Other' (Said, 2003). It should be noted that the lack of research on Christian youth and their experiences in combining religiosity and sports constitutes a knowledge gap and a blind spot in research on sport, youth and religion.

Note

1   The FIFA hijab ban was lifted in 2012 after the FIFA medical committee found no problems with two tested soccer hijab prototypes.

References

Abdelrahman, N.A. (1992). *Women and Sport in the Islamic Society*. Alexandria: Alexandria University.

Ahmad, A. (2011). British football: Where are the Muslim female footballers? Exploring the connections between gender, ethnicity and Islam. *Soccer and Society*, *12*(3): 443–456.

Amara, M. (2008). An introduction to the study of sport in the Muslim world. In Houlihan, B. (ed), *Sport and Society. A Student Introduction* (pp. 532–552). Los Angeles: Sage, 2nd edition.

Amara, M. and Henry, I. (2010). Sport, Muslim identities and cultures in the UK, an emerging policy issue: Case studies of Leicester and Birmingham. *European Sport Management Quarterly*, *10*: 419–443.

Baker, W.J. (2007). *Playing with God. Religion and Modern Sport*. Cambridge: Harvard University Press.

Benn, T., Dagkas, S. and Jawad, H. (2011). Embodied faith: Islam, religious freedom and educational practices in physical education. *Sport, Education and Society*, *16*(1): 17–34.

Benn T., Pfister, G. and Jawad, H. (2011). *Muslim Women and Sport*. New York: Routledge.

Brock, B. (2012). Discipline, Sport and the religion of Winners: Paul on running to win the prize. 1 Corinthians 9: 24–27. *Studies in Christian Ethics*, *25*(1): 4–19.

Burdsey, D. (2010). British Muslim experiences in English first-class cricket. *International Review for the Sociology of Sport*, *45*(3): 315–334.

Coakley, J. (2007). *Sports in Society: Issues and Controversies* (10th ed.) Boston: McGraw Hill.

Dagkas, S., Benn, T. and Jawad, H. (2011). Multiple voices: improving participation of Muslim girls in physical education and school sport. *Sport, Education and Society*, *16*(2): 223–239.

Dahl, D. (2008). Zum Verständnis von Körper, Bewegung und Sport in Christenum, Islam und Buddhismus- Impulse zum interreligiösen Ethikdiskurs zum Spitzensport. Phd dissertation. Oslo: Norges Idrettshøgskole.

Dunn, R. and Stevenson, C. (1998). The paradox of the church hockey league. *International Review for the Sociology of Sport*, *33*(2): 131–141.

Farooq, S. and Parker, A. (2009). Sport, physical education, and Islam: Muslim independent schooling and the social construction of masculinities. *Sociology of Sport Journal*, *26*: 277–295.

Guerin, P. B., Diiriye, R. O., Corrigan, C. and Guerin, B. (2003). Physical activity programs for refugee Somali women: Working out in a new country. *Women and Health*, *38*(1): 83–99.

Hargreaves, J. (2000). *Heroines of Sport: The Politics of Difference and Identity*. London: Routledge.

Hamzeh, M. and Oliver, K. (2012). 'Because I am Muslim, I cannot wear a swimsuit': Muslim girls negotiate participation opportunities for physical activity. *Research Quarterly for Exercise and Sport*, *83*(2): 330–339.

Hoffman, S.J. (1992). *Sport and Religion*. Champaign, Illinois: Human Kinetics Books.

Jawad, H., Al-Sinani, Y. and Benn, T. (2011). Islam, women and sport. In Benn, T., Pfister, G. and Jawad, H. (eds) *Muslim Women and Sport* (pp. 25–40). New York: Routledge.

Jiwani, N. and Rail, G. (2010). Islam, hijab and young Shia Muslim Canadian women's discursive constructions of physical activity. *Sociology of Sport Journal*, *27*(3): 251–267.

Johnston, R.K. (1983). *The Christian at Play*, Grand Rapids, MI: William B. Eerdmans Publishing Company.

Kamrava, M. (2006) *The New Voices of Islam. Rethinking Politics and Modernity. A reader*. Berkely: University of California Press.

Koca, C. and Hacisoftaoglu, I. (2001). Religion and the state: the story of a Turkish athlete. In Benn, T., Pfister, G. and Jawad, H. (eds) *Muslim Women and Sport*. New York: Routledge.

Magdalinski, T. and Chandler, T.J.L.(2002). *With God on Their Side. Sport in the Service of Religion*. London: Routledge.

Messner, M. (1992). Sport, Men, and Gender. In Messner, M. (ed.) *Power at Play* (vol. 1), (pp. 7–23). Boston: Beacon Press.

Navabinejad, S. (1994). Comparative study on athletes' participation in the first Islamic countries Women Sports Solidarity Games. In Schilling, G. (ed.) *Frauen im Sport* (pp. 75–83). Zurich: Studentendruckerei.

Neale, R.E. (1969). *In Praise of Play. Towards a Psychology of Religion*. New York: Harper and Row.

Novak, M. (1994). *The Joy of Sports: End Zones, Bases, Baskets, Ball and Consecration of the American Spirit*. New York: Basic Books.

Palmer, C. (2009). Soccer and the politics of identity for young Muslim refugee women in South Australia. *Soccer and Society*, *10*(1): 27–38.

Pfister, G. (2000). Rekorde im Tschador? Frauen und Sport im Iran. In Deutsches Olympisches Institut (ed.) *Jahrbuch 2000* (pp. 235–249). Aachen: Meyer and Meyer,

Pfister, G. (2000). Doing sport in a headscarf? German sport and Turkish females. *Journal of Sport History*, *27*(3): 401–429.

Pfister, G. (2011). Muslim women and sport in diasporas: theories, discourses and practices – analysing the case of Denmark. In T. Benn, G. Pfister, and H. Jawad (eds), *Muslim Women and Sport* (pp. 41–77). New York: Routledge.

Ramadan, T. (2004). *Western Muslims and the Future of Islam*. Oxford: Oxford University Press.

Ratna, A. (2011). "Who wants to make aloo gobi when you can bend it like Beckham?" British Asian females and their racialised experiences of gender and identity in women's football, *Soccer and Society*, *12*(3): 382–401.

Said, E.W. (2003). *Orientalism*. London: Penguin Books.

Schroeder, P.J. and Scribner, J.P. (2006). To honor and glorify God: The role of religion in one intercollegiate athletics culture. *Sport, Education and Society*, *11*(1): 39–54.

Sehlikoglu, S. (2013). Subjectivity and desire: Members of the women-only gyms in Istanbul. *Anthropology of the Contemporary Middle East and Central Eurasia*, *1*(1).

Sfeir, L. (1985). Conflict between cultural tradition and modernization. *International Review for the Sociology of Sport, 20*(4): 283–306.

Stevenson, C.L. (1991). The Christian athlete: An interactionist-developmental analysis. *Sociology of Sport Journal, 8*(4): 362–379.

Stevenson, C.L. (1997). Christian athletes and the culture of elite sport: Dilemmas and solutions. *Sociology of Sport Journal, 14*(3): 241–62.

Storli, E. (2011). KRIK – What are the reasons KRIK sports camp appear attractive to youth? Masterthesis. Institutt for Husdyr og Akvakulturvitenskap, Universitetet for miljø- og biovitenskap.

Strandbu, Å. and Bakken, A. (2007). *Aktiv Oslo-Ungdom. En Studie av Idrett, Minoritetsbakgrunn og Kjønn.* Report no. 2. Oslo: NOVA.

Strandbu, Å. (2005). Identity, embodied culture and physical exercise. Stories from Muslim girls in Oslo with immigrant background. *Young, 13*(1): 27–45.

Tlili, H. (2010). Women of Arabic-Muslim culture and their involvement in departments of sport and physical education: A comparative study of motor practices of students in France and Tunisia. In Talleu, C. (ed), *Sport and Discrimination in Europe.* Sport policy and practices series (pp. 137–143). Strasbourg: Council of Sport Publishing.

Trysnes, I. (2010). Å campe med Gud: en studie av kristne sommerstevner på Sørlandet. Oslo: Unipub.

Walseth, K, and Fasting, K. (2003). Islam's view on physical activity and sport – Egyptian women interpreting Islam. *International Review for the Sociology of Sport, 38*(1): 45–60.

Walseth, K. (2006). Young Muslim Women and Sport: the Impact of Identity Work. *Leisure Studies, 25*: 75–94.

Walseth, K. (2015). Sport within Muslim organizations in Norway – ethnic segregated activities as an arena for integration. *Leisure Studies.* http://www.tandfonline.com/doi/pdf/10.1080/02614367.2015 1055293

Walsh, A.J. and Guilianotti, R. (2007). *Ethics, Money and Sport: The Sporting Mammon.* London: Routledge.

Watson, N.J. and Parker, A. (2013). Sports and Christianity Mapping the Field. In N.J. Watson and A. Parker (eds), *Sports and Christianity: Historical and Contemporary Perspectives* (pp. 9–88). London: Routledge.

Wray, S. (2002). Connecting ethnicity, gender and physicality: Muslim Pakistani women, physical activity and health. In S. Scraton and A. Flintoff (eds), *Gender and Sport: A Reader* (pp. 127–140). London: Routledge.

Zaman, H. (1997). Islam, well-being and physical activity: Perceptions of Muslim young women. In G. Clarke and B. Humberstone (eds), *Researching Women and Sport* (pp. 50–67). London: Macmillan.

Qaradawy, Y. al. (1992). *The Status of Women in Islam.* Cairo: Islamic Home Publishing and Distribution.

Internet reference. www.islamonline.net:www.onislam.net/english/ask-the-scholar/sports-and-games/175408-sports-definition-etiquette-and-ruling.html?Games. Retrieved 29.01.2014.

29

YOUTH SPORT AND DIS/ABILITY

Donna Goodwin

Youth Sport and Dis/ability

Physical activity patterns developed during youth appear to be critical for developing long-term physical activity habits (Robertson-Wilson *et al.*, 2003; Shephard, 1991; Zick *et al.*, 2007). The psychosocial benefits of sport and physical activity are similar for both non–disabled and disabled populations (Dattilo *et al.*, 1998; Malone *et al.*, 2012). These benefits include enhanced self-esteem (Kosma *et al.*, 2002), reduced clinical depression (Hutchinson *et al.*, 2003; Kleiber *et al.*, 2002), improved family and social interactions, and a sense of community belonging (Dattilo *et al.*, 1998; Goodwin and Staples, 2005; Goodwin, *et al.*, 2011, Levins *et al.*, 2004).

Regrettably, youth experiencing disability[1] are significantly less active and more obese than their non–disabled peers (Bult *et al.*, 2011; Rimmer and Rowland, 2008). Physical inactivity places youth experiencing disability at risk of acquiring secondary health conditions that may lead to decreased functional capacity and quality of life. Health conditions include such concerns as fatigue, skin breakdown, obesity, diabetes, heart disease, osteoporosis and respiratory problems (Ditor *et al.*, 2003; Hetz *et al.*, 2011; Martin Ginis *et al.*, 2010; Shephard, 1991; Wilhite, and Shank, 2009).

When undertaken within appropriate training environments (e.g. clear expectations, facilities, positive social climate of belonging, psychological safety), youth sport, whether it leads to recreational or competitive involvement, provides opportunities for physical, personal and social skill development (Strachan *et al.*, 2011). The same can be said for disability sport. In this chapter, sport is being interpreted broadly to include recreational and competitive versions, as well as physical education and physical activity within community settings. The aim is to think critically about how *disability* youth sport can contribute or constrain behaviours, attitudes and self-efficacy toward lifelong physical activity and wellness. I will focus primarily on experiences of physical impairment,[2] not because other experiences of disablement are not of equal importance, but rather the relationship between physical impairment and sport is the most widely-researched and understood (Howe, 2008a, 2008b; Thomas and Smith, 2009).[3]

The chapter is organized into three parts or frames.[4] Frames are conceptualised as mental structures that shape the way we see the world – the goals we seek, the plans we make, the way we act and what counts as a good or bad outcome of our actions. Reframing is changing the way the public sees the world (Lakoff, 2004, p. xv). The first section provides a brief overview of two models that have framed disability sport – the so-called medical and social models of disability (Howe, 2008b). The next section provides a reflective overview of selected literature framed by youth sport, physical education and community-based physical activity. The final section highlights potential strategies for reframing disability sport as a potentially transformational force for contesting social inequality and promoting progressive human discourses (Lakoff, 2004).

Disability frames

It has been argued that the medical model remains the primary frame through which disability is understood in society:

> The medical model is a clinical approach to disability which focuses on the use of diagnostic tools to identify pathology and make interventions in that pathology in order to cure or minimize it. Under this framework, disability is based in the body, normal is constructed as idea, disabled people are dependent and our identities are tragedies in need of intervention.
>
> *(Withers, 2012, p. 31)*

As a domain of the *expert* (i.e. physician), disability becomes ableistically value-laden (Silvers, 2003). 'Ableism constructs bodies as "impaired" and positions these as "Other": different, lesser, undesirable, in need of repair or modification and de-humanised' (Hodge and Runswick-Cole, 2013, p. 312). The features of the ableistic medical model of disability are:

- disability is a personal tragedy based on impairment (biological) and defined by people who do not experience disability;
- the inability to conform to normative understandings of the body is characterised as of weakness, dependency and vulnerability;
- disability is to be diminished, adapted or concealed as much as possible through technological and medical means; and,
- disability becomes the primary point through which all other information about the person is viewed.

(Shakespeare, 2006; Withers, 2012)[5]

Social models of disability emerged in resistance to the alleged moral authority of others (e.g. medical practitioners) constructing people with disabilities' identities (Oliver, 1990). Led predominately by people experiencing disability, the social model reframed the understanding of disability (Oliver, 1990; Thomas, 2006; Wendell, 1996). Although a number of social models have emerged for the last thirty years (Withers, 2012), socio-cultural structures – be they attitudes, policies or inaccessible built environments – are deemed to be oppressive and contribute to the disablement of people (Shakespeare, 2006). The key features of social models are:

- social and environmental structures constructed by and for non-impaired people create barriers that can result in a loss or the limitation of full participation in society;
- disability being the social oppression that people with impairments face (i.e. disabled people);
- disability not being perceived as illness or something to be cured; and,
- a community of united people experiencing disability emerged to challenge and resist oppressive social structures.

(Shakespeare, 2006; Withers, 2012)

309

While the medical model tells people what constitutes a good life, the social model targeted community-building as a way to challenge oppressive social structures while striving for socioeconomic, identity and political progressiveness. The social model led to a declining interest among theorists, researchers, policy-makers and service providers in an individualized and medicalized understanding of disability (Withers, 2012). It is important to note that 'rejecting the medical model, however, does not necessitate a rejection of medicine or medical care' (Withers, 2012, p. 55).

What is the relevance of the medical or social models to disability sport? Put another way, 'To what extent is the definition of disability a fundamentally significant issue?' (Barton, 2009, p. 48). Withers (2012) answers this question from a social model perspective, 'Who is disabled? People are disabled. We are disabled if those in power say we are . . . Self-defining as "disabled" enables us to take ourselves seriously and demand others do also' (pp. 113–114).

A tension exists around the provision of social programmes under both models. From a medical model frame, it is immoral to give people things they have not earned as they may not develop self-discipline and may become dependent. From the social model, it is immoral to provide social programmes as it removes responsibility to change the social structures that oppress people and keep them dependent upon the state (Oliver, 1993, 2013; Oliver and Barnes, 1991; Withers, 2012). Guaranteed incomes for people experiencing disability, for example, removes the focus from underemployment and the need to gain access to paid employment (Withers, 2012).

Scholars who adhere to the social model regard the body as a source of oppression, thereby explaining why sport, which is practised through the body, has been underexplored within disability studies research (Howe, 2008b). Dominant discussions specific to policy matters and everyday practical issues (e.g. employment, access, rights) may further explain the atheoretical criticism waged against disability studies (Gleeson, 1999) and lack of interest by disability social scientists in sport-related narratives. Arguably, disability embodiment is at the heart of sport processes and the unique social spaces it creates.

Some suggest that the structural fallacy of the abandonment of embodiment limits how the disability experience is informed (Anastasiou and Kauffman, 2013; Gleeson, 1999; Holt, 2007): 'Because many disabled people find pride in our disabled mind and bodies, this doesn't mean that we don't have difficulty with them . . . not because we are disabled [but] . . . because we are human' (Withers, 2012, p. 115). It can be argued that the lived or phenemonologically understood body provides a means by which to explore the place of the 'imperfect' body in sport (Paterson and Hughes, 1999). Others suggest that the distinction between impairment and disability is itself a social construction as there is no biological reality of impairment that is not socially created (Withers, 2012). Irrespective of which position is held, 'social scientists, all agree that biological reductionism is to be avoided at all costs' (Thomas, 2006, p. 181).

Disability sport frames

Sport is central to Western cultural identity (Coakley and Donnelly, 2009). It is an institution that involves social status, social roles, ritual and achievement, and comes with ideals such as dedication, sacrifice, excellence and rewards. The relationship between sport and such social dynamics as class, gender, sexuality, ethnicity, age and dis/ability has been extensively researched (Coakley and Donnelly, 2009). The social dynamics of disability sport – 'sport that has been designed for or is specifically practiced by athletes with disabilities' (DePauw and Gavron, 2005, p. 8) – has, however, received less attention (DePauw, 1997; Howe, 2008b).

The shift away from the medical model of disability corresponded with a shift away from exercise and sport as therapy, and sport for sport's sake, with all of its benefits and ills (Fitzgerald,

2009; Goodwin and Peers, 2012, Martin, 2010). In a review of selected research, Martin (2011) documented the beneficial and deleterious effects of disability sports participation among youth. The health benefits included increased functional abilities, enhanced cardiovascular fitness and gains in muscular strength and endurance. The energy demands of sport were also a factor in offsetting the caloric imbalances that lead to obesity. Decreased loneliness and enhanced self-esteem and friendships also resulted from sports engagement. The articulated risks of sport included overuse injuries and psychological harm resulting from exclusion, threatened self-esteem and teasing (Martin, 2013; Martin and Whalen, 2012; Shapiro and Martin, 2014).

Sport represents ideas and beliefs about the body and ability that can exclude youth experiencing disability. Involvement in sport has less to do with ability and impairment (i.e. ableism of the medical model) than with social institutions associated with environmental, social, attitudinal and regulatory factors (Goodwin and Peers, 2012; Howe, 2008b; Peers, 2009). Sport can serve two purposes. It can be a site for the reproduction of social inequity or it can be a site for cultural transformation. Cultural transformation is possible when a critical perspective is brought to bear on the structural power, privilege and traditions of sport that can marginalize athletes based upon perceptions of ability (DePauw, 1997).

DePauw (1997, p. 424) argued that sport has tended to view individuals with disabilities in three ways:

1   They have been invisible or excluded from sport (invisibility of disability in sport);
2   They have become visible in sport as disabled athletes (visibility of disability in sport);
3   They are increasingly becoming visible in sport as athletes [(in)Visibility of disAbility in sport].

At first glance, the Paralympics might be seen as representative of the visibility of disability in sport (DePauw, 1997). On the other hand, Purdue and Howe (2012, p. 203) present a compelling argument for 'seeing all bodies in the context of sport in which they compete. All bodies possess limitations, even so-called able bodies. It is important to appreciate elite disability sport on its own merits'. In other words, there is a tension (the 'Paralympic paradox') created in the representation of the Paralympian as 'either an impaired athlete or an athlete (with a disability)' (Purdue and Howe, 2012, p. 190). In the terms of DePauw's (1997) typology, a tension exists between visibility of disability in sport and the (in)visibility of disability in sport.

Purdue and Howe (2012) argue that the Paralympic paradox is framed by Paralympian as athlete or Paralympian as *impaired* athlete. They argue that viewing impairment as incidental to the Paralympic identity (as an athlete first and foremost) may serve to dispel 'tragic overcoming' stories and reinforce respect for excellence and athletic prowess. In uncoupling impairment from the athlete they may, however, be decreasing their credibility as role models for members of the disability community. Purdue and Howe further suggest that the elevated status of athlete may narrow the range of impaired bodies that would fit the Paralympic athlete identity, thereby excluding some athletes.

On the other side of the paradox are Paralympians who embrace impaired embodiment as central to their identity (impaired athlete), maintaining their credibility as role models for others with similar impairments (Purdue and Howe, 2012). Impaired athlete identity is also 'a possible way out of the trap of negative identification' (Huang and Brittain, 2006, p. 372). Under both Paralympic frames (i.e. athlete and impaired athlete), there is an effort to avoid associations of disability with deficit and marginalization of opportunities but from different perspectives. As *athlete*, impairment is secondary to elite performance and not the frame by which the athletes chose to be identified (i.e. the medical model). As impaired athlete, impairment is a central frame to Paralympic identity.

Visibility and invisibility in sport is a complex question for youth to negotiate. DePauw (1997, p. 438) places the challenge before coaches, athletes, teachers and instructors in stating that the future lies in being able to 'see sport and athlete with a disability without any contradiction'. A recent article by Fitzgerald (2012b) is a case in point. English high-school aged youngsters without disabilities were asked how they understood Paralympic athletes and disability sport. Their responses reflected individual deficit perceptions of disability in which disability embodiment was 'not normal' (p. 248), nor was disability sport as it did not follow the 'right rules' (p. 249). Disability sport was undervalued as 'lazy' as in the case of sitting volleyball, 'unskilful' (p. 251) in the case of basketball, but worth a go as it would be 'funny' and 'easier' (p. 252). Sporting habituses framed the students' perceptions of disability athletes and disability sport, even in light of the increasing media coverage and debate surrounding the Paralympics (e.g. Howe, 2008a; Thomas and Smith, 2003). While the Paralympics is viewed by some as the pinnacle of the visibility of ability in sport (DePauw, 1997), it did not resonate as such with the students in this study.

Physical education

There is theoretical and empirical support for the claims of physical, social, cognitive and affective benefits to engagement in physical education and school sport (Bailey *et al.*, 2009). Whether these benefits are accrued by students experiencing disability is less clear. Well-established and intuitively sound best practices in inclusive physical education such as use of peer tutors, adaptations of rules and equipment, and providing choice are often viewed uncritically (Goodwin, 2009). While they may ease the challenges that inclusive physical education contexts present, they may also create 'special education damage' (Allen, 2005, p. 286) in the form of dependency, perceptions of incompetence, and stigmatization (Goodwin, 2000, 2001; Hutzler, 2008; Lindemann, 2003; Rossow-Kimball and Goodwin, 2009; Standal and Jespersen, 2009). The ethical work of inclusive physical education involves the critical reflection of values such as autonomy, integrity, influence and participation. In fairness to teachers, they themselves fall victim to arguably ethically questionable practices such as inadequate preparation (Hodge *et al.*, 2004), inadequate classroom support (Lienert, Sherrill and Myers, 2001) and administrative abandonment (Goodwin, 2009).

The socialization of children with and without impairments in inclusive (physical) education contexts is presented as a means for decreasing negative representations of disability. How children (re)produce or (re)construct sameness or otherness is 'somewhat of a black box, however (Holt, 2007, p. 783). In-depth research into the everyday relational and experiential understanding of the corporeal body sameness and difference (inclusion and exclusion) is not well understood. Fitzgerald (2012b) argued that school based physical education may be the key to transforming medicalized conceptualizations of disability. Teachers, coaches, and students can disrupt narrowly defined *knowing* of disability. The challenges are great, however. In physical education curricula – based upon typical motor development, fundamental motor skills acquisition, and the application of motor skills in normative physical activity and sport – students experiencing disability seldom play with or alongside non-disabled classmates in equitable or self-enhancing ways (Goodwin, 2003, 2009). In contrast to Fitzgerald's optimism, others have contended that school sites are specific and contextual and are spaces where negative sociocultural representations of disability tend to be reproduced (Anderson and Goodey, 1998; Holt, 2007).

Reverse integration may be one pedagogical strategy for reconceptualising disability through school curricula (Stevenson, 2009). Demonstration disability sports parallel curricular sport, or are unique to disability sport, such as wheelchair basketball and goal ball respectively. These sessions can be of relatively short duration (one or two weeks) and occur once throughout the entire curriculum, however. The nature and intensity of reverse integration experiences needed to bring about conceptual shifts is not well understood. Although not within an educational setting, a study of reverse integration in female wheelchair basketball (nine classified wheelchair athletes, four non-classified athletes) suggests that extended involvement in reverse integration sport contexts has the potential to enhance physical and social participation benefits of sport where disability athlete numbers are low (Spencer-Cavaliere and Peers, 2011). Viewed through a social model of disability, the significance of this pedagogical approach becomes visible. All players in the study expressed a strong athletic identity, not as athletes with or without disability. Wheelchair basketball itself was not viewed as a disability sport as the wheelchair gave everyone the same functional ability, dissolving the ability-disability distinction. The lack of (dis)ability distinction also occurred off the court as social relationships developed, dispelling the perceived role of non-disabled players being disability and sport helpers. Couched in DePauw's (1997) terms, reverse integration provides an example of the (in)visibility of disability sport.

Physical literacy is an increasingly popular concept (e.g. Canada, Australia, UK, USA) and has been adopted by educators, coaches and physical activity professions as a new *game plan* for addressing physical inactivity and sedentary lifestyles (Keegan *et al.*, 2013; Whitehead, 2001). It is purported to be of relevance to all children and youth

> as appropriate to each individual's endowment, physical literacy can be described as a disposition to capitalize on the human embodied capability, wherein the individual has the motivation, confidence, physical competence, knowledge and understanding to value and take responsibility for maintaining purposeful physical pursuits/activities throughout the lifecourse.
>
> *(Whitehead, 2010)*[6]

Primary schools have been targeted as the most influential for the delivery of physical literacy given their ability to reach every child (Mandigo *et al.*, 2009). At first glance, the notion of physical literacy is one that promotes participation and inclusion. By definition, however, it is stated in terms of individual responsibility. At the risk of being sceptical, the challenges individuals experiencing disability face negotiating the ableistic norms of physical activity and sport suggest that physical literacy is a concept that is exclusionary in its basic premise. It remains to be seen if youth, their parents, instructors, coaches, facility managers and fellow participants are available to support individuals (i.e. medical model frame) in this pursuit within the social milieu of sport, schools and community (i.e. social model frame) (Martin and Choi, 2009).

Community physical activity

One of the largest challenges for youth experiencing disability and their families is to find ways to engage in physical activity and exercise activities in community settings (Rimmer and Rowland, 2008). The barriers to participation (professional and environmental) are lengthy, complex and well-documented. Environmental barriers include physically inaccessible facilities and exercise equipment, poor transportation, economic barriers, under-trained staff, administrative resistance to inclusive programming, safety, programme procedures and policies, informational barriers and limited resources (e.g. Anaby *et al.*, 2013; Arbour-Nicitopoulos and Martin Ginis, 2011;

Bedini, 2000; French and Hainsworth, 2001; Kehn and Kroll, 2009; Law *et al.*, 2007; Rimmer, 2002; Rimmer *et al.*, 2004; Shields, Synnot, and Barr, 2012). Parents of youth with disabilities may also be apprehensive about social isolation for their children in mainstream programmes, perceiving that friendships developed in specialized programmes will be severed or that inclusive environments will accentuate differences between youth with and without disabilities (Devine and Parr, 2008; Thompson and Emira, 2012).

Community professionals who are insecure in their role in inclusion in the community may revert to a medical model frame for guidance, with the result that youth experiencing disability and their families become 'clients' who are, 'subjected to professional determinations from powerful disciplines . . . that construct socio-ethical identities based on labels, limitations and loss' (Clapton, 2003, p. 542). These professionals range from rehabilitation professionals, kinesiologists, recreation therapists and social workers. Stigma, perceptions of dependence, unsolicited help and underprepared professionals may become too much to address on an ongoing basis. Managing and educating others requires energy to manage and is a moderator to community physical activity and exercise engagement (e.g. Goodwin *et al.*, 2004; Martin, 2013; Mulligan *et al.*, 2012; Rolfe *et al.*, 2009). Social and psychological factors may be as important as environmental barriers in explaining physically inactive lifestyles.

To address the social and environmental barriers to the structure of facility-based, registration-driven community physical activity programmes, an internet-based personalized physical activity programme was developed. Rimmer and Rowland (2008) outlined an intervention model aimed at youth experiencing disability who find it difficult to participate in school or community-based sport and recreation programmes. Wellness coaches complete a needs-assessment with the youth and develop an individualized programme that takes into consideration interests and circumstances, readiness, health concerns, family input and barriers to participation. A programme that is built by the youth and their families may provide flexibility not previously possible and encourage graduated participation. Successful participants can ultimately be linked to community programmes for long-term maintenance.

Reframing youth disability sport: identifying the way forward

Professional practice is defined as 'a coherent, socially organized activity with notions of good practice within the practitioners' understanding and skilful comportment. A practice has shared understandings about goals, skills and equipment and is continually being worked out in new contexts' (Benner, 1997, p. 50). Without ethical self-reflection, our work becomes merely technical, allowing judgements regarding whether it is well or badly performed but seldom enabling us to judge whether it is right or wrong. This brings our professional integrity into question (Fernandez-Balboa, 2009). Exploring the intersection of coaching and instructional practice and issues of daily ethical concern in sport may assist us to understand how ethical issues arise, how they are structured, and how they are or should be managed.

Information technology may be a promising approach to addressing physical inactivity among youth experiencing challenging circumstances (e.g. limited opportunities, difficulty engaging with school or sport settings) (Rimmer and Rowland, 2008).

There is pressing need for research that is empirically grounded in the past and present social experiences of youth experiencing disability, in order to understand the oppressive forces within youth sport and social arrangements that are non-disabling. Research approaches that embrace lived experiences provide insights into first person perspectives, that although frowned upon by some as mere subjectivism, or at their worst, symbolic violence of outsiders trying to empathize with that which they have played a role in creating, can serve as a critical lens to view the experiences of ability and disability (Anderson, 2006; Jespersen and McNamee, 2008). Reflexive athlete ethnographies from youth sporting contexts provide a unique vantage point for uncovering and understanding disablement practices (Howe, 2009). Understanding of counter-stories constructed from the lived experiences of persons experiencing disability may offer an ethical platform from which to engage in crucial discussions (Clapton, 2003). A counter-story is a 'story that contributes to the moral self-definition of its teller by undermining the dominant story, undoing it and retelling it in such a way as to invite new interpretations and conclusions . . . Counter-stories are real lived and relational experiences with, and of, people with disability' (Clapton, 2003, p. 545).

Much of the disability sport research has been labelled as awareness raising or cognitive emancipation (Fitzgerald *et al.*, 2003; Kitchen, 2000). Emancipatory research is a form of political action that explores and identifies avenues for change based upon questions of relevance to the disability community. Control in all aspects of the research, from the formulation of research questions to the dissemination of the findings, is given to those with impairments (Walmsley, 2001). Bringing imagination and creativity to methodological frameworks of emancipatory research for youth opens avenues for capturing ideas, strategies and practices of most relevance to youth. Photography, timeline generation, drawings and youth generated questionnaires are but a few examples (Fitzgerald, 2011a; Goodwin, Krohn and Kuhnle, 2004).

'Critical pedagogy refers to a constellation of educational theories, teaching, and learning practices that raise critical consciousness about oppressive social conditions' (Anderson, 2006, p. 372). Sport is a place where the historically invisible can be made visible. For youth experiencing disability, sport can play a role in promoting dignity, equality and belonging to those cultural values of most importance and relevance to their chosen identity. Bringing together understanding of the socio-structural constraints of society and culture with disability youth athletes' experiences and practices in a dialectical way may provide a platform from which to transform them together (Bourdieu, 1990).

Notes

1 Disability has both a historical and socially produced identity. Readers will be familiar with the terms 'people with disabilities' and 'disabled people'. The first term is intented to humanize and respect the rights of all people. The latter term serves a political function by foregrounding socially imposed oppression that disables people with impairments. I use the term people experiencing disability (Peers, 2009) to acknowledge those 'who have been subjected to medical diagnoses of disability, disabling social conditions, and/or who have claimed a disability-related identity' (Goodwin and Peers, 2012, p. 187).

2 Although beyond the space limitations of this chapter, disableism is also intersected by racism, sexism, homophobia, ageism and economic stratification (Thomas, 2006; Wendell, 2006).

3 The chapter is further bound by literature produced by Western English-speaking countries. There may be some transference of the information to other disability experiences and cultural contexts, however, it will be of a theoretical, or tacit nature rather than an empirical one.

4 I am writing this chapter as a non-disabled, white, well-educated, upper-class female. I do not directly experience the social discrimination, marginality or oppression of people with impairments. This limits my ability to understand and explain embodied disablement in sporting contexts. As a disability ally, I have worked to listen with care and critically reflect upon professional practice in adapted physical activity (Thomas, 2006). It is from this humble position as non-disabled outsider that I bring the ideas in this chapter forward, contributing to our understanding as the base of disability researchers in this area continues to grow (Kitchener, 2000; Macbeth, 2010): 'Social justice can never be achieved without working with disabled people and on disability issues' (Withers, 2012, p. 11).

5 I have attempted to give voice to disability theorists who have contributed to my thinking (e.g. Bredahl, Oliver, Peers, Shakespeare, Wendall, Withers). Weaknesses in the chapter are solely attributable to me.

6 www.physical-literacty.org.uk/definitions.php

References

Allen, J. (2005). Inclusion as an ethical project. In S. Termain (ed.), *Foucault and the Government of Disability* (pp. 281–297). Ann Arbor, MI: University of Michigan Press.

Anaby, D., Hand, C., Bradly, L., DiRezze, B., Forhan, M., DiGiamcomo, A. and Law, M. (2013). The effect of the environment on participation on children and youth with disabilities: A scoping review. *Disability and Rehabilitation, 35*, 1589–1598.

Anastasiou, D. and Kauffaman, J. M. (2013). The social model of disability: Dichotomy between impairment and disability. *Journal of Medicine and Philosophy, 38*, 441–459.

Anderson, (2006). Teaching (with) disability: Pedagogies of lived experience. *The Review of Education, Pedagogy, and Cultural Studies, 28*, 367–379.

Anderson, P. and Goodey, C. (1998). *Enabling Education: Experiences in Special and Ordinary Schools*. London: Tufnell Press.

Arbour-Nicitopoulos, K. P. and Martin Ginis, K. (2011). Universal accessibility of "accessible" fitness and recreational facilities for persons with mobility disabilities. *Adapted Physical Activity, 28*, 1–15.

Austin, W. (2007). The ethics of everyday practice: Healthcare environments as moral communities. *Advances in Nursing Science, 30*, 81–88.

Bailey, R., Armur, K., Kirk, D., Jess, M., Pickup, I, Sandford, R. and BERA Physical Education and Sport Pedgogy Special Interest Group (2009). The educational benefits claimed for physical education and school sport: An academic review. *Research Papers in Education, 24*, 1–27.

Barton, L. (2009). Disability, physical education and sport. In H. Fitzgerald (ed.). *Disability and Youth Sport* (pp. 39–50). New York, NY: Routledge.

Bedini, L. A. (2000). "Just sit down so we can talk": Perceived stigma and community recreation pursuits of people with disabilities. *Therapeutic Recreation Journal, 1*, 55–68.

Benner P. (1997). A dialogue between virtue ethics and care ethics. *Theoretical Medicine: An International Journal for the Philosophy and Methodology of Medical Research and Practice. 18*, 47–61.

Bergum, V. (2013). Relational ethics in nursing. In J. L. Storch, P. A. Rodney and R. C. Starzomski (eds). *Toward a Moral Horizon: Nursing Ethics for Leadership and Practice* (pp. 485–503, 2nd ed.). Toronto, ON: Pearson.

Bergum, V. and Dossetor, J. B. (2005). *Relational Ethics: The Full Meaning of Respect*. Hagerstown, MD: University Pub. Group.

Blinde, M. E. and McAllister, S. G. (1998). Listening to the voices of students with disabilities. *Journal of Physical Education, Recreation and Dance, 69*, 64–68.

Blinde M. E. and McClung, L. R. (1997). Enhancing the physical and social self through recreational activity: Accounts of individuals. *Adapted Physical Activity Quarterly, 14*, 327–344.

Bourdieu, P. (1990). *The Logic of Practice*. Cambridge, UK: Polity Press.

Bredahl, A. M. (2011). Coaching ethics and Paralympic sport. In A. R. Hardman and C. Jones (eds). *The Ethics of Coaching* (pp. 134–146). New York, NY: Routledge.

Bult, M. K., Verschuren, O., Jongmans, M. J., Lindeman, E. and Ketelaar, M. (2011). What influences participation in leisure activities of children and youth with physical disabilities? A systematic review. *Research in Developmental Disabilities, 32*, 1521–1529.

Clapton, J. (2003). Tragedy and catastrophe: Contentious discourses of ethics and disability. *Journal of Intellectual Disability Research, 47*, 540–547.

Coakley, J. and Donnelly, P. (2009). *Issues and Controversies: Sport in Society* (2nd ed.). Toronto, ON: McGraw Hill.

Dattilo, J., Caldwell, L., Lee, Y. and Kleiber, D. A. (1998). Returning to the community with a spinal cord injury: Implications for therapeutic recreation specialiss. *Therapeutic Recreation Journal, 32*, 13–27.

DePauw, K. P. (1997). The (in)visibility of disability: cultural contexts and 'sporting bodies'. Quest, 49, 416–430.

DePauw, K. (2009a). Disability sport: Historical context. In H. Fitzgerald (ed.). *Disability and Youth Sport* (pp. 11–23). New York, NY: Routledge.

DePauw, K. (2009b). Ethics, professional expectations, and graduate education: Advancing research in kinesiology. *Quest, 61*, 52–58.

DePauw, K. and Gavron, S. J. (2005). *Disability Sport* (2nd ed.). Champaign, IL: Human Kinetics.

Devine, M.A. and Parr, M.G. (2008). "Come on in, but not too far:" Social capital in an inclusive leisure setting. *Leisure Sciences, 30*, 391–408.

Ditor, D. S., Latimer, A. E., Martin Ginis, K., Arbour, K. P., McCartney, N. and Hicks, A. L. (2003). Maintenance of exercise participation in individuals with spinal cord injury: Effects on quality of life, stress and pain. *Spinal Cord, 41,* 446–450.

Doubt, L. and McCall, M. (2003). A secondary guy: Physically disabled teenagers in secondary schools. *The Canadian Journal of Occupational Therapy, 70,* 139–151.

Fernandez-Balboa, J. (2009). Bio-pedagogical self-reflection in PETE: Reawakening the ethical conscience and purpose in pedagogy and research. *Sport, Education and Society, 14,* 147–163.

Fitzgerald, H. (2009). *Disability and Youth Sport.* London: Routledge.

Fitzgerald, H. (2012a). 'Drawing' on disabled students' experiences of physical education and stakeholder responses. *Sport, Education and Society, 17,* 443–462.

Fitzgerald, H. (2012b). Paralympic athletes and "knowing disability." *International Journal of Disability, Development and Education, 59,* 243–255.

Fitzgerald, H., Joblin, A. and Kirk, D. (2003). Valuing the voices of young disabled people: Exploring experience of physical education and sport. *European Journal of Physical Education, 8,* 175–200.

French, D. and Hainsworth, J. (2001). 'There aren't any buses and the swimming pool is always cold!': Obstacles and opportunities in the provision of sport for disabled people. *Managing Leisure, 6,* 35–49.

Gaz, D. V. and Smith, A. M. (2012). Psychosocial benefits and implications of exercise. *Physical Medication and Rehabilitation, 4,* 812–817.

Gleeson, B. (1999). *Geographies of Disability.* London: Routledge.

Goodwin, D. L. and Watkinson, E. J. (2000). Inclusive physical education from the perspective of students with physical disabilities. *Adapted Physical Activity Quarterly, 17,* 144–160.

Goodwin, D. L. (2001). The meaning of help in PE: Perceptions of students with physical disabilities. *Adapted Physical Activity Quarterly, 18,* 289–303.

Goodwin, D. L. (2003). Instructional approaches to the teaching of motor skills. In R. D. Steadward, G. D. Wheeler, and E. J. Watkinson (eds), *Adapted Physical Activity.* (pp. 255–284) Edmonton, AB: University of Alberta Press.

Goodwin, D. L. (2008). Self-regulated dependency: Ethical reflections on interdependence and help in adapted physical activity. *Sport, Ethics and Philosophy, 2,* 172–184.

Goodwin, D. L. (2009). The voices of students with disabilities: Are they informing inclusive physical education practice? In H. Fitzgerald (ed.). *Disability and Youth Sport* (pp. 53–75). London: Routledge.

Goodwin, D. L., Krohn, J. and Kuhnle, A. (2004). Beyond the wheelchair: The experience of dance. *Adapted Physical Activity Quarterly, 21,* 229–247.

Goodwin, D. L., Lieberman, L. J., Johnston, K. and Leo, J. (2011). Connecting through summer camp: Youth with visual impairments find a sense of community. *Adapted Physical Activity Quarterly, 28,* 40–55.

Goodwin, D. L. and Staples, K. (2005). Meaning of summer camp experiences to youths with disabilities. *Adapted Physical Activity Quarterly, 22,* 160–178.

Goodwin, D. L., Thurmeier, R. and Gustafson, P. (2004). Reactions to the metaphors of disability: The mediating effects of physical activity. *Adapted Physical Activity Quarterly, 21,* 379–398.

Goodwin, D. L. and Peers, D. (2012). Disability, sport and inclusion. In S. Dagkas and Armour, K. (eds). *Inclusion and Exclusion Through Youth* (pp. 186–202). London: Routledge.

Hetz, S. P., Latimer, A. E., Abour-Nicitopoulos, K. and Martin Ginis, K. (2011). Secondary complications and subjective well-being in individuals with chronic spinal cord injury: Associations with self-reported adiposity. *Spinal Cord, 49,* 266–272.

Hodge, N. and Runswick-Cole, K. (2013). 'They never pass me the ball': Exposing ableism through leisure experienes of disabled children, young people and their families. *Children's Geographies, 11,* 311–325.

Hodge, S., Ammah, J., Casebolt, K., Lamaster, K. and O'Sullivan, M. (2004). High school general physical education teachers' behaviors and beliefs associated with inclusion. *Sport, Education and Society, 9,* 395–419.

Holt, L. (2007). Children's sociospatial (re)production of disability within primary school. *Environmental and Planing D: Society and Space, 25,* 783–802.

Howe, P. D. (2008a). From inside the rewsroom: Paralympic media and the 'production' of elite disability. *International Review for the Sociology of Sport, 43,* 135–150.

Howe, P. D. (2008b). *The Cultural Politics of the Paralympic Movement Through an Anthropological Lens.* London: Routledge.

Howe, P. D. (2009). Reflexive ethnography, impairment and the pub. *Leisure Studies, 28,* 489–496.

Huang, C. and Brittain, I. (2006). Negotating identities through disability sport. *Sociology of Sport Journal, 23,* 352–375.

Hutchison, S. L., Loy, D. P., Kleiber, D. A. and Dattilo, J. (2003). Leisure as a coping resource:Variations in coping with traumatic injury and illness. *Leisure Sciences, 25*, 143 –161.

Hutzler, Y. (2008). Ethical considerations in adapted physical activity practices.*Sports Ethics and Philosophy, 2*, 158–171.

Hutzler, Y., Fliess, O., Chacham, A. and Van den Auweele, Y. (2002). Perspective of children with physical disabilities on inclusion and empowerment supporting the limiting factors. *Adapted Physical Activity Quarterly, 19*, 300–317.

Jespersen, E. and McNamee, M. (2008). Philosophy, adapted physical education and dis/ability. *Sport, Ethics and Philosophy, 2*, 87–96.

Keegan, R. J., Keegan S. L., Daley, S., Ordway, C. and Edwards, A. (2013). *Getting Austrailia Moving: Establishing a Physically Literate and Active Nation (Game Plan).* Canberra, Australia: University of Canberra.

Kehn, M. and Kroll, T. (2009). Staying physically active after spinal cord injury: A qualitative exploration of barriers and facilitators to exercise participation. *BMC Public Health, 9*, 168–168.

Kleiber, D. A., Hutchison, S. L. and Williams, R. (2002). Leisure as a resource in transcending negative life events: Self-protection, self-restoration, and personal transformation. *Leisure Sciences, 224*, 219–235.

Kitchen, R. (2000). The researched opinions on research Disabled people and disability research. *Disability and Society, 15*, 25–47.

Kosma, M., Cardinal, B. J. and Rintala, P. (2002). Motivating individuals with disabilities to be physically active. *Quest, 24*, 144–159.

Kristen, L., Patriksson, G. and Fridlund, B. (2003). Parents' conceptions of the influences of participation in a sport programmes on their children and adolescent with physical disabilities. *European Physical Education Review, 9*, 23–41.

Lakoff, G. (2004). *Don't Think of an Elephant: Know Your Values and Frame the Debate.* White River Junction, VT: Chelsea Green.

Law, M., Petrenchik, T., King, G. and Hurley, P. (2007). Perceived environmental barriers to recreational, community, and school participation for children and youth with physical disabilities. *Archives of Physical Medicine and Rehabilitation, 88*, 1636–1642.

Levins, S. M., Redenbach, D. M. and Dyck, I. (2004). Individual and societal influences on participation in physical activity following spinal cord injury: A qualitative study. *Physical Therapy, 84*, 496–509.

Lienert, C., Sherrill, C. and Myers, B. (2001). Physical educators' concerns about integrating children with disabilities: A cross-cultural comparison. *Adapted Physical Activity Quarterly, 18*, 1–17.

Lindemann, K. (2003). The ethics of receiving. *Theoretical medicine and bioethics, 24*, 501–509.

Macbeth, J. L. (2010). Reflecting on disability reseach in sport and leisure settings. *Leisure Studies, 29*, 477–485.

Mandigo, J., Francis, N., Lodewyk, K. and Lopez, R. (2009). *Position Paper: Physical Literacy for Educators.* Ottawa, ON: Physical and Health Education Canada.

Malone, L. A., Barfiedl, J. P. and Brasher, J. D. (2012). Perceived benefits and barriers to exercise among person with physical disabilities or chronic health conditions within action or maintenance stages of exercise. *Disability Health Journal, 5*, 254–260.

Martin, J. (2010). The psychosocial dynamics of youth disability sport. *Sport Science Review, XIX*, 49–69.

Martin, J. (2011). Disability youth sport participation: Health benefits, injuries, and psychological effects. In A. D. Farelli (ed.), *Sport Participation*, (pp. 105–121). Hauppauge, NY: Nova Science Publishers.

Martin, J. (2013). Benefits and barriers to physical activity for individuals with disabilities: A social–relational model of disability perspective. *Disability and Rehabilitation, Early Online:* 1–8.

Martin, J. (2013). Peer relationships in youth disability sport. In S. Kaufmann and V. Meyer (eds), *Friendships: Cultural Variations, Developmental Issues and Impact on Health,* (pp. 169–176). Hauppauge, NY: Nova Science Publishers

Martin, J. and Choi, Y. S. (2009). Parents' physical activity – related perceptions of their children with disabilities. *Disability and Health Journal, 2*, 9–14.

Martin, J. and Whalen, L. (2012). Self-concept and physical activity in athletes with physical disabilities. *Disability and Health Journal, 5*, 197–200.

Martin Ginis, K., Jetha, A., Mack, D. E. and Hetz, S. (2010). Physical activity and subjective well being among people with spinal cord injury: A meta-analysis. *Spinal Cord, 48*, 65–72.

McNamee, M. J. (2008). *Sports, Virtues and Vices: Morality Plays.* London, Routledge.

Mulligan, H. F., Hale, L. A., Whitehead, L. and Baxter, G. D. (2012). Barriers to physical activity for people with long-term neurological conditions: A review study. *Adapted Physical Activity Quarterly, 29*, 243–265.

Oliver, M. (1990). *The Politics of Disablement.* Houndsmills, UK: McMillan Press.

Oliver, M. (1993). Disability and dependency: A creation of industrial societies? In L. Barton (ed.), *Disability and Dependency*, (pp. 7–22). London: Routlege.

Oliver, M. (2013). The social model of disability: Thirty years on. *Disability and Society, 28*, 1024–1026.

Oliver, M. and Barnes, C. (1991). Discrimination, disability, and welfare: From needs to rights. In M. Oliver and C. Barnes (ed.), *Equal Rights for Disabled People*, (pp. 9–17). London: Public Policy Institute.

Paterson, K. and Hughes, B. (1999). Disability studies and phenomenology: The carnal politics of everyday life. *Disability and Society, 14*, 597–610.

Peers, D. (2009). (Dis)empowering Paralympic histories: Absent athlete and disabling discourses. *Disability and Society, 24*, 653–665.

Purdue, D. E. J. and Howe, P. D. (2013). Who's in and who is out? Legitimate bodies within the Paralympic games. *Sociology of Sport Journal, 30*, 24–40.

Rimmer, J. H. (2002). Health promotion for individuals with disabilities: The need for a transitional model in service delivery. *Disease Management and Health Outcomes, 10*, 337–343.

Rimmer, J. H., Riley, B., Wang, E., Rauworth, A. and Jurkowski, J. (2004). Physical activity participation among persons with disabilities: Barriers and facilitators. *American Journal of Preventative Medicine, 26*, 419–425.

Rimmer, J. H. and Rowland, J. L. (2008). Physical activity for youth with disabilities: A critical need in an underserved population. *Developmental Neurorehabilitiation, 11*, 141–148.

Roberston-Wilson, J., Baker, J., Derbyshire, E. and Coté, J (2003). Childhood physical activity involvement in active and inactive female adults. *Avante, 9*, 1–8.

Rolfe, D. E., Yoshida, K., Renwick, R. and Bailey, C. (2012). Balancing safety and autonomy: Structural and social barriers affecting the exercise participation of women with disabilities in community recreation and fitness facilities. *Qualitative Research in Sport, Exercise and Health, 4*, 265–283.

Rossow-Kimball, B. and Goodwin, D. (2009). Self-determination and leisure experiences of women living in two group homes. *Adapted Physical Activity Quarterly, 26*, 1–20.

Shakespeare, T. (2006). *Disability Rights and Wrongs.* London: Routledge.

Shapiro, D. and Martin, J. (2014). The relationships among sport self-perceptions and social well-being in athletes with physical disabilities. *Disability and Health Journal, 7*, 42–48.

Shephard, R. J. (1991). Benefits of sport and physical activity for the disabled: Implications for the individual and for society. *Scandinavian Journal of Rehabiltiation Medicine, 23*, 233–241.

Shields, N., Synnot, A. J. and Barr, M. (2012). Perceived barriers and facilitators to physical activity for children with disability: A systematic review. *British Journal of Sports Medicine, 46*, 989–997.

Silvers, A. (2003). On the possibility and desirability of constructing a neutral conception of disability. *Theoretical Medicine, 24*, 471–487.

Simons, H. and Usher, R. (2000). Introduction: Ethics in the practice of research. In H. Simons and R. Usher (eds). *Situated Ethics in Educational Research,* (pp. 1–11). London: Routledge.

Spencer-Cavaliere, N. and Peers, D. (2011). "What's the difference?" Women's wheelchair basketball, reverse integration and the question(ing) of disability. *Adapted Physical Activity Quarterly, 28*, 291–309.

Spencer-Cavaliere, N. and Watkinson, E. J. (2010). Inclusion understood from the perspectives of children with disability. *Adapted Physical Activity Quarterly, 27*, 275–293.

Standal, O. F. and Jespersen, E. (2008). Peers as resources for learning: A situated learning approach to adapted physical activity in rehabilitation. *Adapted Physical Activity Quarterly, 25*, 208–227.

Stevenson, P. (2009). The pedagogy of inclusive youth sport: Working towards real solutions. In H. Fitzgerald (ed). *Disability and Youth Sport* (pp. 119–131). London: Routledge.

Strachan, L., Côté, J. and Deakin, J. (2011). A new view: Exploring positive youth development in elite sport contexts. *Qualitative Research in Sport, Exercise and Health, 3*, 9–32.

Thomas, C. (2006). Disability and gender: Reflections on theory and research. *Scandinavian Journal of Disability Research, 2–3*, 177–185.

Thomas, N. and Smith, A. (2003). Preoccupied w;ith able-bodiedness? An analysis of the British media coverage of the 2000 Paralympic Games. *Adapted Physical Activity Quarterly, 20*, 166–181.

Thompson, D. and Emira, M. (2011). "They say every child matters, but they don't": An investigation into parental and carer perceptions of access to leisure facilities and respite care for children and young people with autistic spectrum disorder (ASD) or attention deficit, hyperactivity disorder (ADHD). *Disability and Society, 26*, 65–78.

Walmsley, J. (2001). Normalisation, emancipatory research and inclusive research in learning disability. *Disability and Society, 16*, 187–205.

Wendell, S. (1996). *The Rejected Body*. London: Routledge.

Wilhite, B. and Shank, J. (2009). In praise of sport: Promoting sport participation as a mechanism of health among person with a disability. *Disability and Health Journal, 2*, 116–127.

Whitehead, M. (2001). The concept of physical literacy. *European Journal of Physical Education, 6*, 127–138.

Whitehead, M. (ed.). (2010). *Physical Literacy: Throughout the Lifecourse*. London: Routledge.

Withers, A. J. (2012). *Disability Politics and Theory*. Halifax, NS: Fernwood Publishing.

Zick, C. D., Smith, K. R., Brown, B. B., Fan, J. X. and Kowaleski-Jones, L. (2007). Physical activity during the transition from adolescence to adulthood. *Journal of physical activity and health, 4*, 125–137.

30

UNPACKING GENDER/ SEXUALITY/RACE/ DISABILITY/SOCIAL CLASS TO UNDERSTAND THE EMBODIED EXPERIENCES OF YOUNG PEOPLE IN CONTEMPORARY PHYSICAL CULTURE

Laura Azzarito and Doune Macdonald

Introduction

At the beginning of the twenty-first century, a new wave of critical scholars suggested more nuanced conceptualizations of young people in sports, viewing young people as active agents who negotiate norms of gender/sex, race/ethnicity, disability and social class established in and through sport, and thus, situating the intersectionality of those categories at the African American of understanding young people's embodied identities (Anderson and McCormack, 2010; Azzarito and Solomon, 2005; Benet-Weiser, 1999; Brayton, 2005; Flintoff, Fitzgerald, and Scraton, 2008; Thorpe, 2010; van Sterkenburg and Knoppers, 2004; Wright and Macdonald, 2010). From this critical standpoint, young people's ways of performing, practicing and expressing masculinities and femininities are viewed as plural and fluid, informed by race and social class relations, as produced by and negotiated in specific sport contexts. Simply put, young women and men perform multidimensional identities that they cultivate differently across sport practices based on the complex ways they view, experience, negotiate and embody dominant discourses around the body (Brayton, 2005). Examining the contradictions and fluidity of gender/sex relations at the intersection of race, disability and social class can offer fresh insights into young women's and young men's subjective experiences in physical culture (Thorpe, 2010). With this chapter, we thus suggest that the ways in which the institution of sport impacts young people's embodied experiences in their daily lives need to be unpacked with careful and critical attention to the complex articulation of gender/sex, race/ethnicity, social class and disability.

Drawing from third-wave feminist theories (i.e. poststructuralism, feminism and queer theory), gender/sex, race/ethnicity, social class and disability are regarded as merely social categories that impact identities in various ways, producing, inscribing and placing bodies into hierarchies (Butler, 1990). From this theoretical view, young girls and boys in sport contexts are heterogeneous groups that fluidly perform femininities and masculinities in a wide range of ways and at the intersection of other social categories, impacting their positionality from marginal to African American. This, in turn, informs their identity development, and thus their decision to participate in or resist sport practices. First, we suggest that sport has a powerful influence on young people, impacting their embodied experiences in significant ways. Drawing from a review of literature informed by third-wave feminist theories, we then present key issues, re-framing gender/sexuality/social class/(dis)ability as intersecting, fluid and contradictory social constructs that young people embody, negotiate and perform in predominantly North American sport contexts. In this context, intersectionality is employed as a theoretical tool to understand the complex and fluid dimensions of difference while noting the theoretical weaknesses that can occur where intersectionality is limited in the scope of differences being considered and where differences (e.g. gender, race, disability) are approached as 'fixed', cumulative variables (Flintoff, Fitzgerald and Scraton, 2008; Hylton, 2009). In the last section, we conclude with some implications for future research on intersectionality and young people in sport through the lens of strengths-based and identity-work approaches.

Sport and the (re)production of racialized, heteronormative masculinities

Sport represents a contested terrain for young people (Van Sterkenburg and Knoppers, 2004, p. 303), a context in which dominant forms of normative femininity and masculinity, as well as racial, social class and disability stereotypes, are articulated, circulated and sustained, yet contested (Brayton, 2005). Sport then creates and mobilizes a set of ideological beliefs and practices that aim, implicitly and explicitly, to sustain power structures (Kane, 1996). Historically, ideological beliefs around gender, sexuality and race have produced a 'culture of racism' (Lawrence, 2005) as well as 'ableism', 'sexism', disability and 'homophobia' (McDonald, 2002) that have become deeply ingrained in the institution of sport. Young people's constructions and performances of identity are intimately connected to social categories, such as race/ethnicity, gender/sex, social class and (dis)ability, and their negotiation of power relations is produced in specific contexts of sports (Azzarito and Katzew, 2010). Further, other scholars have suggested that sport continues to be a male-dominated social space (Hanis-Martin, 2006, p. 265) that reproduces a gender order (Messner and Sabo, 1990), functions to marginalize and underrepresent women's sport (McDonald, 2002), and does very little to encourage the interrogation of racial relations. Sport and sport media remain a White male-dominated institution that embraces colour-blind ideologies implicitly sustaining White supremacy and racial inequalities (Ferber, 2007; Van Stenkenburg and Knoppers, 2004).

As sport also has the potential to create a sense of belonging, inclusion and emotional connection, it has become a site of empowerment for young people, as well as a site for social change (Azzarito and Solmon, 2005). The transformative aspect of sport can bridge differences and potentially enable and encourage young women and men to experience their bodies and construct their identities in positive, confident, and affirmative ways (Hanis-Martin, 2006). Given that sport is a powerful site for young people's body construction, performance and making sense of the self, young people embody, present and express gender as well as racial athletic identities in multiple, intersecting ways (Louis, 2003). Young people's embodied practices in sport cannot only be understood through experiences of oppression, domination and/or binaries, but rather, their practices involve more complex processes of identity investment, resistance and negotiation of power-relations in contexts of physical culture (Thorpe, 2010). In Ferber's (2007) words, 'sport is a particularly powerful institution, a cultural text central to American identity' (p. 19). In line with Ferber's (2007) argument, Bimper and Harrison (2011) have contended that sport is not simply a game to play and enjoy but rather 'a means of defining self' (p. 275) for young men and women.

Numerous scholars have suggested, for instance, that the social construction of race has important implications for young boys' constitution of their self-concept, their masculinity and how they view themselves in society (Azzarito and Harrison, 2008; Bimper and Harrison, 2011; Harrison, Azzarito and Burden, 2004; Ferber, 2007; Nelson, 2012). According to Bimper and Harrison (2011, p. 280), 'Race and sport have become inseparable'. In the context of North America, for example, developing an athletic identity is a salient factor in young African American boys making sense of themselves and their lives as well as a means of expressing the self in positive, affirming and culturally relevant ways. For many African American boys, 'The game is my life', especially basketball and football, represent sites for cultural identification, management of race, construction of self-concept and pursuit of their dreams to become 'somebody' in society (Bier and Harrison, 2011, p. 277). Developing a strong athletic identity is often linked to a lack of investment in education pursuits, significantly limiting African American young boys' career options beyond professional sport (Harrison *et al.*, 2004).

Race also plays an important role in explaining the over-representation of African Americans in certain sports because it informs the pervasive stereotypical construction of African Americans' physical superiority and intellectual inferiority (Harrison, 2011), fuelling their 'hoop dreams' and 'football fantasies' to become successful in society through professional sport. As Harrison *et al.* (2004) eloquently explained: 'Race is so often stereotypically associated with different ethnic groups' performance of specific sports, that quite often this stereotypical thinking can mislead people to believe that those racial differences in sport participation are "biological" or "natural"' (p. 160). This means that African Americans' success in certain sports often is used as evidence – the *fact* that proves their innate racial ability or genetic advantage. Similar assumptions racialize sport elsewhere in the world such as particular football codes for Maoris, Australian Aborigines and Pacifica boys (e.g. Eruti and Palmer, 2014; Hallinan and Judd, 2012; Hokowhitu, 2003).

To explain African Americans' overrepresentation in certain sports, Entine (2000) has provided a controversial explanation endorsing the Black natural athleticism discourse. In particular, Entine (2000) has attempted to attribute African Americans' overrepresentation in basketball, track and field, and football to natural genetic racial differences, aiming to establish a link between racial genetic inheritance and athletic achievement. From an educational perspective, in line with Entine's argument, Murray and Hernstein (1996) have argued that Blacks have inferior intellectual abilities compared to Whites and Asians. Entine's (2000) view, as well as Murray and Hernstein's (1996), mark Black young boys as being 'different' and/or the 'other' compared to the normative Whites. Both of these positions implicitly produce stereotypical constructions of the African American body that are fallacious and thus can have serious detrimental effects on both African American and white young people.

In contrast to such positions, some sociologists in physical culture have argued that the overrepresentation of blacks in certain sports is the result of cultural tradition as well as historical, educational, and social factors that, in complicated ways, have channelled African Americans' participation into certain sports (Azzarito and Harrison, 2008; Binger and Harrison, 2011;

Harrison, Azzarito, and Burden, 2004; Ferber, 2007; Nelson, 2012). The dominant discourse of Blacks' innate physical edge reflects a form of cultural racism that positions African Americans as the *other*, implicitly suggesting their intellectual inferiority compared to Whites. Black bodies are marked as the *other* in opposition to White bodies, which in turn, are 'constructed as the neutral body that contains no difference and, thus, does not feel the effects of normalization' (Erickson, 2005, p. 384). While invisible, however, whiteness as a material classification of skin informs the ways the body is viewed, constructed and experienced. For instance, several researchers have demonstrated how the 'White men can't jump' discourse on the one hand, and the 'black edge' discourse on the other, are intimately attached to both White and African American boys' bodies and the construction of hegemonic (hyper)masculinity. For both White and African American boys, racialized discourses of dominant masculinities might have detrimental effects on their embodied identities (Azzarito and Harrison, 2008; Binger and Harrison, 2011; Harrison, Azzarito and Burden, 2004; Lawrence, 2005; Louis, 2003). For example, as a result of such racialized discourses, Black male youths are often channelled by coaches and physical education (PE) teachers into certain sports, encouraging them to embody the *hoop dreams* discourse at the expense of academics, while discouraging White youth from pursuing their dreams of becoming professional athletes. This is problematic for both White and African American young boys' construction of their masculinity in their negotiations of racial power relations embedded in certain sports.

Resisting black sport and the restoration of heteronormative white masculinity: the *white negro* in alternative sports

Each sport symbolizes a different way of being, thus producing a wide range of cultural expressions and experiences of masculinities. 'White men can't jump', for example, reproduces the rhetoric of Black physical superiority on the basketball court, while attempting to restore White heteronormative masculinity, staging the possibility that 'White men can finally dunk' (Brayton, 2010, p. 67). While sustaining Black male physical superiority (and intellectual inferiority), Entine's argument, however, reflects an increasing anxiety about White racial inferiority in sport, aiming implicitly and explicitly, to re-establish White male power. Because sport intrinsically ties to the construction of boys' masculinity, alternative sports have become a context of subversion of Black's domination of certain sports to manage insecurities about Whiteness and masculinity, and thus to re-African American and re-establish White male power. In the context of North America, hegemonic forms of masculinity naturalized by traditional, heavy contact, male-dominated sports such as American football and basketball are contested by young White boys' engagement in alternative sports.

In line with other forms of masculine sporting bodies for instance, the climbing body in extreme and alternative sports is a strategic use of the body that hides the weaknesses and insecurities of White masculinity, thus re-establishing the heterosexual 'real man' (Erickson, 2005). Thorpe (2010), for instance, offers insights into the different forms of heteronormative masculinities created in the context of snowboarding, identifying 'the grommets', 'the bros', 'the real men' and 'the old guys'. As demonstrated in Thorpe's study, male snowboarders' gendered identities are dynamic, fluid, contradictory and multidimensional, established based on the configuration of power relations and young people's negotiation of gender/sex power relations embedded in this specific sport context. Masculinities operate in young boys' lives differently based on how they decide to negotiate gender/sex, race, and social class power relations and expectations, competitive culture, body appearance and performance, ideals of masculinity, and desire.

In particular, the displacement of White boys from traditional popular sports, such as basketball and football, has produced subcultural representations of White youths in alternative and/or extreme sports (e.g. snowboarding, skateboarding, rock climbing, BMX), establishing the rebirth of both White masculinity and White male resistance to Black-dominated sports (Brayton, 2005; Erickson, 2005; Thorpe, 2010). Different from American football and basketball, alternative sports, such as skateboarding, snowboarding, and rockclimbing, which tend to be dominated by young White and middle and upper class young men, might simultaneously represent a homosocial escape from normative hegemonic forms of hypermasculinity in more popular sports, such as football and basketball, and/or a form of refusal to participate in sports dominated by the 'other' (Erickson, 2005; Thorpe, 2010).

As Brayton (2005) suggested, to restore 'insecurities of Whiteness and masculinity [that] are reflected and articulated through popular culture' (p. 357), alternative sports present nonconformist and transgressive, yet empowering sites for young White boys to confidently perform the athletic body as well as to rebel against White normative masculinity constructed upon middle-class norms and grounded in White suburbia. Alternative sports, in this case, symbolize the rebirth of White masculinity as well as White resistance to Black-dominated sports, yet a compliance to aspects of Black body performance. Resisting mainstream norms, alternative sports offer an unconventional physical culture context for celebrating a new form of White heteromasculinity – a White masculinity that is confident, strong, brave and athletic. Through and in alternative sport, White boys re-construct themselves, expressing new forms of sporting bodies: bodies that refuse to comply to mainstream norms and escape the traditional space of popular sports and that repudiate a form of heteromasculinity informed by White middle-class norms. Rather, through their engagement in alternative sports, those sporting bodies espouse a new form of heteronormative performance of masculinity characterized by cool features of the Black *other*.

While the 'insecurity of Whiteness and masculinity are reflected and articulated through popular culture' (Brayton, 2005, p. 357), alternative sports offer sites of physical culture for the performance of the athletic 'Black Negro'. Such subcultures reject the middle-class White norms and values that traditional sports often embrace, and thus they seek to represent a 'strong, proud, confident, unconstrained, and unapologetic White athletic masculinity' (p. 359), constructing, re-articulating and borrowing aspects of Black physicality, thus becoming the *White Negro*. The image of the athletic *White Negro* functions as a means to repair a damaged White masculinity by adhering to some hypermasculine performative aspects of the *other* – sexual and athletic prowess – in unconventional sports contexts. For many White male youth, investing in the athletic *White Negro* in extreme and alternative sports distance themselves from traditional sports (dominated by the *other*), while simultaneously compensating for insecurities of White normative identity by restoring a confident, strong, masculine identity that complies with the *other*.

Young people's identities, both Black and White, are precarious and contestable rather than fixed and stable. While traditional, alternative and extreme sports produce different kinds of masculinities, all these sport-driven sites of physical culture can be violently homophobic and sexist (Azzarito and Solomon, 2004; Azzarito and Harrison, 2010; Thorpe, 2010), sustaining and legitimating *real men's* behaviour at the expense of women and gay male athletes. Sports that are strictly male-dominated produce and maintain male bonding experiences, which in turn, reinforce gendered ideals about sporting behaviour that can become exclusionary and discriminatory. Certain subcultures in alternative sports, however, welcome women who demonstrate physical prowess rather than qualities associated with the traditional construction of femininity in sport (e.g. lack of skilfulness and assertive behaviour). Snowboarding culture, for example, accepts women who can display physical prowess, courage, confidence, skilfulness and strength – all needed physicality traits to become a skilled snowboarder (Thorpe, 2010). These traits are based on expectations and values imprinted on snowboarding male bodies. Yet, the underlying assumption that informs the snowboarding culture is hierarchical: men are *naturally* physical superior and women snowboarders are accepted into the heteronormative snowboarding culture only if they fit in, thus stabilizing the gender/sex binary.

Sporting bodies that disturb compulsory heteronormativity in sport: a 'gender trouble'

Snowboarding and/or other performances of sporting bodies that are implicitly heteronormative can contribute to discrimination against, and cultural subjugation of, gay young people (Anderson and McCormack, 2010; McDonald, 2002). The rigid boundaries put up and dictated by male sports create a compulsory heterosexuality culture, which, in turn, has a material impact on the body, keeping out *queer* performances of athleticism (Anderson and McCormack, 2010). As a result, sporting young boys learn how to self-monitor and self-manage to strictly adhere to acceptable forms of compulsory masculine heterosexuality, carefully disavowing other forms of masculinity that can be categorized as different and thus repressed in the context of sport. Homophobia has material, real effects on gay young boys by labelling their bodies as abnormal bodies that need to be punished, treated and normalized. Homophobia, which is deeply rooted in sport contexts, produces social exclusion, and moreover, has the potential to seriously damage the embodiment of young boys who self-identify as gay. Historically, in the United States (US), Black and White gay men have faced significant persecution and experienced physical violence (McDonald, 2002). In the context of the United Kingdom (UK), 'It was not until 1967 that male homosexuality was decriminalized in Great Britain and it took a further seven years before the American Psychiatric Association ruled that homosexuality should be taken off the list of diseases and no longer regarded as a mental disorder' (Clarke, 2006). Because sport still sustains a strictly heterosexual culture, as Anderson and McCormack (2010) asserted: 'It is obvious that overt, cultural, and institutional oppression of gay boys and men leads to more athletes remaining closeted compared to non-athletes' (p. 959). As long as homophobia permeates sporting culture, gay boys in sport will continue to experience discrimination, and oppression and they will be more likely to self-segregate, stay closeted and create different, safe sporting subcultures.

Homophobia impacts young girls in sport as well. Dominant discourses of compulsory heterosexuality validate and reinforce 'morally appropriate' behaviour dictating what constitutes acceptable/normal sexual identities (Clarke, 2006). Recognizing that the 'hoop dream comes through for millions of American girls' (Banet-Weser, 1999, p. 415), young girls (as well as young boys) feel pressure to use strategies to demonstrate feminine, heterosexual qualities to reassure their families, peers, coaches and teachers that they are not butch but real women. Indeed, other sports, such as figure skating, gymnastics, golf and tennis, remain predominantly White-dominated, reproducing White female ideals of agility, elegance, grace and feminine beauty (Azzarito and Solmon, 2005). Maintaining a feminine appearance means constructing a body that is in opposition to a masculine look. It is important to recall that the normative gender/sex category is constructed upon exclusion, hierarchical classification and repudiation of the *other*. Butch, lesbian bodies are marked as other, abnormal and/or deviant bodies that represent sites of disruption of the gender/sex heteronormative alignment that disturb the normative landscape of sports (Azzarito and Katzew, 2010). Girls might experience significant distress in their efforts to reconcile sexual identity with sport for fear of harassment and negative labelling (Clarke, 2006). Like for boys, girls are often pressured to self-manage a body performance that is accepted and legitimated in society. Homophobia thus works to stabilize the gender/sex alignment, functioning as a means to monitor, scrutinize and control heteronormative femininity, pathologizing and classifying female bodies that are too masculine as threats to the ideal of athletic, heterosexual, female bodies (Hannis-Martin, 2006).

The world of sport for young girls is not easy to negotiate, though there has been progress over the past forty years in terms of gender equity and equality. Dominant homophobic stereotypes and normative gendered and racialized social beliefs remain and they are difficult to eradicate from Western societies. Since the 1970s and 1980s, however, second-wave feminism has helped young women to gain significant access into the male-dominated world of sport both in and outside of school, as well as male-dominated professions (Azzarito and Solmon, 2005). In the US, as a result of the second-wave feminist movement and the passage of Title IX legislation in 1972, young women have been able to enter more thoroughly into the world of professional and amateur sports and have had more access to sport opportunities and athletic facilities in school contexts (Azzarito and Solomon, 2005; Hanis-Martin, 2006). The UK, as well as the US, aims to affirm women's achievement of gender equality and social change and has witnessed a significant increase of young women's participation in sport over the past two decades (Scraton *et al.*, 2005). Although second-wave feminism challenged the gendered social construction of sport, opening up more opportunities and choices for women's entrance into previously inaccessible male-dominated arenas of sport, inequalities and inequities still persist (Kane, 1996; Walseth, 2006).

To continue working toward gender equality, today's gender(s) agenda aims to destabilize the gender/sex binary at the intersection of other social categories and thus disrupt the gender order of sports, in an effort to re-construct sport as a more inclusive and equitable space for young girls (McDonald, 2002). Another goal of the new gender(s) agenda is to reveal the ways dominant discourses of race/gender and social class construct stereotypical construction of young girls' bodies that put them into hierarchies, from low- to high-status sporting bodies. In the construction of heteronormative femininity, for instance, differences related to race, social class and disability play a crucial role (Azzarito, 2010), producing a wide range of femininities and masculinities that are accepted and/or rejected in society, differing based on sport, cultural context and political-economic power relations. While young boys invest in the construction of traditional masculinity through sport in their efforts to become *real men*, the construction of the female sporting body is not tied to traditional ideals of femininity. Rather, female sporting bodies are fabricated in opposition to ideals of femininity, disturbing the conventionally male-dominated space of sport. The binary of gender/sex aims to cement muscularity, competition and athletic prowess – all conventionally masculine traits – in opposition to feminine characteristics, such as slenderness and the lack of skillfulness and athleticism. When sex and gender are aligned, heteronormative discourses around womanhood embedded in whiteness inform the construction of the good White girl (McDonald, 2002). In the North American context, White middle-class women have been viewed historically as central figures in the creation of the heteronormative family, child rearing and devotion to home and husband, expecting to perform gendered physicality and engage in morally appropriate behaviour. Sport was not viewed as encouraging lady-like behaviour but instead as being potentially damaging to vulnerable, frail women's bodies and reproductive systems (Cahn, 1998; Vertinsky, 1990).

As a result, while the White middle-class woman has traditionally signified ideals of womanhood, in the American fantasy of gender hierarchy, female African American young women's bodies have been viewed as disrupting the ideal of womanhood. In the sport context, the image of the mannish lesbian can be as threatening as the Black woman. Similar to lesbians, or women's bodies that look too masculine, African American women are positioned by discourses of Whiteness and compulsory heterosexuality as *other* women, having bodies that deviate from the heteronormative fantasy of White ideal womanhood (Hannis-Martin, 2006). The image of ideal middle-class White womanhood is positioned in opposition to the Black women's engagement in strenuous sport given their experience of hard physical labor, excessive exertion and low socio-economic class. Images of African American women have been constructed historically as being potentially detrimental to women's devotion to fostering a stable home and child rearing. African American women have been presented culturally as strong, erotic, athletic bodies – bodies different and deviant from *real* White women (Azzarito and Solomon, 2005).

The intersection of Whiteness and heteronormative discourses creates gendered, socially classed and racialized codes, hierarchical systems of difference that become inscribed on young girls' bodies. African American sporting women and their *excessive* muscularity displayed in the Women's National Basketball Association (WNBA), for instance, have been constructed as threatening bodies that create cultural anxiety with regard to the ideal White girl construct (Hannis-Martin, 2006). Another dominant discourse discussed in the literature, naked female aggression, circulates and celebrates women's basketball while simultaneously marking African American women's bodies as overtly and excessively masculine (Banet-Weiser, 1999). Such discourses damage the representation of Black women in sport, positioning and objectifying their bodies as deviant from normative, maternal, and morally appropriate. The naked female aggression discourse implicitly fixates social meanings of true women who demonstrate that they are morally superior and morally guardians of the game, not to African American but to White female women in sport. Because of the circulation of these racialized and heteronormative discourses around the feminine body, Black women, lesbians and/or young women who deviate from the ideal of feminine heteronormative ideals might suffer from negative labels and stereotypes that portray them as not being real women. Recently, however, the ideal of being a girl in sport has become increasingly complicated by global trends that put forward new heteronormative ideals of future girls, who display powerful, strong bodies and are as successful as boys in sport, transcending barriers of social class and race with self-determination, self-esteem and confidence (Azzarito, 2010).

Re-centering young people experiencing disability in sport

Through their engagement in sport, young people might be coded and code themselves in categorical and/or disparaging terms, such as feminine, masculine, Black, White, straight, butch, real men, wimp, faggots, and disabled, seeing and constituting themselves through stereotypical discourses of gender, sexuality, race, class and disability (Sterkenburg and Knoppers, 2004). In Western society, race/ethnicity, gender/sexuality and (dis)ability have been used historically in categorical terms to give meanings to experiences and the body, classifying normative bodies in opposition to other ways of being in sport (Flintoff, Fitzgerald and Scraton, 2008). The process of *othering* also has been applied to disabled young peoples' bodies, marking them as bodies with disadvantage or deficit (McPhail and Freeman, 2005). With regard to the ways the intersectionality of gender/race/sexuality/social class impacts young people's physicality in sport, Fitzgerald (2006) argued that issues of disability are often excluded from such socio-cultural analysis and that they need to be re-centered to fully understand intersectionality and youth in sport.

In Western society, dualistic ways of thinking or naturalistic categories of the normal/ abnormal body historically have been applied to the construction of disability as well. Informed by a medical model, young people's disabled bodies continue to be treated as belonging to a homogeneous group and excluded from the context of normative sport. Similar to other bodies in sport, the medical model has defined and framed disabled bodies as being deficient, an abnormal body that is hierarchically inferior to the able body. In particular, the medicalization of the disabled body has informed the construction of disabled young people as being flawed – sick, spoilt, non-conforming – compared to able, normative bodies. Several scholars (Fitzgerald, 2006; Goodwin, 2009; McPhail and Freeman, 2005) have pointed out that the medicalization of the disabled body can result in a significantly narrow and restricted understanding of the experiences of young people's disabled bodies in the context of sports.

The meanings of disability cannot be interrogated as long as disability continues to be framed within a deficit-based medical paradigm (Goodwin, 2009). Young people who are framed as a problem will make sense of their embodiment within that frame. Within disability and sport, to challenge the deficit-based model, Goodwin and Peers (2012) suggest that the term disabled young people be re-defined as young people experiencing disability to reconceptualize disability as a social condition, as well as to legitimate young people who claim a disability-related identity. Sport that is constructed upon able-body norms excludes young people experiencing disability. Scholars thus have called for research that challenges paradigms of normativity, re-articulating disability from an embodied perspective (Goodwin, 2009; McPhail and Freeman, 2005). Because such binaries and normative ways of thinking about the body can impact the bodies of young people experiencing disability in a detrimental way, there is a need to enable them to experience their sporting bodies in a positive light (Fitzgerald, 2006, p. 757). Thus, researchers need to explore the insights and meaning-making of young people experiencing disability in sports. Spaces of sport constructed upon alternative sporting values could potentially enable young people experiencing disability to construct their bodies in new ways, taking down able-bodied walls cemented on the court.

Conclusion

Intersectionality makes an important theoretical and methodological contribution to understanding the complexity of sport, identity and opportunity. In this chapter, it has informed how, for example, gender, sexuality, race and class intersect to *other* and exclude many young people. In some senses, it is a meta-framework as its breadth and complexity invite multiple ways of understanding specific dimensions of difference using their own theoretical tools such as could occur when the place of race in intersectional research is further examined through critical race theory (e.g. Hylton, 2009). Intersectionality also lends itself to driving methodologies in which empirical data is generated at the intersections of dimensions of difference as well as generating understanding of nuanced, lived experiences of young people. However, aspirations to capture complexity through intersectionality are necessarily limited as the interplay of a young person's biography, social and geographical location, identity, biology etc., is infinite in what together work as barriers to sporting engagement. As researchers and practitioners we can be left with the challenge of disrupting dominant discourses and practices such that all young people have the opportunity to experience positive outcomes from sport.

It is here that strengths-based or identity-work approaches to sport, education, health and human services and so forth (e.g. Azzarito *et al.*, 2014; Holt, 2008; McCuaig, Quennerstedt and Macdonald, 2013; Seligman *et al.*, 2009; Seidler, 2010) can be a useful complement to intersectionality as the focus moves from accounting for the interplay of gender, sexuality, ability, race, ethnicity, geographical location, class, colour, body shape and so on and focuses on young people's strengths. The questions become: *how do young people successfully engage in sport?* And, *what personal, social and community resources do young people have upon which we can build?* regardless of the constellation of their positionality as others. This flipped way of thinking can risk privileging a focus on the individual and not structural problems, many of which have been outlined in this chapter. Nevertheless, in our view, they do offer an inclusive approach that challenges binaries, and consequentially othering, and values all young people and the fluidity of their contexts and preferences (Macdonald *et al.*, 2012). They also accounts for questions of power that can arise in equity research and interventions as the young people themselves become empowered rather than being objects of others' scholarship interests (e.g. Rossi, Rynne and Nelson, 2013). The complementarity of intersectionality and strengths-based or identity-work approaches to youth sport offers the field exciting ways to understand complexity and promote positive sporting experiences for all young people.

References

Anderson, E. and McCormack, M. (2010). Intersectionality, critical race theory, and American sporting oppression: Examining black and gay male athletes. *Journal of Homosexuality*, *57*, 949–967.

Azzarito, L. (2010). Future girls, transcendent femininities and new pedagogies: Toward girls' hybrid bodies. *Sport. Education and Society*, *15*, 261–275.

Azzarito, L. and Harrison, L. (2008). 'White men can't jump.' Race, gender and natural athleticism. *International Review for the Sociology of Sport*, *43*, 347–364.

Azzarito, L. and Katzew, A. (2010). Performing identities in physical education: (En)gendering fluid selves. *Research Quarterly for Exercise and Sport*, *81*(1), 25–37.

Azzarito, L. and Solomon, M.A. (2005). A reconceptualization of physical education:The intersection of gender/race/social class. *Sport, Education and Society*, *10*, 25–47.

Azzarito, L., Marttinen, R., Simon, M., Markiewiez, R. (2014). "I'm beautiful": A case for adopting a sociocultural perspective in physical education teacher education. In S.B. Flory, S. Sanders, and A. Tishler (eds), *Sociocultural issues in physical education. Case Studies for teachers*. New York, Rowman and Littlefiled.

Benet-Weiser, S. (1999). Hoop dreams. Professional basketball and the politics of race and gender. *Journal of Sport and Social Issues*, *23*, 403–420.

Bimper, A.Y., Harrison, L. (2011). Meet me at the crossroads: African American athletic and racial identity. *Quest*, *63*, 275–288.

Brayton, S. (2005). "Black-lash": Revisiting the "White Negro" through skateboarding. *Sociology of Sport Journal*, *22*, 356–372.

Butler, J. (1990). *Gender trouble: Feminism and the subversion of identity*. New york: Routledge.

Cahn, S. (1998). From the 'muscle moll' to the 'butch' ballplayer: Mannishness, lesbianism, and homophobia in US women's sports. In R. Weitz (ed), *The politics of women's bodies: Sexuality, appearance, and behaviour* (pp. 67–81). Oxford: Oxford University Press.

Carrington, B. and Wood, E. (1995). Body talk: Images of sport in a multi-racial school. In C. Critcher, P. Bramham, and A. Tomlinson (eds), *Sociology of Leisure: A reader* (55–72). London: E. and F.N. Spon.

Carrington, B., Chivers, T. and Williams, T. (1987). Gender, leisure and sport: A case-study of young people of South Asian descent. *Leisure Studies*, *6*, 265–279.

Clarke, G. (2006). Sexuality and physical education. In D. Kirk, Macdonald, D. and O'Sullivan, M. (eds), *Handbook of Physical Education* (pp. 723–736). London: Sage Publications.

Erickson, B. (2005). Style matters: Explorations of bodies, Whiteness, and identity in rock climbing. *Sociology of Sport Journal*, *22*, 373–396.

Erueti, B. and Palmer, F. (2014). *Te Whariki Tuakiri* (the identity mat): Māori elite athletes and the expression of ethno-cultural identity in global sport. *Sport in Society*, *17*(8), 1061–1075.

Ferber, A.L. (2007). The construction of black masculinity: White supremacy now and then. *Journal of Sport and Social Issues*, *31*, 11–24.

Fitzgerald, H. (2006). Disability and physical education. In D. Kirk, Macdonald, D. and O'Sullivan, M. (eds), *Handbook of Physical Education* (pp. 752–766). London: Sage Publications.

Flintoff, A. Fitzgerald, H. and Scraton, S. (2008). The challenges of intersectionality: researching difference in physical education. *International Studies in Sociology of Education*, *2*, 73–85.

Goodwin, D. and Peers, D. (2012). Disability, sport and inclusion. In S. Dagkas and K. Armour (eds), *Inclusion and exclusion through youth sport* (pp. 186–202). Champaign, Illinois: Human Kinetics.

Hallinan, C. and Judd, B. (2012). Duelling paradigms: Australian Aborigines, marn-gook and football histories. *Sport in Society*, *15*(7), 975–986.

Hokowhitu, B. (2003). 'Physical beings': Stereotypes, sport and the 'physical education' of New Zealand Maori. *Culture, Sport, Society, 6* (2–3), 192–218.

Hanis-Martin, J. (2006). Embodying contradictions: The case of professional women's basketball. *Journal of Sport and Social Issues, 30,* 265–288.

Harrison, L. (2011). Athletes' rights and justice issues: It's not business, it's personal. *Journal of Intercollegiate Sport, 4,* 14–17.

Harrison, L., Azzarito, L. and Burden, J. (2004). Perceptions of athletic superiority: A view from the other side. *Race, Ethnicity and Education, 7,* 149–166.

Holt, N.L. (2008). *Positive youth development through sport.* London: Routledge.

Hylton, K. (2009). *"Race" and sport: critical race theory.* London: Routledge.

Kane, M.J. (1996). Media coverage of the post Title IX female athlete: A feminist analysis of sport, gender, and power. *Duke Journal of Gender Law and Policy, 3,* 95–127.

Lawrence, S.M. (2005). African American athletes' experiences of race in sport. *International Review for the Sociology of Sport, 40,* 99–110.

Macdonald, D., Pang, B., Knez, K., Nelson, A. and McCuaig, L. (2012). The will for inclusion: bothering the inclusion/exclusion discourses of sport. In S. Dagkas and K. Armour (eds), *Inclusion and exclusion through youth sport* (pp. 9–23). London: Routledge.

McDonald, M.G. (2002). Queering Whiteness: The peculiar case of the women's national basketball association. *Sociological Perspectives, 45,* 379–396.

McCuaig, L., Quennerstedt, M. and Macdonald, D. (2013). A salutogenic, strengths-based approach as a theory to guide HPE curriculum change. *Asia-Pacific Journal of Health, Sport and Physical Education, 4(2),* 109–125.

McPhail, J.C. and Freeman, J.G. (2005). Beyond prejudice: thinking toward genuine inclusion. *Learning Disabilities Practice, 20(4),* 254–267.

Messner, M.A. and Sabo, D.F. (1990). Toward a critical feminist reappraisal of sport, men, and the gender order. In M.A. Messner and D.F. Sabo (eds), *Sport, men, and the gender order. Critical feminist perspectives* (pp. 1–16). Champaign, Illinois: Human Kinetics.

Millington. B., Vertinsky, P., Boyle, E. and Wilson, B. (2008). Making Chinese-Canadian masculinities in Vancouver's physical education curriculum. *Sport, Education and Society, 13,* 195–214.

Nelson, A. (2012). 'You don't have to be black skinned to be black': Indigenous young people's bodily practices. *Sport, Education and Society, 17,* 57–75.

Rossi, A., Rynne, S. and Nelson, A. (2013) 'Doing whitefella research in blackfella communities in Australia: Decolonizing method in sports related research', *Quest, 65,* 116–131.

Scraton, S., Caudwell, J. and Holland, S. (2005). 'Bend it like Patel'. Centering race, ethnicity and gender in feminist analysis of women's football in England. *International Review for the Sociology of Sport, 40,* 71–88.

Seidler, V.J. (2010). *Embodying identities. Culture, differences and social theory.* Bristol; The Policy Press.

Seligman, M., Ernst, R., Gillham, J., Reivich, K. and Linkins, M. (2009). Positive education: positive psychology and classroom interventions. *Oxford Review of Education, 35(3),* 293–311.

St Louis, B. (2003). Sport, genetics and the 'natural athlete': the resurgence of racial science. *Body and Society, 9,* 75–95.

Thorpe, H. (2010). Bourdieu, gender reflexivity, and physical culture: A case of masculinities in the snowboarding field. *Journal of Sport and Social Issues, 34,* 176–214.

van Sterkenburg, J. and Knoppers, A. (2004). Dominant discourses about race/ethnicity and gender in sport practice and performance. *International Review for the Sociology of Sport, 39,* 301–321.

Vertinsky, P. (1990). *The eternally wounded woman: Woman, doctors and exercise in the late nineteenth century.* Manchester: Manchester University Press.

Vogler, P. (2003). Students with disabilities in physical education: possibilities and problems. In S.J. Silverman and C.D. Ennis (eds), *Student learning in physical education: Applying research to enhance instruction* (pp. 227–241). Champaign, Illinois: Human Kinetics.

Walseth, K. (2006). Sport and belonging. *International review for the Sociology of Sport, 41,* 447–464.

Wright, J. and Macdonald, D. (eds). (2010). *Young people, physical activity and the everyday.* London: Routledge.

31

YOUTHS' PARTICIPATION RIGHTS IN RELATION TO DOMINANT MOVEMENT CULTURES

Karin Redelius and Håkan Larsson

Introduction

Participating in sport is a vital aspect of many young people's lives. Since the 1970s, increased participation among young people have been reported across the developed world (Green, 2010). While child and youth sport is primarily taking place in schools in countries such as the USA, Canada and UK, voluntary sports clubs have an important role in this respect in the Scandinavian countries (Ibsen and Seippel, 2010). In Sweden, around ninety per cent participate in a sport club at one time or another during their youth (Thedin Jakobsson, 2015). During adolescence, however, many are dropping out of sport, which is also an international trend that has been highlighted in a number of studies (Coakley and Pike, 2009; De Knop *et al.*, 1996; Findlay *et al.*, 2009; Pilgaard, 2013; Seabra *et al.*, 2007; Scheerder *et al.*, 2006). A variety of causes for dropping out (Fraser-Thomas *et al.*, this volume) have been examined; for example conflicts of interest, lack of fun and perception of low abilities (Weiss and Amorose, 2008); conflicts with coaches, and the need for more playing time (Weiss and Williams, 2004); as well as negative factors related to early specialization (Wall and Côté, 2007).

Research also indicates that children and youth who do not feel that they can influence their sporting practice and whose views are not taken into account tend to stop earlier than others. A study that focused on youth's participation rights showed that far from all young people feel they can make their voices heard (Trondman, 2011). On the contrary, the results suggest that more than eight out of ten young club sport participants do not feel they have any kind of influence over their own training and competition activities. Many young people seemed pleased with that situation and did not wish to have more to say about their sporting practice. The question is rather complex, however. The ones who did feel that they had the possibility to influence their sport were not satisfied either; in short, they wished they had even greater opportunities to influence. An important finding in the study was that the young athletes who did not feel so involved in decision-making, which they in themselves were happy with, tended to drop-out earlier than the youth who felt more involved. Apparently the perceived degree of involvement was related to the willingness or unwillingness to remain in club sports. Working to increase children's and young people's influence is therefore important in the endeavours to get more youth to want to continue longer. Siedentop (2002: 397) comments thus:

> I am convinced that junior sport must increasingly allow for decision-making and foster independence as youth grow through their teens. [. . .] If we are to have adults to choose to participate in sports, we must take more seriously the goal of helping youngsters to become more independent and make good choices in sport. Unfortunately, models of coaching throughout the world tend to emphasize coach control of athletes that limits their independence and decision-making.

In the above quote, Siedentop draws our attention to prevailing coaching practices that make little space for young athletes' decision making. In a Swedish study, a majority of the coaches said that there was nothing, or at least nothing they could think of, that youth could decide on in the sporting context (Redelius, 2011). A number of questions can thus be raised: Do children who participate in sport have any rights? What can children decide for themselves in sport? Do they ever get a chance to be heard? Why is the coach at the centre of sport (Parameswara, 1985) and not youth?

Children and youth certainly have rights, rights that are articulated in the United Nation's Convention on the Rights of the Child, which has been ratified by all but two of the world's nations (United Nations, 1989). A child is regarded a person up to eighteen years of age, which means that the convention covers those we also call youth. In this chapter, we will discuss the possibilities for children and young people to have something to say about their participation in sport as a part of a wider physical culture. We are thus interested in illuminating their chances to be subjects in their own thinking and acting when participating in sport. This endeavour is tantamount to the intentions in the Convention on the Rights of the Child.

The Convention on the Rights of the Child

According to the United Nation, the Convention on the Rights of the Child (CRC) sets out the rights that must be realized for children to develop their full potential, free from hunger and want, neglect and abuse. It reflects a new vision of the child. Children are neither the property of their parents nor helpless objects of charity. They are human beings and, as human beings, have their own rights. The CRC offers a vision of the child as an individual and as a member of a family and community, with rights and responsibilities appropriate to his or her age and stage of development. By recognizing children's rights in this way, the CRC firmly places the focus on the whole child. Human rights apply to all age groups. If children have the same general human rights as adults, why do they then need an extra Convention? The CRC was launched in 1989 and it is a result of the recognition that children and youth are particularly vulnerable. Therefore, they also have particular rights that recognize their special need for protection, but protection is only one of the three Ps mentioned in the CRC. The others are provision and participation. In other words, a child has the right to:

- provision (health and education)
- protection (against discrimination, abuse, neglect)
- participation (the right to be heard in decisions that affect his or her life).

The CRC recognizes the human rights of children and is without doubt the most powerful child rights instrument. Its starting point is not that children are passive and vulnerable objects in need of protection, but that they are active subjects who can and want to exercise their rights. The principles that are considered the most important, the so-called core principles, are Article 2, which states that all children have equal rights and equal value and should not be discriminated; Article 3, which indicates that it is the child who must be a primary consideration in all decisions affecting the child (what is the child's best interest must be resolved in each case); Article 6, which says that every child has the right to survive, live and develop (physically and spiritually, morally, mentally and socially); and, finally, Article 12, concerning the child's right to express his or her views and to have them taken into account in all matters that concern them. Perhaps the most important article is number 3: In all actions concerning children, the best interest of the child shall be the major consideration. But what does this have to do with sport?

The rights of the child in relation to sport

The CRC does not say anything explicit about sport, although researchers maintain that most of its substantive articles have a bearing on youth's participation in sport (Donnelly, 2008) Are sporting activities not designed with the child's best interests in mind? Do sports organizations and coaches not follow the principles of the CRC? According to the two Canadian researchers, Donnelly and Petherick (2004), who have conducted extensive studies of children's rights in sport, this is not always the case. Instead, they argue that children's rights are violated in many of the countries that organise youth sport. They believe that violations occur, occasionally or routinely and directly and indirectly, in about half of the forty articles of the Convention. In an attempt to provide a larger picture of the ethical issues surrounding youth's engagement in sport from a human rights perspective, David (2005) broke new and important ground. His book *Human Rights in Youth Sport: A Critical Review of Children's Rights in Competitive Sport* demonstrates that human rights and competitive sport are closely interwoven, despite the fact that, as David himself says, 'they have ignored each other for decades' (David, 2005: 3). There is indeed a growing interest in issues concerning children's rights and child protection in sport. Research acknowledges the role of overtraining, sexual abuse, burnout, dropout and the exploitation of child athletes, for example, the trafficking of young male football players. These issues have prompted a number of academics, concerned parents and former athletes to speak out against severe training regimes and to call for investigations into the balance between individual rights and adult and state responsibilities in sport. In short, the issue is whether children and young people are regarded as athletes first and children second in the sporting context.

In the next section, we will discuss children and young people's opportunities to have something to say about their participation in sport from a cultural sociological perspective. In other words, we are interested in the prerequisites for youths to exercise the right to express their views freely and to have them accounted for in the sporting context of different movement cultures. Essentially, having something to say about one's participation is closely related to whether the participants are primarily constructed as subjects of experience and willingness, or as objects of external forces and demands, and this is in turn largely affected by cultural norms and values that dominates sporting practices of physical culture.

Movement cultures, practical sense and logics of practice

When children grow up, they face an already existing physical culture, which consists of different movement cultures, where the term 'movement culture' designates the ways in which social groups deal 'with the need and desire for movement beyond labor or maintaining life (Crum, 1993: 341). Different movement cultures are characterised by different norms, values and practices. As children and young people interact in different movement cultures, they (learn to) make use of different collections of cultural 'tools' that serve as the means for the performance of action (Sewell, 2005: 46). These tools are not to be seen as coherent systems of symbols and meanings, they are to differing degrees contingent and, as such, they enable actors 'to play on the multiple meanings of symbols – thereby redefining situations in ways that they believe will favour their purposes' (Sewell, 2005: 51).

According to the French cultural sociologist Pierre Bourdieu, the actor's, or in Bourdieu's words, the agent's possibilities for using cultural tools to effectively favour their purposes depends on their 'practical sense' (Bourdieu, 1990). Practical sense, or to use Bourdieu's own metaphor *the feel for the game*, represents 'what gives the game a subjective sense – a meaning and a *raison d'etre*, but also a direction, an orientation, an impending outcome for those who take part and therefore acknowledge what is at stake' (Bourdieu, 1990: 66). The practical sense, however, 'is not so much a state of the mind as a state of the body, a state of being' (Thompson, 1991: 13). The participants' 'considerations' are to be seen as *corporal* rather than mental: 'It feels right' – or not right. Hence, it becomes difficult to address the culture critically; at least should it not by itself include particular tools for criticism. In order to be able to participate in any movement culture, not to say to be able to *change* the practice of that movement culture, the rising generation has to practically learn to make sense of the norms, values and practices of the culture, that is, to develop an appropriate practical sense. The practical sense of the participants, and indeed the possibilities to change or even to make their voices heard and having something to say about the practice of a certain culture is related to the logic of practice that dominates the culture.

The *logic of practice* is, according to Bourdieu, not to be seen as a way of projecting a rational logic on practice, but rather as a way of understanding practice on its own practical terms (Bourdieu, 1990). The world of practice, which is not the same as the world of rational logic, is corporal. Here, time and space is the essence: 'Practice unfolds in time and it has all the correlative properties, such as irreversibility [. . .] Its temporal structure, that is, its rhythm, its tempo, and above all its directionality, is constitutive of its meaning' (Bourdieu, 1990: 81). Bourdieu adds that:

> A player who is involved and caught up in the game adjusts not to what he sees but to what he fore-sees, sees in advance in the directly perceived present; he passes the ball not to the spot where his team-mate is but to the spot he will reach – before his opponent – a moment later.
>
> *(Bourdieu, 1990: 81)*

Characteristic of the logic of practice is that the actor of a practice – the practitioner – is dwelling in his or her practice, deciding what to do next, not from the point of view of a rational logic, but from the point of view of what is required from him or her to do in order to fulfil the logic of practice. The primary question for a practitioner is not to ask 'why do I do this or that?' but 'what do I do next in order to reach a convenient end?' This is where the concept of logics of practice fits neatly with the concept practical sense. An agent must develop a practical sense in order to master the logic of practice. As children grow up, they (must) learn to master the logics of practice of the different movement cultures in which they participate. But what are these movement cultures, what characterises them and, importantly, what possibilities have children and young people to make their voices heard and influence the conditions under which they participate?

Children, young people and sporting practices

In the article, *Who is physically active? Cultural capital and sports participation from adolescence to middle age – a 38-year follow-up study*, Swedish researcher Lars-Magnus Engström (2008), inspired by Pierre Bourdieu's toolbox, outlines a number of sporting practices occurring in movement culture. It is important to note that these sporting practices are not to be confused with the purposes or motives that people suggest inform their decision to participate in physical activity. Rather, the sporting practices include the logics of practice that govern how the activity unfolds in time and space, and consequently, they condition the practical sense that an individual must develop in order to successfully participate in the practice. In physical culture more broadly, Engström (2008) identifies a number of sporting practices, including competition and ranking, physical training, play and recreation, learning of skills, and *friluftsliv*, many of which he argues are particularly influential during childhood and adolescence.

Among small children, play and recreation is the dominant practice (Huizinga, 1955; Caillois, 1961; Kretschmar, 1973) with play being commonly regarded as a voluntary activity that should be fun, spontaneous and rarely involves thinking about the meaning or purpose of the game (Engström 2008). In this practice, children do not play because they want to accomplish particular objectives, but because they want to play. This way of viewing play emphasises the *process* of playing, and it is based on the perspective of the player and his or her *agency*. Play in this way may well include elements of struggle or physical challenges, but important here is not the outcome of the struggle or what benefits, economically or otherwise symbolically, the individual can cash in as a result of overcoming the physical challenge. Struggling and taking on challenges is primary, not what happens afterwards. Playing is fun here and now. Sometimes, however, and especially in sports, play is dealt with not as a process but rather as an activity – a play. Then the focus shifts easily from the process to the product, or the (intended) outcome of the activity. This is common when coaches use a play in a training regimen in order to achieve certain training objectives. With this comes, arguably, that children may exert less agency over the activity. Agency is transferred from the children to the coach. Looking at children participating in a play means that it might look *as if* the children are playing – they are participating in a play or a game, but are they really playing in terms of exerting agency?

Another significant practice during childhood and adolescence is *learning skills*. The learning of movement skills can take place both in organised and un-organised settings, the central objective of which, for Engström (2008), is the improvement and performance of motor (sport) skills through practice and systematic training in which the performance of the activity, rather than the body's physical condition, is prioritised. This practice is characterised by practitioners testing and practising, and evaluating and re-evaluating the result of their moving (Aggerholm, 2015). The corporeal character of physical culture means that the results of the movements are often self-evaluative and autodidactic; that is, the mover can immediately evaluate the level of success based on the outcome of the movement and try a new way of moving. Also when it comes to the learning of skills, the level of organisation may condition the agency of the participants. In less organised settings, the participants can choose for example, what to practice, the level of difficulty, the duration, and so on with a relatively higher grade of autonomy as compared to more organised settings. On the other hand, in organised settings, or in communities of practice (Lave and Wenger, 1991), there might be experts (who can be coaches but also skilled practitioners) who introduce and guide beginners, or legitimate peripheral participants, facilitating effective learning trajectories.

A third practice, which is also the dominating organised sporting practice among children and young people, is competition and ranking. The central objective here is to win, or to defeat the opponents, or at least to perform the best possible results. This practice might resemble play but it differs in the sense that here, winning, or the outcome of the activity, is more important than the activity itself. According to Engström (2008), this practice is often linked to certain values, including the use of the body as an instrument and the adoption of a particular way of life to assist in the achievement of desired goals through competition. He also adds that practice is crucial because:

> it is important to win, perform, be systematic and specialized, follow the rules and abide by the judge's decision, be law-abiding, dependent on authority and not oppositional, follow through on agreements, be loyal, display physical and psychological courage, take on challenges, remain 'cool' in moments of truth, to fight and never give up – even when faced with setbacks and extreme fatigue – and so on. [. . .] In sum, the central lesson involved in competition and ranking can be expressed as follows: it is essential to be capable and deliver positive results compared with others of the same gender.
>
> *(Engström, 2008: 340)*

Much of the above – pointing, for instance, to the need for the participants to follow the rules, be law-abiding, dependent on authority and not oppositional – is appropriate in relation to the opportunities to produce comparable results. Unlike in play, the practice of competition and ranking presupposes stable contest conditions, otherwise comparison of the produced results is rendered impossible. In a way, the subject has to choose to subordinate him- or herself to the contest conditions in order to be able to compete successfully, that is, in order to develop the appropriate feel for the game.

Arguably, the practice of competition and ranking takes a dominant position in physical culture in the sense that it exerts influence over other practices. For example, and as mentioned above, play – or what is at least designated 'play' – is utilised for training purposes. The relationship between play and competition is also seen in the propensity to view competition as *for real* while playing is merely *for fun*. Further, the practice of learning skills is often framed within a competition and ranking culture, as it is to a large extent in club sports, for which the learning of skills is a prerequisite. Then the value of the particular skill transforms from being valued in itself to being valued as means in order to win the contest, the match or the game.

Conclusion

In Sweden, the most influential organised leisure time form of physical activity is club sport. And the dominating practice of club sport is competition and ranking, although most of the time it may not be devoted to competitions *per se*. Much time is devoted to practising (learning of skills) and, as the participants grows older, physical training. The practice is however, as mentioned above, often heavily influenced by the practice of competition and ranking. Swedish children typically join sports clubs when they are between five and ten years old, boys generally somewhat earlier than girls. Participation is highest around the age of twelve, and then it drops again (Jakobsson *et al.*, 2014).

This pattern means, arguably, that small children are in the main faced with a physical culture characterised by the practices of play and recreation and the learning of skills. When they are five to ten years old, they join sport clubs and become faced with the practice of competition and ranking. During adolescence, the practice of physical training also grows important; however this is also, as was the case with play and the learning of skills, practiced within the frames of competition and ranking. The adolescent years are thus almost entirely dominated by the practice of competition and ranking, arguably with the consequence that many young people experience physical activities to be tantamount to competition. This might explain the large drop-out rates from club sport, as well as the gradually lower physical activity rates among adolescents and young adults.

Children and young people make up a large proportion of the participants in competitive sport, but competitive sport seems not primarily to be organised considering the children and the young (a primary focus on play/individual agency and the learning of skills). Rather, competitive/club sport is often organised on the basis of élite sport (a focus on producing objectively comparable results). With this follows that children and young people are not valued as *beings*, but as what they *might* become (should they be equipped with the appropriate talent and ability or willpower). In other words, children are regarded as raw materials that with proper processing can be developed into future elite athletes. In this sense, their sports participation has no intrinsic value, but is an investment for the future. The value lies in the athletic performance they may carry out or the money they might generate. Tied to this way of reasoning is the propensity among coaches and other sport representatives to emphasise if young people are equipped with talent and a desire to improve. This way of looking at youth is sometimes so strong that sport coaches feel that what they take to be talent and a desire to improve legitimises taking decisions concerning the children above the heads of the children. Coaches might even experience taking such decisions as being in the best interest of the child. The spirit of the CRC, however, is quite different. Childhood has a value in itself – it is not only a preparatory phase for what is to come. Also, regardless of development and potential talent, every child is precious and has the right to be treated as such here and now.

Finally, there is a widespread tendency to present sport as essentially positive with regard to the development of children and young people. According to Houlihan (2010), 'the magic dust of sport' has more broadly been seen as the solution to a range of problems relating to health, education, social cohesion, and so forth. Bailey and colleagues (2009) list a number of benefits that have been attributed to physical education and school sport. Rather than seeing sport as a social construction, which is then given meaning by the agents of the field, participants as well as more powerful defining agents, sport in itself the solution to different kinds of problem. As was the case with talent and the desire to improve, *a priori* notions about the benefits of sport might increase the tendency to decide what the best is for children above their heads. We believe that sport *might* be beneficial for lots of reasons. However, it is not a given fact. The benefits of sport do not come automatically but must be planned for. Sport for children has no intrinsic value, unless we construct it this way. To construct sport in the spirit of what is best for the child is every sporting child's right, and this includes actively involving children and young people in all decision making that concerns them.

References

Aggerholm, K. (2015). *Talent development in sport. On becoming an elite athlete*. London: Routledge.

Bailey, R., Armour, K., Kirk, D., Jess, M., Pickup, I., Sandford, R. and the BERA Physical Education and Sport Pedagogy Special Interest Group (2009). The educational benefits claimed for physical education and school sport: An academic review. *Research Papers in Education*, (24)1, 1–27.

Bourdieu, P. (1990). *The logic of practice*. Palo Alto, CA: Stanford University Press.

Caillois, R. (1961). *Men, play and games*. New York: The Free Press of Glencoe.

Coakley, J. and Pike, E. (2009). *Sport in society: issues and controversies*. Maidenhead: McGraw-Hill Education.

Crum, B. (1993). Conventional thought and practice in physical education: problems of teaching and implications for change. *Quest*, 45(3), 339–56.

David, P. (2005). *Human rights in youth sport: a critical review of children's rights in competitive sports*. London: Routledge.

De Knop, P., Engström L.-M. and Skirstad, B. (1996). Worldwide trends in youth sport. In P. De Knop, L.-M. Engström, B. Skirstad and M.R. Weiss (eds) *Worldwide trends in youth sport*. Champaign, Illinois: Human Kinetics.

Donnelly, P. (2008). Sport and human rights. *Sport in Society*, 11(4), 381–394.

Donnelly, P. and Petherick, L. (2004). Workers' playtime? Child labour at the extremes of the sporting spectrum. *Sport in Society*, 7(3), 301–321.

Engström, L.-M. (2008). Who is physically active? Cultural capital and sports participation from adolescence to middle age – a 38-year follow-up study. *Physical Education and Sport Pedagogy*, 13(4), 319–43.

Findlay, L., Garner, R. and Kohen, D. (2009). Children s organized physical activity patterns from childhood into adolescence. *Journal of Physical Activity and Health*, 6: 708–716.

Green, K. (2010). *Key themes in youth sport*. London: Routledge.

Houlihan, B. (2010) *Policy convergence in elite sport development: A critical review of the evidence*. Keynote presentation at the European Association for Sport Management conference, Prague, 2010.

Huizinga, J. (1955). *Homo ludens*. Boston, MA.: Beacon Press.

Ibsen, B. and Seippel, Ö. (2010). Voluntary organized sport in Denmark and Norway. *Sport in Society*, 13(4), 593–608.

Kretschmar, C.M. (1973). Ontological possibilities. sport as play. *The Philosophy of Sport*, 64–78.

Lave, J. and Wenger, E. (1991). *Situated learning: legitimate peripheral participation*. Cambridge, MA: Cambridge University Press.

Parameswara Ram, N. (1985) Coach is the centre of sports: philosophical perspective. *International Journal of Physical Education*, 1(1): 16–20.

Petlichkoff, L.M. (1993). Coaching children: understanding the motivational process. *Sport Science Review*, 2(1), 48–61.

Pilgaard, M. (2013). Age specific differences in sport participation in Denmark: Is development caused by generation, life phase or time period effects? *European Journal for Sport and Society*, 1(1): 31–52.

Redelius, K. (2011). Idrottsledarna och barnkonventionen: *Om idrottande barns rättigheter*. [*Coaches views' on the Convention on the Rights of the Child*]. Stockholm: Riksidrottsförbundet.

Seabra, A.F., Mendonca, D.M., Thomis, M.A., Malina, R.M. and Maia, J.A. (2007). Sports participation among Portuguese youth 10 to 18 years. *Journal of Physical Activity and Health*, 4()3), 370–380.

Scheerder, J., Thomis, M., Vanreusel, B., Lefevre, J., Renson, R., Vanden Eynde, B. and Beunen, G.P. (2006). Sports Participation among female from adolescence to adulthood. A longitudinal study. *International Review for the Sociology of Sport*, 41(3–4), 413–430.

Sewell, W. (2005). The concept(s) of culture. In G. Spiegel (ed). *Practicing history. New directions in historical writing after the linguistic turn*. London: Routledge.

Siedentop, D. (2002). Junior Sport and the Evaluation of Sport Cultures. *Journal of Teaching in Physical Education*, 21(4), 392–401.

Thedin Jakobsson, B., Lundvall, S., Redelius, K. and Engström, L.-M. (2012). Almost all start but who continue? A longitudinal study of youth participation in Swedish club sports. *European Physical Education Review*, 18(1), 3–18.

Thedin Jakobsson, B. (2015). *Vilka stannar kvar och varför?* [*Who continue with club sport and why?*] (diss.), Stockholm: Gymnastik- och idrottshögskolan.

Thompson, J.B. (1991). Editor's introduction. In: P. Bourdieu (ed), *Language and symbolic power*. Cambridge, MA: Harvard University Press.

Trondman, M. (2011). *Ett idrottspolitiskt dilemma: Unga, föreningsidrotten och delaktigheten*, [*A political dilemma in sport: Youth, club sport and participation*]. Stockholm: Centrum för idrottsforskning.

United Nations (1989). *Convention on the Rights of the Child*, UN General Assembly resolution 44/25 on 20 November 1989. New York: UN.

Wall, M. and Côté, J. (2007). Developmental activities that lead to dropout and investment in sport. *Physical Education and Sport Pedagogy*, 12(1), 77–87.

Weiss, M.R. and Amorose, A. (2008). Motivational orientations and sport behaviour. In T.S. Horn (ed.) *Advances in sport psychology*. Champaign Illinois: Human Kinetics.

Weiss, M.R. and Williams, L. (2004). The why of youth sport involvement: A developmental perspective on motivational processes. In M.R. Weiss (ed). *Developmental sport and exercise psychology: A life span perspective. morgantown*, WV: Fitness Information Technology.

SECTION 6

Youth sport, physical activity and health

32

INTRODUCTION

Andy Smith

For well over a century, much ink has been spilt on the health of young people and how this is related to their engagement in activities such as sport and physical activity, as well as other popular uses of leisure. Since the nineteenth century, concern with the health of young people (and other groups) found expression in the emergence of the *'mens sana in corpore sano* ethos, a process which was bolstered in the wider society by the emergence, on the one hand of the so-called "rational recreation" movement, and on the other, of what might be called the "sport/health" ideology' (Dunning and Waddington, 2003: 355). The development of school subjects such as physical education has also variously been associated with largely uncritically accepted claims about its alleged positive contribution to the health of young people, while discussions about the ways in which young people spend their leisure has repeatedly attracted the attention of many concerned with crime, community cohesion and civil order. Discussions of child poverty, malnutrition, mental health and well-being, and experience of sexual abuse and violence are among the many other subjects that have been examined in the almost innumerable studies that have been published on young people and health.

In the period since the 1970s, particular attention has been focused on the development of non-communicable or so-called lifestyle diseases (e.g. coronary heart disease, some cancers, obesity, hypertension, type two diabetes) among the general population (e.g. Hardman and Stensel, 2009), the corrosive impact of growing wealth and income inequalities on individual and population health and well-being (e.g. Dorling, 2014; Pickett and Wilkinson, 2015; Wilkinson and Pickett, 2010), and the growing trend towards the adoption of sedentary and physically inactive lifestyles (e.g. Biddle *et al.*, 2015). Writing of the health costs of physical inactivity, in 2010 the World Health Organization (WHO) (2010) noted that physical inactivity is the fourth leading risk factor for global mortality (six per cent of deaths globally), and that levels of physical inactivity:

> are rising in many countries with major implications for the general health of people worldwide and for the prevalence of NCDs [noncommunicable diseases] such as cardiovascular disease, diabetes and cancer and their risk factors such as raised blood pressure, raised blood sugar and overweight . . . It is estimated currently that of every 10 deaths 6 are attributable to noncommunicable conditions.
>
> *(WHO, 2010: 10)*

More recently, Public Health England (2014: 6) has similarly noted that physical inactivity directly contributes to 'one in six deaths in the UK: the same number as smoking', and they add that 'around a quarter of us are still classified as inactive, failing to achieve a minimum of 30 minutes of activity a week. In some communities only one in ten adults are active enough to stay healthy'. For young people and other population groups, this is especially significant since engagement in regular physical activity can contribute to the prevention and reduction of non-communicable diseases and incidence of mental illness (e.g. depression, anxiety), can assist in the control of body weight and help prevent osteoporosis (Department of Health, Physical Activity, Health Improvement and Protection [DHPAHIP], 2011; Public Health England, 2014).

In the light of these comments, the chapters that comprise Section 6 of the Handbook examine the complex relationships that exist between young people's participation in sport and physical activity and their physical, mental and social health. In the first chapter, entitled *Physical activity and sedentary behaviour in youth*, Mai Chin A Paw, Amika Singh, Saskia te Velde, Maïté Verloigne, Willem van Mechelen and Johannes Brug report on survey data from a large-scale cross-European cross-sectional study – known as the ENERGY study – conducted with 10–12-year-olds in Norway, the Netherlands, Belgium, Spain, Greece, Hungary, Slovenia and Switzerland. The study revealed notable differences in the amount of physical activity and sedentary behaviour reported by young people, but on the whole physical activity levels were described as 'alarmingly low' and sedentary activities such as TV viewing and computer-time were considerably common across the sample of European nations. Although schools were identified as critical sites of youth health promotion, the authors also noted that while schools in four countries (Belgium, Greece, Hungary and the Netherlands) provided young people with between two to three hours of PE per week and an average of forty to seventy minutes of break time (recess) per day, the majority of school children in the sample failed to meet the recommended daily guideline of engaging in thirty minutes of moderate to vigorous physical activity.

Robert Malina, Sean Cumming and Manuel Coelho-e-Silva further develop several of these themes in their chapter, *The health-enhancing effects of physical activity among youth*. Malina and colleagues explore the ways in which multi-dimensional behaviours such as physical activity, sport participation, and physical inactivity and sedentary behaviour impact on the health of young people, including adiposity, skeletal/bone health and psycho-behavioural health. In discussing major trends in physical activity and the tracking of physical activity between youth and adulthood, Malina *et al.* emphasize the importance of understanding the shifting social contexts in which sport and physical activity are performed, the meanings this has for young people, and how associations with sport and physical activity change throughout the life course. They conclude that physical activity during adolescence is 'at best moderately related to activity in young adulthood', and that 'participation in sport during adolescence is reasonably predictive of physical activity in young adulthood'. More detailed longitudinal studies of youth that spans adolescence through young adulthood is needed, Malina *et al.* argue, if we are to better understand the links between participation during youth and subsequent life-stages.

In the following chapter, *Measuring physical activity among youth*, Maria Hildebrand and Ulf Ekelund take as their starting point the observation that despite the advances that have been made in relation to 'the assessment of physical activity and sedentary behaviour, limitations related to measurement accuracy still exist'. Maximizing the accuracy of these assessments, they add, is vital 'to establish a dose-response relationship between physical activity, sedentary behaviour and various health outcomes'. Having reviewed definitions of physical activity, exercise, fitness and sedentary behaviour, Hildebrand and Ekelund consider some of the major methods of assessing habitual physical activity and sedentary behaviour (including the role of new technologies), the strength and limitations of these methods and some of the key issues that need to be borne in mind when interpreting objective and subjective physical activity data. They helpfully remind readers that the selection of methods used for the assessment of youth physical activity and sedentary behaviour needs to be informed by considerations of validity, reliability and responsiveness, as well as the purpose of the study and the outcome of interest.

The second half of Section 6 investigates some of the potential health 'costs' of young people's participation in sport and physical activity, including the risk of injury that provides the basis of the chapter by Evan James, Roald Bahr and Robert F. LaPrade. In *Youth sport, health and physical activity*, Evans *et al.* examine the frequency and severity of injuries in youth sport, the associated risk factors of injury and some of the prevention strategies that should be considered to mitigate against the risk to young people of injury from engaging in sport and physical activity. Since Evans *et al.* observe that the 'rapid growth and developmental changes that occur during adolescence and early adulthood present unique physiological and psychological conditions that may influence athletic performance and increase the risk of injury', it is perhaps not surprising that data on the frequency and severity of acute and overuse injuries indicate that significant proportions of young people are treated annually for sports-related injuries. They describe the burden of injury among those under nineteen-years old as significant, and cite data that estimates that two million athletes in this population are treated annually for sports-related injuries in the United States, 500,000 of which require a visit to a doctor and 30,000 result in hospital-izations. Following a comprehensive review of data on different classifications of youth sports injury, Evans *et al.* outline some of the injury prevention strategies that require careful consideration as part of the future practice of sports medicine, which, it is held, will be required as the trend towards 'increasing specialization and the field of play becomes more competitive and global', and as 'athletes aim to achieve ever higher levels of achievement'.

The next chapter by Guy Faulkner and Katherine Tamminen, entitled *Youth sport and mental health*, provides an important corrective to the dominant tendency in existing studies to focus on adults and on the relationship between exercise and mental health. Much less emphasis, Faulkner and Tamminen note, 'has been placed on exploring sport participation and mental health' and that where research does exist on this relationship it is predominantly cross-sectional in nature. Based on a systematic search for longitudinal studies (at least one year in length) that examined whether sport participation predicted a mental health outcome at a later point in time, Faulkner and Tamminen conclude that it is 'difficult to draw clear conclusions regarding youth sport participation and mental health based on the existing evidence'. They also report that while there is good evidence that sport participation, particularly team sport participation, may have a protective effect against depressive symptoms, the evidence regarding the impact of sport participation on self-esteem is inconsistent. They conclude that future programme 'evaluations are needed to identify the processes involved within sporting contexts that maximise the likelihood that children and youth will experience mental health benefit', and that such evaluations – together with research on the mental health of competitive youth athletes – should take greater account of 'the many influences of parents, peers, coaches, and the structure and delivery of sport programmes'.

Other features of the relationship between sport, physical activity and mental health are examined in the next two chapters. Nanna Meyer, Jorunn Sundgot-Borgen and Alba Reguant Closa explore eating disorders and disordered eating among young athletes, and especially the three clinical eating disorders of anorexia nervosa, bulimia nervosa and binge eating disorder. Reviewing evidence on the prevalence of eating disorders and disordered eating behaviour, Meyer *et al.* conclude that these behaviours are common among young people and often first emerge around nine years old and may develop from 'adolescence to adulthood with rising rates of extreme weight control methods and binge eating episodes'. They also note that while eating disorders (ED) and disordered eating (DE) are more prevalent among women and among those competing in weight sensitive sports, they are also common among men and among participants of other types of sport. Significantly, however, Meyer *et al.* point out that 'it is currently unknown whether the prevalence of EDs and DE is higher among adolescent elite athletes than athletes at lower competitive levels or non-athletes'. It is likely, however, that the generic (e.g. low self-esteem, depression, body image concerns) and sport-specific risk factors (e.g. weight management and training practices) for both types of behaviours will help explain their prevalence among young athletes.

In *Everyday distortions: youth sport and body images*, Michael Gard makes a powerful case for his contention that 'the body images generated by and associated with sport and physical activity are now a dominant, perhaps pre-eminent, cultural economy through which young bodies are understood, experienced and consumed'. Gard argues that focusing on the concept of body image not only raises important questions about their 'healthiness', but it also helps us understand the ways in which youth sport and physical activity is variously experienced by young people in diverse social contexts and sporting situations. No less importantly, the methods of internal and external surveillance to which Gard refers are also central to explanations of how young people experience their bodies, how they and others perceive their bodies, and the cumulative impact this has on the management of their bodies in sporting contexts. For Gard, the participation of many young people in sport and physical activity is essentially an exercise in body image management, where perceptions and experiences of various body images are grounded in increasingly narrow and limited notions of what constitute acceptable bodies.

The final chapter, *Youth sport, cigarettes, alcohol and illicit drugs*, is by Patrick Peretti-Watel, Fabrice Lorenté and Laurent Grélot who explore the links between sport participation and the use by young people of legal and illegal drugs. The evidence reviewed by the authors suggest that, at its most simplest, sport participation tends to be positively associated with alcohol use by young people, but is negatively associated with cigarette smoking and illicit drug use. Since sport, like any other activity, is context-specific the use of legal and illegal drugs will vary (perhaps considerably so) in those contexts. As Perretti-Watel *et al.* point out, a more nuanced explanation of the relationship between sport participation and the consumption of drugs depends on the kind of use being considered, the subcultures surrounding sport in which people compete at various levels of seriousness, and other participant-related characteristics (e.g. gender, age, ethnicity and social class). For young people, initiation into drug use associated with their participation in sport (especially during adolescence) may be a fleeting activity undertaken during periods of experimentation that are subsequently dropped, while for others the consumption of drugs (particularly alcohol) may become more established features of their socialization practices in sport which are pursued for a myriad of reasons. Perretti-Watel *et al.* also rightly note that, in higher levels of sport, young athletes may also use both recreational and performance-enhancing drugs in ways that are intended to improve sports performance, as well as for managing diverse experiences such as competitive stress and anxiety.

References

Biddle, S., Mutrie, N. and Gorely, T. (2015). *Psychology of physical activity: determinants, well-being and interventions*. (3rd edition). London: Routledge.

Department of Health, Physical Activity, Health Improvement and Protection (2011). *Start active, stay active: a report on physical activity for health from the four home countries' Chief Medical Officers*. London: Department of Health, Physical Activity, Health Improvement and Protection.

Dorling, D. (2014). *Inequality and the 1 per cent*. London: Verso.

Dunning, E. and Waddington, I. (2003). Sport as a drug and drugs in sport: some exploratory comments. *International Review for the Sociology of Sport*, 38(3), 351–68.

Hardman, A. and Stensel, D. (2009). *Physical activity and health: the evidence explained*. (2nd edition). London: Routledge.

Pickett, K. and Wilkinson, R. (2015). Income inequality and health: a causal review, *Social Science and Medicine*, 128 (March), 316–26.

Public Health England (2014). *Everybody active, every day. An evidence-based approach to physical activity*. London: Public Health England.

Wilkinson, R. and Pickett, K. (2010). *The spirit level*. London: Penguin.

33

PHYSICAL ACTIVITY AND SEDENTARY BEHAVIOUR IN YOUTH

Mai Chin A Paw, Amika Singh, Saskia te Velde, Maïté Verloigne, Willem van Mechelen and Johannes Brug

Introduction

A low level of daily physical activity is one of the main causes for the avoidable burden of non-communicable disease and premature death (Lee *et al.*, 2012). Sedentary behaviour (low-energy activities performed while sitting during waking time, such as TV viewing, computer use, reading) is not synonymous with physical inactivity. Recent research has shown that highly active children can also participate in high levels of sedentary behaviour (De Bourdeaudhuij *et al.*, 2013; te Velde *et al.*, 2007). In adults, excessive sedentary behaviour has been shown to have adverse health effects, independent of moderate to vigorous physical activity (Grontved and Hu, 2011; Proper *et al.*, 2011; van der Ploeg *et al.*, 2012). Physical activity levels decline and sedentary behaviour increases throughout childhood into older age (Van Mechelen, *et al.*, 2000). Therefore, promoting physical activity and limiting sedentary behaviour are important health policy priorities in Europe and beyond.

Data on participation in these behaviours is needed in order to:

1   identify risk groups and specific risk behaviours that need specific attention
2   monitor trends
3   evaluate the effectiveness of preventive interventions.

To be able to compare differences according to country, ethnicity and sex, standardized measurement procedures are essential. Within the European Commission-funded ENERGY (*EuropeaN Energy balance Research to prevent excessive weight Gain among Youth*) project, we conducted a large-scale cross-European cross-sectional study (Brug *et al.*, 2010). The ENERGY project was conducted by a consortium cooperation of fifteen partners across Europe and Australia. The overall aim of the ENERGY project was to promote healthy energy balance-related behaviours in children across Europe.

Schools are considered to be an important setting for promoting time spent in physical activity and for tackling time spent sedentary at school. Large numbers of children from differing backgrounds, including children from lower social economic or ethnic minority families, can be accessed through schools. Besides the fact that children spend a large part of their day at school, schools also have the opportunities and capacity to engage in physical activity during school hours (i.e. recess or break time and physical education (PE) lessons). To direct future school-based physical activity promotion interventions, it is important to monitor the prevalence and distribution of physical activity and sedentary time at school.

This chapter presents results and conclusions from the ENERGY cross-sectional study which included a survey of children aged 10–12 years from eight European countries: Norway, the Netherlands, Belgium, Spain, Greece, Hungary, Slovenia and Switzerland. These results have been published before in international scientific journals (Brug *et al.*, 2012a; Brug *et al.*, 2012b; van Stralen *et al.*, 2013; Verloigne *et al.*, 2012). The survey was conducted in 2010 according to a standardized measurement protocol. This chapter describes:

1   Self-reported engagement in sport activities, active commuting to school, TV and PC time (Figure 33.1);
2   Differences in self-reported physical activity and sedentary activities according to sex, parental education and ethnicity (Figure 33.2);
3   Objectively assessed physical activity and sitting time;
4   School time physical activity and sitting time.

Methods

Seven countries from the ENERGY consortium, Belgium, Greece, Hungary, the Netherlands, Norway, Slovenia and Spain, participated in the cross-sectional survey (van Stralen *et al.*, 2011). An eighth country, Switzerland, joined in a later phase (Herzig *et al.*, 2012). The standardized procedure for sampling, data collection and data handling for the survey was the same in all countries. The cross-sectional survey was carried out in primary schools among 10–12 year-old children. The recruitment and data collection took place from March–July 2010. Recruitment methods are described in more detail elsewhere (van Stralen *et al.*, 2011). The total sample comprised 7234 children (fifty-two per cent girls; mean age 11.6 ± 0.7). Accelerometer data was collected in 1082 children of whom 686 children (fifty-three per cent girls) provided valid accelerometer data. Adolescents from parents that were both born in the country of administration (i.e. native ethnic group) were distinguished from those for whom at least one parent was born in another country (i.e. non-native ethnic group).

The ENERGY child questionnaire included questions on various energy balance-related behaviours and their potential determinants and was developed based on existing measures (Singh *et al.*, 2012). The ENERGY child questionnaire is available via the ENERGY website in English and all the languages in which the questionnaire was administered: www.projectenergy.eu. Actigraph accelerometer (GT1M, GT3X and Actitrainer) data was collected among subsamples in Belgium, Greece, Hungary, the Netherlands, and Switzerland according to standardized protocols (Yildirim *et al.*, 2011). Children were asked to wear an accelerometer during all waking hours – except during water-based activities – for seven consecutive days, including two weekend days. Children were included in the analyses if they had had at least two weekdays with a minimum of 10-hours wearing time and one weekend day with minimum of 8-hours wearing time. The following cut-off points were used: less than 100 counts per minute (cpm) for sedentary activities (Fischer *et al.*, 2012; Treuth *et al.*, 2004), 101–2999 cpm for light intensity physical activity and more than 3000 for moderate to vigorous intensity physical activity (MVPA) (Treuth *et al.*, 2004).

Exact school-time for each school was recorded by the school director or his/her equivalent. By means of time filters (including the exact school-time per school), percentages and minutes of sedentary time, and MVPA were calculated during school time. International guidelines suggest that children should engage each day in at least 60 minutes of MVPA of which at least 30 minutes should be at school, including PE classes (Biddle, Sallis and Cavill, 1998). Based on the MVPA data, the percentage of children who met these recommendations was calculated.

How do European children do?

Physical activities

Figure 33.1 shows the mean minutes of active transport, sports participation and screen time per day in native and non-native children. Boys reported from 300 minutes/week for sport activities in Norway to less than 200 minutes/week in Greece. Girls spent less time in sports, ranging from 250 minutes/week in Slovenia to less than 150 minutes/week in Greece. This difference between boys and girls was consistent in all countries. Children of higher educated parents and children from native ethnic groups participated significantly more often in sports than those from lower educated parents and the non-native ethnic group, in the total sample and in the separate countries (Brug *et al.*, 2012a; Brug *et al.*, 2012b).

Regarding active commuting to school, there were large differences between the countries, ranging from 111 minutes per week in Norwegian girls to 40 minutes in Greek girls. Walking to school was the main mode of active transportation to school, but in Norway, the Netherlands and Belgium cycling was also relevant. Girls reported statistically significantly more weekly minutes of walking to school than boys. No significant differences according to parental education in total active commuting time were observed, but children with lower parental education were less likely to cycle and more likely to walk to school. In the total sample, children from non-native ethnic groups reported spending more time on active commuting to school

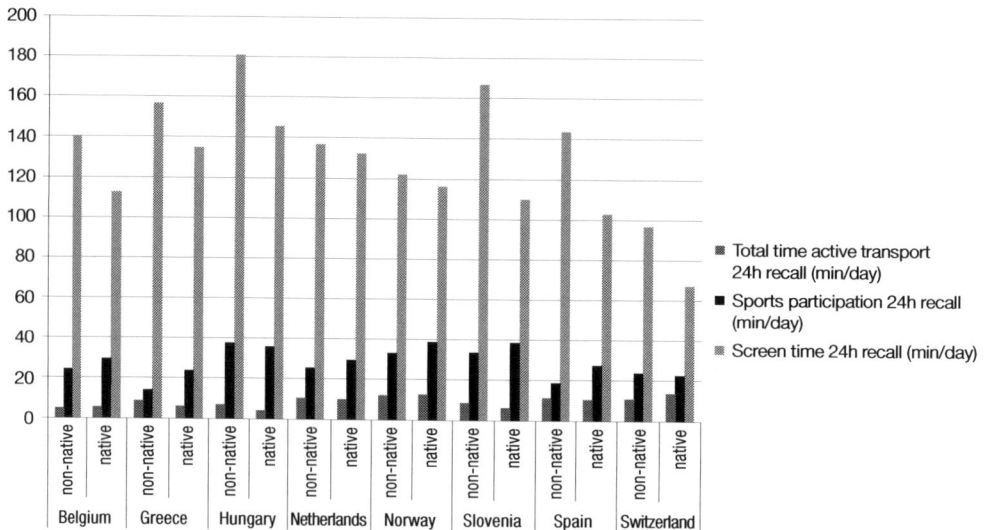

Figure 33.1 Active transport, sports participation and screen time (minutes/day) in native and non-native children – The ENERGY project

than native children, and similar patterns were found in most individual countries (Brug *et al.*, 2012a; Brug *et al.*, 2012b).

Screen time

Across the countries, boys reported spending about 2½ hours per day and girls somewhat less than 2 hours on screen-based activities (TV and computer-time combined); ranging from more than 230 minutes per day in Hungarian boys to 160 minutes per day in Spanish girls. In all countries, mean total screen time as well as TV and computer time were higher for boys than girls. Children of higher educated parents and children from native ethnicity reported less screen time than those from lower educated parents and non-native ethnicity, respectively (Brug *et al.*, 2012a; Brug *et al.*, 2012b).

These results indicate that children from Southern and Eastern European countries, children from lower educated parents and children from non-native ethnic groups are less likely to engage in physical activities and more likely to engage in screen-based behaviours than their peers from Northern European countries and from families with higher educated parents and families from native ethnicity.

Objectively assessed physical activity and sedentary time

Figure 33.2 provides an overview of the mean levels of sedentary time, light intensity physical activity and MVPA. Results showed that the mean level among European children was far below the recommended 60 minutes of MVPA per day. Only five per cent of girls and seventeen per

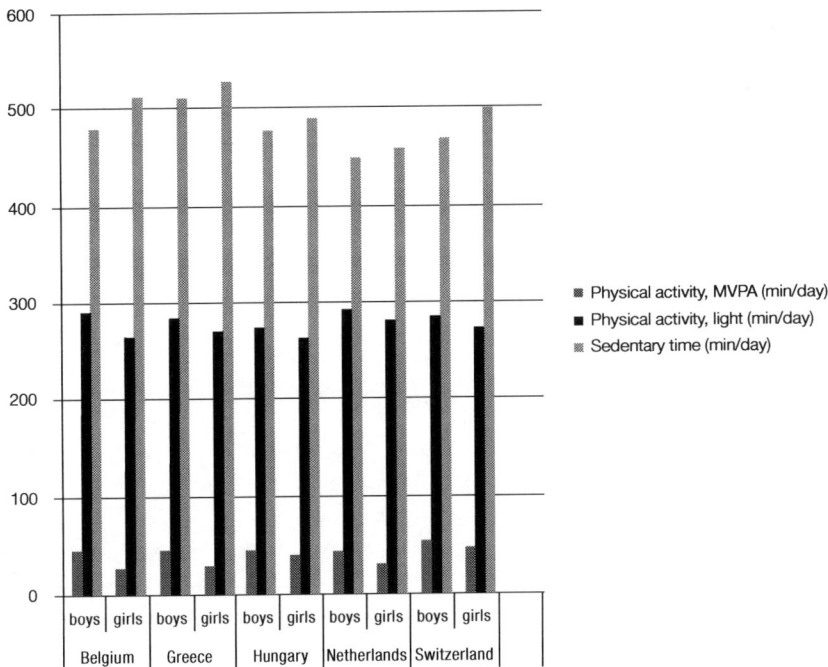

Figure 33.2 Mean levels of sedentary time, light intensity physical activity and MVPA in European boys and girls – the ENERGY Project

cent of boys reached this recommendation. These percentages are alarming and emphasize the need for continuous and further intensified efforts to promote physical activity behaviour in children. The average level of sedentary time was high in boys and girls across all five countries with approximately eight hours per day spent sedentary. The high levels of sedentary time demonstrated in the present study urge the need to develop intervention programmes focusing particularly on reducing the total sedentary time in this age group (Verloigne *et al.*, 2012).

These low levels of physical activity urge the need for effective programmes that promote MVPA in 10–12-year-old European children. In line with previous studies (Basterfield *et al.*, 2011; Trost *et al.*, 2002), sex differences were found for both sedentary time and physical activity across all countries. Girls spent significantly more time being sedentary (500 minutes per day) compared to boys (474 minutes per day). Moreover, girls also engaged in less light intensity physical activity (267 minutes per day) and in less MVPA (32 minutes per day) than boys (284 minutes per day and 43 minutes per day, respectively) (Verloigne *et al.*, 2012). These sex differences at the age of 10–12 are the precursors of even larger differences in adolescence, making girls an important target group for intervention programmes.

Sedentary time and MVPA levels also differed between countries. Greek children had the highest levels of sedentary time compared to the other children. Greek boys were significantly more sedentary (510 minutes per day) than all other boys and Greek girls also spent the most time sedentary (526 minutes per day), although they did not differ significantly from Belgian (511 minutes per day) and Swiss girls (498 minutes per day). Children from the Netherlands on the other hand had the lowest levels of sedentary time of all European children. Dutch girls spent on average 457 minutes per day being sedentary and Dutch boys 447 minutes per day (Verloigne *et al.*, 2012).

Concerning MVPA, it was apparent that Swiss children spent generally more time in MVPA than other European children. Swiss girls engaged in significantly more MVPA (43 minutes per day) than all other girls and Swiss boys had the highest levels of MVPA (50 minutes per day) in comparison with the other boys, although they did not significantly differ from Belgian (42 minutes per day) and Greek boys (41 minutes per day). With regard to light intensity physical activity, no significant country differences were observed (Verloigne *et al.*, 2012).

The difference in MVPA levels between countries may be attributable to differences in policy and organization of physical activity and sports: for example, financial issues and policy priorities in the field of sport. However, this needs further research.

Physical activity and sitting time at school

The results showed that the mean sedentary time at school ranged from 182 minutes per day in Greece to 231 minutes per day in Belgium. On average, children spent sixty-five per cent of their school-time being sedentary, ranging from sixty-three per cent in Belgium to sixty-seven per cent in Hungary. The percentage of school time spent sedentary was slightly but significantly higher in Hungary and the Netherlands (sixty-six per cent) versus Belgium, Greece (sixty-three per cent) and Switzerland (sixty-three per cent) (van Stralen *et al.*, 2013).

MVPA time at school ranged from 13 minutes in the Netherlands to 21 minutes in Switzerland. On average, children spent five per cent of their school time in MVPA, with small differences between countries. On average seven per cent of the children met the recommendation of at least 30 minutes of MVPA during a school day, ranging from two per cent in the Netherlands to fourteen per cent in Switzerland (van Stralen *et al.*, 2013). These differences might be due to political, physical and social cultural environmental differences between the different countries. Although the evidence for school environmental influences on school-time physical activity and sedentary time is limited and ambiguous, there are indications that a supportive school environment is associated with increased levels of physical activity.

Differences between girls and boys were small but statically significant: girls spent more time sedentary during school-time (sixty-seven per cent) than boys (sixty-three per cent; p < 0.001), and less time in MVPA (four per cent in girls vs five per cent in boys; p < 0.001), which was consistent in all countries (van Stralen *et al.*, 2013).

Thus European schoolchildren spent small amounts of their school-time in MVPA and large amounts of their school-time being sedentary. Current guidelines propose that children should accumulate at least 30 minutes of MVPA during school-time (Pate *et al.*, 2006). Only seven per cent of the children, ranging from two per cent in the Netherlands to fourteen per cent in Switzerland achieved this goal. These small amounts of school-time spent in MVPA and large amounts being sedentary are alarming and should serve as a call to action for current school systems.

Implications and recommendations

Physical activity levels were alarmingly low while sedentary activities such as TV viewing and computer-time were abundant across Europe. Generally, children of more highly educated parents and native ethnicity tended to engage in more physical activity and less sedentary behaviour.

As children spend a large part of their day at school, schools have many opportunities to target physical activity as well as sedentary activities, not only during PE and recess but also in regular lessons. First, the frequency, content and intensity of PE lessons and recess time should be critically addressed. Data from the ENERGY school management questionnaire among Belgium, Greek, Hungarian and Dutch schools showed that schools provided between 2–3 hours of PE per week and provided on average between 40 minutes and 70 minutes of recess per day. Thus, despite the fact that schools provided opportunities to be moderately to vigorously active for more than 30 minutes per day, the majority of children did not meet this guideline. Future interventions may target the content and intensity of PE lessons, for example by including a large variety of activities or games that require vigorous intensity activities, involving all children. Additional physical activity options that compliment but do not replace PE lessons could be provided, targeting especially the least active children. In addition, children's activity levels during recess periods could be increased, for example by providing game equipment during recess (Verstraete *et al.*, 2006) or playground markings (Janssen *et al.*, 2013; Ridgers *et al.*, 2007). To reduce sedentary time at school, physical activity breaks during class time, sitting on stability balls or physically active learning modules are potential interventions.

Another approach is to adjust the physical school environment. In general, today's schools are insufficiently designed in a way that stimulates children to be physically active. Today's school systems often demand children to sit still, in order to concentrate. Adding physical activity breaks may also improve school performance (Singh *et al.*, 2012). Additionally, previous studies have demonstrated that light intensity physical activity in children is also associated with overweight (Kwon *et al.*, 2011; Pate *et al.*, 2006; Treuth *et al.*, 2009). Future research should further investigate the impact of the transition from sedentary activities to light intensity physical activities as well as MVPA on children's physical as well as mental health, including school performance.

Acknowledgements

This chapter is based on the ENERGY-project, which is funded by the Seventh Framework Programme (CORDIS FP7) of the European Commission, HEALTH (FP7-HEALTH-2007-B), Grant agreement no. 223254. In the Netherlands, the ENERGY-project was additionally supported by a grant from the Netherlands Organization for Health Research and Development (Grant number 50–50150–98–002).

References

Basterfield, L., Adamson, A.J., Frary, J.K., Parkinson, K.N., Pearce, M.S. and Reilly, J.J. (2011). Longitudinal study of physical activity and sedentary behavior in children. *Pediatrics*, 127 (1), e24 –e30.

Brug, J., te Velde, S.J., Chin A Paw, M.J., Bere, E., De Bourdeaudhuij, I., Moore, H., Maes, L., Jensen, J., Manios, Y., Lien, N., Klepp, K.I., Lobstein, T., Martens, M., Salmon, J. and Singh, A.S. (2010). Evidence-based development of school-based and family-involved prevention of overweight across Europe: the ENERGY-project's design and conceptual framework. *BMC Public Health*, 10, 276.

Brug, J., van Stralen, M.M., Chin A Paw, M.J., De Bourdeaudhuij, I., Lien, N., Bere, E., Singh, A.S., Maes, L., Moreno, L., Jan, N., Kovacs, E., Lobstein, T., Manios, Y. and Te Velde, S.J. (2012a). Differences in weight status and energy-balance related behaviours according to ethnic background among adolescents in seven countries in Europe: the ENERGY-project. *Pediatric Obesity*, 7 (5), 399–411.

Brug, J., van Stralen, M.M., te Velde, S.J., Chin A Paw, M.J., De Bourdeaudhuij, I., Lien, Bere, E., Maskini, V., Singh A.S., Maes, L., Moreno, L., Jan, N., Kovacs, E., Lobstein, T. and Manios, Y. (2012b). Differences in Weight Status and Energy-Balance Related Behaviors among Schoolchildren across Europe: The ENERGY-Project. *PLoS One*, 7 (4), e34742.

De Bourdeaudhuij, I., Verloigne, M., Maes, L., Van Lippevelde W., Chin A Paw, M.J., te Velde, S.J., Manios, Y. Androutsos. O., Kovacs, E., Dossegger, A. and Brug, J. (2013). Associations of physical activity and sedentary time with weight and weight status among 10- to 12-year-old boys and girls in Europe: a cluster analysis within the ENERGY project. *Pediatric Obesity*, 8 (5), 367–375.

Ferreira, I., van der Horst, K., Wendel-Vos, W., Kremers., Van Lenthe, F.J. and Brug, J. (2007). Environmental correlates of physical activity in youth – a review and update. *Obesity Reviews*, 8, 129–54.

Fischer CC, Yildirim M, Salmon J and Chin A Paw, M. (2012). Comparing different accelerometer cut points for sedentary time in children. *Pediatric Exercise Science* 24, 220–228.

Grontved, A. and Hu, F.B. (2011). Television viewing and risk of type 2 diabetes, cardiovascular disease, and all-cause mortality: a meta-analysis. *Journal of the American Medical Association*, 305 (23), 2448–2455.

Herzig, M., Dossegger, A., Mader, U., Kriemler, S., Wunderlin, T., Grize, L., Brug, J., Manios, Y., Braun-Fahrlander, C. and Bringolf-Isler, B. (2012). Differences in weight status and energy-balance related behaviors among schoolchildren in German-speaking Switzerland compared to seven countries in Europe. *International Journal of Behavioral Nutrition and Physical Activity*, 9, 139.

Janssen, M., Twisk, J.W., Toussaint, H.M., van Mechelen W. and Verhagen, E.A. (2013). Effectiveness of the PLAYgrounds programme on PA levels during recess in 6-year-old to twelve-year-old children. *British Journal of Sports Medicine*, Jan 4 [Epub ahead of print].

Kwon, S., Janz, K.F., Burns, T.L. and Levy, S.M. (2011). Association between light-intensity physical activity and adiposity in childhood. *Pediatric Exercise Science*, 23 (2), 218–229.

Lee, I.M., Shiroma, E.J., Lobelo, F., Puska, P., Blair, S.N. and Katzmarzyk, P.T. (2012). Effect of physical inactivity on major non-communicable diseases worldwide: an analysis of burden of disease and life expectancy. *Lancet*, 380 (9838), 219–229.

Pate, R.R., Davis, M.G., Robinson, T.N., Stone, E.J., McKenzie, T.L. and Young, J.C. (2006). Promoting physical activity in children and youth: a leadership role for schools: a scientific statement from the American Heart Association Council on Nutrition, Physical Activity, and Metabolism (Physical Activity Committee) in collaboration with the Councils on Cardiovascular Disease in the Young and Cardiovascular Nursing. *Circulation*, 114 (11), 1214–1224.

Proper, K.I., Singh, A.S., van Mechelen W. and Chin A Paw, M.J. (2011). Sedentary behaviors and health outcomes among adults: a systematic review of prospective studies. *American Journal of Preventive Medicine*, 40 (2), 174–182.

Ridgers, N.D., Stratton, G., Fairclough, S.J. and Twisk, J.W. (2007). Long-term effects of a playground markings and physical structures on children's recess physical activity levels. *Preventive Medicine*, 44 (5), 393–397.

Singh, A., Uijtdewilligen, L., Twisk, J.W., van Mechelen W. and Chin A Paw, M.J. (2012). Physical activity and performance at school: a systematic review of the literature including a methodological quality assessment. *Archives of Pediatrics and Adolescent Medicine*, 166 (1), 49–55.

te Velde S.J., de Bourdeaudhuij I., Thorsdottir I., Rasmussen M., Hagströmer M., Klepp K.I. and Brug J. (2007). Patterns in sedentary and exercise behaviors and associations with overweight in 9–14-year-old boys and girls–a cross-sectional study. *BMC Public Health*, 31 (7), 16.

Treuth, M.S., Schmitz, K., Catellier, D.J., McMurray, R.G., Murray, D.M., Almeida, M.J., Going, S., Norman, J.E. and Pate, R. (2004). Defining accelerometer thresholds for activity intensities in adolescent girls. *Medicine and Science in Sports and Exercise*, 36 (7), 1259–1266.

Treuth, M.S., Baggett, C.D., Pratt, C.A., Going, S.B., Elder, J.P., Charneco, E.Y. and Webber, L.S. (2009). A longitudinal study of sedentary behavior and overweight in adolescent girls. *Obesity*, 17 (5), 1003–1008.

Trost, S.G., Pate, R.R., Sallis, J.F., Freedson, P.S., Taylor, W.C., Dowda, M. and Sirard, J. (2002). Age and gender differences in objectively measured physical activity in youth. *Medicine and Science in Sports and Exercise*, 34 (2), 350–355.

van der Ploeg, H.P., Chey, T., Korda, R.J., Banks, E. and Bauman A. (2012). Sitting time and all-cause mortality risk in 222 497 Australian adults. *Archives of Internal Medicine*, 172 (6), 494–500.

van Mechelen, W., Twisk, J.W.R., Post, G.B., Snel, J. and Kemper, H.C.G. (2000). Physical activity of young people: the Amsterdam Longitudinal Growth and Health Study. *Medicine and Science in Sports and Exercise*, 32 (9), 1610–1616.

van Stralen, M.M., te Velde, S.J., Singh, A.S., De Bourdeaudhuij, I., Martens, M.K., van der Sluis M., Manios, Y., Grammatikaki, E., Chin A Paw, M.J., Maes, L., Bere, E., Jensen, J., Moreno, L., Jan, N., Molnar, D., Moore, H. and Brug, J. (2011). EuropeaN Energy balance Research to prevent excessive weight Gain among Youth (ENERGY) project: Design and methodology of the ENERGY cross-sectional survey. *BMC Public Health*, 11, 65.

van Stralen, M.M., Yildirim, M., Wulp, A., Te Velde, S.J., Verloigne, M., Doessegger, A. androutsos, O., Kovacs, E., Brug, J. and Chin A Paw, M.J. (2013). Measured sedentary time and physical activity during the school day of European 10- to 12-year-old children: The ENERGY project. *Journal of Science and Medicine in Sport*. 17 (2), 201–206.

Verloigne, M., Van Lippevelde W., Maes, L., Yildirim, M., Chin A Paw, M., Manios, Y. Androutsos, O., Kovacs, E., Bringolf-Isler, B., Brug, J. and De Bourdeaudhuij, I. (2012). Levels of physical activity and sedentary time among 10- to 12-year-old boys and girls across 5 European countries using accelerometers: an observational study within the ENERGY-project. *International Journal of Behavioral Nutrition and Physical Activity*, 9, 34.

Verstraete, S.J., Cardon, G.M., de Clercq, D.L. and de Bourdeaudhuij, I.M. (2006). Increasing children's physical activity levels during recess periods in elementary schools: the effects of providing game equipment. *European Journal of Public Health*, 16 (4), 415–419.

Yildirim, M., Verloigne, M., De Bourdeaudhuij, I., Androutsos, O., Manios, Y., Felso, R., Kovacs, E., Doessegger, A., Bringolf-Isler, B., Te Velde S., Brug, J. and Chin A Paw, M.J. (2011). Study protocol of physical activity and sedentary behaviour measurement among schoolchildren by accelerometry – Cross-sectional survey as part of the ENERGY-project. *BMC Public Health*, 11 (1), 182.

34

THE HEALTH-ENHANCING EFFECTS OF PHYSICAL ACTIVITY AMONG YOUTH

Robert Malina, Sean Cumming and Manuel Coelho-e-Silva

Introduction

Youth is a variably defined descriptor of the life stage between childhood and adulthood. In the context of the present volume, the age range 16–25 years has been suggested as a guide to evaluating health benefits of physical activity. From the perspective of growth and maturation, the proposed age range encompasses late adolescence and young adulthood in the majority of youth. Individual differences in timing and tempo of biological growth and maturation and behavioural development associated with puberty and the adolescent growth spurt occur in most youth before 16 years, but the impact may persist into later adolescence and young adulthood. The need to consider both biological and psycho-behavioural characteristics of youth is essential and highlights the need for researchers to adopt a biocultural perspective.

The proposed age range comprising youth, 16–25 years, should be viewed in terms of temporally arranged transitions that precede and include this interval. Required schooling and many associated socially sanctioned and valued forms of physical inactivity dominate childhood and adolescence. Biological and social demands associated with the transition into and through adolescence entail additional biosocial interactions and adaptations. The college years prolong adolescence in many cultures, while additional stresses are associated with the transition into the work force. Youth also move into social relationships. A survey of Americans 18–25 years of age indicated the following: no relationship, 25 per cent; casual dating, 8 per cent; dating exclusively, 27 per cent; cohabitating relationship, 20 per cent; and married, 20 per cent (Scott *et al.*, 2011). The period of youth is thus complex with many demands associated with school, work, friends, family, social relationships and perhaps child rearing.

Available research does not necessarily overlap the proposed age range. Discussions of health benefits of physical activity on youth commonly focus on individuals of school age, that is, 6–18 years (Centers for Disease Control and Prevention, expert panel, Strong *et al.*, 2005) and 5–19 years (Physical Activity Guidelines Advisory Committee, 2008), while young adulthood is often extended to 30 years.

Allowing for these caveats, this chapter evaluates health benefits of physical activity in youth. Three general topical issues are considered:

1   dimensions of physical activity and inactivity;
2   potential benefits of physical activity on several indicators of health status among youth;
3   tracking of activity and health indicators from adolescence into adulthood.

Physical activity and inactivity

Physical activity is a multi-dimensional behaviour that occurs in multiple contexts. Although activity is an important avenue for learning, physical and psychological development, enjoyment, social interactions and self-understanding, it is currently viewed most often in terms of potential health benefits associated with regular energy expenditure in moderate-to-vigorous physical activity (MVPA) and the stresses and strains associated with weight bearing and ground reaction forces. Proficiency in a variety of movement skills and physical fitness (performance- and health-related) is important dimensions of activity. Context is an additional dimension of physical activity that is often overlooked; it refers to types, purposes and settings of activity and includes play, physical education, exercise, sport, dance, physical labour, among others. Contexts per se and meanings attached to them vary with age among adolescents and young adults, and among and within different cultural groups (Malina, 2008).

Physical inactivity or sedentary behaviour is independent of physical activity and is also multi-dimensional. Although the biomedical view of physical activity is critical of excessive inactivity, many sedentary behaviours are highly valued by societies – school, studying, reading, music, art, television viewing, computer games and the like, and have benefits for the individual. Engagement in computer/video games, for example, has been associated with a number of benefits including superior performance on a number of cognitive and motor tasks, improved eyesight, hand eye coordination, and pain relief. Motorized transport is also a form of inactivity that is valued by major segments of society, including youth.

Physical activity and inactivity are independent behaviours performed in a societal context, and both have high valence in society. There is a need for better understanding of the meanings attached to and motivations for physical activities and sedentary behaviours by adolescents and young adults. These behaviours are of interest to education and to public health and medicine. Education highlights activity in the context of physical education as a component of overall school experiences. However, many in the profession would equate physical education with physical activity or sport, and in so doing reduce the educational relevance of physical education. The public health and biomedical views focus on physical activity in the context of health promotion and disease prevention and physical inactivity as a major risk factor for, among others, cardiometabolic diseases. It remains to be established, however, whether youth view physical activity in terms of the current biomedical/public health model.

School and non-school sport, both formal (organized) and informal, are major contexts of physical activity for youth, while many youth perceive physical activity as equivalent with sport. Participation in sport has the potential to contribute to the objectives of physical activity, but formal and informal sport, and specific sports vary in intensity of activity. Sport activities can include warm-up, instruction and practice (drills, repetitions), rest, scrimmages, games, among others. Team sports such as soccer, basketball, ice and field hockey involve reasonably continuous activity that varies in intensity during practices or a match, whereas baseball and American football involve intermittent activities among frequent periods of relative inactivity. Intermittent activities are also characteristic of gymnastics, diving, racket sports and some field events in athletics, while continuous activity is a more likely feature of swimming and running events.

Trends in physical activity

Studies of physical activity have historically been based on questionnaires among adolescents and young adults. On average, level of physical activity tends to reach a peak circa 12–14 years, and subsequently declines. Boys are, on average, more active and less sedentary than girls, though the sex difference is attenuated when maturity status is controlled in adolescents (Thompson *et al.*, 2003; Machado Rodrigues *et al.*, 2010), that is, girls tend to be less active and more sedentary than boys of the same age due to their advanced biological maturation. Nevertheless, age trends in activity vary among studies and with measurement instrument and context.

More recent surveys are based on accelerometry and often focus on epochs of MVPA, the intensity of activity that is most often associated with health benefits (Strong *et al.*, 2005). Observations derived from 4–7 days of accelerometry in a nationally representative sample of US youth indicated a decline in MVPA from 9 –15 years of age in both sexes, higher levels of MVPA in boys than in girls, and higher levels of MVPA on weekdays compared to weekend days in both sexes (Nader *et al.*, 2008). Boys exceeded the recommended 60 minutes of MVPA at all ages except 15 years, while girls exceeded the recommendation from 9–13 years when levels of MVPA fell below 60 minutes. In 2005–2006, only 36 per cent of American young adults 18–29 years (males 39 per cent, females 32 per cent) reported regular participation in leisure time physical activity (National Center for Health Statistics, 2009).

Decline in sport participation with age parallels trends in physical activity. In the United States, participation in school sport in 2010 ('all students who have participated to any degree in school athletic teams' during the school year) declined from eighth (~14 years) to twelfth (~18 years) grades, 67 per cent to 61 per cent in males and 61 per cent to 51 per cent in females (Child Trends Data Bank, 2013). The decline across grade levels probably reflects differential drop-out and persistence in sport and also the selectivity of sport. Trends collated by the sporting goods industry indicate a decline in participation in team sports from 12–26 years and an increase in participation in fitness activities and individual sports from 18–24 years of age (Physical Activity Council, 2012).

Sport programmes, trends in participation and methods of reporting vary among countries. Among English youth 5–16 years, 57 per cent participated in organized sport outside of school for at least one hour, while 35 per cent and 21 per cent, respectively, participated in at least 2 or 3 hours of sport (Fraser and Ziff, 2009). Among Finnish youth, daily participation in sport club training declined from 9 to 21 years, while participation twice per week declined from 12–18 years (Telama and Yang, 2000). Portuguese youth under 17 years of age comprised 50 per cent of sport participants in 2003, whereas youth 17–19 years comprised only 11 per cent of participants (Instituto do Desporto de Portugal, 2005). The percentage of Italian youth in 2000 who regularly practised sport declined from 45 per cent at 17–19 years to 34 per cent at 18–24 years (Istituto Nazionale di Statistica, 2005). Among Canadian youth in 2005, regular sport participation declined from 59 per cent at 15–18 years to 43 per cent at 19–24 years (Ifedi, 2008). In all countries and within each age group, males participated more in sport than females.

Systematic reviews (Sallis *et al.*, 2000; Van der Horst *et al.*, 2007) indicate a variety of factors that influence physical activity among adolescents 13–18 years of age. Correlates of physical activity noted in the reviews are limited to those included in surveys of activity habits and levels: sociodemographic factors (age, sex, ethnicity, socioeconomic status); specific beliefs, motives and behaviours (achievement orientations, self-determined motivations, intention to be active, perceived competence); parental and peer support; previous activity and community sports among others. Motor proficiency and level of physical fitness have not been included among correlates of activity, although the concept of physical literacy is emerging in the literature (Tremblay and Lloyd, 2010). Except for the BMI, other potential biological correlates of activity, including growth and maturity status, have also not been considered. The latter is especially relevant as inter-individual variation in biological maturity status has been increasingly noted as a factor that may contribute both directly and indirectly to physical activity among adolescents through self-perceptions and the evaluations and reactions of others (Sherar *et al.*, 2010). Further, twin and family studies show familial aggregation of physical activity-related traits suggesting potential influence of genotypic, common environmental and/or both factors (Bouchard *et al.*, 1997; Teran-Garcia *et al.*, 2008). In contrast to physical activity, there is limited information of correlates of physical inactivity (Van der Horst *et al.*, 2007).

Participation in youth sports is influenced by an equally diverse range of biological, psycho-behavioral and sociocultural factors. More positive perceptions of the self, in particular body image and athletic competence, peer and familial support, and coach encouragement have been noted as important predictors of sport participation in girls (Biddle *et al.*, 2005a; Snyder and Spreitzer, 1976). Parental engagement in exercise is also associated with increased sport involvement in youth (Cleland *et al.*, 2005). Conversely, health risk behaviours, for example, smoking and drinking, are generally associated with less involvement in sport (Biddle *et al.*, 2005b). Relative age and maturity timing have also been documented as important predictors of participation in a number of sports, in particular those sports where a specific physique or body size affords an athletic advantage. With regard to sociocultural factors, socioeconomic status and ethnicity have also been shown to impact youth engagement in sport, with certain groups being more or less likely to engage in specific sports, and sport in general (Biddle *et al.*, 2005b; Gottlieb and Chen, 1985).

Health-related benefits of physical activity

The subsequent discussion considers comparisons of active and less active youth based on cross-sectional and longitudinal studies, and on the influence of specific intervention or activity programmes on a variety of health indicators. Comprehensive summaries of two review panels (Physical Activity Guidelines Advisory Committee, 2008; Strong *et al.*, 2005) provide the basis for a good part of the discussion. More recent data dealing with clustered indicators of cardiovascular and metabolic health and complications of obesity in youth are also considered. It should be noted, however, that the study of relationships between physical activity and health status in youth is especially challenging in that many of the health risks associated with inactivity in childhood may not present themselves until later in adult life (Cumming and Riddoch, 2008).

Adiposity

Common indicators of adiposity are skinfold thicknesses and percentage body fat (per cent fat), although the BMI is increasingly used as such in many studies. The BMI is an indicator of weight-for-height and is not a measure of body composition. It is significantly correlated with both fat-free mass and fat mass in normal weight youth (Malina and Katzmarzyk, 1999) and is perhaps more closely associated with lean rather than fat mass among relatively thin youth (Freedman *et al.*, 2005). Nevertheless, the BMI may not accurately predict body fat in individuals while percentages fat associated with cut-offs for overweight and obesity vary with age (Taylor *et al.*, 2002).

Results of correlation and regression analyses in youth of mixed weight status (normal weight, overweight, obese) indicate a low and at best moderate relationship between habitual physical activity and adiposity. Although most of the variance in adiposity is not explained by physical activity, youth who engage in more activity tend to have less adiposity than those who engage in less activity.

Enhanced activity programmes in normal weight youth appear to have a minimal effect on adiposity. The issue of activity dose, however, has not been systematically addressed. It is possible that normal weight youth require a greater activity volume. In contrast to normal weight youth, physical activity interventions with overweight and obese youth result in reductions in overall adiposity and in visceral (abdominal) adiposity. These programmes include a variety of activities, largely aerobic, of moderate and vigorous intensity, 3–5 times per week, for 30–60 minutes. The most consistent favourable effects of activity on adiposity were found in studies that used more direct estimates of body composition, specifically dual X-ray absorptiometry (DEXA) estimates of per cent Fat and magnetic resonance imaging of visceral adiposity, in contrast to the BMI, skinfolds per se estimates or percentage Fat predicted from skinfold thicknesses (Malina *et al.*, 2007).

Skeletal/bone health

Bone is a feature of body composition that is currently a focus of attention specifically in the context of preventing osteoporosis later in life. In general, the more mineral accumulated in the skeleton during growth and maturation, the better off the individual several decades later when mineral content of the skeleton begins to decline. Regular physical activity has a beneficial effect on bone mineral content and bone mineral density. Evidence from a variety of cross-sectional and longitudinal studies indicates a beneficial effect of regular physical activity on bone mineral content in youth. Most data are derived from pre-pubertal children of both sexes and youth in the early stages of puberty, girls more often than boys. Among post-pubertal youth or those nearing maturity, the influence of physical activity, though generally positive, is more variable. In a longitudinal series of Canadian youth followed through the adolescent growth spurt, youth who are active during the interval of maximal growth accrue more bone mineral compared to less active youth (Bailey *et al.*, 1999). This would suggest an enhanced effect of physical activity on bone mineral accrual during the period of rapid growth in both boys and girls.

Activity interventions aimed at augmenting bone mineral are consistent with observations based on comparisons of active and less active youth. The programmes generally met 2 to 3 times per week for moderate-to-high intensity activities, weight bearing activities of a longer duration (45–60 minutes) and/or high impact activities over a shorter duration (10 minutes). More recent data based on three-dimensional imaging suggest a positive role of physical activity in enhancing bone strength in youth. Accordingly, changes in bone geometry indicate a substantial increase in bone strength. Bone strength is related to habitual physical activity and short bouts of activity may be as effective as sustained activity in youth (MacDonald *et al.*, 2006).

Cardiometabolic risk factors

A variety of cardiovascular and metabolic indicators have been surveyed among youth, including lipids and lipoproteins and blood pressures, among others. Cross-sectional and longitudinal studies indicate relatively weak associations between level of physical activity and total cholesterol, HDL–C, LDL–C and triglycerides. Relationships, though weak, are best for physical activity and HDL–C and triglycerides. The observational data are consistent with a variety of intervention studies that show a weak, beneficial influence of MVPA on HDL–C and triglycerides; on the other hand, such programmes have no influence on total cholesterol and LDL–C. School-based intervention programmes were generally not effective in improving lipid and lipoprotein profiles of youth. As with adiposity, it is possible that a more sustained volume of activity may be needed to beneficially influence lipids and lipoproteins. School-based programmes may be confounded in part by youth who had relatively normal values of lipids and lipoproteins at the start of interventions.

There is no clear association between physical activity and blood pressures in youth with normal blood pressures, that is, normotensive. Aerobic training programmes, however, beneficially influence blood pressures of hypertensive youth, and may also reduce blood pressures in youth with mild essential hypertension. Limited data for resistance (strength) training indicate no effect on blood pressures of hypertensive youth.

Risk factors for cardiovascular and metabolic complications commonly cluster in individuals. These include low HDL-C, high triglycerides, elevated blood pressures, impaired glucose metabolism, insulin resistance, obesity and abdominal obesity. The clustering of these risk factors is often labeled the metabolic syndrome and increases risk for type two diabetes and cardiovascular morbidity (Grundy, 2007). Of relevance to the present discussion, these risk factors are increasingly documented in youth (Cook *et al.*, 2003, 2008).

In largely non-obese samples of youth, a favourable metabolic profile (lower blood pressures, total cholesterol, triglycerides and glycemia; higher HDL-C; lower skinfolds) is independently associated with high physical activity and low physical inactivity and with high aerobic fitness (Katzmarzyk *et al.*, 1999). Evidence from the European Youth Heart Study, a multi-centre, international, cross-sectional study, shows consistent associations between physical activity (accelerometry) and aerobic fitness (cardiorespiratory fitness, maximal power output on a cycle ergometer), on one hand, and a better cardiometabolic profile, on the other (Andersen *et al.*, 2006, 2008; Anderssen *et al.*, 2007; Brage *et al.*, 2004; Rizzo *et al.*, 2007; Ekelund *et al.*, 2007). The European Youth Heart Study also indicates interactions between physical activity and cardiorespiratory fitness affecting the cardiometabolic profile (Brage *et al.*, 2004), stronger relationships between cardiorespiratory fitness and reduced metabolic risk than between physical activity and risk (Rizzo *et al.*, 2007), and independent inverse associations between aerobic fitness and cardiometabolic risk and between habitual physical activity and cardiometabolic risk (Ekelund *et al.*, 2007). Overall, youth who are regularly active and/or who have good aerobic fitness tend to present a favourable metabolic risk profile. Adiposity is an additional independent risk factor for cardiometabolic risk; youth who are leaner and with less central adiposity (measured indirectly as waist circumference) tend to present a more favourable risk profile. Fitness and adiposity are also independently related with clustered cardiometabolic risk among late adolescent youth (Buchan *et al.*, 2012, 2013).

The preceding studies demonstrate important associations between physical activity and cardiometabolic risk. What is the influence of physical activity programmes on risk factors individually or clustered? Trends in studies of several individual risk factors were noted above, for example, adiposity, lipids and lipoproteins and blood pressures. Increasingly, evidence shows that experimental physical activity programmes improve the cardiometabolic risk profile of overweight and obese youth – reduction in adiposity, insulin and triglycerides; improved insulin sensitivity, lipid profile and cardiorespiratory fitness; increased heart rate variability; and reduction in inflammation indicators (Gutin *et al.*, 2000; 2008; Bell *et al.*, 2007; Carrel *et al.*, 2005; Nassis *et al.*, 2005). However, the favourable responses to regular activity are lost when obese youth are no longer involved in regular physical activity (Carrel *et al.*, 2007), that is, youth relapse to a lifestyle without or with reduced physical activity. The results highlight the need for physical activity on a regular basis and raise further questions. For example, how much activity is needed to maintain the beneficial effects associated with intervention programmes?

Aerobic fitness

Data from both cross-sectional and longitudinal studies indicate higher levels of aerobic fitness, measured as maximal aerobic power (VO_2 max) or endurance runs, in active youth than in less active youth. Some longitudinal data suggest an enhanced effect of physical activity during the interval of maximal growth of VO_2 max, which occurs coincidentally with peak height velocity during the adolescent spurt (Mirwald and Bailey, 1986). In experimental studies of youth, 8 years through late adolescence, continuous, vigorous physical activity has a favourable effect on maximal aerobic power. Programmes generally involved continuous, vigorous activity (e.g. 80 per cent of maximal heart rate) for 3 days per week at 30–45 minutes per session. The associated gain in VO_2 max was about 10 per cent (3–4 ml/kg/min).

Muscular strength and endurance

Cross-sectional and longitudinal data are equivocal regarding the association of physical activity with indicators of muscular strength and endurance among youth with one exception. Evidence from a longitudinal study of Belgian boys indicated better upper body muscular strength and endurance (flexed arm hang) in active compared to less active youth (Beunen et al., 1992). On the other hand, experimental data show significant gains in muscular strength and endurance in youth with resistance training programs involving a variety of progressive activities that incorporate reciprocal and large muscle groups. Most programmes involved sessions of 30–45 minutes duration 2–3 days per week with a rest day between sessions, and were 8–12 weeks in duration (Malina, 2006). The results also show some degree of specificity. Larger strength gains are associated with protocols of relatively high resistance and low repetitions, while greater muscular endurance gains are associated with protocols of relatively low resistance and high repetitions. An essential ingredient in the safety of strength training protocols is adult supervision.

Psycho-behavioural health

Evidence dealing with psychological and behavioural health benefits of physical activity is mixed with certain outcomes receiving more or less attention than others. The available data are limited by the variety of outcome measures that can limit comparison across studies. Sample sizes also tend to be small and largely of convenience, and many are limited to adolescents. The bias toward adolescents may reflect biological and behavioural interactions as youth adjust to or cope with the physiological changes and social demands of the transition into and progress through puberty. This being said, indicators of biological growth and maturation are rarely considered in such studies. Research addressing potential influences of physical activity is largely associational, although some quasi-experimental and longitudinal data are available for certain outcomes. Variable modes of physical activity are also considered, for example, sport, aerobic and dance separately or in combination. Activity together with cognitive behavioural modification is also considered.

A positive association between physical activity and self-concept is a consistent finding that has been documented in cross-sectional and longitudinal studies (Garza et al., 2008). Physical activity is positively associated with measures of global self-concept and two sub-domains, physical self-concept and perceived sport competence. The influence of physical activity on perceived sport competence is generally positive, but there is considerable variation that is likely associated with winning (positive) and losing (negative) and the quality of adult supervision and involvement in sport. In contrast, associations between physical activity and the appearance, social/emotional and academic domains of self-concept are not consistent. Physical activity is strongly associated with higher perceptions of self-efficacy. Body image and self-esteem are also positively associated with physical activity, though the evidence is somewhat less conclusive (Garza *et al.*, 2008).

More recently, research has demonstrated that both acute and chronic exercise can result in improvements in cognitive function and, potentially, academic performance (Hillman *et al.*, 2008; Pontifex *et al.*, 2011). Much of this interest has been fuelled by a perceived need to justify the inclusion of physical education and sport in schools. Although research on this topic is limited and has many confounding factors, emerging evidence suggests that more physically active youth perform better on tests of cognitive functioning and academic performance. Nevertheless, comparatively little is known about the processes and mechanisms that explain the effects, or about the mode, frequency, intensity or duration of activity necessary to obtain the benefits.

Data are less extensive for the potential influence of physical activity on emotional health, and the trends are variable. Overall, sport, aerobic and aerobic plus other activities have a small positive effect on well-being and quality of life and on anxiety and depression symptoms in youth, but physical activity in conjunction with cognitive behavioural modification tends to have a stronger positive effect on anxiety and depression symptoms. Accordingly, there is a growing need to study the role of physical activity in the prevention and treatment of general and more specific forms of mental health in youth, including conditions such as attention deficit hyperactivity disorder (ADHD) where physical activity appears to alleviate some of the symptoms and associated problems (Smith *et al.*, 2013; Verret *et al.*, 2012).

Overview

Several factors merit consideration in evaluating the effects of physical activity on youth. First, individual differences in normal growth and maturation are the rule rather than the exception. Variables of interest generally change with normal growth and maturation and are influenced by individual differences in the timing and tempo of sexual maturation and the adolescent spurt. Moreover, several (e.g. bone mineral content, aerobic fitness, HDL-C, adipose tissue) have their own growth patterns and some have adolescent spurts that vary in timing (Malina, Bouchard and Bar-Or, 2004).

Second, inter-individual variation in responses to activity intervention and experimental protocols needs further study. For example, peak VO2 increased, on average, from 44.7– 47.6 ml/kg/min after a twelve-week aerobic training protocol in a sample of thirty-five boys and girls 10.9–12.8 years of age (Rowland and Boyajian, 1995). The mean relative gain was 6.5 per cent, but changes in individuals ranged from −2.4 per cent to +19.7 per cent. Six youngsters showed relative changes in peak VO2 between 0 per cent and −2.4 per cent. Similarly, twelve weeks of aerobic training in 15 obese girls (13.1±1.8 years) resulted in improved insulin sensitivity without significant changes in body mass and percentage fat (Nassis *et al.*, 2005). Insulin sensitivity improved in 11 girls, showed a negligible change in one girl, and declined in three girls. Similar variation among individual girls was also evident for the glucose area under the curve.

Third, the beneficial effects of physical activity on indicators of health appear to differentiate to some extent between healthy and unhealthy youth. Among healthy children and adolescents (i.e. normal weight, normotensive blood pressure), the evidence base is strongest for skeletal health, aerobic fitness, and muscular strength and endurance, with relatively small effects on lipids, adiposity and blood pressures. It is possible that a greater volume of activity is needed to induce effects in healthy youth. On the other hand, physical activity programmes have a beneficial effect in unhealthy youth – on adiposity in the obese, blood pressures in the hypertensive, and insulin, triglycerides and adiposity in obese youth with clustered cardiometabolic risk factors.

Fourth, intervention and experimental studies of the influence of physical activity on indicators of health are generally focused on outcomes of the respective programmes. However, beneficial effects associated with activity are lost or markedly reduced when programmes stop. There is a need to address the amount and intensity of activity needed to maintain the beneficial effects on the health and fitness indicators in question.

Fifth and finally, many indicators of health and fitness, in particular cardiometabolic risk factors, are affected by obesity. A key issue, therefore, is the prevention of unhealthy weight gain in youth. Given the individuality of growth rate and the timing and tempo of growth and maturation during the adolescent growth spurt, it may be difficult to specify unhealthy weight gain. Limited longitudinal data indicate smaller gains in the BMI in physically active youth (Berkey *et al.*, 2003), while an increase in physical activity during adolescence may limit the accrual of fat mass in males though not females (Mundt *et al.*, 2006). The maintenance of smaller gains in the BMI through physical activity over time may help to prevent unhealthy weight gain and in turn reduce risk of overweight/obesity.

Potential health benefits of participation in organized sports

Participation in organized sports is a feature of the lives of significant numbers of adolescents. As such, potential health-related benefits of sport participation merit consideration.

Regulation of body weight and composition

Regular physical activity associated with sport has the potential to favourably influence body weight and composition. Much of the focus, however, is on adiposity and there are more data for relatively elite young athletes in contrast to youth sport participants. Youth athletes in a variety of sports, however, tend to have less adiposity (Malina and Geithner, 2011). The contrast between athletes and non-athletes in percentage body fat is more apparent among females than males. There is variation among sports and some positions or disciplines within a sport, for example, throwing events in track and field, linemen in American football.

Organized sport is increasingly indicated as a potentially important context of physical activity to combat the epidemic of obesity among youth. However, are sports as presently offered and practiced suitable for the obese? A major issue is getting overweight and obese youth involved in sport programmes. Limited movement proficiencies and capacities may be major constraints. Obese youth are often less proficient in motor skills and components of fitness, which reduce the likelihood of experiencing success in a sport. Excess body mass and fatness have a negative influence upon performances of a variety of motor and fitness tests, especially those which require movement or projection of the body. However, isometric and isokinetic strength are greater in obese compared to non-obese youth, reflecting the absolute size advantage of the obese (Malina *et al.*, 2004).

Most youth sports as presently offered are not user-friendly for the overweight and obese, which highlights a need for potential modification of sports to meet their needs. American football, wrestling and weight events in track and field athletics are exceptions. These sports have a place for boys (and girls in track and field), who may be overweight and/or obese. However, given the value placed upon large size and mass per se, it is possible that these sports may place some participants at risk for persistent overweight/obesity.

Skeletal health

Beneficial effects of regular physical activity on bone mineral content are apparent in many studies comparing youth athletes and non-athletes and retrospective studies of adolescent sport activity relative to adult bone mineral content (Malina and Geithner, 2011). Data for youth and adult tennis players highlight the beneficial effects of participating in the sport during growth and maturation and of maintaining the sport activity into adulthood on enhanced bone mineral accrual and prevention of fractures later in life (Ducher *et al.*, 2006). There is, however, variation among sports. Adolescent female soccer players 15–16 years had, for example, significantly greater bone strength (reflected in measures of hip geometry) than swimmers of the same age (Ferry *et al.*, 2011). Of interest, the swimmers had lower scores for bone strength compared to reference values for control subjects.

Cardiometabolic health

Data relating cardiovascular and metabolic risk indicators to training in young athletes are not extensive. Young athletes ~9–18 years in several sports that included a significant endurance component show, on average, a better profile of blood lipids and lipoproteins than the general population. The profiles of athletes, however, are heterogeneous, including some trained athletes with dyslipidaemia. Regular endurance training was not associated with a more favourable HDL-cholesterol profile in adolescent athletes (Eisenmann, 2007). On the other hand, a study of female athletes 9–15 years of age indicates higher levels of HDL-cholesterol and a higher HDL-cholesterol/total cholesterol ratio in gymnasts compared to runners and non-athletes (Vasankari *et al.*, 2000).

Improved fitness

Aerobic fitness is especially well developed in adolescent athletes in sports with a high endurance component, for example, distance running, swimming, cycling, soccer, ice hockey (Malina *et al.*, 2004; Eisenmann, Drenowatz and Malina, 2012).

Psychosocial outcomes

Social interactions with teammates, opponents and adults in and through sport experiences are generally assumed to benefit the psychosocial development of participants. Although there is considerable discussion of psychosocial outcomes associated with participation in youth sports, a good deal of the literature does not deal with outcomes per se. Much of the emphasis is on social influences of parents, coaches and peers in contrast to the influence of sport on psychosocial development of sport participants, for example, self-concept and self-esteem, peer interactions, perceived competence and social interactions, parent-child and coach-child relationships, values of fair play and so on.

Self-concept and its different domains is a behavioural outcome that has received most attention. Although sport activities are positively associated with global self-concept and perceived sport competence, they also have the potential for negative influences. Two key factors in this context are outcome (i.e. winning or losing) and quality of adult involvement, specifically coaches per se and coaching styles (Smoll and Smith, 2003).

Youth evaluations of the sport experience are more closely associated with behaviours of the coach than outcomes of competition (Cumming *et al.*, 2007; Smoll *et al.*, 1993). Coaches trained to adopt a positive approach to coaching young athletes – where behaviours such as reinforcement, encouragement, instruction are emphasized, and punishment is minimized – are more likely to have positive impacts on sport enjoyment, motivation and retention (Smith *et al.*, 1979, 2007). The benefits of the coach education program also have an influence outside of sport, with children applying lessons and values from sport to other achievement domains (Smoll *et al.*, 2007).

Other social outcomes with implications for health

Other benefits have been attributed to sport participation, especially interscholastic sport, though the evidence is variable in quality. These include greater likelihood of staying in school and fewer absences from school (Marsh, 1993), reduced likelihood of being involved in delinquent behaviour (Segrave and Hastad, 1982) and fewer risk-taking sexual behaviours and pregnancies (Sabo *et al.*, 1998; Savage and Holcomb, 1999). Sport participation among youth is associated with a reduction in suicide ideation and suicide attempts (Brown *et al.*, 2007; Oler *et al.*, 1994; Sabo *et al.*, 2005; Women's Sports Foundation, 2000). Though interesting, the evidence varies in quality and is derived largely from interscholastic sport participants in the United States. The associations need to be more critically evaluated relative to the many factors that influence youth behaviours.

Stability of activity and health indicators from adolescence into adulthood

It is generally assumed that habits of physical activity during youth will favorably influence habits of physical activity in adulthood and in turn continue to favourably influence health status. The assumption implies that habits of physical activity track from childhood through adolescence, from adolescence into adulthood, and through adulthood. Tracking refers to the relative stability of a characteristic, or the maintenance of relative position or rank in a group, over time (Malina, 1996). Longitudinal observations for at least two points in time are needed to study tracking. Correlations between observations at two or more age points are used most often to estimate tracking or stability over time. Other approaches include risk analysis, which permit estimates of the odds of maintaining a specific behaviour or characteristic over time, and linear models, which can use data over unequally spaced intervals and can account for missing values.

Presently available data suggest at best moderate relationships between physical activity during youth and activity in adulthood (Malina, 1996, 2001a, 2001b, 2001c). Associations should be considered in the context of different meanings attached to activity by children, adolescents and adults. Indicators of activity in youth do not reflect the same contexts or attributes of activity as in adulthood. Many youth, for example, view activity as equivalent to sport which is not a primary outlet for activity in adulthood.

Several issues need to be considered in the evaluation of tracking. What factors, biological, behavioural or cultural, influence the tracking of activity from youth into adulthood? What is unique about those individuals in whom activity and related variables track compared to those in whom they do not track? What are the determinants of tracking and non-tracking? Over a 26-year span from 14–40 years, for example, adolescent anthropometric characteristics, fitness and sport participation, and parental socioeconomic status and sport participation accounted for only a small portion of the variance in physical activity among adult males, although they accounted for larger proportion of the variance when men with low and high activity levels were contrasted (Beunen *et al.*, 2004).

The discussion also extends to cardiovascular and metabolic risk factors. Data suggest moderate stability of indicators of cardiometabolic health from childhood and adolescence into adulthood (Eisenmann *et al.*, 2004; Katzmarzyk *et al.*, 2001), but activity and fitness during youth do not account for a large portion of the variance in adult physical activity, fitness and health (Eisenmann *et al.*, 2005; Sacker and Cable, 2006; Hancox *et al.*, 2004; Hernelahti *et al.*, 2004). Relationships between physical activity and/or fitness and the tracking of cardiometabolic risk factors from adolescence into adulthood need more detailed study. For example, if activity and fitness are independent risk factors, what are the pathways, biological and/or cultural, through which they operate to influence cardiometabolic health?

The influence of inter-individual variation in biological maturation on growth, performance and physical fitness is reasonably well documented (Malina *et al.*, 2004). Studies of tracking, however, do not ordinarily have access to such information. Nevertheless, what is the implication of maturity-associated variation during adolescence for activity and fitness in adulthood? Do differences apparent during adolescence continue into adulthood? Data are limited. Differences in strength and motor performance among the maturity groups of Belgian boys were eliminated or reversed at 30 years of age (Lefevre *et al.*, 1990), while later maturation was associated with better muscular function at 45–49 years of age in this sample (Beunen *et al.*, 2009). Comparisons of adult females by adolescent maturity status are lacking.

A corollary of the preceding is the persistence or non-persistence of maturity-associated variation in body composition beyond adolescence into adulthood. An early age at PHV was associated with an elevated BMI, fat mass and central adiposity in males 18–20 years of age (Kindblom *et al.*, 2006). The BMI differed significantly among early, average and late maturing adolescent boys during adolescence, but did not differ among the maturity groups at 30 years of age although early maturing boys had relatively more subcutaneous fat on the trunk through adolescence and at 30 years of age (Beunen *et al.*, 1994). In contrast, subcutaneous fat distribution indicated no clear maturity-related pattern in early and late maturing boys and girls at 13–16 and 21–27 years of age (Van Lenthe *et al.*, 1996). The contrasting maturity groups, however, were defined by a difference of only three months between skeletal and chronological ages, which is well within the error associated with assessments of skeletal age.

Interactions between biological maturation and behaviour among adolescents have long been a topic of interest (e.g., Jones *et al.*, 1971). Physical activity is a behaviour, and inter-individual variation in biological maturation is increasingly receiving attention as a factor affecting activity during childhood and especially adolescence (Eisenman and Wickel, 2009; Sherar *et al.*, 2010). Both direct and indirect effects of biological maturation are indicated. Gender per se and advanced maturation of girls compared with boys contribute to sex differences in physical activity among children and adolescents (Cumming *et al.*, 2008; Eaton and Yu, 1989; Machado Rodrigues *et al.*, 2010; Thompson *et al.*, 2003). Indirect effects on activity during adolescence are mediated by beliefs, self-perceptions, social interactions and social expectations, and also by more subtle societal and cultural factors (Cumming *et al.*, 2012; Pindus *et al.*, 2013).

Tracking sport participation

Organized sport provides opportunity for physical activity on a regular basis and in a safe environment. Children and adolescents involved in sports are more physically active than those not involved, and spend more time in MVPA (Katzmarzyk and Malina, 1998; Machado Rodrigues *et al.*, 2012; Wickel and Eisenmann, 2007). Adolescent athletes 16–19 years of both sexes had greater daily energy expenditure and energy expenditure in physical activity than non-athletes (Ribeyre *et al.*, 2000). Although limited to questionnaire-based information, sport participants were also more physically active than non-participants among U.S. (Trost *et al.*, 1997; Pfeiffer *et al.*, 2006) and Mexican (Siegel *et al.*, 2013) youth and Finnish twins 16–18 years (Aarnio *et al.*, 2002).

Participation in sport during adolescence also tends to track at higher levels than other indicators of physical activity (Malina, 2001a, 2001b). Can adult physical activity be predicted from activity or sport participation during childhood and youth? Sport club membership (and by inference, participation) tracks at a higher level than other indices of physical activity among Finnish adolescents and young adults (Telama *et al.*, 1994, 1997). Moreover, frequency of participation in sports at 14 years of age (Tammelin *et al.*, 2003), membership in sport clubs at 16 years of age (Barnekow-Bergkvist *et al.*, 2001) and sport club training and competition during adolescence (Telama *et al.*, 2006) significantly predict physical activity in young adults of both sexes (late 20s-early 30s). The process of how participation in sport during adolescence translates into an active lifestyle in young adults needs study. An association between sport participation during adolescence and psychological readiness for physical activity in adulthood has been proposed (Engström, 1986, 1991).

The preceding is derived from Scandinavian countries. Sport programmes vary across countries, in accessibility and cost, and in degree of sport specialization and participant selectivity (Heinemann, 1999). Many European countries have adopted a sport-for-all theme that contrasts youth and interscholastic sport programs in the United States, which become quite exclusive during adolescence. Sport offerings for youth with lesser skill or with less interest in elite competition are often limited in many communities in the United States. Nevertheless, evidence from a survey of Michigan youth at 12, 17 and 25 years of age indicated sport participation in childhood (time spent on sports) and adolescence (time in sports, kinds of after school activities) as a significant predictor of sport and physical fitness activities in young adulthood (Perkins *et al.*, 2004).

Maturity-associated variation in size, strength and performance is a factor associated with success in sport among youth (Malina, 2002) and may be a factor in continued participation in sport and other physical activities. Prior to adolescence, male and female youth athletes span the spectrum from late through early maturation. Differential persistence or drop out, and/or sport specific selection practices, among others, alter the composition of participants in specific sports as youth progress through adolescence. Advanced and average maturity status within an age group is characteristic of adolescent male athletes, while average and late maturity status within an age group is characteristic of female athletes (Malina, 1983, 1998, 2011; Malina *et al.*, 2013). The changing make-up of youth sport participants as they pass from childhood into and through adolescence merits further study. There is also a need to consider the physical characteristics and sporting habits of those who drop-out of or who are excluded (i.e. cut) from conventional organized sports and take up less formal and informal sport activities, or perhaps become inactive.

Conclusion

Regular physical activity, including participation in sport, has the potential to enhance a variety of indicators of physical and psycho-behavioural health of youth. With the exception of bone mineral content, the persistence of health benefits requires regular participation in activity. Given the available data, there is need for further study of the type and amount (frequency, intensity, duration) of physical activity associated with health benefits during childhood, puberty and the growth spurt, late adolescence and young adulthood. There is also a need to evaluate the amount of activity needed to maintain health benefits.

Physical activity during adolescence is at best moderately related to activity in young adulthood. There is a need to complement available tracking information with more detailed longitudinal study of youth that spans adolescence through young adulthood. In contrast to physical activity per se, limited evidence suggests that participation in sport during adolescence is reasonably predictive of physical activity in young adulthood. The process of how participation in sport during adolescence translates into an active lifestyle in young adults needs elaboration.

References

Aarnio, M., Winter, T., Peltonen, J., Kujala, U.M. and Kaprio, J. (2002). Stability of leisure-time physical activity during adolescence-a longitudinal study among 16-, 17- and 18-year-old Finnish youth. Scandinavian Journal of Medicine and Science in Sports, 12: 179–185.

Andersen, L.B., Harro, M., Sardinha, L.B., Froberg, K., Ekelund, U., Brage, S. and Anderssen, S.A. (2006). Physical activity and clustered cardiovascular risk in children: A cross-sectional study (The European Heart Study). The Lancet, 368: 299–304.

Andersen, L.B., Sardinha, L.B., Froberg, K., Riddoch, C.J., Page, A.S. and Anderssen, S.A. (2008). Fitness, fatness and clustering of cardiovascular risk factors in children from Denmark, Estonia and Portugal: The European Youth Heart Study. International Journal of Pediatric Obesity, 3: 58–66.

Anderssen, S.A., Cooper, A.R., Riddoch, C., Sardinha, L.B., Harro, M., Brage, S. and Andersen, L.B. (2007). Low cardiorespiratory fitness is a strong predictor for clustering of cardiovascular disease risk factors in children independent of country, age and sex. European Journal of Cardiovascular Prevevention and Rehabilitation, 14: 526–531.

Bailey, D.A., McKay, H.A., Mirwald, R.L., Crocker, P.R.E. and Faulkner, R.A. (1999). A six year longitudinal study of the relationship of physical activity to bone mineral accrual in growing children: The University of Saskatchewan Bone Mineral Accrual Study. Journal of Bone Mineral Research, 14: 1672–1679.

Barnekow-Bergkvist, M., Hedberg, G., Janlert, U. and Jansson, E. (2001). Adolescent determinants of cardiovascular risk factors in adult men and women. Scandinavian Journal of Public Health, 29: 208–217.

Bell, L.M., Watts, K., Siafarikas, A., Thompson, A., Ratnam, N. (2007). Exercise alone reduces insulin resistance in obese children independently of changes in body composition. Journal of Clinical Endocrinology and Metabolism, 92: 4230–4235.

Berkey, C.A., Rockett, H.R.H., Gillman, M.W. and Colditz, G.A. (2003). One-year changes in activity and inactivity among 10- to 15-year-old boys and girls: Relationship to change in body mass index. Pediatrics, 111: 836–843.

Beunen, G.P., Lefevre, J., Philippaerts, R.M., Delvaux, K., Thomis, M., Claessens, A.L. (2004). Adolescent correlates of adult physical activity: A 26-year follow-up. Medicine and Science in Sports and Exercise, 36: 1930–1936.

Beunen, G.P., Malina, R.M., Lefevre, J., Claessens, A.L., Renson, R., Simons, J., Maes, H., Vanreusel, B. and Lysens, R (1994). Size, fatness and relative fat distribution of males of contrasting maturity status during adolescence and as adults. International Journal of Obesity, 18: 670–678.

Beunen, G.P., Malina, R.M., Renson, R., Simons, J., Ostyn, M. and Lefevre, J. (1992). Physical activity and growth, maturation and performance: A longitudinal study. Medicine and Science in Sports and Exercise, 24: 576–585.

Beunen, G.P., Peeters, M.W., Matton, L., Claessens, A.L., Thomis, M.A. and Lefevre, J.A. (2009). Timing of adolescent somatic maturity and midlife muscle function: A 34-yr follow-up. Medicine and Science in Exercise and Sports, 41: 1729–1734.

Biddle, S., Coalter, F., O'Donovan, T., Macbeth, J., Nevill M. and Whitehead, S. (2005a). Increasing demand for sport and physical activity by girls. Research Report no. 100. Edinburgh: SportScotland (www.sportscotland.org.uk).

Biddle, S.J., Whitehead, S.H., O'Donovan, T.M. and Nevill, M.E. (2005b). Correlates of participation in physical activity for adolescent girls: A systematic review of recent literature. Journal of Physical Activity and Health, 2: 421–432.

Bouchard, C., Malina, R.M. and Perusse, L. (1997). Genetics of Fitness and Physical Performance. Champaign, Illinois: Human Kinetics.

Brage, S., Wedderkopp, N., Ekelund, U., Franks, P.A., Wareham, N.J. Andersen, L.B. and Froberg, K. (2004). Features of the metabolic syndrome are associated with objectively measured physical activity and fitness in Danish children. Diabetes Care, 27: 2141–2148.

Brown, D.R., Galuska, D.A., Zhang, J., Eaton, D.K., Fulton, J.E., Lowry, R. and Maynard, L.M. (2007). Physical activity, sport participation, and suicidal behavior: US high school students. Medicine and Science in Sports and Exercise, 39: 2248–2257.

Buchan, D.S., Young, J.D., Boddy, L.M., Malina, R.M. and Baker, J.S. (2013). Fitness and adiposity are independently associated with cardiometabolic risk in youth. BioMed Research International, 261698, Champaign, Epub 2013 July 31.

Buchan, D.S., Young, J.D., Cooper, S-M., Malina, R.M., Cockcroft, J. and Baker, J.S. (2012). Relationships among indicators of fitness, fatness and cardiovascular disease risk factors in adolescents. OnLine Journal of Biological Sciences, 12(3): 89–95.

Carrel, A.L., Clark, R.R., Peterseon, S., Eickhoff, J. and Allen, D.B. (2007). School-based fitness changes are lost during the summer vacation. Archives of Pediatric and Adolescent Medicine, 161: 561–564.

Carrel, A.L., Clark, R.R., Peterson, S.E., Nemeth, B.A., Sullivan, J. and Allen, D.B. (2005). Improvement of fitness, body composition, and insulin sensitivity in overweight children in a school-based exercise program. Archives of Pediatric and Adolescent Medicine, 159: 963–968.

Child Trends Data Bank. (2013). Participation in School Athletics. Washington, DC: Child Trends.

Cleland, V., Venn, A., Fryer, J., Dwyer, T. and Blizzard, L. (2005). Parental exercise is associated with Australian children's extracurricular sports participation and cardiorespiratory fitness: A cross-sectional study. International Journal of Behavioural Nutrition and Physical Activity, 2, 3. doi: 10.1186/1479–5868–2–3.

Cook, S., Aunger, P., Li, C. and Ford, E.S. (2008). Metabolic syndrome rates in United States adolescents, from the National Health and Nutrition Examination Survey, 1999–2002. Journal of Pediatrics, 152: 165–170.

Cook, S., Weitzman, M., Auinger, P., Nguyen, M. and Dietz, W.H. (2003). Prevalence of a metabolic syndrome phenotype in adolescence: findings from the third National Health and Nutrition Examination Survey, 1988–1994. Archives of Pediatric and Adolescent Medicine, 157: 821–827.

Cumming, S.P. and Riddoch, C. (2009). Physical activity, fitness and children's health: current concepts. In N. Armstrong and W. van Mechelen (eds), Paediatric Exercise Science and Medicine. (pp. 327–338). Oxford: Oxford University Press.

Cumming S.P., Sherar, L.B., Gammon, C., Standage, M. and Malina, R.M. (2012). Physical activity and self-concept in adolescence: A comparison of girls at the extremes of the biological maturation continuum. Journal of Research on Adolescence, 22: 746–757.

Cumming, S.P., Sherar, L.B., Pindus, D.M., Coelho-e-Silva, M.J., Malina, R.M. and Jardine, P.R. (2012). A biocultural model of maturity-associated variance in adolescent physical activity. International Review of Sport and Exercise Psychology, 5: 22–43.

Cumming, S.P., Smoll, F.L., Smith, R.E. and Grossbard, J.R. (2007). Is winning everything? The relative contributions of motivational climate and won-lost percentage in youth sports. Journal of Applied Sport Psychology, 19: 322–336.

Cumming, S.P., Standage, M., Gillison, F. and Malina, R.M. (2008). Sex differences in exercise behavior during adolescence: Is biological maturation a confounding factor? Journal of Adolescent Health, 42: 480–485.

Cumming, S.P., Standage, M., Gillison, F.B., Dompier, T.P. and Malina, R.M. (2009). Biological maturity status, body size, and exercise behaviour in British youth: A pilot study. Journal of Sports Sciences, 27, 677–686.

Ducher, G., Tournaire, N., Meddahi-Pellé, A., Benhamou, C-L. and Courteix, D. (2006). Short-term and long-term site-specific effects of tennis playing on trabecular and cortical bone at the distal radius. Journal of Bone Mineral Metabolism, 24: 484–490.

Eaton, W.O. and Yu, A.P. (1989). Are sex differences in child motor activity level a function of sex differences in maturational status? Child Development, 60: 1005–1011.

Eisenmann, J.C. (2002). Blood lipids and lipoproteins in child and adolescent athletes. Sports Medicine, 32: 297–307.

Eisenmann, J.C., Drenowatz, C. and Malina, R.M. (2012). Endurance training in children and adolescents. In I. Mujika (ed): Endurance Training: Science and Practice. Vitoria-Gasteiz, Basque Country: Iñigo Mujika S.L.U.

Eisenmann, J.C., Welk, G.J., Wickel, E.E. and Blair, S.N. (2004). Stability of variables associated with the metabolic syndrome from adolescence to adulthood: the Aerobics Center Longitudinal Study. American Journal of Human Biology, 16: 690–696.

Eisenmann, J.C., Wickel, E.E., Welk, G.J. and Blair, S.N. (2005). Relationship between adolescent fitness and fatness and cardiovascular disease risk factors in adulthood: the Aerobics Center Longitudinal Study. American Heart Journal, 149: 46–53.

Ekelund, U. anderssen, S.A., Froberg, K., Sardinha, L.B. andersen, LB. and Brage, S. (2007), Independent associations of physical activity and cardiorespiratory fitness with metabolic risk factors in children: The European Youth Heart Study. Diabetologia, 50: 1832–1840.

Engström, L.-M. (1986). The process of socialization into keep fit activities. Journal of Sports Science, 8: 89–97.

Engström, L.-M. (1991). Exercise adherence in sport for all from youth to adulthood. In P. Oja and R. Telama (eds): Sport for All. (pp. 473–483). Amsterdam: Elsevier Press.

Ferry, B., Duclos, M., Burt, L., Therre, P., Le Gall, F., Jaffré, C. and Courteix, D. (2011). Bone geometry and strength adaptations to physical constraints inherent in different sports: comparison between elite female soccer players and swimmers. Journal of Bone Mineral Metabolism, 29: 342–351

Fraser, J. and Ziff, A. (2009). Children and Young People's Participation in Organised Sport. Omnibus Survey, Ipsos MORI: Department for Children, Schools and Families, Research Report DCSF-RR135 (www.dcsf.gov.uk/research).

Freedman, D.S., Wang, J., Maynard, L.M., Thornton, J.C., Mei, Z., Pierson, R.N., et al. (2005). Relation of BMI to fat and fat-free mass among children and adolescents. International Journal of Obesity, 29: 1–8.

Garza, J.C, Murray, N.G., Sharma, S., Drenner, K.L., Tortolero, S.R. and Taylor, W.C. (2009). Physical activity, physical fitness, and social, psychological, and emotional health. In N. Armstrong and W. van Mechelen (eds), Paediatric Exercise Science and Medicine. Oxford: Oxford University Press, pp. 375–396.

Gottlieb, N.H. and Chen, M.S. (1985). Sociocultural correlates of childhood sporting activities: their implications for heart health. Social Science and Medicine, 21: 533–539.

Grundy, S.M. (2007). Metabolic syndrome: A multiplex cardiovascular risk factor. Journal of Clinical Endocrinology and Metabolism, 92: 399–404.

Gutin, B., Barbeau, P., Litaker, M.S., Ferguson, M. and Owens, S. (2000). Heart rate variability in obese children: relations to total body and visceral adiposity, and changes with physical training and detraining. Obesity Research, 8: 12–19.

Gutin, B., Yin, Z., Johnson, M. and Barbeau, P. (2008). Preliminary findings of the effect of a 3-year after-school physical activity intervention on fitness and body fat: The Medical College of Georgia Fitkid Project. International Journal of Pediatric Obesity, 3: 3–9.

Hancox, R.J., Milne, B.J. and Poulton, R. (2004). Association between child and adolescent television viewing and adult health: a longitudinal birth cohort study. The Lancet, 364: 257–262.

Heinemann, K. (1999). Sport clubs in Europe. In K. Heinemann (ed): Sport Clubs in Various European Countries. Schorndorf, Germany: Karl Hofmann, pp. 13–32.

Hernelahti, M., Levalahti, E., Simonen, R.L., Kaprio, J., Kujala, U.M., Uusitalo-Koskinen, A.L., et al. (2004). Relative roles of heredity and physical activity in adolescence and adulthood on blood pressure. Journal of Applied Physiology, 97: 1046–1052.

Hillman, C.H., Erickson, K.I. and Kramer, A.F. (2008). Be smart, exercise your heart: exercise effects on brain and cognition. Nature Reviews Neuroscience, 9: 58–65.

Ifedi, F. (2008). Sport Participation in Canada, 2005. Ottawa: Culture, Tourism and the Centre for Education Statistics.

Instituto do Desporto de Portugal (2005). Estatística do Associativismo em Portugal 1996–2003. Lisbon: Instituto do Deporto de Portugal.

Istituto Nazionale di Statistica. (2005). Lo sport che cambia: I comportamenti emergenti e le nuove tendenze della pratica sportiva in Italia. Roma: Istituto Nazionale di Statistica.

Jones, M.C., Bayley, N., MacFarlane, J.W. and Honzik, M.P., editors. (1971). The Course of Human Development: Selected Papers from the Longitudinal Studies, Institute of Human Development, the University of California, Berkeley. Waltham, MA: Xerox College Publishing.

Katzmarzyk, P.T. and Malina, R.M. (1998). Contributions of organized sports participation to estimated daily energy expenditure in youth. Pediatric Exercise Science, 10: 378–386.

Katzmarzyk, P.T., Malina, R.M. and Bouchard, C. (1999). Physical activity, physical fitness, and coronary heart disease risk factors in youth: The Quebec Family Study. Preventive Medicine, 29: 555–562.

Katzmarzyk, P.T., Perusse, L. Malina, R.M., Bergeron, J., Despres, J-P. and Bouchard, C. (2001). Stability of indicators of the metabolic syndrome from childhood and adolescence to young adulthood: the Quebec Family Study. Journal of Clinical Epidemiology, 54: 190–195.

Kindblom, J.M., Lorentzon, M., Norjavaara, E., Lonn, L., Brandberg, J., Angelhed, J-E., et al. (2006). Pubertal timing is an independent predictor of central adiposity in young adult males: The Gothenburg Osteoporosis and Obesity Determinants Study. Diabetes, 55, 3047–3052.

Lefevre, J., Beunen, G., Steens, G., Claessens, A. and Renson, R. (1990). Motor performance during adolescence and age thirty as related to age at peak height velocity. Annals of Human Biology, 17, 423–435.

MacDonald, H., Kontulainen, S., Petit, M., Janssen, P. and McKay, H. (2006). Bone strength and its determinants in pre- and early pubertal boys and girls. Bone, 39: 598–608.

Machado Rodrigues, A.M., Coelho-e-Silva, M.J., Mota, J., Cumming, S.P., Shearer, L.B., Neville, H. and Malina, R.M. (2010). Confounding effects of biologic maturation on sex differences in physical activity and sedentary behavior in adolescents. Pediatric Exercise Science, 22: 442–453.

Machado Rodrigues, A.M., Coelho-e-Silva, M.J., Mota, J., Santos, R.M., Cumming, S.P. and Malina, R.M. (2012). Physical activity and energy expenditure in adolescent male sport participants and nonparticipants aged 13 to 16 years. Journal of Physical Activity and Health, 9: 626–633.

Malina, R.M. (1983). Menarche in athletes: A synthesis and hypothesis. Annals of Human Biology, 10: 1–24.

Malina, R.M. (1996). Tracking physical activity and fitness across the lifespan. Research Quarterly for Exercise and Sport, 67: 48–57.

Malina, R.M. (1998). Growth and maturation of young athletes – Is training for sport a factor? In K-M. Chan and L.J. Micheli (eds), Sports and Children. (pp. 133–161). Hong Kong: Williams and Wilkins Asia-Pacific.

Malina, R.M. (2001a). Physical activity and fitness: Pathways from childhood to adulthood. American Journal of Human Biology, 13: 162–172.

Malina, R.M. (2001b). Tracking of physical activity across the lifespan. Research Digest: President's council on Physical Fitness and Sports, series 3, no 14.

Malina, R.M. (2001c). Adherence to physical activity from childhood to adulthood: A perspective from tracking studies. Quest, 53: 346–355.

Malina, R.M. (2002). The young athlete: Biological growth and maturation in a biocultural context. In F.L. Smoll and R.E. Smith (eds): Children and Youth in Sports: A Biopsychosocial Perspective, 2nd edition. (pp. 261–292). Dubuque, IA: Kendall Hunt.

Malina, R.M. (2006). Weight training in youth – growth, maturation, and safety: An evidence based review. Clinical Journal of Sports Medicine, 16: 478–487.

Malina, R.M. (2008). Biocultural factors in developing physical activity levels. In A.L. Smith and S.J.H. Biddle (eds), Youth Physical Activity and Sedentary Behavior: Challenges and Solutions. Champaign, Illinois: Human Kinetics, pp. 141–166.

Malina, R.M. (2011). Skeletal age and age verification in youth sport. Sports Medicine, 41: 925–947.

Malina, R.M. and Geithner, C.A. (2011). Body composition of young athletes. American Journal of Lifestyle Medicine, 5: 262–278.

Malina, R.M. and Katzmarzyk, P.T. (1999). Validity of the body mass index as an indicator of the risk and presence of overweight in adolescents. American Journal of Clinical Nutrition, 70, 131S–136S.

Malina, R.M., Baxter-Jones, A.D.G., Armstrong, N., Beunen, G.P., Caine, D., Daly, R.M., et al. (2013). Role of intensive training in the growth and maturation of artistic gymnasts. Sports Medicine, 43: 783–802.

Malina, R.M., Bouchard, C. and Bar-Or, O. (2004). Growth, Maturation, and Physical Activity (2nd edition). Champaign, Illinois: Human Kinetics.

Malina, R.M., Howley, E. and Gutin, B. (2007). Body mass and composition. Report prepared for the Youth Health subcommittee, Physical Activity Guidelines Advisory Committee.

Marsh, H.W. (1993). The effects of participation in sport during the last two years of high school. Sociology of Sport Journal, 10: 18–43.

Mirwald, R.L. and Bailey, D.A. (1986). Maximal Aerobic Power. London, Ontario: Sport Dynamics.

Mundt, C.A., Baxter-Jones, A.D.G., Whiting, S.J., Bailey, D.A., Faulkner, R.A. and Mirwald, R.L. (2006). Relationships of activity and sugar drink intake on fat mass development in youths. Medicine and Science in Sports and Exercise, 38: 1245–1254.

Nader, P.R., Bradley, R.H., Houts, R.M., McRitchie, S.L. and O'Brien, M. (2008). Moderate-to-vigorous physical activity from ages 9 to 15 years. Journal of the American Medical Association, 300: 295–305.

Nassis, G.P., Papantakou, K., Skenderi, K., Triandafillopoulou, M., Kavouras, S.A., Yannakoulia, M., et al. (2005) Aerobic exercise training improves insulin sensitivity without changes in body weight, body fat, adiponectin, and inflammatory markers in overweight and obese girls. Metabolism, 54: 1472–1479.

National Center for Health Statistics. (2009). Health, United States, 2008, with Special Feature on the Health of Young Adults. Hyattsville, MD: National Center for Health Statistics.

Oler, M.J., Mainous, A.G., Martin, C.A., Richardson, E., Haney, A., Wilson, D. and Adam, T. (1994). Depression, suicidal ideation, and substance abuse among adolescents. Are athletes at less risk? Archives of Family Medicine, 3: 781–785.

Omnibus Survey (2013). School Omnibus Survey: Physical Education. UK: Department of Education (www.deni.gov.uk/physical_education.pdf).

Perkins, D.F., Jacobs, J.E., Barber, B.L. and Eccles, J.S. (2004). Childhood and adolescent sports participation as predictors of participation in sports and physical fitness activities during young adulthood. Youth and Society, 35: 495–520.

Pfeiffer, K.A., Dowda, M., Dishman, R.K., McIver, K.L., Sirard, J.R., Ward, D.S. and Pate, R.R. (2006). Sport participation and physical activity in adolescent females across a four year period. Journal of Adolescent Health, 39: 523–529.

Physical Activity Council (2012). 2012 Participation Report. Jupiter, Fl: Sports Marketing Surveys USA.

Physical Activity Guidelines Advisory Committee (2008) Physical Activity Guidelines Advisory Committee Report, 2008. Washington, DC: US Department of Health and Human Services.

Pindus, D.M., Cumming, S.P., Sherar, L.B., Gammon, C., Coelho-e-Silva, M.J. and Malina, R.M. (2013). Maturity-associated variation in physical activity and health-related quality of life in British adolescent girls: Moderating effects of peer acceptance. International Journal of Behavioral Medicine, Epub ahead of print, 28 September.

Pontifex, M.B., Raine, L.B., Johnson, C.R., Chaddock, L., Voss, M.W., Cohen, N.J., et al. (2011). Cardiorespiratory fitness and the flexible modulation of cognitive control in preadolescent children. Journal of Cognitive Neuroscience, 23: 1332–1345.

Ribeyre, J., Fellmann, N., Montaurier, C., Delaitre, M., Vernet, J., Coudert, J. and Vermorel, M. (2000). Daily energy expenditure and its main components as measured by whole-body indirect calorimetry in athletic and non-athletic adolescents. British Journal of Nutrition, 83: 355–362.

Rizzo, N.S., Ruiz, J.R., Hurtig-Wennlof, A., Ortega, F.B. and Sjostrom, M. (2007). Relationship of physical activity, fitness, and fatness with clustered metabolic risk in children and adolescents: The European Youth Heart Study. Journal of Pediatrics, 150: 388–394.

Rowland, T.W. and Boyajian, A. (1995). Aerobic response to endurance exercise training in children. Pediatrics, 96: 654–658.

Sabo, D., Miler, K., Farrell, M., Barnes, G. and Melnick, M. (1998). The Women's Sports Foundation Report: Sport and Teen Pregnancy. East Meadows, NY: Women's Sports Foundation.

Sabo, D., Miller, K.E., Melnick, M.J., Farrell, M.P. and Barnes, G.M. (2005) High school athletic participation and adolescent suicide. International Review for the Sociology of Sport, 40: 5–23.

Sacker, A. and Cable, N. (2006). Do adolescent leisure-time physical activities foster health and well-being in adulthood? Evidence from two British birth cohorts. European Journal of Public Health, 16: 331–335.

Sallis, J.F., Prochaska, J.J. and Taylor, W.C. (2000). A review of correlates of physical activity of children and adolescents. Medicine and Science in Sports and Exercise, 32: 963–975.

Savage, M.P. and Holcomb, D.R. (1999). Adolescent female athlete's sexual risk-taking behaviors. Journal of Youth and Adolescence, 28, 595–602.

Scott, M.E., Steward-Streng, N.R., Manlove, J., Schelar, E. and Cui, C. (2011). Characteristics of Young Adult Sexual Relationships: Diverse, Sometimes Violent, Often Loving. Washington, DC: Child Trends, Research Brief (publication #2011–01).

Segrave, J.O. and Hastad, D.N. (1982). Delinquent behavior and interscholastic athletic participation. Journal of Sport Behavior, 5: 96–111.

Sherar, L.B., Cumming, S.P., Eisenmann, J.C., Baxter-Jones, A.D.G. and Malina, R.M. (2010). Adolescent biological maturity and physical activity: Biology meets behavior. Pediatric Exercise Science, 22: 332–349.

Sherar, L.B., Esliger, D.W., Baxter-Jones, A.D.G. and Tremblay, M.A. (2007). Age and gender differences in youth physical activity: Does physical maturity matter? Medicine and Science in Sports and Exercise, 39: 830–835.

Sherar, L.B., Gyurcsik, N.C., Humbert, M.L., Dyck, R.G., Fowler-Kerry, S. and Baxter-Jones, A.D.G. (2009). Activity and barriers in girls (8–16 yr) based on grade and maturity status. Medicine and Science in Sports and Exercise, 41: 87–95.

Siegel, S.R., Cumming, S.P., Peña Reyes, M.E., Cárdenas Barahona, E.E. and Malina, R.M. (2013). Characteristics of youth sport participants and non-participants in Mexico City. In P.T. Katzmarzyk and M.J. Coelho-e-Silva (eds), Growth and Maturation in Human Biology and Sports: Festschrift Honoring Robert M. Malina by Fellows and Colleagues. Coimbra: University of Coimbra Press, pp. 217–231.

Smith, A.L., Hoza, B., Linnea, K., McQuade, J.D., Tomb, M., Vaughn, A.J., Shoulberg, E.K. and Hook, H. (2013). Pilot physical activity intervntion reduces severity of ADHD symtoms in young children. Journal of Attention Disorders, 17: 70–82.

Smith, R.E., Smoll, F.L. and Curtis, B. (1979). Coach effectiveness training: A cognitive-behavioral approach to enhancing relationship skills in youth sport coaches. Journal of Sport Psychology, 1: 59–75.

Smith, R.E., Smoll, F.L. and Cumming, S.P. (2007). Effects of a motivational climate intervention for coaches on young athletes' sport performance anxiety. Journal of Sport and Exercise Psychology, 29: 39–59.

Smoll, F.L. and Smith, R.E. (2003). Enhancing coaching effectiveness in youth sports: theory, research, and intervention. In R.M. Malina and M.A. Clark (eds): Youth Sports: Perspectives for a New Century. Monterey, CA; Coaches Choice, pp. 227–239.

Smoll, F.L., Smith, R.E., Barnett, N.P. and Everett, J.J. (1993). Enhancement of children's self-esteem through social support training for youth sport coaches. Journal of Applied Psychology, 78: 602–610.

Smoll, F.L., Smith, R.E. and Cumming, S.P. (2007). Effects of a psychoeducational intervention for coaches on motivational climate and changes in young athletes' achievement goals. Journal of Clinical Sport Psychology, 1: 23–46.

Snyder, E.E. and Spreitzer, E. (1976). Correlates of sport participation among adolescent girls. Research Quarterly, 47: 804–809.

Strong, W.B., Malina, R.M., Blimkie, C.J.R., Daniels, S.R., Dishman, R,K., Gutin, B., et al. (2005). Evidence based physical activity for school youth. Journal of Pediatrics, 146: 732–737.

Tammelin, T., Nayha, S., Hills, A.P. and Jarvelin, M-R. (2003). Adolescent participation in sports and adult physical activity. American Journal of Preventive Medicine, 24: 22–28.

Taylor, R.W., Jones, I.E., Williams, S.M. and Goulding, A. (2002). Body fat percentages measured by dual X-ray absorptiometry corresponding to recently recommended body mass index cut-offs for overweight and obesity in children and adolescents aged 3–18 y. American Journal of Clinical Nutrition, 76: 1416–1421.

Telama, R. and Yang, X. (2000). Decline of physical activity from youth to young adulthood in Finland. Medicine and Science in Sports and Exercise, 32: 1617–1622.

Telama, R., Laakso, L. and Yang, X. (1994). Physical activity and participation in sports of young people in Finland. Scandinavian Journal of Medicine and Science in Sports, 4: 65–74.

Telama, R., Laakso, L., Yang, X. and Vikari, J. (1997). Physical activity in childhood and adolescents as predictor of physical activity in young adulthood. American Journal of Preventive Medicine, 13: 317–323.

Telama, R., Yang, X., Hirvensalo, M. and Raitakari, O. (2006). Participation in organized youth sport as a predictor of adult physical activity: A 21-year longitudinal study. Pediatric Exercise Science, 17: 76–88.

Teran-Garcia, M., Rankinen, T. and Bouchard, C. (2008). Genes, exercise, growth, and the sedentary, obese child. Journal of Applied Physiology, 105: 988–1001.

Thompson, A. M., Baxter-Jones, A. D. G., Mirwald, R. L. and Bailey, D. A. (2003). Comparison of physical activity in male and female children: Does maturation matter? Medicine and Science in Sports and Exercise, 35: 1684–1690.

Tremblay, M. and Lloyd, M. (2010). Physical literacy measurement: The missing piece. Physical and Health Education, Spring: 26–30.

Trost, S.G., Pate, R.R., Saunders, R.P., Ward, D.S., Dowda, M. and Felton, G. (1997). A prospective study of the determinants of physical activity in rural fifth-grade children. Preventive Medicine, 26: 257–263.

van der Horst, K., Paw, M.J.C.A, Twisk, J.W.R. and van Mechelen, W. (2007). A brief review on correlates of physical activity and sedentariness in youth. Medicine and Science in Sports and Exercise, 39: 1241–1250.

van Lenthe, F.J., Kemper, H.C.G., Van Mechelen, W., Post, G.B., Twisk, J.W.R., Welten, D.C. and Snel, J. (1996). Biological maturation and the distribution of subcutaneous fat from adolescence into adulthood: The Amsterdam Growth and Health Study. International Journal of Obesity, 20: 121–129.

Vasankari, T., Lehtonen-Veromaa, M., Möttönen, T., Aholupa, M., Irjala, K., Heinonen, O. et al. (2000) Reduced mildly oxidized LDL in young female athletes. Atherosclerosis 151: 399–405.

Verret, C., Guay, M.C., Berthiaume, C., Gardiner, P. and Béliveau, L. (2012). A physical activity program improves behavior and cognitive functions in children with ADHD an exploratory study. Journal of Attention Disorders, 16: 71–80.

Wickel, E.E. and Eisenmann, J.C. (2007). Contribution of youth sport to total daily physical activity among 6- to twelve-yr-old boys. Medicine and Science in Sports and Exercise, 39: 1493–1500.

Women's Sports Foundation. (2000). Health Risks and the Teen Athlete. East Meadow, NY: Women's Sports Foundation.

35

MEASURING PHYSICAL ACTIVITY AMONG YOUTH

Maria Hildebrand and Ulf Ekelund

Introduction

It is clearly established that physical activity is associated with health benefits and well-being (Kesaniemi *et al.*, 2001; Kruk, 2007), while physical inactivity and sedentary behaviour are main risk factors for premature death (Kokkinos *et al.*, 2011; Lee *et al.*, 2012). Hence, physical activity is one of the most important lifestyle factors for improving public health and disease prevention in children, youth and adults. Accurate assessment of physical activity and sedentary behaviour is necessary to establish a dose-response relationship between physical activity, sedentary behaviour and various health outcomes as an inaccurate assessment of physical activity and sedentary behaviour may weaken the true association between the exposure and outcome. Further, valid and reliable methods for assessing physical activity and sedentary behaviour are essential when monitoring the effect of interventions to make cross-cultural comparisons: and to determine trends in physical activity and sedentary behaviour (Wareham *et al.*, 1998).

Despite much progress in the assessment of physical activity and sedentary behaviour, limitations related to measurement accuracy still exist. These limitations are often amplified in youth and some are unique for this age group as young people's physical activity and sedentary behaviour is different from adults due to alterations in physiology, changes that occur during natural growth and development, as well as the nature of their physical activity pattern. Young people's physical activity is often sporadic, including less organized activity and characterized by intermittent movements with variable intensities with activity bouts only lasting a few seconds (Hoos *et al.*, 2004). In addition, the associations between subcomponents of physical activity and different health outcomes in youth may be weaker than in adults and therefore more difficult to establish (Janssen and LeBlanc 2010), possibly explained by higher activity levels in youth and also a longer lifetime of exposure in adults, with more time for disorders to develop. Subsequently, this has consequences for the assessment of physical activity and for the interpretation of physical activity data in youth. Although many methodological considerations can be generalized between adults and youth the assessment of physical activity in youth is not synonymous with that in adults and should be considered as a separate entity.

In this chapter, we aim to discuss the assessment of physical activity and sedentary behaviour in young people. The first section of the chapter includes definitions of different terminologies commonly used in the field of physical activity research. Thereafter, we will describe different methods used for the assessment of habitual physical activity and sedentary behaviour, the strength and limitations of these methods as well as discuss the most important issues regarding interpretation of physical activity data.

Definitions

Physical activity, exercise, fitness and sedentary behaviour

Physical activity, exercise and physical fitness are different concepts, however often used interchangeably. It is important to define terms often used in physical activity research, and for clarity we refer to these terms as defined by Caspersen and co-workers (Caspersen *et al.*, 1985). Physical activity is 'any bodily movement produced by skeletal muscles that result in energy expenditure'. Exercise is 'a subset of physical activity that is planned, structured, and repetitive and has as a final or an intermediate objective the improvement or maintenance of physical fitness'. Physical fitness is 'a set of attributes either health- or skill related'.

Physical activity is a complex behaviour, according to the definition above, comprising activities such as clapping hands to running a marathon. In general, physical activity is defined in the terms of frequency, duration and intensity, which together make up the total volume of physical activity. *Frequency* is the number of physical activity bouts during a specific period of time, while duration is the time of participation in a single bout of physical activity. *Intensity* is the physiological effort involved in performing physical activity and can be defined in absolute and relative terms and can also be normalized for different body sizes. A widely used absolute physiological term for expressing the intensity of physical activities is multiples of resting metabolic rate, where the traditionally accepted value for 1 MET is 3.5 and 4.0 $mLO_2 kg^{-1} min^{-1}$ for adults and children respectively. However, there is evidence suggesting that the commonly adopted definition of 1 MET overestimates resting energy expenditure (REE) by 20–30 per cent in adults (Byrne *et al.*, 2005; Savage *et al.*, 2007). Further, REE expressed in relation to body weight is substantially higher in young children and decreases by age and maturity, and is influenced by the body composition. Nevertheless, public health recommendations on physical activity intensity are expressed as METs and moderate intensity physical activity refers to 3–6 METs (Ainsworth *et al.*, 2000). These levels correspond to approximately 40–55 per cent of maximal oxygen uptake or 60–70 per cent of maximal heart rate (HR) in adolescents, which are examples of intensity expressed in relative terms (i.e. in relation to an individuals' maximal oxygen uptake or maximal heart rate) (Ekelund *et al.*, 2001).

Other important dimensions of physical activity are the type or mode of activity. Type or mode of physical activity concerns the specific physical activity being performed, and is usually assessed with self-report methods or by direct observation. The domain of physical activity is the context in which the activity takes place, for example at home, at school, during work or during sports and leisure time.

The word sedentary originates from the Latin word *sedere*, which means to sit. Sedentary behaviour and sedentary time are often used interchangeably and is most commonly defined as seated or recline postures characterized by low energy expenditure < 1.5 METs (Owen *et al.*, 2010). This definition consists of two different types of concepts, including posture allocation and metabolic rate. The same posture allocation can serve many different types of sedentary behaviour for example sitting watching TV or sitting at work whereas other types of sitting activities with a higher metabolic rate (e.g. cycling and rowing) are appropriately defined as physical activities.

In physical activity research, it is common to distinguish between an individual that is sedentary, that is, engaging in a large amount of daily sedentary behaviour, and an individual that is physically inactive, that is, not meeting the recommended dose of physical activity according to public health recommendations (Hardy *et al.*, 2013).

Physical activity and energy expenditure

Since physical activity is bodily movement that produces an increase in energy expenditure, physiological energy expenditure above rest can be used as a measure for physical activity or physical activity intensity. Total energy expenditure *(TEE)* is the total amount of energy required by an individual measured in joules or calories typically expressed per day, and consists of four sub components, including:

- basal metabolic rate (BMR)
- resting energy expenditure (REE)
- thermic effect of food intake (TEF)
- physical activity energy expenditure (PAEE)

(Westerterp, 2013)

BMR is the amount of energy needed to sustain the functioning of vital organs in an individual when at complete rest. It is measured in a post absorptive state (immediately after waking in the morning), supine and at least twelve hours after the last meal, expressed in joules or calories per day (Butte *et al.*, 2012). REE is often used synonymously with BMR, but it is the amount of energy required at rest and is not subject to such a rigorous protocol as when measuring BMR. REE is often slightly higher (10–20 per cent) than BMR because of increased energy expenditure due to food intake or physical activity preceding the measurement (Butte *et al.*, 2012).

TEF or diet-induced thermogenesis (DIF) is the increase in energy expenditure above BMR associated with the digestion of food and is determined primarily by the amount and composition of the food consumed. PAEE is the most variable component of TEE and defined as the amount of energy expenditure above the resting level, usually calculated as PAEE = TEE-BMR or PAEE = (0.9xTEE)-BMR to account for the TEF. Physical activity intensity (PAI) is equal to PAEE per unit of time, while the Physical activity level (PAL) is calculated as PAL = TEE/RMR.

Validity, reliability and responsiveness of methods

Validity, reliability and responsiveness are essential concepts for all types of measurements. Validity refers to the degree the method measures what it is intended to measure, in other words, the accuracy of the method (Thomas *et al.*, 2005). There are several different types of validity described in the literature, the strongest one being the *criterion validity* where the measurement from a specific method is compared to a criterion method usually referred to 'gold standard' (Tudor-Locke *et al.*, 2002). If comparison with a gold standard is not possible, a comparison with other methods measuring the same construct can be performed: *convergent validity* (Macfarlane *et al.*, 2006). *Absolute validity* is when the absolute outcome (e.g. PAEE) is compared to another method (usually a criterion method), which provides the same outcome measure expressed in the same unit (e.g. min of MVPA per day). *Relative validity* refers to the agreement between two similar instruments, for example, agreement between two different questionnaires. Caution is warranted when interpreting relative validity, as the two methods can be prone to correlated errors, hence producing an unreasonably high correlation. Preferably, the degree of agreement method described by Bland and Altman should be used to define the magnitude of the bias or agreement between two methods of measurement, however correlation coefficients are often used despite that they might be misleading (Bland and Altman, 2003).

Reliability refers to the methods, precision, accuracy and stability over time, in other words, the consistency of the method (Thomas *et al.*, 2005). A reliable method must give the same results under different conditions in which it is likely to be used. Reliability is a requirement for validity. *Intra-class reliability (test-retest)* indicates the degree of coherence between two or more measurements of the same phenomenon, and is mainly used for self-report physical activity assessment methods. It is often calculated as the intra-class coefficient (ICC), but also the standard error of measurements, coefficient of variation and limits of agreement are used (Atkinson and Nevill, 1998). Inter-class reliability refers to the agreement between different observers and this is relevant to methods such as direct observation or interviews where several investigators perform the measurements.

Responsiveness refers to the methods, capability to capture changes over time and both validity and reliability are prerequisites. For example, a method used for classifying individuals as inactive or physically active may not be suited to use to identify changes in activity levels after an intervention.

Methods of physical activity and sedentary behaviour assessment

There are numerous methods for assessing physical activity and sedentary behaviour and generally these methods are divided into subjective and objective methods. Subjective methods obtain information from the individual by questionnaires, diaries, logs or recalls and data is often collected retrospectively and depends on the individual's cognitive function. Objective measurement methods are not influenced by the individual's self-assessment of physical activity and sedentary behaviour, and may thus be less prone to recall and social desirability bias. Accelerometers, inclinometers, heart rate (HR) monitoring, combined HR and movement sensing and indirect calorimetry are all examples of objective measures for physical activity and sedentary behaviour. When choosing a method for assessing physical activity and sedentary behaviour, several factors need to be considered, not only validity, reliability and responsiveness. Different methods will only be able to assess specific dimensions and therefore the choice of an appropriate assessment method will depend on the research question and the dimensions of activity required for addressing the research question (Table 35.1).

It may not be possible to assess all dimensions of physical activity and sedentary behaviour in one study and not with only one assessment method. Other aspects affecting the choice of method are sample size, budget and resources, time limitations and personnel available.

Criterion methods

Double labelled water (DLW) and calorimetry are often regarded as criterion methods, for assessing TEE and PAEE. DLW and calorimetry both derive their energy expenditure from oxygen consumption and/or carbon dioxide production, but from different sources. The DLW method requires calculation of carbon dioxide production from the differences in elimination rates of stable isotopes obtained by urine or saliva samples, while calorimetry relies on the measurement of oxygen consumption and expired carbon dioxide. Direct observation may be a more practical criterion measure for physical activity and sedentary behaviour since it in theory can validate all dimensions and domains of physical activity and sedentary behaviour.

Table 35.1 Characteristics of Physical Activity and Sedentary Behaviour Assessments Methods

	DLW	Indirect calorimetry	Accelerometry	Inclinometers	Pedometers	Combined heart rate and movement	Subjective methods	Direct observation
Measured dimensions of PA	TEE	TEE, intensity, frequency, duration	Intensity, frequency, duration. EE can be predicted	Posture (sitting, standing and walking).	Total steps	Intensity, frequency, duration. EE can be predicted	Intensity, frequency, duration, type, domain. EE can be predicted	Intensity, frequency, duration, type, domain. EE can be predicted
Suited for assessing free living sedentary behaviour	No	No	Yes	Yes	No	Yes	Yes	Yes
Outcome	Joule, kcal	Joule, kcal	g (m/s^2) or counts per unit time	Minutes in different postures	Total number of steps	Estimate of PAEE, heart rate per minute	Minutes in PA type, domain or intensity. Categorize by PA level and estimate PAEE	Minutes in PA type, domain or intensity
Accuracy	Very accurate	Very accurate	Accurate for ambulatory activities and sedentary behaviour	Accurate for positions and sedentary behaviour	Accurate during walking (>4km/h)	Accurate during all intensity levels	Accurate in short periods and in children over 10 years old	Accurate in short periods
Cost Ease of use	Very expensive Quit easy, but complicated analyses for the investigator	Very expensive Invasive for the participant	Expensive Easy, but participants can forget to wear the monitor	Expensive Easy	Inexpensive Very easy	Expensive Easy, but needs individual calibration	Inexpensive Very easy, but can be time consuming for participants	Expensive Substantial investigator burden
Measurement period	Usually 7–14 days	A few hours	1–14 days, usually 5–7 days	1–7 days	1–14 days	1–14 days	1 day to habitual	Short term, < 24h

TEE – Total energy expenditure, EE – Energy expenditure, PA – Physical activity

Doubly labelled water (DLW)

The DLW method was developed in the late 1940s and early 1950s by Lifson *et al.* (1955). With this method, a known amount of the stable isotopes ^2H and ^{18}O are ingested orally, which over a few hours will be distributed throughout the body water pool. The ^2H-isotope is eliminated as water in perspiration and urine, while ^{18}O will be eliminated as both water and CO_2 in perspiration, urine and expired air. Hence, the difference in concentration of the two isotopes over time represents the elimination rate of CO_2, which is proportional to energy expenditure. This method requires collection of urine or saliva samples, usually daily over 7–14 days, to be able to calculated energy expenditure (Westerterp, 2013). As TEE is assessed using DLW method, the amount of energy required for activity (PAEE) can be calculated by subtracting the measured or predicted BMR or REE from TEE (see above). Despite the several advantages with this method, including high accuracy, non-invasive measurement over prolonged period of time and that it doesn't affect the individual's behaviour, the method is usually limited to small samples due to the high cost of isotopes and analyses of isotopes. In addition, the method does only provide information about the total amount of energy expenditure (i.e. TEE), and does not capture hourly or daily patterns of physical activity and sedentary behaviours, including duration, intensity and frequency (Table 35.1).

Calorimetry

Direct and indirect room calorimetry is able to very accurately estimate energy expenditure but unfortunately associated with very high cost and an unnatural environment. Direct room calorimetry measures the heat transfer from the body to the environment, while indirect room calorimetry relies on measurements of expired gases to calculate energy expenditure. These methods are not suitable for assessing habitual physical activity as they require confinement to a metabolic chamber (Levine, 2005). Indirect calorimetry using a stationary or portable measurement system is more feasible and is frequently used as a criterion method to validate heart rate monitors, pedometers and accelerometers in laboratory and free-living settings for a limited time period. The method is also used to determine the energy cost of different specific activities. Expired air is collected through a face mask, or mouthpiece. The gas analysers are stationed next to the individual or a portable system is mounted on the individual's body. Portable indirect calorimetry systems are lightweight and have been used successfully during structured laboratory activities in young children (Ekblom *et al.*, 2012; Pate *et al.*, 2006). However, the equipment is still too cumbersome to use during prolonged period of times and therefore the method is not suited to measure habitual physical activity for several days.

Direct observation

Direct observation is the most applied method for assessing patterns of physical activity and sedentary behaviour and is by some considered the gold standard for physical activity assessment (Sirard and Pate, 2001). A trained observer observes an individual and uses one of many observational systems available to record physical activity and sedentary behaviour in time intervals, for example, every minute. Direct observation is suitable for assessment in controlled environments, such as during school break-times, and can provide detailed information, including type of behaviour being performed, position, domain, duration and the frequency of the behaviour (Hardy *et al.*, 2013). In addition, it has been shown that direct observation compared to indirect calorimetry provides a valid estimate for absolute intensity in free-living adults (Lyden *et al.*,

2013). However, one could argue that this method is not suited for assessing activity intensity due to the subjective nature of classification. Other limitations with this method include the substantial investigator burden which makes is unsuitable for the assessment of habitual free-living physical activity, the invasion of the individual's privacy, in addition to reactivity and consequently altered behaviour (Hawthorne effect).

Objective methods

Objective assessment methods provide a measure of physical activity and sedentary behaviour that is not dependent of the individual's memory or understanding of the concepts being measured. Commonly used objective methods are accelerometers, inclinometers, heart rate (HR) monitoring, combined HR and movement sensors (Table 35.1).

Heart rate monitoring

Heart rate (HR) monitors are portable and non-restraining devices, generally watches, which display and record HR from a chest-band transmitter. The method relies on the linear relationship between HR and energy expenditure during activity and can be used to estimate PAEE, intensity, frequency and duration of physical activity, both in controlled and free-living settings. However, the method has several limitations. The relationship between HR and energy expenditure is weak during sedentary and low intensity activities because HR at low intensities is affected by factors other than body movement such as age, emotions, food intake, nicotine and medications (Shepherd and Aoyagi, 2012). In addition, there is a substantial inter-individual variance for the relationship between HR and energy expenditure in terms of slope, intercept and curve characteristics due to variation in resting HR and cardiorespiratory fitness. Therefore, some sort of individual calibration is generally necessary and a 'flex point' is often established during laboratory testing used to define above which HR the linear relationship between HR and energy expenditure can be used for energy expenditure calculations (Leonard, 2003). In addition, the lag of the HR response to activity in combination with intermittent activity patterns, may affect assessment of sporadic free-living physical activity. Despite that validations studies of HR monitoring for assessing physical activity in both youth and adults have showed good agreement with PAEE from the DLW method (Allor and Pivarnik, 2001; Eston *et al.*, 1998; Leonard, 2003) research using HR data has not been anywhere as prolific as the use of movement sensors. This is likely due to the complex individual calibration needed and a higher proportion of missing and erroneous data.

Movement sensor

Different types of movement sensors have emerged as the most commonly used objective methods for assessing physical activity and sedentary behaviours. A movement sensor measures body movement using devices attached to the human body at one or more locations. Pedometry and accelerometry are frequently used in physical activity research and the general principles and issues associated with these two methods will be discussed.

Pedometry

Pedometers are small, lightweight, portable and relatively inexpensive monitors that provide an estimate of the number of steps taken or mileage walked over a period of time. Many different pedometers exist but generally electronic pedometers consist of a horizontal spring-suspended lever arm that moves with the vertical acceleration of the hips during ambulation, while newer versions often involve an accelerometer with a horizontal beam and a piezoelectric crystal (Schneider *et al.*, 2004). The use and validity of pedometers has been extensively examined in youth and adults (Beets *et al.*, 2001; Clemes and Biddle, 2013; Schneider *et al.*, 2004), and the two main advantages with this method is that the monitors offer an objective measure of step counts and are of low cost. However, the monitors are only able to accurately measure ambulatory activities and do not record horizontal or upper body movement and they may be susceptible to noise during activities such as cycling or driving on uneven surfaces. In addition, many pedometers only store the total number of steps over the observational time period and cannot assess the intensity or pattern of activities performed. Other weaknesses include insensitivity to gait differences such as stride length, hence reducing comparability of pedometer data across age groups, less accurate in capturing steps during low walking speeds (<4km/h) and outputs from different pedometer brands are not comparable (Clemes and Biddle, 2013). Consequently, pedometers are suitable for measuring and comparing levels of walking in large-scale studies when limitations in resources prevent the use of other more advanced objective methods. Additionally, pedometers have successfully been used as a motivational tool in intervention studies in adolescent and adults (Bravata *et al.*, 2007; Lee *et al.*, 2012).

Inclinometers

Inclinometers are small, lightweight electronic devices consisting of a uniaxial accelerometer that are normally worn on the anterior mid–line of the thigh and have recently received increased attention as a suitable assessment method for assessing duration and types of sedentary behaviour in addition to physical activity (Table 35.1). The device uses accelerometer-derived information to assess thigh orientation with respect to gravity to determine posture allocation, including lying, sitting, standing, postural changes (sit-to-stand) and activity-related acceleration (20 Hz). The main advantages with an inclinometer is that it provides a valid and reliable measurement of time spent in different positions, however it is unable to distinguish between lying and sitting and that it can be used in all age groups, including young children (Aminian and Hinckson, 2012; Davies *et al.*, 2012; Dowd *et al.*, 2012). However, the method may be somewhat limited in accurately categorising postures apart from those standardized (e.g. lying, standing and ambulatory), is expensive to use and does not provide contextual information. In addition, postural misclassification of sitting as standing has been reported (Davies *et al.*, 2012), possibly explained by the set degree used by the proprietary algorithms to distinguish between the horizontal and vertical position of the thigh.

Accelerometry

Acceleration is a change in velocity over time (m/s^{-2}) and can be measured by small, lightweight and portable devices that record movement in one or several planes of the body segment to which it is attached. Uniaxial accelerometers measure acceleration in one direction, biaxial in two directions, while tri-axial measure the acceleration in three directions. The acceleration produced during movement is proportional to the net internal muscular forces used (Godfrey *et al.*, 2008; Kavanagh and Menz, 2008). Therefore, the acceleration can be used as an estimate of the energy cost of the movement and the monitor provides an indication of the frequency, duration and intensity of physical activity and sedentary behaviour (Chen and Bassett, 2005; Corder *et al.*, 2008). The newer versions of monitors use an integrated chip sensor instead of a beam, and the sample frequency can be set at a user-specified rate usually ranging from 30–100 Hz (John and Freedson, 2012). Advantages include the possibility to obtain detailed information about patterns of physical activity and sedentary behaviour (Matthews *et al.*, 2012). Moreover, the monitors are small, easy to wear and not too expensive to be used in large sample sizes (Table 35.1). However, there are several issues associated with this method that need consideration for the user.

Although protocols varies between studies, it has been suggested that accelerometers should be worn during the waking hours for seven continuous days, hence including both weekdays and weekends (Cain *et al.*, 2013). This is important as activity patterns differ between week- and weekend days (Comte *et al.*, 2013; Trost *et al.*, 2000). In addition, a minimum of 10 hours per day of registered movement is usually required to reflect the entire day (Matthews *et al.*, 2012). The placement of the monitor is another issue that needs to be considered when assessing physical activity by accelerometry. This is because the monitor only records acceleration of the body part it is attached to and because movement varies between body segments according to activity type. The accelerometer is normally attached to the body with a strap and several different locations have been used, including the hip, lower back, ankle, wrist or thigh. A hip placement is commonly used as this is the closest place to the centre of gravity of the body. However, recently there has been a shift towards a wrist placement since it has numerous advantages (Nyberg *et al.*, 2009; van Hees *et al.*, 2011). The one most obvious being its greater user acceptability among individuals, leading to greater compliance and less loss of data. However, the output from an accelerometer placed at the hip and the wrist is not directly comparable even for the same activity type (Ekblom *et al.*, 2012; Hildebrand *et al.*, 2014; Rosenberger *et al.*, 2013; Routen *et al.*, 2013).

The primary outcome from accelerometers is acceleration (m/sec^2); however, the majority of accelerometers expresses their outcome as counts, an arbitrary value that is not comparable between monitor brands and influenced by the amplitude and frequency of acceleration (Matthew, 2005; Reilly *et al.*, 2008). The counts are thereafter translated into energy expenditure and physical activity intensities using data from calibration studies. However, there are several issues regarding the conversion of the raw acceleration signal into activity counts and energy expenditure. The vast majority of calibration studies conducted to derive intensity thresholds for intensity, that is, sedentary, light, moderate and vigorous physical activity from accelerometer counts have used treadmill walking and running and/or a combination of lifestyle activities performed in the laboratory (Welk, 2005). However, it is unlikely that specific activities performed during a limited time in the laboratory accurately reflect all activities performed during free-living and therefore calibration studies have also been performed during free-living activities. Since the included activities in a calibration study affect the relationship between accelerometer counts and energy expenditure, this has resulted in a wide variety in intensity thresholds for activity intensities and unfortunately affects the comparability between studies. In youth for example, the upper limits for sedentary behaviour range from 100–1100 counts per minute (cpm) (Puyau *et al.*, 2004; Treuth *et al.*, 2004) and the lower cut-points for moderate intensity activity from 615–3581 cpm (Mattocks *et al.*, 2007; Puyau *et al.*, 2004). When used in the same population; the diverse cut-points can give substantially different results regarding activity level and estimates of energy expenditure (Alhassan *et al.*, 2012; Lyden *et al.*, 2011; Trost *et al.*, 2011; van Cauwenberghe *et al.*, 2011). Unfortunately, there is no consensus on which cut-points to use and consequently, the field of accelerometry has been fragmented by inconsistency in data calibration and the conversion of accelerometer raw output into counts.

In general, accelerometers have been shown to provide a reasonably accurate assessment of ambulatory activities, including time spent in different activity intensities and time spent sedentary (Ekblom *et al.*, 2012; Phillips *et al.*, 2013; Plasqui *et al.*, 2013; Robusto and Trost, 2012; Rosenberger *et al.*, 2013). Compared to the DLW, the accelerometer shows a large variability in output and is less accurate in predicting energy expenditure (Plasqui *et al.*, 2013; Plasqui and Westerterp, 2007). Often energy expenditure is underestimated during activity due to the monitor's inadequate capability to capture activity with little or no movement of the body segment where the monitor is attached, and external work.

New technology and combined methods

Emerging developments in technology have contributed to new generation of methods to assess physical activity, sedentary behaviour and energy expenditure. The newer models of accelerometers allow the user to collect and store data in its raw format (m·s^{-2}), over several days and at high frequency, that is, 100 Hz. Expressing activity data from accelerometry as raw acceleration, instead of counts, may increase the comparability between monitor brands. In addition, the more detailed data enables novel methods to predict PAEE with greater precision, including the use of pattern recognition, neural networks and machine learning (Bonomi, 2013; Lyden *et al.*, 2014; Trost *et al.*, 2012). However, limitations with these methods are that data managing is sophisticated and the methods need a large number of annotated examples of activities to develop the algorithms.

Another method that provides more accurate prediction of PAEE combines accelerometry with a physiological parameter in a single device, including combined heart rate and movement sensors and combined movement and temperature sensors (Butte *et al.*, 2012) (Table 35.1). Combined methods (e.g. HR and movement sensing by accelerometry) capture more variance in PAEE than either method used alone (Corder *et al.*, 2005). However, the increase in accuracy needs to be balanced against the increased cost and feasibility of the method. In addition to the cost, the complexity of data processing and participant burden may limit their use in large scale epidemiological studies but they can nevertheless provide useful information in clinical populations (Corder *et al.*, 2008). Additional novel methods including the use of global positioning systems (GPS) have recently been used to map movement, environmental characteristics and correlates of physical activity (Oreskovic *et al.*, 2012; Troped *et al.*, 2008; Wieters *et al.*, 2012). Taken together, the development of new technologies has great potential in the field of physical activity research and will increase our understanding on where and when people are physically active.

Subjective methods

Subjective assessment methods, also called self-report methods, are the most commonly used method for measuring physical activity and sedentary behaviour and it includes questionnaires, activity diaries and activity logs (Warren *et al.*, 2010). Commonly for all subjective methods are that they relay on self-reported information and may therefore be influenced by opinion and perception from the participants.

Questionnaires

Questionnaires are the most used and arguably simplest and cheapest methods of assessment of physical activity and sedentary behaviour in a large number of people in a short time. In general, questionnaires can be categorised into three different types: global, recall and quantitative questionnaires (Warren *et al.*, 2010). A global questionnaire usually consists of one to four items which aim to stratify the population into broad categories of activity (e.g. inactive, moderately active and active groups) and are often used for epidemiological studies or as a screening tool (Milton *et al.*, 2013). A recall questionnaire is an instrument including 5–15 items that are used to stratify the population into finer categories of physical activity, in addition to quantify physical activity. These types of questionnaires are often used in descriptive epidemiology and for surveillance studies. Quantitative questionnaires usually consists of 15–60 items aimed to capture information on physical activity and sedentary behaviour in various domains (home, work, transportation, leisure, caring for others) and according to several dimensions (intensity, frequency, duration), in addition to derive variables on patterns of physical activity and sedentary behaviour and energy expenditure. This method is often used for etiological studies (Chin A Paw *et al.*, 2010).

Questionnaires have several advantages, including practical to use, low cost, easy to administer, can capture several dimensions of physical activity and sedentary behaviour and can be used in large samples sizes. Compared with objective methods, subjective methods can assess physical activity and sedentary behaviour in specific domains. However, these methods have some unavoidable limitations (Chin A Paw *et al.*, 2010). Recollection of physical activity and sedentary behaviour is a highly complex cognitive task and therefore prone to recall bias. This can either be intentional (social desirability bias) or accidental false recall, missed recall or differential reporting accuracy of different intensities, dimensions and domains of activity. Questionnaires that only measure one aspect of physical activity such as for example sport participation is generally more accurate because it is easier to recall activities that include a conscious decision of a specific behaviour for a defined period of time. However, habitual or usual activity is much more difficult to capture accurately with subjective methods and the subjective classification of intensity contributes to the large variation in error in individual estimates of PAEE. In addition, some questionnaires do not include questions about light intensity activities and sedentary behaviour, and behaviours that are spontaneous and of short duration of time (Tudor-Locke and Myers, 2001). As a result, the methods suffer from floor effect, in other words, the lowest score available is too high for the most sedentary individuals.

Subjective methods are, as opposed to objective methods, usually developed to be used in specific groups and are therefore age and cultural specific. Questionnaires developed for adults may not be suited to assess physical activity and sedentary behaviour among youth. In addition, children below 10–12 years of age are less likely to provide accurate self-report data and therefore parental or teacher-reported questionnaires or proxy-reports are often used. However, recollection of children's physical activity is difficult for adults (Bringolf-Isler *et al.*, 2012), and there are distinctive limitations and errors associated with this method as neither a parent nor a teacher will be able to continuously monitor one child for extended periods of time.

Validation studies comparing the output from a criterion method and subjective methods indicate that questionnaires have limited ability to accurately assess and quantify physical activity, PAEE and sedentary behaviour (Chin A Paw *et al.*, 2010; Helmerhorst *et al.*, 2012; Lubans *et al.*, 2011). However, for certain types of activity, such as MVPA, the correlations between methods can be quite respectable (i.e. r >0.5) (Chin A Paw *et al.*, 2010; Helmerhorst *et al.*, 2012). Some questionnaires may be appropriate to rank young people's physical activity but their absolute validity is likely to be poor. Therefore, the use of subjective methods may mask or distort the true underlying relationship between physical activity and health (Celis-Morales *et al.*, 2012).

Activity diaries

Activity diaries are inexpensive, can be used in large sample sizes and can assess TEE and PAEE. Unlike questionnaires that are retrospective, an activity diary requires the participant to continuously record the activity or the intensity of the activity being carried out in specific time segments of the day, for example every 15 minutes. Hence, the nature of a diary will most likely reduce recall bias. Activity diaries can provide detailed information about patterns of physical activity and sedentary behaviour and energy expenditure and it has been shown to be valid to assess PAEE and EE in adolescents (Machado-Rodrigues *et al.*, 2012; Martinez-Gomez *et al.*, 2009), levels of physical activity compared to accelerometer (Bringolf-Isler *et al.*, 2012; Wickel *et al.*, 2006), and also physical activity type. However, these instruments are associated with high participant burden which may limit compliance, and they may also affect habitual behaviour (Hawthorne effect). In addition, an activity diary only assesses activity in pre-determined time segment and short-term activities will therefore inevitably be omitted or misclassified. Nonetheless, recall periods shorter than fifteen minutes have been found to be too cumbersome with low compliance (Bratteby *et al.*, 1997). Activity diaries have been successfully used in adolescents but are not recommended to be used in children. Increased compliance by using cell phone-based diaries demonstrates promising results (Dunton *et al.*, 2011; Sternfeld *et al.*, 2012).

Conclusion

Physical activity and sedentary behaviour are complex human behaviours comprising several dimensions. To be able to understand the relationship between physical activity, sedentary behaviour and health accurate assessment methods for physical activity and sedentary behaviour is essential. Subjective methods are often easy to use and cost-effective and can capture type of activity, conceptual context and rank individuals into broader categories of physical activity. However they are prone to several limitations and are not able to provide accurate estimates of PAEE or physical activity intensity. Objective methods provide a reasonable accurate quantification of intensity, frequency, duration and PAEE, and newly developed assessment instruments, data processing techniques and statistical methods hold great potential for increased accuracy of physical activity measurements. When choosing a method for assessing physical activity and sedentary behaviour several factors need to be considered, including validity, reliability and responsiveness, as well as the purpose of the study, the population being studied and the outcome of interest.

References

Ainsworth, B. E., W. L. Haskell, M. C. Whitt, M. L. Irwin, A. M. Swartz, S. J. Strath, W. L. O'Brien, D. R. Bassett, Jr., K. H. Schmitz, P. O. Emplaincourt, D. R. Jacobs, Jr. and A. S. Leon. Compendium of physical activities: an update of activity codes and MET intensities. *Medicine & Science in Sports & Exercise* 32:498–504, 2000.

Alhassan, S., K. Lyden, C. Howe, K. S. Kozey, O. Nwaokelemeh, and P. S. Freedson. Accuracy of accelerometer regression models in predicting energy expenditure and METs in children and youth. *Pediatric Exercise Science* 24:519–536, 2012.

Allor, K. M. and J. M. Pivarnik. Stability and convergent validity of three physical activity assessments. *Medicine & Science in Sports & Exercise* 33:671–676, 2001.

Aminian, S. and E. A. Hinckson. Examining the validity of the ActivPAL monitor in measuring posture and ambulatory movement in children. *International Journal of Bevioral Nutrition and Physical Activity* 9:119, 2012.

Atkinson, G. and A. M. Nevill. Statistical methods for assessing measurement error (reliability) in variables relevant to sports medicine. *Sports Medicine* 26:217–238, 1998.

Beets, M. W., C. F. Morgan, J. A. Banda, D. Bornstein, W. Byun, J. Mitchell, L. Munselle, L. Rooney, A. Beighle, and H. Erwin. Convergent validity of pedometer and accelerometer estimates of moderate-to-vigorous physical activity of youth. *Journal of Physical Activity & Health* 8 Suppl 2:295–305, 2011.

Bland, J. M. and D. G. Altman. Applying the right statistics: analyses of measurement studies. *Ultrasound in Obstetrics and Gynecology* 22:85–93, 2003.

Bonomi, A. G. Towards valid estimates of activity energy expenditure using an accelerometer: searching for a proper analytical strategy and big data. *Journal of Applied Physiology (1985).* 115(9):1227–8, 2013.

Bratteby, L. E., B. Sandhagen, H. Fan, and G. Samuelson. A 7-day activity diary for assessment of daily energy expenditure validated by the doubly labelled water method in adolescents. *European Journal of Clinical Nutrition* 51:585–591, 1997.

Bravata, D. M., C. Smith-Spangler, V. Sundaram, A. L. Gienger, N. Lin, R. Lewis, C. D. Stave, I. Olkin, and J. R. Sirard. Using pedometers to increase physical activity and improve health: a systematic review. *Journal of the American Medical Association* 298:2296–2304, 2007.

Bringolf-Isler, B., U. Mader, N. Ruch, S. Kriemler, L. Grize, and C. Braun-Fahrlander. Measuring and validating physical activity and sedentary behavior comparing a parental questionnaire to accelerometer data and diaries. *Pediatric Exercise Science* 24:229–245, 2012.

Butte, N. F., U. Ekelund, and K. R. Westerterp. Assessing physical activity using wearable monitors: measures of physical activity. *Medicine & Science in Sports & Exercise* 44:S5–12, 2012.

Byrne, N. M., A. P. Hills, G. R. Hunter, R. L. Weinsier, and Y. Schutz. Metabolic equivalent: one size does not fit all. *Journal of Applied Physiology (1985.)* 99:1112–1119, 2005.

Cain, K. L., J. F. Sallis, T. L. Conway, D. D. Van, and L. Calhoon. Using accelerometers in youth physical activity studies: a review of methods. *Journal of Physical Activity & Health* 10:437–450, 2013.

Caspersen, C. J., K. E. Powell, and G. M. Christenson. Physical activity, exercise, and physical fitness: definitions and distinctions for health-related research. *Public Health Reports* 100:126–131, 1985.

Celis-Morales, C. A., F. Perez-Bravo, L. Ibanez, C. Salas, M. E. Bailey, and J. M. Gill. Objective vs. self-reported physical activity and sedentary time: effects of measurement method on relationships with risk biomarkers. *PLoS One* 7:e36345, 2012.

Chen, K. Y. and D. R. Bassett, Jr. The technology of accelerometry-based activity monitors: current and future. *Medicine & Science in Sports & Exercise* 37:S490-S500, 2005.

Chin A Paw, M. J., L. B. Mokkink, M. N. van Poppel, M. W. van, and C. B. Terwee. Physical activity questionnaires for youth: a systematic review of measurement properties. *Sports Medicine* 40:539–563, 2010.

Clemes, S. A. and S. J. Biddle. The use of pedometers for monitoring physical activity in children and adolescents: measurement considerations. *Journal of Physical Activity & Health* 10:249–262, 2013.

Comte, M., E. Hobin, S. R. Majumdar, R. C. Plotnikoff, G. D. Ball, and J. McGavock. Patterns of weekday and weekend physical activity in youth in 2 Canadian provinces. *Applied Physiology, Nutrition and Metabolism* 38:115–119, 2013.

Corder, K., S. Brage, N. J. Wareham, and U. Ekelund. Comparison of PAEE from combined and separate heart rate and movement models in children. *Medicine & Science in Sports & Exercise* 37:1761–1767, 2005.

Corder, K., U. Ekelund, R. M. Steele, N. J. Wareham, and S. Brage. Assessment of physical activity in youth. *Journal of Applied Physiology* 105:977–987, 2008.

Davies, G., J. J. Reilly, A. J. McGowan, P. M. Dall, M. H. Granat, and J. Y. Paton. Validity, practical utility, and reliability of the activPAL in preschool children. *Medicine & Science in Sports & Exercise* 44:761–768, 2012.

Dowd, K. P., D. M. Harrington, A. K. Bourke, J. Nelson, and A. E. Donnelly. The measurement of sedentary patterns and behaviors using the activPAL Professional physical activity monitor. *Physiological Measurement* 33:1887–1899, 2012.

Dunton, G. F., Y. Liao, S. S. Intille, D. Spruijt-Metz, and M. Pentz. Investigating children's physical activity and sedentary behavior using ecological momentary assessment with mobile phones. *Obesity. (Silver. Spring)* 19:1205–1212, 2011.

Ekblom, O., G. Nyberg, E. E. Bak, U. Ekelund, and C. Marcus. Validity and comparability of a wrist-worn accelerometer in children. *Journal of Physical Activity & Health* 9:389–393, 2012.

Ekelund, U., E. Poortvliet, A. Yngve, A. Hurtig-Wennlov, A. Nilsson, and M. Sjöström. Heart rate as an indicator of the intensity of physical activity in human adolescents. *European Journal of Applied Physiology* 85:244–249, 2001.

Eston, R. G., A. V. Rowlands, and D. K. Ingledew. Validity of heart rate, pedometry, and accelerometry for predicting the energy cost of children's activities. *Journal of Applied Physiology* 84:362–371, 1998.

Godfrey, A., R. Conway, D. Meagher, and G. ÓLaighin. Direct measurement of human movement by accelerometry. *Journal of Science and Medicine in Sport* 30:1364–1386, 2008.

Hardy, L. L., A. P. Hills, A. Timperio, D. Cliff, D. Lubans, P. J. Morgan, B. J. Taylor, and H. Brown. A hitchhiker's guide to assessing sedentary behaviour among young people: deciding what method to use. *Journal of Science and Medicine in Sport* 16:28–35, 2013.

Helmerhorst, H. J., S. Brage, J. Warren, H. Besson, and U. Ekelund. A systematic review of reliability and objective criterion-related validity of physical activity questionnaires. *International Journal of Behavioral Nutrition and Physical Activity* 9:103, 2012.

Hildebrand, M., V. T. van Hees, B. H. Hansen, and U. Ekelund. Age-group Comparability of Raw Accelerometer Output from Wrist- and Hip-Worn Monitors. *Medicine & Science in Sports & Exercise* 46(9):1816–24, 2014.

Hoos, M. B., H. Kuipers, W. J. Gerver, and K. R. Westerterp. Physical activity pattern of children assessed by triaxial accelerometry. *European Journal of Clinical Nutrition* 58:1425–1428, 2004.

Janssen, I. and A. G. LeBlanc. Systematic review of the health benefits of physical activity and fitness in school-aged children and youth. *International Journal of Behavioral Nutrition and Physical Activity* 7:40, 2010.

John, D. and P. Freedson. ActiGraph and Actical physical activity monitors: a peek under the hood. *Medicine & Science in Sports & Exercise* 44:S86-S89, 2012.

Kavanagh, J. J. and H. B. Menz. Accelerometry: a technique for quantifying movement patterns during walking. *Gait & Posture*. 28:1–15, 2008.

Kesaniemi, Y. K., Danforth E. Jr, M. D. Jensen, P. G. Kopelman, P. Lefebvre, and B. A. Reeder. Dose-response issues concerning physical activity and health: an evidence-based symposium. *Medicine & Science in Sports & Exercise* 33:S351-S358, 2001.

Kokkinos, P., H. Sheriff, and R. Kheirbek. Physical inactivity and mortality risk. *Cardiology Research and Practice* 2011:924945, 2011.

Kruk, J. Physical activity in the prevention of the most frequent chronic diseases: an analysis of the recent evidence. *Asian Pacific Journal of Cancer Prevention* 8:325–338, 2007.

Lee, I. M., E. J. Shiroma, F. Lobelo, P. Puska, S. N. Blair, and P. T. Katzmarzyk. Effect of physical inactivity on major non-communicable diseases worldwide: an analysis of burden of disease and life expectancy. *The Lancet* 380:219–229, 2012.

Lee, L. L., Y. C. Kuo, D. Fanaw, S. J. Perng, and I. F. Juang. The effect of an intervention combining self-efficacy theory and pedometers on promoting physical activity among adolescents. *Journal of Clinical Nursing* 21:914–922, 2012.

Leonard, W. R. Measuring human energy expenditure: what have we learned from the flex-heart rate method? *American Journal of Human Biology* 15:479–489, 2003.

Levine, J. A. Measurement of energy expenditure. *Public Health Nutrition* 8:1123–1132, 2005.

Lifson, N., G. B. Gordon, and R. McClintock. Measurement of total carbon dioxide production by means of D2O18. *Journal of Applied Physiology* 7:704–710, 1955.

Lubans, D. R., K. Hesketh, D. P. Cliff, L. M. Barnett, J. Salmon, J. Dollman, P. J. Morgan, A. P. Hills, and L. L. Hardy. A systematic review of the validity and reliability of sedentary behaviour measures used with children and adolescents. *Obesity Review* 12(10):781–99, 2011.

Lyden, K., S. K. Keadle, J. Staudenmayer, and P. S. Freedson. A Method to Estimate Free-Living Active and Sedentary Behavior from an Accelerometer. *Medicine & Science in Sports & Exercise* 46(2):386–97, 2014.

Lyden, K., S. L. Kozey, J. W. Staudenmeyer, and P. S. Freedson. A comprehensive evaluation of commonly used accelerometer energy expenditure and MET prediction equations. *European Journal of Applied Physiology* 111:187–201, 2011.

Lyden, K., N. Petruski, S. Mix, J. Staudenmayer, and P. Freedson. Direct Observation is a Valid Criterion for Estimating Physical Activity and Sedentary Behavior. *Journal of Physical Activity & Health*. 11(4):860–3, 2013.

Macfarlane, D. J., C. C. Lee, E. Y. Ho, K. L. Chan, and D. Chan. Convergent validity of six methods to assess physical activity in daily life. *Journal of Applied Physiology (1985)*. 101:1328–1334, 2006.

Machado-Rodrigues, A. M., A. J. Figueiredo, J. Mota, S. P. Cumming, J. C. Eisenmann, R. M. Malina, and Coelho-E-Silva MJ. Concurrent validation of estimated activity energy expenditure using a 3-day diary and accelerometry in adolescents. *Scandinavian Journal of Medicine & Science in Sports* 22:259–264, 2012.

Martinez-Gomez, D., M. A. Puertollano, J. Warnberg, M. A. Calabro, G. J. Welk, M. Sjostrom, O. L. Veiga, and A. Marcos. Comparison of the ActiGraph accelerometer and Bouchard diary to estimate energy expenditure in Spanish adolescents. *Nutrición Hospitalaria* 24:701–710, 2009.

Matthew, C. E. Calibration of accelerometer output for adults. *Medicine & Science in Sports & Exercise* 37:512–522, 2005.

Matthews, C. E., M. Hagstromer, D. M. Pober, and H. R. Bowles. Best practices for using physical activity monitors in population-based research. *Medicine & Science in Sports & Exercise* 44:68–76, 2012.

Mattocks, C., S. Leary, A. Ness, K. Deere, J. Saunders, K. Tilling, J. Kirkby, S. N. Blair, and C. Riddoch. Calibration of an accelerometer during free-living activities in children. *International Journal of Pediatric Obesity* 2:218–226, 2007.

Milton, K., S. Clemes, and F. Bull. Can a single question provide an accurate measure of physical activity? *British Journal of Sports Medicine* 47:44–48, 2013.

Nyberg, G. A., A. M. Nordenfelt, U. Ekelund, and C. Marcus. Physical activity patterns measured by accelerometry in 6- to 10-yr-old children. *Medicine & Science in Sports & Exercise* 41:1842–1848, 2009.

Oreskovic, N. M., J. Blossom, A. E. Field, S. R. Chiang, J. P. Winickoff, and R. E. Kleinman. Combining global positioning system and accelerometer data to determine the locations of physical activity in children. *Geospatial Health* 6:263–272, 2012.

Owen, N., G. N. Healy, C. E. Matthews, and D. W. Dunstan. Too much sitting: the population health science of sedentary behavior. *Exercise and Sport Sciences Reviews* 38:105–113, 2010.

Pate, R. R., M. J. Almeida, K. L. McIver, K. A. Pfeiffer, and M. Dowda. Validation and calibration of an accelerometer in preschool children. *Obesity. (Silver. Spring)* 14:2000–2006, 2006.

Phillips, L. R., G. Parfitt, and A. V. Rowlands. Calibration of the GENEA accelerometer for assessment of physical activity intensity in children. *Journal of Science and Medicine in Sport* 16:124–8, 2013.

Plasqui, G., A. G. Bonomi, and K. R. Westerterp. Daily physical activity assessment with accelerometers: new insights and validation studies. *Obesity Reviews* 14:451–462, 2013.

Plasqui, G. and K. R. Westerterp. Physical activity assessment with accelerometers: an evaluation against doubly labeled water. *Obesity. (Silver. Spring)* 15:2371–2379, 2007.

Puyau, M. R., A. L. Adolph, F. A. Vohra, I. Zakeri, and N. F. Butte. Prediction of activity energy expenditure using accelerometers in children. *Medicine & Science in Sports & Exercise* 36:1625–1631, 2004.

Reilly, J. J., V. Penpraze, J. Hislop, G. Davies, S. Grant, and J. Y. Paton. Objective measurement of physical activity and sedentary behaviour: review with new data. *Archives of Disease in Childhood* 93:614–619, 2008.

Robusto, K. M. and S. G. Trost. Comparison of three generations of ActiGraph activity monitors in children and adolescents. *Journal of Sports Sciences* 30:1429–35, 2012.

Rosenberger, M. E., W. L. Haskell, F. Albinali, S. Mota, J. Nawyn, and S. Intille. Estimating activity and sedentary behavior from an accelerometer on the hip or wrist. *Medicine & Science in Sports & Exercise* 45:964–975, 2013.

Routen, A. C., D. Upton, M. G. Edwards, and D. M. Peters. Discrepancies in accelerometer-measured physical activity in children due to cut-point non-equivalence and placement site. *Journal of Sports Sciences* 30:1303–1310, 2012.

Savage, P. D., M. J. Toth, and P. A. Ades. A re-examination of the metabolic equivalent concept in individuals with coronary heart disease. *Journal of Cardiopulmonary Rehabilitation and Prevention* 27:143–148, 2007.

Schneider, P. L., S. Crouter, and D. R. Bassett. Pedometer measures of free-living physical activity: comparison of 13 models. *Medicine & Science in Sports & Exercise* 36:331–335, 2004.

Sedentary Behaviour, R. N. Letter to the editor: standardized use of the terms "sedentary" and "sedentary behaviours". *Applied Physiology, Nutrition and Metabolism* 37:540–542, 2012.

Shephard, R. J. and Y. Aoyagi. Measurement of human energy expenditure, with particular reference to field studies: an historical perspective. *European Journal of Applied Physiology* 112:2785–2815, 2012.

Sirard, J. R. and R. R. Pate. Physical activity assessment in children and adolescents. *Sports Medicine* 31:439–454, 2001.

Sternfeld, B., S. F. Jiang, T. Picchi, L. Chasan-Taber, B. Ainsworth, and C. P. Quesenberry, Jr. Evaluation of a cell phone-based physical activity diary. *Medicine & Science in Sports & Exercise* 44:487–495, 2012.

Thomas, J. R., S. J. Silverman, and J. K. Nelson. *Research methods in physical activity.* Champaign, Illinois.: Human Kinetics, 2005.

Treuth, M. S., K. Schmitz, D. J. Catellier, R. G. McMurray, D. M. Murray, M. J. Almeida, S. Going, J. E. Norman, and R. Pate. Defining accelerometer thresholds for activity intensities in adolescent girls. *Medicine & Science in Sports & Exercise* 36:1259–1266, 2004.

Troped, P. J., M. S. Oliveira, C. E. Matthews, E. K. Cromley, S. J. Melly, and B. A. Craig. Prediction of activity mode with global positioning system and accelerometer data. *Medicine & Science in Sports & Exercise* 40:972–978, 2008.

Trost, S. G., P. D. Loprinzi, R. Moore, and K. A. Pfeiffer. Comparison of accelerometer cut points for predicting activity intensity in youth. *Medicine & Science in Sports & Exercise* 43:1360–1368, 2011.

Trost, S. G., R. R. Pate, P. S. Freedson, J. F. Sallis, and W. C. Taylor. Using objective physical activity measures with youth: how many days of monitoring are needed? *Medicine & Science in Sports & Exercise* 32:426–431, 2000.

Trost, S. G., W. K. Wong, K. A. Pfeiffer, and Y. Zheng. Artificial neural networks to predict activity type and energy expenditure in youth. *Medicine & Science in Sports & Exercise* 44:1801–1809, 2012.

Tudor-Locke, C., J. E. Williams, J. P. Reis, and D. Pluto. Utility of pedometers for assessing physical activity: convergent validity. *Sports Medicine* 32:795–808, 2002.

Tudor-Locke, C. E. and A. M. Myers. Challenges and opportunities for measuring physical activity in sedentary adults. *Sports Medicine* 31:91–100, 2001.

van Hees, V. T., F. Renstrom, A. Wright, A. Gradmark, M. Catt, K. Y. Chen, M. Lof, L. Bluck, J. Pomeroy, N. J. Wareham, U. Ekelund, S. Brage, and P. W. Franks. Estimation of daily energy expenditure in pregnant and non-pregnant women using a wrist-worn tri-axial accelerometer. *PLoS One.* 6:e22922, 2011.

van Cauwenberghe, E., V. Labarque, S. G. Trost, B. De, I, and G. Cardon. Calibration and comparison of accelerometer cut points in preschool children. *International Journal of Pediatric Obesity* 6:e582–e589, 2011.

Wareham, N. J. and K. L. Rennie. The assessment of physical activity in individuals and populations: why try to be more precise about how physical activity is assessed? *International Journal of Obesity and Related Metabolic Disorders* 22 Suppl 2:30–38, 1998.

Warren, J. M., U. Ekelund, H. Besson, A. Mezzani, N. Geladas, and L. Vanhees. Assessment of physical activity – a review of methodologies with reference to epidemiological research: a report of the exercise physiology section of the European Association of Cardiovascular Prevention and Rehabilitation. *European Journal of Cardiovascular Prevention and Rehabilitation* 17:127–139, 2010.

Welk, G. J. Principles of design and analyses for the calibration of accelerometry-based activity monitors. *Medicine & Science in Sports & Exercise* 37:501–511, 2005.

Westerterp, K. R. Physical activity and physical activity induced energy expenditure in humans: measurement, determinants, and effects. *Frontiers in Physiology* 4:90, 2013.

Wickel, E. E., G. J. Welk, and J. C. Eisenmann. Concurrent validation of the Bouchard Diary with an accelerometry-based monitor. *Medicine & Science in Sports & Exercise* 38:373–379, 2006.

Wieters, K. M., J. H. Kim, and C. Lee. Assessment of wearable global positioning system units for physical activity research. *Journal of Physical Activity & Health* 9:913–923, 2012.

36

YOUTH SPORT, HEALTH AND PHYSICAL ACTIVITY

Evan James, Roald Bahr and Robert F. LaPrade

Introduction

While recreational and organized youth sports present abundant opportunities to increase fitness, share in competition and build camaraderie, participation may also increase risk of injury. The rapid growth and developmental changes that occur during adolescence and early adulthood present unique physiological and psychological conditions that may influence athletic performance and increase the risk of injury. In recent years, the field of sports medicine has placed added emphasis on the development of injury prevention measures (Adirim, 2003; Bahr, 2011). This shift is especially pertinent to youth sports injuries because injuries suffered in the early years of life may have profound long-term consequences later in life. Thus, injury prevention is fast becoming a central focus of sports medicine research in youth sports. Programmes in sports injury prevention research begin by outlining the frequency and severity of injury, continue with identifying the mechanisms of injury and associated risk factors and conclude by implementing measures to mitigate risk while tracking the efficacy of interventions (Bahr, 2009; van Mechelen, 1992). This chapter will follow a similar sequence to highlight the frequency and severity of youth sports injuries, associated risk factors and general injury prevention strategies.

Injury in youth sports may be caused by an acute traumatic event or repetitive microtrauma that accumulates over time leading to overuse injury. In the acute setting, a wide array of injuries such as lacerations, fractures, muscle strains, sprains or concussion are commonly seen. The incidence and severity of injuries tend to be sport-, sex- and exposure-specific and often vary between youth and adult participants. In addition, chronic injuries are becoming common as young athletes increasingly specialize in one sport year round. In cases of chronic injury, subclinical microtrauma builds over time without adequate time to heal, leading to a situation where the athlete is at an increased risk for injury. A subsequent acute traumatic event, which in an otherwise healthy athlete may be inconsequential, may precipitate a symptomatic injury and presentation for treatment in these athletes. Finally, acute exacerbation of medical conditions such as heat stroke, exercise induced hyponatremia, asthma or congenital cardiovascular disease may lead to injury, loss of playing time or even death in the youth athlete. Thus, injury prevention research is essential to keep young athletes safe and active in both recreational and organized sports.

Frequency and severity of injury in youth sports

In order to develop appropriate treatment and prevention strategies, it is first important to understand the frequency and severity of acute and overuse injuries in youth sports. In the United States, for example, approximately 30–45 million youth participate in organized sports each year (Gottschalk, 2011; Pate, 2000). Approximately 2.6 million patients less than nineteen-years old are treated annually for sports- and recreation-related injuries in the United States (CDC, 2009). Each year at the high school level, an estimated 2 million athletes are treated for sports-related injuries, leading to 500,000 doctor visits and 30,000 hospitalizations (Darrow 2009; Powell, 1997). By other accounts, the number of young athletes treated in the United States may be as high as 3.5 million patients (Worldwide Safe Kids, 2012). The burden of injury in this age group is significant. This section will highlight the frequency and severity of acute injuries, chronic overuse injuries and exacerbation of medical conditions commonly seen in youth sports.

Head, neck and spinal cord injuries

Sports-related head, neck and spine injuries in youth sports have received increased attention in recent years. This is especially the case regarding concussion. There has been growing concern regarding long-term sequelae, such as chronic traumatic encephalopathy and chronic neuro-cognitive impairment, associated with concussive and subconcussive head trauma sustained during an athlete's developmental years (Harmon, 2013). Compared to adults, young athletes are at a greater risk for sustaining traumatic brain injuries with increased severity and often must endure a longer recovery (McCrory, 2009). According to a report by the Centers for Disease Control and Prevention (CDC), 6.5 per cent of all sports- and recreation-related injuries treated from 2001 to 2009 were traumatic brain injuries (CDC, 2009). Of these patients, males accounted for 71 per cent of those treated and patients between the ages of 10–19-years old accounted for 70.5 per cent.

Concussions are the most common of all traumatic brain injuries suffered by young athletes. These injuries are defined as any transient trauma-induced disturbance in brain function and mental status (Harmon, 2013; Marar, 2012). Over the last decade, the incidence of concussions in youth sports has increased (Harmon, 2013; Hootman, 2007). However, rather than an absolute increase in the number of concussions annually, it is likely that the increased incidence represents improved recognition and reporting of the symptoms associated with these injuries. For this reason, it is likely that the reported incidence of concussions in youth sports will continue to rise as team healthcare personnel and coaches become more attuned to the signs and symptoms of these injuries.

In a review of six epidemiological surveys of injuries in high school and college level athletes, Harmon *et al.* reported that the majority of concussions in organized sports occured in American football, wrestling, girls' basketball, and boys' and girls' soccer (Harmon, 2013). In a recent survey by Marar *et al.* of U.S. high school athletes across twenty sports, the highest concussion rates were reported in American football, boys' hockey and boys' lacrosse (Marar, 2012). The overall concussion rate was 2.5 per 10,000 athletic exposures. Comparing gender, girls had a higher concussion rate (RR 1.7) than boys (RR 1.0) and player-player contact accounted for nearly four times the concussions compared to player-playing surface contact. Overall, the study demonstrated that concussions suffered in youth athletics vary by sport, gender and type of exposure.

Neck and spinal cord injuries also occur in youth sports, though compared to concussions these are rare. Among all spinal cord injuries, the National Spinal Cord Injury Statistical Center reports that 9.2 per cent of all injuries are attributable to sports-related causes (National Spinal

Cord Injury Statistical Center, 2006). Typically, the mechanism of injury is an axial compressive load exerted on the crown of the head with the neck slightly flexed. These injuries primarily affect young adults with nearly half of all injuries occurring in those between the ages of 16 and 30. A study by Katoh *et al.* documented sports-related spinal cord injuries in Japan over a three year period (Katoh, 1996). The results demonstrated an incidence of 1.95 spinal injuries per million individuals, a mean age at injury of 28.5 years, and 88.1 per cent of injuries in males. On a sport-specific basis, traumatic spinal cord injuries are most common in contact and high velocity sports including football, ice hockey, wrestling, diving, skiing, snowboarding, rugby, cheerleading and baseball (Boden, 2008; Gottshalk, 2011). The highest incidence of cervical spine injuries in high school level sports is in American football (Boden, 2008). Taken together, these data indicate that sports-related head, neck and spinal cord injuries are a significant concern in youth sports.

Upper extremity injuries

Upper extremity injuries in young athletes occur primarily in overhead throwing activities. Examples include baseball and softball, which are among the most popular sports at the high school and club levels (Lawson, 2009). The spectrum of injuries observed in pediatric athletes includes proximal humerus and clavicle fractures, physeal injuries, shoulder instability and brachial plexus injuries (Dasche, 2013). Proximal humerus fractures reportedly account for 0.45 per cent of all paediatric fractures (Di Gennaro, 2008) and less than 5 per cent of adolescent fractures (Taylor, 2009). The incidence of proximal humerus fractures caused by sports-related activities in skeletally immature patients has been reported from 13 per cent to 20 per cent (Dasche, 2013; Kocher, 2000; Leonard, 2010; Taylor, 2009). By contrast, clavicle fractures are the most common paediatric long bone fracture accounting for 5 per cent to 15 per cent of all fractures in this age group (Dasche, 2013). Fracture in the midportion of the clavicle is far more common than acromioclavicular or sternoclavicular injuries in this patient population because the ligamentous connections are much stronger than the clavicular physes. Closure of the medial clavicle physes often does not occur until 22–25 years of age, rendering this region at risk for injury (Caird, 2012; Dasche, 2013).

In addition, overuse injuries are becoming increasingly common in the upper extremity as young athletes tend to specialize in one sport year round (Leonard, 2010). In youth baseball, 'Little League shoulder' consisting of a traction physiolysis of the proximal humerus is common when throwing volume or intensity is increased (Dasche, 2013). In addition, injury to the elbow ulnar collateral ligament injury or, more commonly, injury to the medial epicondyle physis where the ulnar collateral ligament attaches is common (Shanley, 2013). Approximately 28 per cent of all youth baseball pitchers report experiencing elbow pain (Lyman, 2002).

Across the general population, 40 per cent of primary shoulder dislocations occur in patients younger than 22-years of age and predominantly consist of anterior dislocations (Dasche, 2013). In one study investigating shoulder injuries in high school athletes, dislocations and shoulder separations accounted for just fewer than 30 per cent of injuries sustained during a seven-year period (Robinson, 2014). Therefore, shoulder instability is a significant cause of injury in young athletes. Finally, brachial plexus injuries can occur in high velocity sports but are rare; only 10 per cent of all brachial plexus injuries are caused by sports-related activities (Pham, 2011).

Hip injuries

Hip injuries in adolescent athletes have gained increased attention in recent years with the advent of hip arthroscopy and advanced diagnostic techniques using magnetic resonance imaging

(Kovacevic, 2011). The incidence of hip injuries and disorders varies with the age of the athlete and can be divided in traumatic and atraumatic etiologies. Legg–Calve-Perthes' disease is often found in children aged 4–10, slipped capital femoral epiphysis in obese teens and acetabular labral tears in late adolescence (Berend, 2001). Several studies have shown a correlation between congenital hip disorders such as Legg–Calve-Perthes' disease or slipped capital femoral epiphysis and development of femoral acetabular impingement (FAI) later in life (Philippon, 2013). Since FAI is most commonly found in athletes, this may be an important consideration in managing congenital hip conditions in young athletes. An example of FAI in an elite youth ice hockey goalie is presented in Figure 36.1.

Other hip injuries in adolescent athletes include coxa saltans in which the iliotibial band catches and snaps along the greater trochanter of the femur, apophyseal avulsion fractures at physeal plates, hip subluxation or dislocation, and athletic pubalgia consisting of osteitis pubis, adductor muscle injuries, and sports hernias (Frank, 2013). With respect to avulsion fractures, Rossi *et al.* described 203 avulsion fractures documented over a twenty-two-year period and found that 54 per cent of fractures were located at the ischial tuberosity, 22 per cent at the anterior inferior iliac spine and 19 per cent at the anterior superior iliac spine (Rossi, 2001).

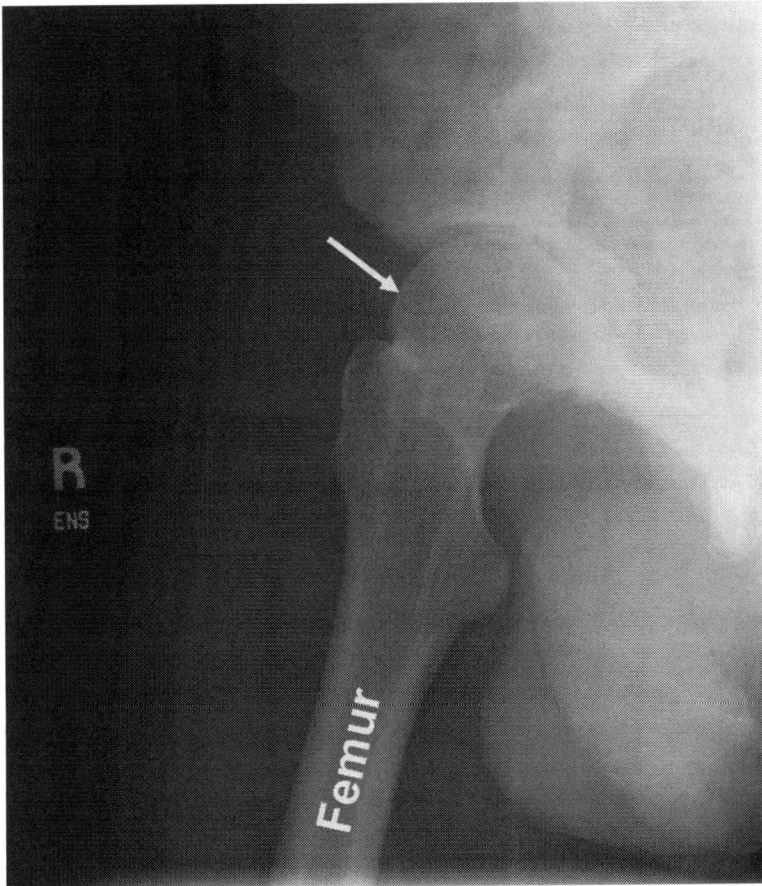

Figure 36.1 Radiograph of femoral acetabular impingement with cam impingement (arrow) in a high level youth hockey goalie (right hip)

Knee injuries

Knee injuries are very common in young athletes. In one study of high school athletic injuries, knee injuries accounted for 29.0 per cent of all injuries, followed by the ankle (12.3 per cent) and shoulder (10.9 per cent) (Darrow, 2009). The spectrum of knee injuries in young athletes includes chondral, meniscal, ligamentous, tendinous and bony pathology. Anterior knee pain is a common complaint in young athletes and may be caused by synovial impingement syndromes, tendinopathy, patellar instability, patellar malalignment, osteochondritis dissecans and tumors (Kodali 2011). Tendinopathy and Osgood-Schlatter's disease is common in young athletes (Kodali 2011). Osgood-Schlatter's disease is caused by traction placed on the tibial tuberosity via the patellar tendon leading to gradual separation of the apophysis. In addition to tendinopathy, ligament and tendon injuries are common in pediatric athletes. Since ligamentous tissue is comparatively stronger in young athletes compared to bone, bony avulsions such as at the tibial attachment of the anterior cruciate ligament are more common in adolescent athletes than midsubstance tears (Kocher, 2003) (Figure 36.2).

Anterior cruciate ligament (ACL) injuries present a significant burden for athletes in general, as nearly 250,000 athletes per year tear their ACL (Schub, 2011). Of these, 0.5 per cent to 3 per cent of these athletes have open physes.

Patellofemoral instability including acute dislocation is the most common acute knee injury in pediatric and adolescent patients (Hennrikus, 2013). Among this group, females aged

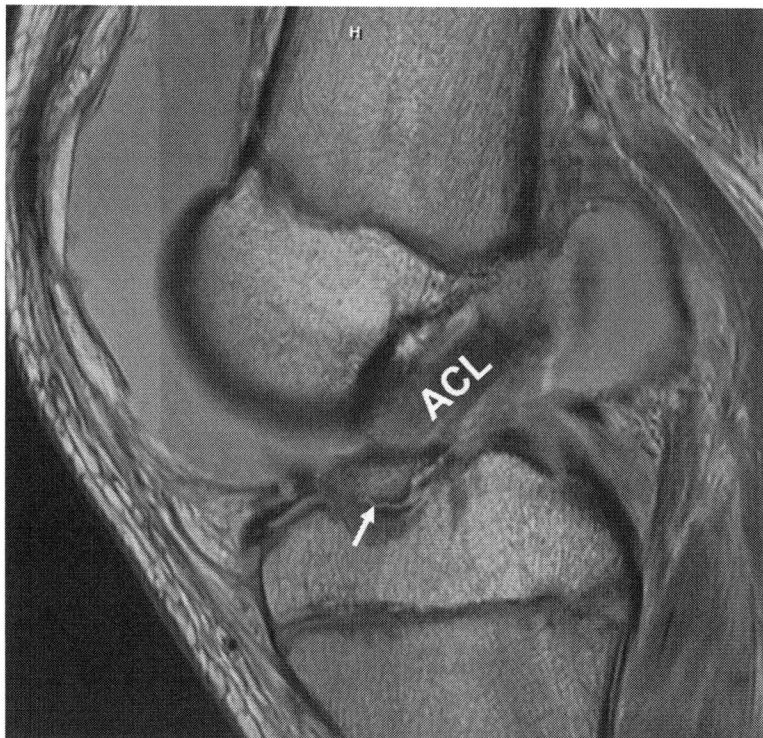

Figure 36.2 Anterior curciate ligament (ACL) avulsion fractures at the tibial spine (arrow) are far more common in pediatric patients than adults where midsubstance ACL tears are more common (left knee)

10–17 years old most commonly experience a primary dislocation event. The incidence of primary dislocations in children has been reported at approximately 43 dislocations per 100,000 individuals (Cash, 1988; Hennrikus, 2013; Nietosvaara, 1994). Following a primary dislocation event, studies have reported redislocation rates ranging from 20 per cent to 44 per cent (Hennrikus, 2013). Recurrent dislocations increase the risk of chondral injuries to the patella or trochlea and associated osteochondral avulsion fractures. In a study of 72 acute patellar dislocations, 28 knees (39 per cent) had a concurrent osteochondral fracture (Nietosvaara, 1994).

Foot and ankle injuries

Along with the knee, foot and ankle injuries are among the most commonly injured sites in young athletes. The presence of open growth plates makes injury patterns observed in adolescents often different than in adults (Malanga, 2008). In a study of high school athletes, Darrow *et al.* (2009) found that ankle injuries represented 12.3 per cent of all injuries documented over a three-year period. Other studies have reported that ankle injuries account for 30 per cent of visits to sports medicine clinics and 10 per cent of all injuries treated in an emergency department setting (Frey 1996; Mahaffey, 1999; Pommering, 2005). In one study, ankle injuries represented 19.1 per cent of all injuries experienced by high school female athletes, while only 9.2 per cent of injuries in male athletes indicating a strong gender bias towards injuries in female athletes (Darrow, 2009). The majority of these injuries are lateral ankle sprains in adolescent athletes. Lateral ankle sprains can be associated with other complications such as talar dome injuries in up to 6.5 per cent of lateral ankle sprains (Malanga, 2008). Overuse and stress injuries are common in adolescent runners, especially in high school and college-level athletes as the demands of training and competition increase (Kennedy, 2005). Due to the high frequency of foot and ankle injuries in young athletes, proper training among coaches and team health care professionals are key to managing these injuries.

Exacerbation of medical conditions

Finally, exacerbation of medical conditions such as heat stroke, exercise induced hyponatremia, asthma or congenital cardiovascular disease are important considerations in young athletes. Depending on the sport-specific demands and season, heat stroke and heat intolerance may cause injury or death and should be monitored in sports including football, basketball, wrestling, track and cross-country (Luckstead, 2002). Exercise induced hyponatremia occurs in as many as 2 per cent to 7 per cent of endurance athletes and is caused by excessive water or hypotonic fluid intake with inadequate water excretion by the kidneys (Rosner, 2009). In some cases, it can be fatal. Asthma is among the most common chronic conditions afflicting children. Prevalence of asthma in 10-year-old children in Oslo, Norway, was reported to be 20.1 per cent and exercise-induced bronchoconstriction to be 8.6 per cent (Lødrup Carlsen, 2006). Since asthma limits participation in physical activity and can lead to an acute respiratory emergency, evaluation and management of asthma in young athletes is imperative to ensure full participation in practice and competition (Carlsen, 2011). Finally, congenital cardiovascular diseases such as heart valve abnormalities, conduction abnormalities and cardiomyopathies are important to screen for as these can lead to sudden death on the field of play (Asif, 2012; De Wolf, 2013; Maron, 2009).

Injury risk factors

In order to develop targeted injury prevention measures for youth sports, it is first necessary to identify risk factors associated with injury. Some injury risk factors are present across nearly all sports, while other injury risk factors are sport specific. Risk factors can be categorized into intrinsic and extrinsic risk factors. Intrinsic risk factors are defined as individual physiological or psychosocial characteristics, while extrinsic risk factors are related to factors external to the athlete including environmental conditions and sport-specific requirements such as workload, technique and equipment. For example, intrinsic risk factors for foot and ankle injuries in adolescent runners have been reported to be anatomic factors such as alignment, gender, stage of development and extent of skeletal maturity (Kennedy, 2005), while external risk factors include overtraining, running shoes, running surface, training load and speed. Overall, differences in sport-athlete interactions lead to risk factors that are highly individualized and may vary considerably between athletes and sports.

Risk factors for acute injury can be categorized as those intrinsic to the athlete such as growth and development status, tissue quality, and strength and conditioning level and those extrinsic to the athlete including, for example, changing weather conditions, intensity of competition or protective equipment use. In the young athlete, growth and development may have a disproportionate impact on injury risk compared to skeletally mature athletes. During rapid periods of growth, tissue quality and bone mineralization may be asynchronous leaving certain joints or tissues more at risk. Soft tissue such as tendons and ligaments are comparatively stronger during development than bone since there is a decrease in bone mineral density that occurs just prior to peak growth velocity. One example of injury patterns observed as a result of these developmental changes is the propensity for skeletally immature athletes to suffer anterior cruciate ligament avulsion fractures, while adults, whose bone is stronger than the ligament, tend to tear the ligament midsubstance. Together, these factors place young athletes at an increased risk for acute injuries.

Risk factors for overuse injuries in young athletes are the result of repetitive behaviours that cause microtrauma to at risk tissue including the muscles, tendons, bones, bursae or physes. Athletes with a prior history of overuse injury are at greater risk for developing subsequent overuse injuries. Overuse injuries are also very common during the adolescent growth spurt and should be monitored closely. This population is particularly at risk due to the vulnerability of rapidly growing physes, apophyses and articular cartilage surfaces, which are highly susceptible to traumatic forces, more so than in the mature or prepubescent state. Finally, the physeal perfusion is vulnerable during rapid growth and may account for the higher rate of physeal stress injuries seen during this phase of development.

Increased training quantity and intensity has been shown to increase the risk of chronic injury across multiple sports (Di Fiori, 2014). As repetitive microtrauma accumulates without adequate healing time, young athletes are at high risk for developing symptomatic injury. Unfortunately, this scenario is becoming increasingly pervasive. Weekend-long tournaments with multiple events each day are common in youth sports such as soccer, baseball or tennis. These athletes are often competing for at least six hours a day and are exposed to the elements for an additional two to three hours between games or matches (Brenner, 2007). Compounding the problem, year round competition on multiple teams is increasing, leading to increased risk of burnout and overuse injuries (Bahr, 2014). Overscheduling is also a serious problem that increases the risk of chronic overuse injuries when the workload-to-recovery time ratio is high. Sometimes seasons even overlap, which can create situations where athletes must compete in multiple sports over consecutive days. However, data has indicated that athletes who play multiple sports throughout the year are less likely to drop out of competition compared to those who specialize in one sport before puberty (American Academy of Pediatrics, 2000).

Finally, special consideration should be given to risk factors in male and female athletes. In highly competitive youth sports, the use of anabolic androgenic steroids may be a concern, especially in young men. Studies have shown that between 4 per cent and 6 per cent of high school males have used anabolic steroids to build muscle bulk and increase athletic performance (Coward, 2013). Use of anabolic steroids places men at increased risk for hypogonadism and azoospermia. As for female young athletes, the female triad, recently referred to as RED-S (Relative Energy Deficiency in Sport) (Mountjoy, 2014), is a widely described phenomenon consisting of amenorrhea, osteoporosis and disordered eating. A history of amenorrhea in sports such as long distance running, ballet, dance or other sports that emphasize leanness is a risk factor for low bone density. It is theorized that inadequate caloric intake leads to hypo-estrogenemia, low bone mineral density and subsequently an increased risk of fracture. The recently proposed entity RED-S encompasses symptoms more indicative of a syndrome than a 'triad', with complex physiological, health and athletic performance consequences that can be found in both males and females. These and other examples illustrate that gender-specific risk factors function as important health determinants in male and female young athletes.

Injury prevention

Once intrinsic and extrinsic risk factors have been identified, injury prevention strategies can be developed to minimize modifiable risks. It is important to note that while the effect of some risks can be minimized, others are not as amenable to change. Implementation of risk mitigation strategies requires education of athletes, coaches, trainers and physicians. For younger athletes, parents also play a pivotal role in providing support for implementing injury prevention strategies. Certain preventative measures such as structured warm-ups, adjusting the rules of the game, better protective equipment, strength and conditioning programmes and pre-participation screening have had a profound impact on decreasing the incidence and severity of youth sports injuries, both minor and severe.

Structured warm-up programmes

The efficacy of structured warm-up programmes prior to practice and competition is well documented. A programme called The 11+ programme (The 11+ Manual 2012) was implemented to evaluate the effect of a comprehensive warm-up programme in 1892 female American youth soccer players and 837 players in a control group (Soligard, 2008). The structured programme consisted of eight minutes of running warm-ups, ten minutes of strength, plymometrics and balance exercises, and concluded with two additional minutes of running exercises. Injuries to the lower extremity were tracked for one league season. Results demonstrated that the group with a structured warm-up programme had a significantly lower risk of injuries overall, overuse injuries and severe injuries. In a separate study, Olsen *et al.* studied the efficacy of exercises to prevent lower limb injuries in 1837 youth handball players (Olsen 2005). A total of 958 players were instructed in a structured warm-up programme that improved technique and focused on neuromuscular control, balance and strength. Results after one season demonstrated that eighty-one injuries occurred in the control group, while only forty-eight injuries occurred in those who participated in the warm-up programme. These and other studies (Emery CA 2010; Herman 2012; Walden 2012) together support the efficacy of structured warm-up programmes in reducing the risk of injury among youngsters during practice and competition.

Conditioning and fitness

Conditioning and fitness decrease risk of injury, increase athletic performance and increase long-term health. Conditioning and fitness programmes should be customized to the demands of a given sport and performed in a supervised environment in youth sports. In young athletes, strength training should focus on development of correct technique, multi-joint exercises and avoiding maximal lifting until Tanner stage 5 is reached (Nettle, 2011). As the field of play becomes increasingly competitive in organized youth sports, athletes are required to maintain peak physical condition to perform optimally in elite-level competition.

Protective equipment

Helmets and padded headgear are ubiquitous across all ability levels of sport and function to diminish the severity of impacts to the head (Figure 36.3).

By and large, helmet design has remained unchanged over the past thirty years. The standard helmet consists of a comfort inner liner, absorptive liner, outer shell and restraint strap. While the efficacy of helmet use remains unproven in some sports, helmets have shown to reduce impact forces to the brain and may help prevent trauma such as skull fractures related to falling on a hard surface (McCrory, 2012). Barriers to helmet use in young athletes include social stigma, cost and sport requirements. Other protective equipment includes mouth guards, which help reduce the risk of dental trauma. Most high speed and contact sports have sport-specific protective equipment that is recommended for practice and competition, for example, a chest protector for catchers in baseball or shoulder pads in American football and rugby.

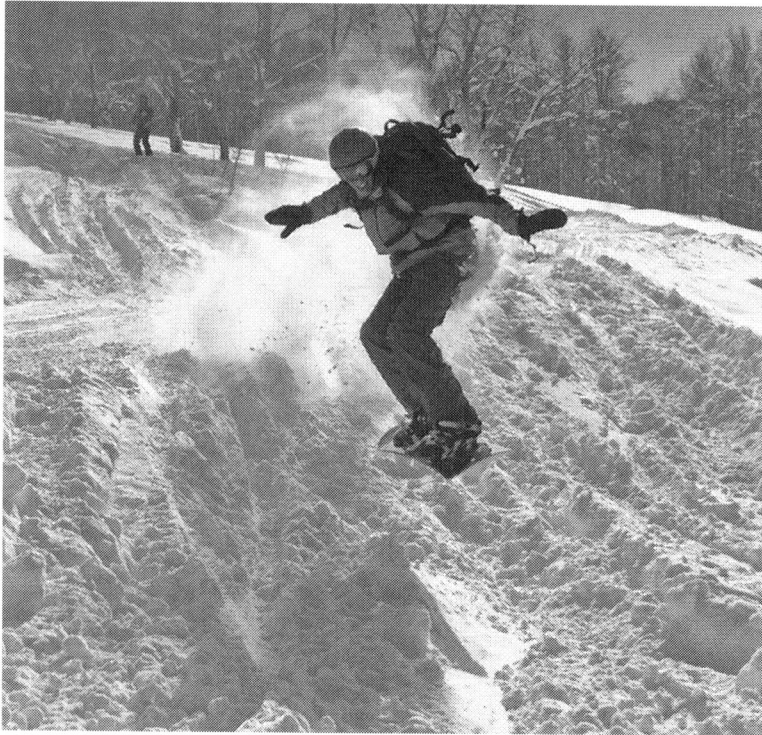

Figure 36.3 Helmet use for high speed sports, such as snowboarding, is an excellent means to minimize risk of concussions and other traumatic brain injuries

Environmental considerations

The demands of youth sports and an athlete's health may be profoundly influenced by environmental factors including heat, cold and high altitude. Certain precautions can help to prevent injuries in extreme environments. For example, strict weather-related match cancellation rules implemented by the national Royal Belgian Football Association led to significant reductions in soccer injuries from 2000 to 2010 (Bollars, 2014). With regard to American football, early season practices for high school, college and professional teams often take place twice a day, sometimes in extreme heat and humidity. Care should be taken to examine athletes for signs of heat exhaustion. Conversely, prevention of cold-related injuries such as hypothermia and frost bite is important in other sports such as alpine or Nordic skiing. Dehydration may still occur in winter sports such as ice hockey or Nordic skiing where the combination of the sport demands, copious precipitation and bulky clothing may cause excessive fluid loss. It is important to remember that the ability to adapt to varying environmental conditions may vary considerably from athlete to athlete. On an individual level, factors that influence the ability to adapt include ability level, past medical history, nutrition and hydration status, acclimatization, sweat loss rate, fitness and psychological status (Bergeron, 2012). For this reason, coaches and medical personnel must monitor athlete adaptation to varying environmental conditions in both heat and cold on an individual by individual basis.

Preventing burnout

Preventing burnout in youth sports is imperative in athletes who compete year-round in multiple sports or on multiple teams. Burnout, or overtraining syndrome, is the result of overtraining and overspecialization in sport and can lead to an athlete either temporarily or permanently dropping out from participation (Di Fiori, 2014; Roberts, 2014). Sports and activities that were once enjoyable become burdensome and stressful. Symptoms of burnout include fatigue, depression, loss of interest, sleep disturbances, lack of motivation and diminished self-confidence. Treating and preventing burnout involves rest and recovery with an emphasis on realistic goals and positive reinforcement of the value of that individual's participation. In some cases, consulting with a sports psychologist or pharmacological agents may be necessary if other methods fail to offer improvement.

Pre-participation screening

In 2009, the International Olympic Committee recommended periodic health evaluation of elite Olympic-level athletes (Ljungqvist, 2009). Preparticipation screening has also been highly recommended for young athletes prior to the start of an athletic season. Some advocate for standard cardiac screening through a thorough screening for symptoms, family medical history, and physical exam. More recently, some have advocated for electrocardiogram screening of young athletes to minimize the incidence of sudden cardiac death in sport.

A landmark study performed in the Veneto region of Italy between 1979 and 2004 reported fifty-five sudden cardiovascular deaths in screened athletes and 265 sudden cardiac deaths in unscreened athletes (Corrado, 2006). Recommended non-cardiac components of an athlete health exam include pulmonary, haematological, allergies, infections, ear, nose, and throat, neurological, dermatological, urological, endocrine, metabolic and psychological (Ljungqvist, 2009). Finally, pre-participation screening provides the opportunity to identify past injuries and develop strategies for future injury prevention.

Nutrition and hydration

Proper nutrition and hydration are essential to keep up with the demands of sport, decrease fatigue, and adjust appropriately to varying environmental conditions. In addition to the demands of sport, young persons in general require special attention to proper nutrition during periods of accelerated growth and development. After sports participation, young athletes should focus on adequate high quality carbohydrate and protein intake (Desbrow, 2014). Caloric intake should appropriately match the calories expended by competition. Furthermore, it is recommended that athlete nutrition be provided primarily through core foods rather than manufactured or artificial supplements (Desbrow, 2014). Fluid intake is essential in children since they are more susceptible to heat stress given their higher surface area to body ratio and lower sweating capacity compared to adults (Nemet, 2009). Dehydration also decreases endurance, strength and power, which are needed for optimal athletic performance.

Conclusion

As youth sports trend towards increasing specialization and the field of play becomes more competitive and global, the practice of sports medicine will likely expand as athletes aim to achieve ever higher levels of achievement. Safe and legal methods of enhancing performance will likely gain wider acceptance, while better screening and safeguards are put in place to detect and discourage illegal performance enhancement. A trend towards injury prevention may well prevail as safety equipment is improved, athletes and coaches are educated and the rules of the game develop to decrease risk of injury. Without question, recreational and organized youth sports represent an integral part of youth culture worldwide. Sports medicine practitioners and researchers are tasked with the critical role of improving understanding of the frequency and severity of youth sports injuries, associated risk factors and injury prevention strategies.

References

Adirim, T.A. and Cheng, T.L. (2003). Overview of injuries in the young athlete. *Sports Medicine* 33(1):75–81.

American Academy of Pediatrics, Committee of Sports Medicine and Fitness (2000). Intensive training and sports specialization in young athletes. *Pediatrics 106*:154–157.

Asif, I.M. and Drezner, J.A. (2012). Sudden cardiac death and preparticipation screening: the debate continues-in support of electrocardiogram-inclusive preparticipation screening. *Progress in Cardiovascular Diseases 54*(5): 445–50.

Bahr, R. (2014). Demise of the fittest: Are we destroying our biggest talents? *British Journal of Sports Medicine* 48 (17): 1265–1267.

Bahr, R. (2011). IOC commitment moves injury prevention to centre stage. *British Journal of Sports Medicine* 45(4):236–7.

Bahr, R. (2009). No injuries, but plenty of pain? On the methodology for recording overuse symptoms in sports. *British Journal of Sports Medicine 43*(13):966–72.

Berend, K.R. and Vail, T.P. (2001). Hip arthroscopy in the adolescent and pediatric athlete. *Clinical Sports Medicine 20*(4):763–78.

Bergeron, M.F., Bahr, R., Bärtsch, P., Bourdon, L., Calbet, J.A., Carlsen, K.H., Castagna, O., González-Alonso, J., Lundby, C., Maughan, R.J., Millet, G., Mountjoy, M., Racinais, S., Rasmussen, P., Singh, D.G., Subudhi, A.W., Young, A.J., Soligard, T. and Engebretsen, L. (2012). International Olympic Committee consensus statement on thermoregulatory and altitude challenges for high-level athletes. *British Journal of Sports Medicine 46*(11):770–9.

Boden, B.P. and Jarvis, C.G. (2008). Spinal injuries in sports. *Neurologic Clinics 26*(1):63–78; viii.

Bollars, P., Claes, S., Vanlommel, L., Van Crombrugge, K., Corten K. and Bellemans, J. (2014). The effectiveness of preventive programmes in decreasing the risk of soccer injuries in Belgium: national trends over a decade. *American Journal of Sports Medicine 42*(3):577–82.

Brenner, J.S. (2007). American Academy of Pediatrics Council on Sports Medicine and Fitness. Overuse injuries, overtraining and burnout in child and adolescent athletes. *Pediatrics 119*(6):1242–5.

Caird, M.S. (2012). Clavicle shaft fractures: are children little adults? *Journal of Pediatric Orthopaedics 32* Suppl 1:S1–4.

Carlsen, K.H. and Hem, E. and Stensrud, T. (2011) Asthma in adolescent athletes. *British Journal of Sports Medicine 45*(16):1266–71.

Cash, J.D. and Hughston, J.C. (1988). Treatment of acute patellar dislocation. *American Journal of Sports Medicine 16*(3):244–9.

Centers for Disease Control and Prevention. (2011). Nonfatal traumatic brain injuries related to sports and recreation activities among persons aged ≤19 years–United States, 2001–2009. *Morbidity and Mortality Weekly Report* 2011 Oct 7; *60*(39):1337–42.

Corrado, D., Basso, C., Pavei, A., Michieli, P., Schiavon, M. and Thiene, G. (2006). Trends in sudden cardiovascular death in young competitive athletes after implementation of a preparticipation screening programme. *Journal of the American Medical Association 296*(13):1593–601.

Coward, R.M., Rajanahally, S., Kovac, J.R., Smith, R.P., Pastuszak, A.W. and Lipshultz, L.I. (2013). Anabolic steroid induced hypogonadism in young men. *Journal of Urology 190*(6):2200–5.

Darrow, C.J., Collins, C.L., Yard, E.E. and Comstock, R.D. (2009). Epidemiology of severe injuries among United States high school athletes: 2005–2007. *American Journal of Sports Medicine 37*(9):1798–805.

Dashe, J., Roocroft, J.H., Bastrom, T.P. and Edmonds, E.W. (2013). Spectrum of shoulder injuries in skeletally immature patients. *Orthopaedic Clinics of North America 44*(4):541–51.

Desbrow, B., McCormack, J., Burke, L.M., Cox, G.R., Fallon, K., Hislop, M., Logan, R., Marino, N., Sawyer, S.M., Shaw, G., Star, A., Vidgen, H. and Leveritt, M. (2014) Sports Dietitians Australia Position Statement: Sports Nutrition for the Adolescent Athlete. *International Journal of Sport Nutrition and Exercise Metabolism* 2014 Mar 25. [Epub ahead of print]

De Wolf, D. and Matthys, D. (2013). Sports preparticipation cardiac screening: what about children? *European Journal of Pediatrics* 2013 Jun 18. [Epub ahead of print]

Di Fiori, J.P., Benjamin, H.J., Brenner, J.S., Gregory, A., Jayanthi, N., Landry, G.L. and Luke, A. (2014). Overuse injuries and burnout in youth sports: a position statement from the American Medical Society for Sports Medicine. *British Journal of Sports Medicine 48*(4):287–8.

Di Gennaro, G.L., Spina, M., Lampasi, M, Libri, R. and Donzelli, O. (2008). Fractures of the proximal humerus in children. *La Chirurgia degli organi di movimento 92*(2):89–95.

Emery, C.A. and Meeuwisse, W.H. (2010). The effectiveness of a neuromuscular prevention strategy to reduce injuries in youth soccer: a cluster-randomised controlled trial. *British Journal of Sports Medicine 44*(8):555–62.

Frank, J.S., Gambacorta, P.L. and Eisner, E.A. (2013) Hip pathology in the adolescent athlete. *Journal of the American Academy of Orthopaedic Surgeons 21*(11):665–74.

Frey, C., Bell, J., Teresi, L., Kerr, R. and Feder, K. (1996). A comparison of MRI and clinical examination of acute lateral ankle sprains. *Foot & Ankle International 17*(9):533–7.

Gottschalk, A.W. and Andrish, J.T. (2011). Epidemiology of sports injury in pediatric athletes. *Sports Medicine and Arthroscopy Review 19*(1):2–6.

Harmon, K.G., Drezner, J.A., Gammons, M., Guskiewicz, K.M., Halstead, M., Herring, S.A., Kutcher, J.S., Pana, A., Putukian, M., and Roberts, W.O. (2013). American Medical Society for Sports Medicine position statement: concussion in sport. *British Journal of Sports Medicine 47*(1): 15–26.

Hennrikus, W. and Pylawka, T. (2013). Patellofemoral instability in skeletally immature athletes. *Instructional Course Lectures 62*: 445–53.

Herman, K., Barton, C., Malliaras, P., and Morrissey, D. (2012). The effectiveness of neuromuscular warm-up strategies, that require no additional equipment, for preventing lower limb injuries during sports participation: a systematic review. *BioMed Central Medicine 10*:75.

Hootman, J.M., Dick, R. and Agel, J. (2007). Epidemiology of collegiate injuries for 15 sports: summary and recommendations for injury prevention initiatives. *Journal of Athletic Training 42*(2): 311–9.

Katoh, S., Shingu, H, Ikata, T. and Iwatsubo, E. (1996). Sports-related spinal cord injury in Japan (from the nationwide spinal cord injury registry between 1990 and 1992). *Spinal Cord 34*(7): 416–21.

Kennedy, J.G., Knowles, B., Dolan, M. and Bohne, W. (2005). Foot and ankle injuries in the adolescent runner. *Current Opinion Pediatrics 17*(1): 34–42.

Kocher, M.S., Micheli, L.J., Gerbino, P. and Hresko, M.T. (2003). Tibial eminence fractures in children: prevalence of meniscal entrapment. *American Journal of Sports Medicine 31*(3): 404–7.

Kocher, M.S., Waters, P.M. and Micheli, L.J. (2012). Upper extremity injuries in the paediatric athlete. *Sports Medicine 30*(2): 117–35.

Kodali, P., Islam, A. and Andrish, J. (2011). Anterior knee pain in the young athlete: diagnosis and treatment. *Sports Medicine and Arthroscopy Review 19*(1): 27–33.

Kovacevic, D., Mariscalco, M. and Goodwin, R.C. (2011). Injuries about the hip in the adolescent athlete. *Sports Medicine and Arthroscopy Review 19*(1): 64–74.

Lawson, B.R., Comstock, R.D. and Smith, G.A. (2009). Baseball-related injuries to children treated in hospital emergency departments in the United States, 1994–2006. *Pediatrics 123*(6): e1028–34.

Leonard, J. and Hutchinson, M.R. (2010). Shoulder injuries in skeletally immature throwers: review and current thoughts. *British Journal of Sports Medicine 44*(5): 306–10.

Lødrup, Carlsen K.C., Håland, G., Devulapalli, C.S., Munthe-Kaas, M., Pettersen, M., Granum, B., Løvik, M. and Carlsen, K.H. (2006). Asthma in every fifth child in Oslo, Norway: a 10-year follow up of a birth cohort study. *Allergy 61*(4): 454–60.

Luckstead, E.F. and Patel, D.R. (2002). Catastrophic pediatric sports injuries. *Pediatric Clinics of North America 49*(3): 581–91.

Ljungqvist, A., Jenoure, P., Engebretsen, L., Alonso, J.M., Bahr, R., Clough, A., De Bondt, G., Dvořák, J., Maloley, R., Matheson, G., Meeuwisse, W., Meijboom, E., Mountjoy, M., Pelliccia, A., Schwellnus, M., Sprumont, D., Schamasch, P., Gauthier, J.B., Dubi, C., Stupp, H. and Thill, C. (2009). The International Olympic Committee (IOC) Consensus Statement on periodic health evaluation of elite athletes. *British Journal of Sports Medicine 43*(9): 631–43.

Lyman, S., Fleisig, G.S., Andrews, J.R. and Osinski, E.D. (2002) Effect of pitch type, pitch count and pitching mechanics on risk of elbow and shoulder pain in youth baseball pitchers. *American Journal of Sports Medicine 30*(4): 463–8.

Mahaffey, D., Hilts, M. and Fields, K.B. (1999). Ankle and foot injuries in sports. *Clinics in Family Practice 1*(1): 2233–50.

Malanga, G.A. and Ramirez-Del Toro, J.A. (2008). Common injuries of the foot and ankle in the child and adolescent athlete. *Physical Medicine & Rehabilitation Clinics of North America 19*(2): 347–71, ix.

Marar, M., McIlvain, N.M., Fields, S.K. and Comstock, R.D. (2012). Epidemiology of concussions among United States high school athletes in 20 sports. *American Journal of Sports Medicine 40*(4): 747–55.

Maron, B.J., Haas, T.S., Doerer, J.J., Thompson, P.D. and Hodges, J.S. (2009). Comparison of US and Italian experiences with sudden cardiac deaths in young competitive athletes and implications for preparticipation screening strategies. *American Journal of Cardiology 104*(2): 276–80.

McCrory, P., Meeuwisse, W.H., Aubry, M., Cantu, R.C., Dvořák, J., Echemendia, R.J., Engebretsen, L., Johnston, K., Kutcher, J.S., Raftery, M., Sills, A., Benson, B.W., Davis, G.A., Ellenbogen, R., Guskiewicz, K.M., Herring, S.A., Iverson, G.L., Jordan, B.D., Kissick, J., McCrea, M., McIntosh, A.S., Maddocks, D., Makdissi, M., Purcell, L., Putukian, M., Schneider, K., Tator, C.H. and Turner, M. (2013). Consensus statement on concussion in sport: the 4th International Conference on Concussion in Sport, Zurich, November 2012. *Journal of Athletic Training 48*(4): 554–75.

McCrory, P., Meeuwisse, W., Johnston, K., Dvořák, J., Aubry, M., Molloy, M. and Cantu, R. (2009). Consensus statement on concussion in sport – the 3rd International Conference on Concussion in Sport, held in Zurich, November 2008. *Journal of Clinical Neuroscience 16*: 755–63.

Mountjoy, M., Sundgot-Borgen, J., Burke, L., Carter, S., Constantini, N., Lebrun, C., Meyer, N., Sherman, R., Steffen, K., Budgett, R. and Ljungqvist, A. (2014). The IOC consensus statement: beyond the Female Athlete Triad – Relative Energy Deficiency in Sport (RED-S). *British Journal of Sports Medicine 48*(7):491–7.

National Spinal Cord Injury Statistical Center. (2006). Spinal cord injury: facts and figures. University of Alabama; 2006. www.nscisc.uab.edu/. [Accessed 5 April, 2014].

Nemet, D. and Eliakim, A. (2009) Pediatric sports nutrition: an update. *Current Opinion in Clinical Nutrition & Metabolic Care 12*(3): 304–9.

Nettle, H. and Sprogis, E. (2011). Pediatric exercise: truth and/or consequences. *Sports Medicine and Arthroscopy Review 19*: 75–80.

Nietosvaara, Y., Aalto, K. and Kallio, P.E. (1994). Acute patellar dislocation in children: incidence and associated osteochondral fractures. *Journal of Pediatric Orthopaedics 14*(4): 513–15.

Olsen, O.E., Myklebust, G., Engebretsen, L., Holme, I. and Bahr, R. (2005). Exercises to prevent lower limb injuries in youth sports: cluster randomised controlled trial. *British Medical Journal 330*(7489): 449.

Pate, R.R., Trost, S.G., Levin, S. and Dowda, M. (2000). Sports participation and health-related behaviors among US youth. *Physical Medicine & Rehabilitation Clinics of North America 154*(9): 904–11.

Pham, C.B., Kratz, J.R., Jelin, A.C. and Gelfand, A.A. (2011). Child neurology: Brachial plexus birth injury: what every neurologist needs to know. *Neurology* 77(7): 695–7.

Philippon, M.J., Patterson, D.C. and Briggs, K.K. (2013). Hip arthroscopy and femoroacetabular impingement in the pediatric patient. *Journal of Pediatric Orthopaedics* Jul-Aug; *33* Suppl 1: S126–30.

Pommering, T.L., Kluchurosky, L. and Hall, S.L. (2005). Ankle and foot injuries in pediatric and adult athletes. *Primary Care* 32(1): 133–61.

Powell, J.W. and Barber-Foss, K.D. (1999). Injury patterns in selected high school sports: a review of the 1995–1997 seasons. *Journal of Athletic Training* 34(3): 277–84.

Roberts ,W.O. (2014) Overuse injuries and burnout in youth sports. *Clinical Journal of Sport Medicine* 24(1): 1–2.

Robinson, T.W. Corlette, J., Collins, C.L. and Comstock, R.D. Shoulder injuries among US high school athletes, 2005/2006–2011/2012. *Pediatrics* 133(2): 272–9.

Rosner, M.H. (2009). Exercise-associated hyponatremia. *Seminars in Nephrology* 29(3):271–81.

Rossi, F. and Dragoni, S. (2001). Acute avulsion fractures of the pelvis in adolescent competitive athletes: Prevalence, location and sports distribution of 203 cases collected. *Skeletal Radiology* 30(3):127–131.

Schub, D. and Saluan, P. (2011). Anterior cruciate ligament injuries in the young athlete: evaluation and treatment. *Sports Medicine and Arthroscopy Review* 19(1):34–43.

Shanley, E. and Thigpen, C. (2013). Throwing injuries in the adolescent athlete. *International Journal of Sports Physical Therapy* 8(5): 630–40.

Soligard, T., Myklebust, G., Steffen, K., Holme, I,. Silvers, H., Bizzini, M., Junge, A., Dvořák, J., Bahr, R. and Andersen, T.E. (2008). Comprehensive warm-up programme to prevent injuries in young female footballers: cluster randomised controlled trial. *British Medical Journal* 337:a2469.

Taylor, D.C. and Krasinski, K.L. (2009). Adolescent shoulder injuries: consensus and controversies. *Journal of Bone & Joint Surgery* 91(2):462–73.

The 11+ manual. FIFA Medical Assessment and Research Centre. www.f-marc.com/downloads/work book/11plus_workbook_e.pdf. Published 2012. [Accessed 19 May, 2014).

van Mechelen, W., Hlobil, H. and Kemper, H.C. (1992). Incidence, severity, aetiology and prevention of sports injuries. A review of concepts. *Sports Medicine* 14(2):82–99.

Waldén, M., Atroshi, I., Magnusson, H., Wagner, P. and Hägglund, M. (2012). Prevention of acute knee injuries in adolescent female football players: cluster randomised controlled trial. *British Medical Journal* 344:e3042.

Worldwide SK: Coaching Our Kids to Fewer Injuries: A Report on Youth Sports Safety, April 2012. Available at: www.safekids.org/sportsresearch. [Accessed 5 April, 2014).

37

YOUTH SPORT AND MENTAL HEALTH

Guy Faulkner and Katherine Tamminen

Youth sport and mental health

Mental health could be described as a type of resilience that enables us to enjoy life and to cope with adversity. More formally, mental health has been defined as a state of well-being in which the individual realizes his or her own potential, can cope with the normal stresses of life, can work productively and fruitfully, and is able to make a contribution to her or his own community (World Health Organization, 2001). There is a convincing evidence base that supports the existence of a relationship between physical activity and a number of dimensions of mental health among children, youth and adults (Ekkekakis, 2013). However, much of this research has concentrated on adults and has tended to focus on exercise – a subset of physical activity in which the activity is structured, often supervised and undertaken with the aim of maintaining or improving physical fitness or health. Less emphasis has been placed on exploring sport participation and mental health. A number of reasons might explain this. First, researchers examining physical activity and mental health are usually focused on controlling the dose of exercise an individual receives while eliminating potential confounding variables (e.g. interacting with others) in order to explore potential associations (Taylor and Faulkner, 2014). Yet this may be difficult if not impossible in a sporting context where sports differ in terms of, for example, the level of competition, whether the sport is an individual or team sport, and whether participation is organized or informal in nature. The influence of parents, peers and coaches is also likely to be highly variable.

Second, sport participation has likely received just as much negative attention for the possibility that it may promote less than optimal health through the experiences of stress (Tamminen and Holt, 2010), injury (Emery *et al.*, 2010), aggression and hazing (Fields *et al.*, 2009), sexual and emotional abuse (Stirling and Kerr, 2007) and exposure to alcohol and drug use (Kwan *et al.*, 2014). Given steep declines in sport participation throughout adolescence (Belanger *et al.*, 2009), it is also possible that there is something about sport that is less appealing than other physical activity options to most youth. Accordingly, research has perhaps focused on the mental health benefits of alternative forms of physical activity and exercise, particularly among girls. The purpose of this chapter is to address some of these issues by first exploring the prospective evidence that sport participation is associated with better mental health. Second, we consider some of the psychosocial concerns faced by adolescent athletes.

Does sport participation promote mental health among youth?

Research to date regarding the mental health benefits of youth sport is predominantly cross-sectional in nature (Eime *et al.*, 2013). Such a design limits causal inferences regarding the temporal relationship between sport and mental health outcomes. In contrast, longitudinal studies have the potential to offer additional insights by uncovering the direction of relationships. This was one of Bradford Hill's (1965) main criteria for judging if a causal link exists between two variables. Specifically, Hill explained that prospective-based studies have the strength to examine the temporal sequence between two variables, which may explain whether baseline levels of sport participation, for example, contribute to mental health outcomes at a later point in time. Thus, from a public health and research perspective, it is important to systematically review prospective studies that examine the protective influence sport may have on mental health for youth.

A systematic search of four electronic databases (Medline, PsychInfo, Scopus and SportDiscus) was conducted between May and June 2014. Key words and search terms included sport, structured sport, organized sport, elite sport, mental health, self-efficacy, happiness, depression, stress, anxiety, mood (affect) and quality of life. Studies had to be longitudinal in nature and at least one year in length and examining whether sport participation predicted a mental health outcome at a later point in time. Exclusion criteria included articles that discussed exercise/physical activity (unstructured activity), adapted sports for individuals with disability, reports addressing sub-populations as well as articles in book chapters and from conference proceedings or thesis dissertations. Article titles and/or abstracts were scanned in order to check for relevance to the research question at hand. Once studies were selected, data was extracted regarding author (yr), country, sample size, age range, length of study, primary mental health outcome, measure of sport participation, key findings and risk of bias assessment. A formal quality assessment for each study was conducted independently using a modified version of the Critical Appraisal Skills Programme (CASP) for prospective studies. The CASP appraises both internal and external validity by addressing four methodological issues:

1   potential selection bias
2   potential bias in the measurement of sport participation
3   potential bias in the measurement of the mental health outcome
4   whether analyses accounted for confounding variables.

Each issue was assessed and each study was assigned a number representing the number of potential biases. Each study then has a composite score ranging from 0 to 4, with a higher number representing more potential sources of bias and a lower quality study: 0 or 1, high quality; 2, modest; and 3 or 4, low quality.

Twenty longitudinal studies were identified (Table 37.1). Time between data collection was generally between one and three years for the majority of studies. The age ranges of the children and adolescents differed considerably across studies with some focusing on children as young as seven (e.g. Dimech and Seiler, 2011) with some looking at sport participation during adolescence and its association with mental health in early adulthood (e.g. Jewett *et al.*, 2014). All but one study looked at both boys and girls. Pederson and Seidman (2004) examined adolescent girls from racially and ethnically diverse backgrounds in the United States. Sample sizes also varied considerably from 176 in the smallest study to 10, 613 in the largest. The majority of studies were conducted in the United States (n=11) and Canada (n=5). Eleven studies were rated high quality with six rated as moderate and three as low quality. There was evidence of selection bias in seven studies using a convenience sample with loss at follow-up. The majority (n=14) of studies were rated as having high potential for bias for sport participation measurement by using categorical measures of sport participation (e.g. participant versus non-participant). Most studies used validated mental health measures (n=16) and most attempted to control for some potential confounding variables such as gender or education (n=14). Self-esteem was the most commonly assessed mental health outcome (n=10) followed by depressive symptoms (n=8).

Self-esteem

Self-esteem has been described as 'the global and relatively stable evaluative construct reflecting the degree to which an individual feels positive about him- or herself' (Fox, 1998, p. 296). High self-esteem is associated with a number of important life adjustment qualities, whereas low self-esteem is associated with poor health behaviour decisions and is characteristic of many mental disorders such as depression (Fox, 1997). In our review, findings were mixed as to whether sport participation improved self-esteem over time. Several studies reported that involvement in sports predicts increased self-esteem over time (e.g. Daniels and Leaper, 2006; Pederson and Seidman, 2004), and social and academic self-concept (Marsh, 1993). One study reported an indirect effect (Slutzky and Simpkins, 2009) while the majority have shown no association (Adachi and Willoughby, 2014; Barber *et al.*, 2001; Brettschneider, 2001; Fredricks and Eccles, 2006; Kort-Butler and Hagewen, 2011; Marsh, 1998). The most recent study, rated high quality, found evidence for a selection effect in that adolescents with higher self-esteem play sports more frequently and enjoy sports more than adolescents with lower self-esteem (Adachi and Willoughby, 2014).

Depression

Mental health problems affect 10 to 20 per cent of children and adolescents worldwide and account for a large portion of the global burden of disease (Kieling *et al.*, 2011). Adolescents with major depression or subthreshold depression report poorer quality of life and impairment of psychosocial function (Judd *et al.*, 2002). Depression is also a risk factor for suicide. Accordingly, identifying modifiable factors that relate to depression early in life is a critical public health need. Five out of eight studies we reviewed reported that sport participation was associated with lower depressive symptoms over time. Two of these studies were rated as having low risk of bias (Gore *et al.*, 2001; Zarrett *et al.*, 2009). Three studies reported no association (Agans and Geldhof, 2012; Barber *et al.*, 2001; Fredricks and Eccles, 2006).

Positive associations were generally weak as was the proportion of variance explained in depression (Brunet *et al.*, 2013; Gore *et al.*, 2001; Jewett *et al.*, 2014). Notably, there was some evidence that team, as opposed to individual, sport participation was a protective factor. In a large Canadian study over two years, lower levels of team sport participation at age 8 was predictive of higher levels of depressive symptoms at age 10. Individual sport participation at age 8 was unrelated to depressive symptoms at age 10 (Perron *et al.*, 2012). Two other studies also found that team sports participation was negatively related to depressive symptoms (Brunet *et al.*, 2013; Gore *et al.*, 2001). The context of collaborative goal striving and the social cohesion of team sports may explain these findings (Vella *et al.*, 2014). Taliaferro *et al.* (2011) found that compared to non-participants, youth involved in sport in both middle and high school had lower odds of suicidal ideation during high school. Additionally, youth who discontinued sport after middle school had higher odds of attempting suicide during high school than non-participants.

Table 37.1 Prospective studies that examine the protective influence sport may have on mental health for youth

Author (yr)	Country	Sample (n)	Age (Mean or Range)	Time	Measure of Mental Health	Measure of Sport Participation	Key Findings	Sources of Bias (0–4)
Marsh 1993	United States	10,613	Last 2 years of high school	2 years	Self-concept; educational outcomes	Sum of responses to 3 items (1=nonparticipant; 2= participant; 3=leader/officer)	Participation in sport positively affected social and academic self-concept and educational aspirations	2
Marsh 1998	Australia	899	Grade 6-12	2 years	Physical self-concept	Elite athletes from a sports high school compared to 'non-athletes'	Physical self-concept is stable through the adolescent period. Elite athletes have higher physical self-concepts than non-athletes.	2
Brettschneider 2001	Germany	500	12-18 years	3 years	Self-esteem	Members of sports clubs versus non-members	Self-esteem improves in both sports club members and non-members alike.	4
Barber et al. 2001	United States	900	Grade 10- to age 24	6 years	Depressed mood; social isolation; self-esteem; academic outcomes	Participation on one or more school teams	Sport participation predicted positive occupational and educational outcomes, lower levels of social isolation as well as higher rates of drinking. Sport participation was not associated with change in self-esteem or depressed mood.	2

continued . . . .

Table 37.1 Continued

Author (yr)	Country	Sample (n)	Age (Mean or Range)	Time	Measure of Mental Health	Measure of Sport Participation	Key Findings	Sources of Bias (0–4)
Gore et al. 2001	United States	1,036	Grades 9–11	1 year	Depression	Self-reported any sports activity	Team sport involvement associated with reduced depressed mood but effect was weak	0
Pederson & Seidman, 2004	United States	247	13–16 yrs	3 years	Self-esteem	Self-reported playing in a league, school team or other organized group, and ever won an award/captained	Sport participation in early adolescence positively related with self-esteem in middle adolescence	1
Daniels & Leaper, 2006	United States	10,500	12–21 yrs	1 year	Self-esteem	Frequency of sport participation in last week. Non-participants excluded from analyses	Peer acceptance mediated the relationship between sport participation and global self-esteem for boys and girls	3
Fredricks & Eccles, 2006	United States	912 at final wave	11th grade at baseline	2 years	Depression; Academic achievement	Member of sport teams or involved in any organized summer or after school sports over past 12 months	11th (eleventh) graders' sport participation predicted number of years of school completed after high school but not depression or self-esteem.	1

Study	Country	N	Age	Duration	Outcome	Measure of participation	Findings	
Findlay & Coplan, 2008	Canada	201	10.1 yrs at baseline	1 year	General well-being; Self-esteem; loneliness	Sport participation based on years and level of participation	Shy children who participated in sport demonstrated a decrease in anxiety over one year.	3
Slutzky & Simpkins, 2009	United States	987	Grades 2–6	1 year	Self-esteem	Parental report of sport participation and time/week. Classified as team or individual	Participation in team (not individual) sports positively predicted sport-concept one year later. In turn, sport self-concept was positively associated with self-esteem.	1
Zarrett et al. 2009	United States	1,357	Grades 5–7	1 year	Depression	Participation in OST (out-of-school activities) activities. Duration of participation in sports. Quantity of participation	After controlling for total time spent in activities, duration, participation in sports and religious activities, or sports alone remained significant predictors of lower depression rates.	0
Dimech & Seiler, 2011	Switzerland	176	7–9-year-olds	12–18 months	Social anxiety	Self-reported extracurricular participation	Reduction in social anxiety over time in children practicing a team sport.	2
Kort-Butler & Hagewen, 2011	United States	5399	14–26 years	8 years	Self-esteem	Self-reported extracurricular participation (sports only; clubs only; mixed; non-participation)	Those who did not participate in any school-based activity and those who had a clubs only portfolio experienced the most growth in self-esteem.	1

continued . . . .

Table 37.1 Continued

Author (yr)	Country	Sample (n)	Age (Mean or Range)	Time	Measure of Mental Health	Measure of Sport Participation	Key Findings	Sources of Bias (0–4)
Taliaferro et al., 2011	United States	739	12.8 years at baseline	5 years	Suicidal ideation	Sport participation in last 12 months	Adolescents involved in sport in both middle and high school were less likely to report suicidal ideation during high school than were youth who never participated in sport.	2
Agans & Geldhof, 2012	United States	710	Grade 10–12	3 years	Depression	Athletic activity participation (individual; team; dance)	No impact on depression symptoms.	2
Perron et al. 2012	Canada	1,250	7–10 years old	2 years	Depression	Frequency of sport participation in team or individuals sports (assessed by mothers)	Lower levels of team sport participation at age 8 was predictive of higher levels of depressive symptoms at age 10. Individual sports participation at age 8 unrelated to depressive symptoms at age 10.	1
Brunet et al., 2013	Canada	–860	Aged 12–13 (at baseline) – data collected at ages 18–24	5 years	Depression	Past involvement in organized team sports (7-day recall checklist). Current involvement in organized team sports	Involvement in team sports negatively related to depressive symptoms but association was weak.	1

Study	Country	N	Age/Grade	Duration	Outcome	Measure	Findings	
Adachi & Willoughby, 2013	Canada	1,492	Grade 9-12	4 years	Self-esteem	Frequency of involvement in sports. Enjoyment of sports	Higher levels of self-esteem predicted increased involvement in sports over time, but increased involvement in sports did not predict higher levels of self-esteem over time.	1
Jewett et al., 2014	Canada	853	Mean age of 20.4 years old	8 years	Depression; Perceived stress; Self-rated mental health	Involvement in school sport	Adolescence involvement in school sport predicted lower rates of depressive symptoms and perceived stress as well as high self-rated mental health in young adulthood.	1
Vella et al., 2014	Australia	4,042	Mean age 8.25	2 years	Parent reported health-related quality of life	Parental report of sport participation (team/individual)	Children who continued to participate in sports between the ages of 8 and 10 had greater health-related quality of life at age 10 compared with those who did not participate in sports.	1

Other outcomes

Findlay and Coplan (2008) did not find significant effects of sport participation over a year on social skills, self-esteem, positive adjustment or externalizing problem behaviours. However, shy children who participated in sport demonstrated a decrease in anxiety over one year. Dimech and Seiler (2011) reported a reduction in social anxiety over time among 7–8-year-old Swiss children practicing a team sport. In a recent Australian study (Vella *et al.*, 2014), children who continued to participate in sports between the ages of 8 and 10 had greater health-related quality of life at age 10 compared with those who did not participate in sports.

Summary: youth sport and mental health

It is difficult to draw clear conclusions regarding youth sport participation and mental health based on the existing evidence. There is good evidence that sport participation, particularly team sport participation, may have a protective effect against depressive symptoms. Evidence is inconsistent regarding impact on self-esteem. Sport participation is itself defined by self-selection. Thus, any positive relationships found may reflect a selective aggregation of individuals who bring fewer problems across many domains of functioning (Taliaferro *et al.*, 2011). Weaknesses in the assessment of sport participation also makes it difficult to understand how such participation is impacting mental health and it likely varies by factors such as level of competition, and intensity and duration of participation. Most studies examine sport participation as a binary variable – participant or non-participant – and this says nothing about the quality of the experience. Future research should incorporate more extensive assessments of sport participation and control for factors that may also explain the relationship between participation and mental health such as education, social support and parental income.

Psychosocial concerns among competitive athletes

As discussed above, sport participation has some positive associations with decreased depressive symptoms, lower anxiety and improved health-related quality of life. In addition to these findings from longitudinal studies, there is additional evidence from cross-sectional research that high levels of sport participation and competition are associated with some positive outcomes. For example, Lam *et al.* (2013) reported that athletes' quality of life scores were higher across all ages for emotional and social functioning compared to a reference group of non-athletes. The athletes were generally less afraid, sad, angry or worried, and they were more likely to get along with peers and less likely to have trouble making friends or getting teased. Athletes also fared better academically and reported fewer problems paying attention in class, keeping up with schoolwork, and missing school. Similar results were reported in a multi-national study by Wold *et al.* (2013), who found that young soccer players (aged 10–14) reported higher life satisfaction than the reference sample even after controlling for age, country, and family wealth. Despite these positive findings, one limitation is that there is little information about 'how much' sport participation is associated with adolescent athletes' positive wellbeing and mental health.

To address this issue, Merglen *et al.* (2013) examined competitive athletes' wellbeing as a function of their total weekly hours of practice per week. The results indicated that competitive sport participation was a protective factor against poor wellbeing: wellbeing scores increased as athletes' time spent in sport increased. Athletes who spent an average of 14 hours per week practicing their sport reported the highest wellbeing scores; however athletes who reported very high levels of sport participation (over 17.5 hours per week) reported lower wellbeing scores.

Merglen *et al.* (2013) demonstrated a U-shaped association between athletes' amount of sport participation and wellbeing scores, which suggests that there is a diminishing return on investment when it comes to adolescent athletes' participation in sport. This is supported by another study examining wellbeing among adolescent athletes (*M* age = 19.2) living and training at an elite sport centre compared to non-elite athletes: elite athletes reported spending more time training and lower psychosocial wellbeing compared to non-elite athletes (Verkooijen *et al.*, 2012). Thus, researchers have suggested that sport participation may be associated with increases in adolescents' functioning; however very high training loads can potentially be detrimental to athletes' physical and emotional wellbeing. While there are several concerns associated with competitive sport participation such as eating disorders, alcohol and drug use, abuse, and increased risk of injury, these are discussed in detail in other chapters within this book. In the next part of this chapter, we will focus on research examining some psychosocial concerns such as burnout and wellbeing among highly competitive athletes.

Burnout

Burnout is defined as a syndrome characterised by emotional and physical exhaustion, sport devaluation and a reduced sense of accomplishment (Raedeke, 1997), and it is typically associated with intensive sport participation and high training demands (Gould and Dieffenbach, 2002). A related concept is overreaching, which is 'an accumulation of training and nontraining stress resulting in a *short-term* decrement in performance capacity with or without psychological signs and symptoms of overtraining' (Kreider *et al.*, 1998, p.vii). Taken together, burnout and overreaching are associated with decreased performance as well as negative psychosocial outcomes for athletes, including higher levels of anger and depression (Schmikli *et al.*, 2012), and decreased motivation to participate and compete in sport (Martinent *et al.*, 2014). While it is difficult to accurately track rates of burnout and overreaching, estimates suggest that 29 per cent of young elite athletes and 20 per cent of sub-elite athletes (local and regional level) have experienced overreaching (Matos *et al.*, 2011), and up to 9 per cent of athletes have suffered from symptoms of burnout (Gustafsson *et al.*, 2007). High training loads are commonly associated with reports of burnout, fatigue and decreased wellbeing (Kennedy *et al.*, 2013; Merglen *et al.*, 2014); however not all athletes report experiencing burnout in sport. Researchers agree that it is not just excessive training load that contributes to burnout among young athletes, and that the problem should be viewed as multidimensional and affected by a variety of factors (Gustafsson *et al.*, 2007; Matos *et al.*, 2011). There are several personality, social and environmental factors within the sport context, which may also influence athlete burnout.

Stress, coping and social support

A primary body of research in the area of burnout among young competitive athletes concerns the impact of perceived stress, coping and social support on athletes' experiences of burnout. Adolescent athletes competing at national and international levels report training and coach stressors more frequently than athletes competing at lower levels (Nicholls *et al.*, 2007), and athletes' first experiences competing at large-scale events can be overwhelming for elite athletes (Kristiansen and Roberts, 2009). Research among competitive adolescent swimmers revealed that perceived stress, coping and perceived levels of social support explained 43 per cent of the variance in athletes' global burnout scores (Raedeke and Smith, 2004). Athletes who reported higher stress also reported greater exhaustion; they valued sport less, and felt they were accomplishing less in their sport compared to athletes who perceived lower levels of stress. Athletes who reported better coping behaviours (e.g. better time management, life management and self-regulation skills) and greater satisfaction with their social support reported lower stress than those athletes who had poorer coping and who were less satisfied with their social support. These findings were corroborated by Matos *et al.* (2011) who reported that young soccer players with symptoms of overreaching perceived significantly greater expectations to perform and they also reported that they did not cope well with school/training demands and tiredness compared to athletes who did not experience overreaching/overtraining.

Personality constructs

Higher perceived stress is consistently associated with higher emotional/physical exhaustion, sport devaluation and reduced accomplishment, as well as lower positive affect and higher negative affect. However, these associations appear to be influenced by athletes' personality dispositions, for example, the extent to which they are optimistic or hopeful about the future. Optimism is a personality trait that reflects an expectation that good things will happen in the future (Scheier and Carver, 1992), and hope represents a positive motivational state based on a sense of successful agency thinking (e.g. goal-directed energy) and pathways to achieve those goals (e.g. planning) (Snyder *et al.*, 1991). It appears that optimistic and hopeful athletes perceive less stress and report greater positive affect, which are associated with lower burnout (Gustafsson and Skoog, 2012; Gustafsson *et al.*, 2013).

While traits such as optimism and hope may help to protect against burnout, there have been mixed results when examining associations between burnout and constructs such as athletic identity, passion and perfectionism. Athletic identity refers to the extent to which individuals identify with the athlete role (Brewer, 1993), and it is suggested to be a predictor of burnout (Gustafsson *et al.*, 2008). On one hand, researchers have found that elite adolescent athletes with a strong athletic identity and who are more strongly committed to their athletic role and who had high levels of perfectionism were considered a high-risk group for accepting physical and psychosocial risks to succeed in their sport (e.g. 'In order to be successful in sports, I am willing to accept chronic pain' and 'I constantly think about practice and competition') (Schnell *et al.*, 2014). This higher level of risk acceptance among elite athletes may put them at risk of experiencing physical and psychological consequences of burnout from pushing to achieve high levels of performance. Conversely, Verkooijen *et al.* (2012) found that elite athletes did not have a higher degree of athletic identity than non-elite athletes, although the elite athletes did have poorer psychosocial wellbeing scores. Thus, the association between athletic identity and athletes' burnout and wellbeing is unclear.

Passion is described as 'a strong inclination towards an activity that individuals enjoy and consider important, and in which they invest considerable time and energy' (Gustafsson *et al.*, 2011, p. 387). There are two dimensions of passion: obsessive passion, which is considered a more inflexible, 'controlling' motivational force to engage in an activity (e.g. 'I have difficulties imagining my life without sport') (Vallerand *et al.*, 2003); and harmonious passion, which drives individuals to engage in an activity autonomously (e.g. 'sport allows me to live a variety of experiences'). In a study of junior elite soccer players, athletes reporting high levels of obsessive passion scored higher on measures of burnout than athletes with high levels of harmonious passion (Gustafsson *et al.*, 2011). Obsessive passion was also positively associated with exhaustion, negative affect and perceived stress, while harmonious passion was negatively associated with perceived stress, negative affect, exhaustion, sport devaluation and reduced sense of accomplishment. Thus, athletes who are passionate about their sport may be at risk of experiencing burnout depending on whether their passion is more harmonious or obsessive.

Similar to passion, perfectionism is another construct that shows mixed associations with burnout. Perfectionism is a multidimensional personality trait reflecting 'the compulsive pursuit of exceedingly high standards and a tendency to engage in overly critical appraisal of accomplishments' (Appleton *et al.*, 2009, p. 458). Aspects of perfectionism are associated with higher perceived burnout among elite adult athletes (Lemyre *et al.*, 2008), and research with adolescent athletes paints a similar picture. Appleton *et al.* (2009) reported a positive association between socially prescribed perfectionism (e.g. the athlete's perception that others have extreme standards and a sense that their achievement striving will be subjected to harsh critical evaluation by others) and all three dimensions of burnout. Conversely, self-oriented perfectionism (e.g. the pursuit of exceedingly high standards in conjunction with harsh self-critical appraisals of performance) was negatively associated with burnout. These findings suggest that athletes' perfectionistic concerns that are associated with social expectations may contribute to their burnout, rather than setting high personal standards for oneself. Thus, there appear to be interactions between features of the sport environment with athletes' personality characteristics that may lead some to be more prone to experiencing burnout in competitive sport.

Social-environmental factors

Considering that competitive sport participation involves high training loads that may put athletes at risk of experiencing burnout and overreaching, it is important to identify aspects of the sport environment that may help prevent burnout and help promote positive psychosocial wellbeing in sport. Some aspects of the sport environment that are potentially modifiable and which show positive associations with athletes' wellbeing include athletes' coach autonomy-supportive behaviours and the coach-initiated motivational climate, transformational leadership behaviours, athletes' peer relationships and the peer motivational climate in the sport environment.

Coaches

Researchers have used theoretical perspectives such as basic needs theory (Deci and Ryan, 2000) and achievement goal theory (Ames, 1992) to examine aspects of the sport environment that contribute to higher wellbeing and lower burnout among adolescent athletes. One line of research examining coach behaviours has found support for coaches' use of autonomy supportive behaviours (e.g. 'I feel that my coach provides me with choices and options') predicting higher levels of wellbeing among competitive adolescent athletes. For example, in a longitudinal study of elite male soccer players Adie *et al.* (2012) found that there was an increase in athletes' emotional and physical exhaustion over the course of a season; however, players' perceptions of coach autonomy support explained between-person differences in emotional and physical exhaustion. Perceived coach autonomy support was also associated with athletes' subjective vitality across two seasons of sport participation. Similarly, Ntoumanis *et al.* (2012) found that athletes' perceptions of a coach-created motivational climate that promotes effort and mastery (i.e. a task-involving motivational climate) was associated with reduced burnout, whereas a coach-created motivational climate that promotes demonstrations of superior ability and intra-team competition (i.e. an ego-involving motivational climate) was a positive predictor of athlete burnout. These findings are consistent with previous research examining coach behaviours and wellbeing among competitive adolescent athletes (Kipp and Weiss, 2013; López-Walle *et al.*, 2012).

Additional research examining coaches' impact on wellbeing in competitive youth sport contexts has focused on coaches' transformational leadership behaviours (Bass and Riggio, 2006). Generally, transformational leadership refers to leader behaviours that positively influence followers' values, needs, awareness and performance (Bass and Riggio, 2006; Hoption *et al.*, 2014). Examples of transformational leadership behaviours include holding high expectations, encouraging athletes to achieve more than they think they can, treating athletes as people and recognizing their accomplishments and improvements, and adopting positive values and 'doing the right thing' to develop trust with athletes. There are positive associations between athletes' perceptions of coaches' transformational leadership behaviours and their need satisfaction and wellbeing. Collectively, it appears that a sport environment that includes coaches' autonomy supportive and transformational leadership behaviours can help to promote positive wellbeing and reduce burnout among competitive adolescent athletes.

Peers and teammates

Peers and teammates may be both helpful and harmful in terms of highly competitive athletes' experiences of burnout. Previous research among university-level swimmers (*M* age = 20) suggested that teammates may be helpful for dealing with burnout, but that teammates and peers also contributed to high perceived performance and training expectations (Kennedy *et al.*, 2013). Ntoumanis *et al.* (2012) reported that perceptions of a peer task climate negatively predicted burnout, suggesting that peer groups in competitive sport that promote effort and mastery may be a protective factor against developing burnout. Thus, it appears that the type of motivational climate emphasized by peers and also by coaches may be protective against burnout among adolescent athletes.

Summary: burnout and wellbeing among competitive athletes

Athlete burnout is associated with high training volumes, high perceived stress, low coping ability and social support, and it may also be predicted by some personality constructs such as hope, optimism, perfectionism and athletic identity; however, the research in these areas is still limited. It appears that a task-involving motivational climate emphasized by coaches and peers may help to protect against burnout, whereas an ego-involving climate may be a risk factor for developing burnout.

Future research examining the development of burnout among male versus female adolescent athletes is warranted. There is some evidence that adult female athletes may report higher burnout than male athletes, although findings are mixed (e.g. Finch, 1999; Heidari, 2013). There is also evidence that female coaches may report greater emotional exhaustion compared to male coaches (Goodger *et al.*, 2007; Vealey *et al.*, 1992). Considering that male and female adolescent athletes may perceive and cope with some social stressors differently than males, particularly with regards to using social support to cope with interpersonal stressors (Hoar *et al.*, 2010; Nicholls *et al.*, 2007), it may be valuable to examine whether adolescent female athletes' experiences of burnout are qualitatively different compared to male athletes.

There is little research examining parental influence on adolescent athletes' experiences of burnout. It is unclear whether parental involvement, pressure and support have associations with athletes' burnout; however, perceptions of pressure to meet parental expectations for success have been implicated as a possible contributor to burnout (Cohn, 1990). As primary sources of support for highly competitive adolescent athletes, parents may also be key agents in the prevention, identification and management of burnout. However at the moment there is no research that has examined parents' perceptions of athlete burnout or how they manage their child's burnout in sport.

Conclusion

Sport represents a likely path to school attachment and belonging as well as social capital (Fredricks and Eccles, 2006; Marsh, 1993). Participation links youth to supportive peers and adults and contributes to their identity as valued members of a community. However, participating in extra-curricular activities in general is likely related to a range of mental health benefits as found in several studies (Kort-Butler and Hagewen, 2011; Zarrett *et al.*, 2009). Extra-curricular activities, including sport, can be seen as 'learning environments with distinct "opportunity structures" for developing personal and interpersonal skills' (Fredricks and Eccles, 2006, p. 712) that may promote mental health. There may be a need to re-orient our language from 'there is a positive association between sport participation and mental health' to the more provisional 'there could be a positive association that is achievable under conducive circumstances' (Whitelaw *et al.*, 2010). Programme evaluations are needed to identify the processes involved within sporting contexts that maximise the likelihood that children and youth will experience mental health benefit. Such benefits are inextricably linked to the many influences of parents, peers, coaches and the structure and delivery of sport programmes (Fraser-Thomas *et al.*, 2005).

Acknowledgements

We thank Dane Mauer-Vakil (University of Toronto) for his assistance in conducting the literature search.

References

Adachi, P.J. and Willoughby, T. (2014). It's not how much you play, but how much you enjoy the game: The longitudinal associations between adolescents' self-esteem and the frequency versus enjoyment of involvement in sports. *Journal of youth and adolescence*, *43*(1): 137–145. Champaign: 10.1007/s10964-013-9988-3

Adie, J.W., Duda, J.L. and Ntoumanis, N. (2012). Perceived coach-autonomy support, basic need satisfaction and the well- and ill-being of elite youth soccer players: A longitudinal investigation. *Psychology of Sport and Exercise*, *13*(1): 51–59. Champaign: 10.1016/j.psychsport.2011.07.008

Agans, J. P. and Geldhof, G.J. (2012). Trajectories of participation in athletics and positive youth development: The influence of sport type. *Applied Developmental Science*, *16*(3): 151–165. Champaign: 10.1080/10888691.2012.697792

Ames, C. (1992). Classrooms, goals, structures, and student motivation. *Journal of Educational Psychology*, *84*(3): 261–271.

Appleton, P.R., Hall, H.K. and Hill, A.P. (2009). Relations between multidimensional perfectionism and burnout in junior–elite male athletes. *Psychology of Sport and Exercise*, *10*(4): 457–465. Champaign: 10.1016/j.psychsport.2008.12.006

Barber, B.L., Eccles, J.S. and Stone, M.R. (2001). Whatever happened to the jock, the brain, and the princess? Young adult pathways linked to adolescent activity involvement and social identity. *Journal of adolescent research*, *16*(5): 429–455. Champaign: 10.1177/0743558401165002

Bass, B.M. and Riggio, R.E. (2006). *Transformational leadership* (2nd edition). Mahwah, NJ: Erlbaum.

Belanger, M., Gray-Donald, K., O'Loughlin, J., Paradis, G. and Hanley, J. (2009). When adolescents drop the ball: Sustainability of physical activity in youth. *American Journal of Preventive Medicine*, *37*(1): 41–49. Champaign: 10.1016/j.amepre.2009.04.002

Brettschneider, W.D. (2001). Effects of sport club activities on adolescent development in Germany. *European Journal of Sport Science*, *1*(2): 1–11. Champaign: 10.1080/17461390100071201

Brewer, B.W. (1993). Self-identity and specific vulnerability to depressed mood. *Journal of Personality*, *61*(3): 343–364. Champaign: 10.1111/j.1467–6494.1993.tb00284.x

Brunet, J. Sabiston, C.M. Chaiton, M. Barnett, T.A. O'Loughlin, E. Low, N.C. and O'Loughlin, J.L. (2013). The association between past and current physical activity and depressive symptoms in young adults: a 10-year prospective study. *Annals of epidemiology*, *23*(1): 25–30. Champaign: http://dx.doi.org/10.1016/j.annepidem.2012.10.006.

Cohn, P.J. (1990). An exploratory study on sources of stress and athlete burnout in youth golf. *The Sport Psychologist*, *4*: 95–106.

Daniels, E. and Leaper, C. (2006). A longitudinal investigation of sport participation, peer acceptance, and self-esteem among adolescent girls and boys. *Sex Roles*, *55*(11–12): 875–880. Champaign: 10.1007/s11199-006-9138-4

Deci, E.L. and Ryan, R.M. (2000). The "what" and "why" of goal pursuits: Human needs and the self-determination of behavior. *Psychological Inquiry*, *11*(4): 227–268. Champaign: 10.1207/S15327965PLI 1104 01

Dimech, A.S. and Seiler, R. (2011). Extra-curricular sport participation: a potential buffer against social anxiety symptoms in primary school children. *Psychology of Sport and Exercise*, *12*(4): 347–354. Champaign: 10.1016/j.psychsport.2011.03.007

Eime, R.M. Young, J.A. Harvey, J.T. Charity, M.J. and Payne, W.R. (2013). A systematic review of the psychological and social benefits of participation in sport for children and adolescents: Informing development of a conceptual model of health through sport. *International Journal of Behavioral Nutrition and Physical Activity*, *10*: 98. Champaign: 10.1186/1479–5868–ten to98

Ekkekakis, P. (2013). *Routledge handbook of physical activity and mental health*. Abingdon, Oxford: Routledge.

Emery, C.A. Kang, J. Shrier, I. Goulet, C. Hagel, B.E. Benson, B.W., A. McAllister, J. and Meeuwisse, W. (2010). Risk of injury associated with body checking among youth ice hockey players. *Journal of the American Medical Association*, *303*(11): 2265–2272. Champaign: *10.1503/cmaj.101540*

Fields, S.K. Collins, C.L. and Comstock, R.D. (2009). Violence in youth sports: Hazing, brawling, and foul play. *British Journal of Sports Medicine*, *44*(1): 32–37. Champaign: 10.1136/bjsm.2009.068320

Finch, S. (1999). Comparison of team and individuals, male and female athletes' potential for burnout, and coping strategies. Unpublished Master's thesis, McGill University.

Findlay, L.C. and Coplan, R.J. (2008). Come out and play: Shyness in childhood and the benefits of organized sports participation. *Canadian Journal of Behavioural Science/Revue canadienne des sciences du comportement*, *40*(3): 153–161. Champaign: 10.1037/0008-400X.40.3.153.

Fox, K. (1997). *The physical self: From motivation to well-being*. Champaign,Illinois: Human Kinetics.

Fox, K. (1998). Advances in the measure of the physical self. In J. L. Duda (ed), *Advances in sport and exercise psychology measurement* (pp. 295–310). Morgantown, WV: Fitness Information Technology, Inc.

Fraser-Thomas, J. Côté, J. and Deakin. J. (2005). Youth sport programs: An avenue to foster positive youth development. *Physical Education and Sport Pedagogy*, *10*(1): 19–40.

Fredricks, J. A. and Eccles, J. S. (2006). Is extracurricular participation associated with beneficial outcomes? Concurrent and longitudinal relations. *Developmental Psychology*, *42*(4): 698–713. Champaign: 10.1037/0012-1649.42.4.698

Goodger, K. Gorely, T. Lavallee, D. and Harwood C. (2007). Burnout in sport: A systematic review. *The Sport Psychologist*, *21*(2): 127–151.

Gore, S. Farrell, F. and Gordon, J. (2001). Sports involvement as protection against depressed mood. *Journal of Research on Adolescence*, *11*(1): 119–130. Champaign: 10.1111/1532–7795.00006

Gould, D. and Dieffenbach, K. (2002). Overtraining, underrecovery and burnout in sport. In M. Kellman (ed), *Enhancing recovery: Preventing underperformance in athletes* (pp. 25–35). Champaign,Illinois: Human Kinetics.

Gustafsson, H. Hassmen, P. and Hassmen, N. (2011). Are athletes burning out with passion? *European Journal of Sport Science*, *11*(6): 387–395. Champaign: 10.1080/17461391.2010.536573

Gustafsson, H. Hassmen, P. Kentta, G. and Johansson, M. (2008). A qualitative analysis of burnout in elite Swedish athletes. *Psychology of Sport and Exercise*, *9*: 800–816. Champaign: 10.1016/j.psychsport.2007.11.004

Gustafsson, H. Kentta, G. Hassmen, P. and Lundqvist, C. (2007). Prevalence of burnout in competitive adolescent athletes. *The Sport Psychologist*, *21*: 21–37.

Gustafsson, H. and Skoog, T. (2012). The mediational role of perceived stress in the relation between optimism and burnout in competitive athletes. *Anxiety, Stress, and Coping*, *25*(2): 183–199. Champaign: 10.1080/10615806.2011.594045

Gustafsson, H. Skoog, T. Podlog, L. Lundqvist, C. and Wagnsson, S. (2013). Hope and athlete burnout: Stress and affect as mediators. *Psychology of Sport and Exercise, 14*(5): 640–649. Champaign: 10.1016/j.psychsport.2013.03.008

Heidari, S. (2013). Gender differences in burnout in individual athletes. *European Journal of Experimental Biology, 3*(3): 583–588.

Hill, A.B. (1965). The environment and disease: association or causation? *Proceedings of the Royal Society of Medicine, 58*(5): 295–300.

Hoar, S. Crocker, P.R.E. Holt, N. L. and Tamminen, K.A. (2010). Gender differences in adolescent athletes' coping with interpersonal stressors in sport: More similarities than differences? *Journal of Applied Sport Psychology, 22*: 134–149. Champaign: 10.1080/10413201003664640

Hoption, C. Phelan, J. and Barling, J. (2014). Transformational leadership in sport. In M. Beauchamp, and M. Eys (eds), *Group dynamics in exercise and sport psychology* (2nd ed. pp. 55–72). New York: Routledge.

Jewett, R. Sabiston, C.M. Brunet, J. O'Loughlin, E.K. Scarapicchia, T. and O' Loughlin, J. (2014). School sport participation during adolescence and mental health in early adulthood. *Journal of Adolescent Health.* Advance online publication. Champaign: 10.1016/j.jadohealth.2014.04.018

Judd, L.L. Schettler, P.J. and Akiskal, H.S. (2002). The prevalence, clinical relevance, and public health significance of subthreshold depressions. *The Psychiatric Clinics of North America, 25*(4): 685–698. Champaign: 10.1016/S0193–953X(02)00026–6

Kennedy, M.D. Tamminen, K.A. and Holt, N.L. (2013). Factors that influence fatigue status in Canadian university swimmers. *Journal of Sports Sciences, 31*(5): 554–564. Champaign: 10.1080/02640414.2012.738927

Kieling, C. Baker-Henningham, H, Belfer, M. Conti, G. Ertem, I. Omigbodun, O. Rohde, L.A. Srinath, S. Ulkuer, N. and Rahman, A. (2011). Child and adolescent mental health worldwide: evidence for action. *Lancet, 378*(9801): 1515–1525. Champaign: 10.1016/S0140–6736(11)60827-1.

Kipp, L.E. and Weiss, M.R. (2013). Social influences, psychological need satisfaction, and well-being among female adolescent gymnasts. *Sport, Exercise, and Performance Psychology, 2*(1): 62–75. Champaign: 10.1037/a0030236

Kort-Butler, L.A. and Hagewen, K.J. (2011). School-based extracurricular activity involvement and adolescent self-esteem: A growth-curve analysis. *Journal of Youth and Adolescence, 40*(x): 568–581. Champaign: 10.1007/s10964–0ten to9551–4

Kreider, R.B. Fry, A.C. and O'Toole, M.L. (1998). *Overtraining in sport.* Champaign, Illinois: Human Kinetics.

Kristiansen, E. and Roberts, G.C. (2009). Young elite athletes and social support: Coping with competitive and organizational stress in "Olympic" competition. *Scandinavian Journal of Medicine and Science in Sport, 20*(4): 686–695. Champaign: 10.1111/j.1600–0838.2009.00950.x

Kwan, M. Bobko, S. Faulkner, G. Donnelly, P. and Cairney, J. (2014). Sport participation and alcohol and illicit drug use in adolescents and young adults: A systematic review of longitudinal studies. *Addictive Behaviors, 39*(3): 497–506. Champaign: 10.1016/j.addbeh.2013.11.006

Lam, K.C. Valier, A.R. Bay, C. and McLeod, T.C. (2013). A unique patient population? Health–related quality of life in adolescent athletes versus general, healthy adolescent individuals. *Journal of Athletic Training, 48*(2): 233–241. Champaign: 10.4085/1062–6050–48.2.12

Lemyre, P.N. Hall, H.K. and Roberts, G.C. (2008). A social cognitive approach to burnout in elite athletes. *Scandinavian Journal of Medicine and Science in Sports, 18*(2): 221–234. Champaign: 10.1111/j.1600–0838.2007.00671.x

López-Walle, J. Balaguer, I. Castillo, I. and Tristán, J. (2012). Autonomy support, basic psychology needs and wellbeing in Mexican athletes. *The Spanish Journal of Psychology, 15*(3): 1283–1292. Champaign: 10.5209/rev_SJOP.2012.v15.n3.39414

Marsh, H. W. (1993). The effects of participation in sport during the last two years of high school. *Sociology of Sport Journal, 10*(1): 18–43.

Marsh, H. W. (1998). Age and gender effects in physical self-concepts for adolescent elite athletes and nonathletes: A multicohort-multioccasion design. *Journal of Sport and Exercise Psychology, 20*(3): 237–259.

Martinent, G. Decret, J.C. Guillet-Descas, E. and Isoard-Gautheur, S. (2014). A reciprocal effects model of the temporal ordering of motivation and burnout among youth table tennis players in intensive training settings. *Journal of Sports Sciences.* Advance online publication. Champaign: 10.1080/02640414.2014.912757

Matos, N.F. Winsley, R.J. and Williams, C.A. (2011). Prevalence of non-functional overreaching/overtraining in young English athletes. *Medicine and Science in Sports and Exercise, 43*(7): 1287–1294. Champaign: 10.1249/MSS.0b013e318207f87b

Merglen, A. Flatz, A. Belanger, R.E. Michaud, P.A. and Suris, J.C. (2013). Weekly sport practice and adolescent well-being. *Archives of Disease in Childhood*, *99*(3): 208–210. Champaign: 10.1136/archdischild-2013-303729

Nicholls, A.R. Polman, R. Levy, A.R. Taylor, J. and Cobley, S. (2007). Stressors, coping, and coping effectiveness: Gender, type of sport, and skill differences. *Journal of Sports Sciences*, *25*(13): 1521–1530. Champaign: 10.1080/02640410701230479

Ntoumanis, N. Taylor, I.M. and Thogersen-Ntoumani, C. (2012). A longitudinal examination of coach and peer motivational climates in youth sport: Implications for moral attitudes, well-being, and behavioral investment. *Developmental Psychology*, *48*(1): 213–223. Champaign: 10.1037/a0024934

Pedersen, S. and Seidman, E. (2004). Team sports achievement and self_esteem development among urban adolescent girls. *Psychology of Women Quarterly*, *28*(4): 412–422. Champaign: 10.1111/j.1471-6402.2004.00158.x

Perron, A. Brendgen, M. Vitaro, F. Côté, S. M. Tremblay, R. E. and Boivin, M. (2012). Moderating effects of team sports participation on the link between peer victimization and mental health problems. *Mental Health and Physical Activity*, *5*(2): 107–115. Champaign: 10.1016/j.mhpa.2012.08.006

Raedeke, T.D. (1997). Is athlete burnout more than just stress? A sport commitment perspective. *Journal of Sport and Exercise Psychology*, *19*(4): 396–417.

Raedeke, T.D. and Smith, A.L. (2004). Coping resources and athlete burnout: An examination of stress mediated and moderation hypotheses. *Journal of Sport and Exercise Psychology*, *26*: 525–541.

Scheier, M.F. and Carver, C.S. (1992). Effects of optimism on psychological and physical wellbeing: Theoretical overview and empirical update. *Cognitive Therapy and Research*, *16*(2): 201–228. Champaign: 10.1007/BF01173489

Schmikli, S.L. de Vries, W.R. Brink, M.S. and Backx, F.J.G. (2012). Monitoring performance, pituitary-adrenal hormones and mood profiles: How to diagnose non-functional overreaching in male elite junior soccer players. *British Journal of Sports Medicine*, *46*(14): 1019–1023. Champaign: 10.1136/bjsports-2011-090492

Schnell, A. Mayer, J. Diehl, K. Zipfel, S. and Thiel, A. (2014). Giving everything for athletic success! Sports-specific risk acceptance of elite adolescent athletes. *Psychology of Sport and Exercise*, *15*(2): 165–172. Champaign: 10.1016/j.psychsport.2013.10.012

Slutzky, C.B. and Simpkins, S.D. (2009). The link between children's sport participation and self-esteem: Exploring the mediating role of sport self-concept. *Psychology of Sport and Exercise*, *10*(3): 381–389. Champaign: 10.1016/j.psychsport.2008.09.006

Snyder, C.R. Irving, L. and Anderson, J.R. (1991). Hope and health: Measuring the will and the ways. In C.R. Snyder and D.R. Forsyth (eds), *Handbook of social and clinical psychology: The health perspective* (pp. 285–305). Elmford, NY: Pergamon.

Stirling, A.E., and Kerr, G.A. (2007). Elite female swimmers' experiences of emotional abuse across time. *Journal of Emotional Abuse*, *7*(4): 89–113. Champaign: 10.1300/J135v07n04_05

Taliaferro, L.A. Eisenberg, M.E. Johnson, K.E. Nelson, T.F. and Neumark-Sztainer, D. (2011). Sport participation during adolescence and suicide ideation and attempts. *International Journal of Adolescent Medicine and Health*, *23*(1): 3–10.

Tamminen, K.A. and Holt, N.L. (2010). A meta-study of qualitative research examining stressor appraisals and coping among adolescents in sport. *Journal of Sports Sciences*, *28* (14): 1563–1580. Champaign: 10.1080/02640414.2010.512642

Taylor, A. and Faulkner, G. (2014). Evidence and theory into practice in different health care contexts: A call for more translational science. *Mental Health and Physical Activity*, *7*(1): 1–5. Champaign: 10.1016/j.mhpa.2013.06.007

Vallerand, R.J. Blanchard, C. Magneau, G.A. Koestner, R. Ratelle, C. Leonard, M. Gagné, M. and Marsolais, J. (2003). Les passions de l'ame: On obsessive and harmonious passion. *Journal of Personality and Social Psychology*, *85*(4): 756–767. Champaign: 10.1037/0022-3514.85.4.756

Vealey, R.S. Udry, E.M. Zimmerman, V. and Soliday, J. (1992). Intrapersonal and situational predictors of coaching burnout. *Journal of Sport and Exercise Psychology*, *14*: 40–58.

Vella, S.A. Cliff, D.P. Magee, C.A. and Okely, A.D. (2014). Sports participation and parent-reported health-related quality of life in children: Longitudinal associations. *The Journal of Pediatrics*, Advance online publication. Champaign: http://dx.doi.org/10.1016/j.jpeds.2014.01.071.

Verkooijen, K.T. van Hove, P. and Dik, G. (2012). Athletic identity and well-being among young talented athletes who live at a dutch elite sport center. *Journal of Applied Sport Psychology*, *24*(1): 106–113. Champaign: 10.1080/10413200.2011.633153

Whitelaw, S. Teuton, J. Swift, J. and Scobie, G. (2010). The physical activity and mental wellbeing association in young people: a case study in dealing with a complex public health topic using a 'realistic evaluation' framework. *Mental Health and Physical Activity, 3*(2): 61–66. Champaign: *10.1016/j.mhpa.2010.06.001*

Wold, B. Duda, J.L. Balaguer, I. Smith, O.R.F. Ommundsen, Y. Hall, H.K. Samdal, O. Heuzé, J.P. Haug, E. Bracey, S. Castillo, I. Ramis, Y. Quested, E. and Krommidas, C. (2013). Comparing self-reported leisure-time physical activity, subjective health, and life satisfaction among youth soccer players and adolescents in a reference sample. *International Journal of Sport and Exercise Psychology, 11*(4): 328–340. Champaign: 10.1080/1612197X.2013.830433

World Health Organization (2001). What is mental health? Retrieved 2nd May 2014 from www.who.int/features/qa/62/en/.

Zarrett, N. Fay, K. Li, Y. Carrano, J. Phelps, E. and Lerner, R. M. (2009). More than child's play: Variable- and pattern-centered approaches for examining effects of sports participation on youth development. *Developmental Psychology, 45*(2): 368– 382. Champaign: 10.1037/a0014577

38

EATING DISORDERS IN YOUNG ATHLETES

Nanna L. Meyer, Jorunn Sundgot-Borgen and
Alba Reguant Closa

Introduction

Eating disorders (EDs) and disordered eating (DE) are most likely to occur in weight–sensitive sports. Both male and female athletes are at risk for developing EDs and DE. Screening, early identification, interdisciplinary treatment approaches and successful prevention strategies are needed to reduce risk and promote performance capacity with minimal health consequences in young people. This chapter includes the science and practice of ED in young athletes and begins with a discussion on the classification of ED/DE, their prevalence, signs and symptoms, health and performance consequences, and concludes with treatment and prevention modalities.

Classification of eating disorders and disordered eating

Eating disorders are classified into clinical and subclinical EDs, the latter commonly referred to as DE. The clinical EDs include the three conditions – anorexia nervosa (AN), bulimia nervosa (BN) and binge eating disorder (BED). These eating disorders are recognized by the American Psychiatric Association (APA) and are described in the Diagnostic Statistical Manual of Mental Disorders (DSM-5; APA, 2013). Classification and diagnosis, however, are challenging due to systematic overlap across a range of EDs. For example, body dissatisfaction, dietary restraint and binge eating can be characteristic of all three categories (Treasure, Claudino and Zucker, 2010).

Clinical eating disorders

The clinical EDs currently classified by the DSM-5 include AN, BN and BED. These three categories may be visualized on a spectrum, upon which individuals may be located at different times of their illness. The spectrum also includes the subclinical or contemporarily termed 'other specified feeding or eating disorder' (OSFED) discussed later. First, we review the DSM-5 for clinical EDs.

Anorexia nervosa

Anorexia nervosa is characterized by a low body weight (i.e. less than minimally normal weight in adults, or less than minimally expected weight in children and adolescents). Patients with AN must state or behaviourally demonstrate that they refuse to gain weight and it is not uncommon for young patients failing to gain sufficient weight to support growth. Further, AN patients are pre-occupied with a fear of gaining weight or becoming fat despite being classified as underweight. Body dissatisfaction – specifically how weight, shape or size are perceived and to what degree this experience undermines self-evaluation and self-worth – are consistent features of AN. A patient with AN may also be in denial, meaning that the patient may not want to accept the seriousness of the problem. Importantly, AN can be of two different types: restricting or binge-eating/purging type (APA, 2013).

Bulimia nervosa

Bulimia Nervosa is characterized by repeated binge eating followed by purging to counteract the binges. Based on DSM-5, to be diagnosed with BN, binge-eating and purging episodes must occur a minimum of one time per week for the duration of at least three months. It is difficult to define the scope of a binge eating episode, as this is highly individual. According to the DSM-5, binge eating refers to eating in a discrete period of time (e.g. within a two-hour time period), a quantity of food that is larger than most people would eat during such a period of time under similar circumstances. In addition, the lack of control associated with the binge eating episode (for example that bingeing cannot be stopped) is also considered a diagnostic criterion for patients with BN. Self-evaluation in patients with BN is unduly influenced by body weight, size and shape. A final diagnostic criterion also specifies that the disturbance does not exclusively occur during episodes of AN.

Binge eating disorder

Binge eating disorder is a new category of DSM-5. Binge eating disorder is defined as frequent binge-eating patterns, differentiated from BN by the absence of recurrent inappropriate compensatory methods such as purging (Treasure *et al.*, 2010). Consistent with the new diagnosis criteria for BN, binge eating episodes have to occur an average of at least once per week for three or more months. Binge eating disorder is often associated with obesity and less common in athletes although it should not be excluded, especially in youth.

Other specified feeding or eating disorder (OSFED)

The term other specified feeding or eating disorder (OSFED) is used by practitioners to classify patients with a feeding or ED of concern; however, the patient does not fully meet all clinical criteria for AN, BN or BED. Individuals with OSFED may also be described as having DE patterns, and these can be physical, psychological and behavioural. Disordered eating is common in athletes and includes various abnormal eating behaviours such as restrictive eating, fasting, frequently skipping meals, using diet pills, laxatives, diuretics or enemas (Nattiv *et al.*, 2007).

The DSM-5 also includes the term ARFID (Avoidant Restrictive Food Intake Disorder), as new diagnostic criteria (APA, 2013). The purpose of this disorder was to differentiate from other EDs with similar signs and symptoms but aiming to avoid classifying this disorder as OSFED (Nicely *et al.*, 2014). ARFID emerges in infancy or childhood but can also be present in older ages. Patients with ARFID will present with eating or feeding disturbances that might lead to reduced food intake and lose weight or develop nutritional deficiencies. Interestingly, ARFID is not related to body shape or weight disturbances.

Here we will define an ED as a clinical mental disorder as published by the DSM-5 and characterized by abnormal eating behaviours, an irrational fear of gaining weight, and false beliefs about eating, weight and body shape (Nattiv *et al.*, 2007) and retain the term DE – including eating patterns of concern due to their subclinical anomaly – on the grounds that they do not demonstrate severe psychopathology nor do they meet the DSM-5 criteria (APA, 2014).

Spectrum of eating disorders and disordered eating

A spectrum of normal to abnormal eating exists that ranges from a healthy body weight, body image and energy balance to abnormal eating, including AN, BN and BED (Nattiv *et al.*, 2007). It is not uncommon for individuals with clinical EDs to move between AN, BN and BED, except for those with BN who develop AN (Fairburn and Harrison, 2003). In athletes, energy restriction or dieting can also occur on a spectrum. There is less concern about athletes gradually reducing energy intake (EI) to reduce weight and optimize body composition, if done in collaboration with a health care professional such as a sports dietitian. However, rapid weight loss (RWL) to meet a specific weight class (e.g. wrestling, light weight rowing, boxing, taekwondo, judo) is of greater risk, especially if unsupervised and using pathogenic weight control methods (e.g. extreme energy restriction and dehydration methods). Furthermore, severe and sustained caloric restriction, often seen in aesthetic and endurance sports, to achieve or maintain a low body mass (e.g. diving, gymnastics, figure skating, endurance sports, ski jumping) is considered more dangerous. Whether or not these athletes meet the DSM-5 criteria for a clinical ED is probably not as critical as the fact that suboptimal nutrition through RWL or chronic energy restriction will eventually interfere with performance improvements, normal growth and health. Taken together, health care professionals must pay attention to the spectrum of abnormal eating in athletes and develop effective approaches for screening, identification, referral, treatment and prevention. Thus, timely and effective treatment as well as prevention can only occur if at-risk athletes are identified early, and this is typically recommended during the pre-participation physical screening process (Nattiv *et al.*, 2007; Sundgot-Borgen *et al.*, 2013).

Recovery from eating disorders

Recovery from an ED is variable. For some, the disease is of short duration, especially for DE, as energy restriction may only be temporary with full recovery after intervention (Sundgot-Borgen, 1996). The best prognosis for full recovery is seen in young individuals with a relatively short history of DE or EDs (Fairburn and Harrison, 2003). In newly diagnosed athletes, average recovery time spanned across a year but varied greatly (Arthur–Cameselle and Quatromoni, 2014). However, EDs can also move along the spectrum of ED for 10–20 years. In AN, the shorter the bout of the disease, the better the recovery prognosis. This finding is in direct contrast to BN, where recovery is more likely the longer the duration of the illness (Von Holle, Pinehiro and Thorton, 2008). Furthermore, AN is characterized by an increased mortality rate and persistent psychiatric complications (Berkman, Lohr and Bulik, 2007). Relapse periods are a common issue in ED and DE, also in athletes. What often helps athletes to recover from ED is the deep aspiration to regain health and energy to participate in sport (Arthur–Cameselle and Quatromoni, 2014).

Prevalence of eating disorders and disordered eating

Eating disorders are common in young people. DE behaviours start as early as 9 years of age in both boys and girls (Neumark-Stzainer and Hannan, 2000), and DE behaviours track from adolescence to adulthood with rising rates of extreme weight control methods and binge eating episodes (Neumark-Sztainer *et al.*, 2011). Eating disorders are also prevalent in emerging societies, including China (Chen and Jackson, 2008) and Brazil (De Souza Ferreira and da Veiga, 2008). Lifetime prevalence of EDs in adults is ~0.6 per cent for AN and ~1 per cent for BN, with women being at greater risk (Jacobi, *et al.*, 2004; Hudson and Pope, 2007).

Women (3 per cent) rather than men (2 per cent) are also at greater risk for BED (Hudson and Pope, 2007). Of ED patients, 22.5 per cent of those previously diagnosed with Eating Disorders Not Otherwise Specified (which was replaced by OSFED in the new DSM-5) met the criteria for ARIFD. The patients with ARIFD were younger (11.1 ± 1.7 y vs 14.2 ± 1.5 y) and more were males (Nicely *et al.*, 2014).

In athletes, studies have shown that DE and EDs are more prevalent in weight-sensitive sports than in sports with less emphasis on leanness or low body weight. Byrne and McLean (2001) showed a 31 per cent prevalence of EDs in athletes competing in thin–built sports, versus controls (5.5 per cent), and Sundgot-Borgen and Torstveit (2004) showed a 25 per cent prevalence in Norwegian elite endurance, aesthetic and weight-class sports versus controls (9 per cent). Among sports, males (17.2 per cent) and females (32 per cent) competing in weight-sensitive sports (e.g. gymnastics and running) had a higher prevalence of EDs than athletes in non–weight sensitive (ball-game and technical sports). Others have shown a broad range in DE and ED prevalence among sports (1–62 per cent) (Brownell and Rodin, 1992; Byrne and McLean, 2002; Melin *et al.*, 2014; Nattiv *et al.*, 2007; Rosendahl *et al.*, 2009; Sundgot-Borgen, 1993; Sundgot-Borgen *et al.*, 1994). Of elite athletes competing in weight-category sports, 70 per cent are dieting and have abnormal eating behaviours (Oppliger *et al.*, 1996; Torstveit and Sundgot-Borgen, 2005).

It is currently unknown whether the prevalence of EDs and DE is higher among adolescent elite athletes than athletes at lower competitive levels or non-athletes. One of the difficulties in providing more accurate and precise estimates of prevalence data is the fact that studies use various methodological approaches (e.g. screening tools and false negatives, n-size, ages, sports, lack of control groups; Beals *et al.*, 2010; Beals and Manore, 2002; Johnson *et al.*, 1999; *et al.*, 2010; Rosendahl *et al.*, 2009; Sundgot-Borgen, 1993; Sundgot-Borgen and Torstveit, 2004, 2010). As previously shown, where controls were included, athletes in weight-class sports and sports in which a high power-to-weight ratio and/or leanness are important have a higher prevalence of EDs and DE than controls (Byrne and McLean, 2001; Sundgot-Borgen and Torstveit, 2004). Thus, health care professionals should expect EDs and DE in weight-sensitive sports. However, they occur in all sports.

Female athletes are at greater risk for developing EDs or DE than males (Bratland-Sanda and Sundgot-Borgen, 2013; Sundgot-Borgen, 1993). However, male athletes are also at risk. In a large Norwegian sample, 59 per cent of young elite male athletes showed body dissatisfaction, 19 per cent were dieting and 11 per cent had DE. When analyzed by sport, the prevalence of DE in male was highest (22 per cent) in anti-gravitational sports (e.g. ski jumping), lower in endurance (9 per cent) and lowest in ball sports (5 per cent; Sundgot-Borgen and Torstveit, 2004).

That risk for EDs and DE in ski-jumping is high is associated with the fact that ski-jump length is directly related to body mass, with lower body mass associated with longer flight phases and better performance. Between 1974 and 2002, ski-jumpers' body mass index (BMI) has decreased from 23.6 to 19.4 kg/m^2 (Müller, 2009), measured with skis, suit, and boots. After much debate, the International Ski Federation (FIS) launched a minimum BMI rule, adjusted recently to 21 kg/m^2 and maximum ski length of 145 per cent of athlete height (www.fis-ski.com). While this rule had a positive impact on extremely low body mass, the problem of underweight in ski jumping is not yet resolved.

In young male athletes, weight-category sports are of greatest concern regarding EDs and DE due to RWL before weigh-in (Artioli *et al.*, 2010). The two most commonly reported RWL methods are excessive exercise and dieting/fasting (Chatterton and Petrie, 2013), but other methods (e.g. sauna, sweat suits during exercise, fluid restriction, laxatives, vomiting, diet pills) are also used (Artioli *et al.*, 2010; *et al.*, 2004). One of the most tragic stories of such abuse is reflected in the three male wrestlers who died in 1997 as a result of what was believed to be extreme dehydration and hyperthermia (Manore *et al.*, 2009). This incident initiated rule changes in U.S. collegiate sports.

To meet weight category, athletes have to diet and this starts young. Data in adolescent athletes show that weight-cuts begin early (12.6±6.1 y) (Artioli *et al.*, 2010). Interestingly, athletes who start weight-cuts early in their career may also use more aggressive weight loss methods (Artioli *et al.*, 2010; Kiningham and Gorenflo, 2001). However, this should not be generalized because recent data on Olympians revealed fewer extreme weight loss methods among the medal winners (Jones *et al.*, 2014). This may be due to sport science support, which has the ability to change sport cultures by educating athletes and coaches of the dangers of RWL, initiating evidence-based approaches to optimize, with the least harm, an athlete's weight class, and developing effective recovery strategies post weigh-in. Unfortunately, adopting safety-related rules tends not to be a priority at the elite level and, thus, the risk of EDs and DE in weight-category sports remains (Sundgot-Borgen *et al.*, 2013).

Eating disorders in male athletes also exist in endurance sports. Riebl *et al.*, (2007) showed higher scores on an ED screening test in elite cyclists than non-athletes. Similar trends are also apparent in young cyclists, of whom 50 per cent met the criteria of EDs (Ferrand and Brunet, 2004).

Studies have also investigated whether risk factors for EDs differ from males to females. A recent study in NCAA Division I male athletes has shown different psychological and personality factors predictive of EDs and DE in men versus women (Galli *et al.*, 2014). Similar to social pressures of thinness in girls, leanness and muscularity appear to characterize at-risk male athletes (Neumark-Stainer and Eisenberg, 2014).

Eating disorder prevalence has increased over the last two decades. Although there are only few data available and the studies are limited to Norway, there is no reason to believe that these trends would be different in athletes of other Westernized countries. From 1990 to 2002, EDs have increased from 20 per cent to 28 per cent and 5 to 21 per cent in athletes and controls, respectively. While methodological issues may confound these data (e.g. improved screening, greater awareness, policy changes within sports), a higher incidence of individuals suffering from EDs may be due to increased societal/media as well as sport-specific factors (Sundgot-Borgen and Torstveit, 2010). Considering the high prevalence and increasing incidence of EDs and DE in athletes, it is important to understand the risk factors.

Risk factors for the development of eating disorders

Risk factors for EDs can be divided into general and sport-specific factors. Dieting to be thin or to win is a common entry point for athletes. There are many factors predisposing individuals for DE and EDs, and the reason why athletes may develop DE and EDs is likely to be multifactorial, with environmental and social factors, psychological predisposition, low self-esteem, family dysfunction, abuse, biological factors and genetics potentially all contributing (Nattiv *et al.*, 2007). While it is recognized that EDs occur due to a variety of general trigger factors (e.g. societal pressure to be thin, comorbidities such as depression, sexual abuse, alcoholism; Treasure *et al.*, 2010), for this chapter, we will focus on sport-specific factors.

Sport-specific risk factors for EDs and DE have been identified by Sundgot-Borgen (1994). Athletes with EDs were found to start sport-specific training and dieting earlier than those without EDs. Sudden increases in training volume and intensity, overtraining and associated injuries were found more often in athletes with EDs. The pressure to reduce body weight or change physique, chronic dieting and weight cycling were also associated with greater risk. An interesting quandary is that certain personality traits in athletes are also those identified in individuals with EDs. These include perfectionism and over-compliance – traits generally desired by coaches (Sundgot-Borgen and Torstveit, 2010). It has also been speculated that athletes may have high achievement orientation and the potential for obsessive-compulsive traits commonly associated with EDs (Leon, 1991). For example, an athlete may not use a recovery day but instead opt to repeat the hard training session of the previous day, thinking more is better. Likewise, this personality trait could interfere with adjusting energy intake to the higher energy demands during periods of high intensity/volume training. Whether or not these aspects of suboptimal recovery and fuelling strategies occur inadvertently or due to a body composition/ mass goal does not really matter because, in the long run, such behaviours will eventually derail performance and may lead to injury. The other difficult aspect in sport is the fact that reducing body fat/mass, maintaining low body fat/mass or not gaining body mass during growth may initially lead to improved performance due to an improved power-to-weight ratio. If this occurs in a team setting – and is encouraged by the coach and observed by other athletes – it may trigger energy restriction in others and prove contagious. Considering that body types and shapes are similar within a sport, the one with extra mass or fat may fall outside the norm and be referred to the sports dietitian for weight loss or gain, while the one at risk may not. In an article by Sundgot-Borgen and Torstveit (2010), this was referred to as a sport's body paradigm. Caloric restriction at times of heavy training rarely goes unnoticed, however. Such problematic approaches are programmed to derail an athlete's career due to the powerful (although highly variable) effects on health and performance.

Consequences of eating disorders in athletes

Disordered eating and EDs have variable effects on an individual's health and performance. Some athletes can endure energy deficits quite well, while in others consequences are noticed within a short time frame. Effects on physiological and psychological function vary by degree of DE and EDs and how long the disorder lasts (Beals *et al.*, 2010).

Medical issues

Medical alterations as a result of an ED vary by disorder. Physical findings for AN include dry skin, hair formation on face and arms, also called lanugo. Further AN symptoms include acrocyanosis, alopecia, low body temperature, dehydration, growth retardation, delayed puberty and low body weight. Physical symptoms for BN include erosion of dental enamel, enlarge-ment of the parotid/salivary glands, callus on back of hands from vomiting, and dehydration. Physique assessments should pinpoint an existing or advancing problem in AN. In BN, however, this is not the case because the individual may maintain or even gain weight. Cardiovascular, gastrointestinal, hematologic, biochemical and endocrine changes for both AN and BN are well known (Sundgot-Borgen *et al.*, 2013). While both AN and BN are life threatening diseases, there are several dangers (some of which are acute) associated with a bulimic athlete participating in sport.

Bingeing and purging can lead to gastric and esophageal complications, some of which are irreversible (Carney and Anderson, 1996; Pomeroy and Mitchell, 1992). Gastro-intestinal symptoms depend on purging method but can affect mouth, throat, stomach and gastrointestinal tract. While dehydration may be a common side effect of daily training, an additional loss of body water due to vomiting or laxatives, diuretics or enemas may cause potassium losses, leading to hypokalemia and cardiac arrhythmias (Carney and Anderson, 1996). Electrolyte imbalances are especially of concern in high intensity sports, where a blackout and fall could have severe consequences. Purging can alter pH levels and lead to metabolic alkalosis, while severe laxative abuse can result in metabolic acidosis (Carney and Anderson, 1996). Both conditions are expected to interfere with the athlete's capacity to manage metabolic challenges during exercise. Dehydration can also occur due to RWL as previously discussed in wrestling. This type of dehydration increases the risk of hyperthermia and exertional heat illness (Opplinger *et al.*, 1996).

Nutritional issues

Disordered eating and ED can also manifest in a multitude of nutrition-related complications that may impact sport performance acutely. In young athletes, EDs and DE can interfere with growth and development and the earlier the ED onset, the longer the disorders might continue until adult ages (Desbrow *et al.*, 2014).

Low EI leads to insufficient macro- and micronutrient intakes with potential risk for short and long term nutrient deficiencies, including anaemia, chronic fatigue, and illness and infection. Low carbohydrate intakes during intense training leads to glycogen depletion, early fatigue and increased risk of injury (Brouns *et al.*, 1986; Burke *et al.*, 2004) and infection (Nieman, 2008). Carbohydrate recommendations for athletes vary from 3 to 12 $g \cdot kg^{-1} \cdot d^{-1}$ depending on training loads (Burke *et al.*, 2011), although there are no specific guidelines for adolescent athletes. Low protein intake can affect growth and development, muscle mass accretion and may lead to muscle wasting, especially if energy and carbohydrate intakes are also low. Athletes need a protein intake ranging from 1.3 $g \cdot kg^{-1} \cdot d^{-1}$ to 1.8 $g \cdot kg^{-1} \cdot d^{-1}$ (Phillips and Van Loon, 2011), although higher amounts are recommended during energy restriction (Mettler *et al.*, 2010). A critical phase for young athletes is the post-exercise period and, if missed due to ED or DE, will likely impair muscle repair and the delivery of additional calories to the body. Very low fat intakes fail to deliver adequate essential fatty acids. Athletes should achieve a fat intake of at least 20–25 per cent of total EI or between 0.8 $g \cdot kg^{-1} \cdot d^{-1}$ and 2.0 $g \cdot kg^{-1} \cdot d^{-1}$ (Burke *et al.*, 2004; Stellingwerff, Maughan and Burke, 2011). Low micronutrient intakes may lead to micronutrient deficiencies, potentially impacting the athlete's health and performance, and the ability to adapt to training (Manore *et al.*, 2009). Low intakes of calcium, vitamin D and iron are of special concern, possibly leading to anemia and compromised musculoskeletal and immune health at early age with continued complications during adulthood (Desbrow *et al.*, 2014). The sports dietitican evaluates an athlete's diet using a dietary assessment contrasted with data on energy expenditure, performance patterns, fatigue, sleep and recovery and mood changes.

The female athlete triad and relative energy deficiency in sport (RED-S)

Long-term health consequences of DE and EDs are best illustrated by the Female Athlete Triad (De Souza *et al.*, 2014) and Relative Energy Deficiency in Sport (RED-S) (Mountjoy *et al.*,

2014). Originally, the Triad centred on DE and an ED leading to amenorrhea and osteoporosis (Otis *et al.*, 1997; Yeager *et al.*, 1993). Today, the Triad emphasizes the concept of energy availability (EA), defined as dietary EI minus exercise energy expenditure (EEE). Energy availability is the amount of energy remaining for other physiologic functions after exercise training (Nattiv *et al.*, 2007). Low EA can occur due to low EI, high EEE or a combination. Energy availability is expressed in kilogram of fat free mass (FFM) per day. A threshold at or below 30 kcal/kgFFM/d or greater has been identified as a level of EA needed to maintain normal menstrual function (Ilhe and Loucks, 2004), and levels of 45 kcal/kgFFM/d and higher may be needed to support daily vigorous training and competition (Nattiv *et al.*, 2007). The Triad exists in active girls and women and integrates one or more of the following: 1) low EA, 2) menstrual dysfunction and 3) low bone mineral density (BMD) (De Souza *et al.*, 2014).

Relative Energy Deficiency in Sport recognizes the importance of EA for optimal health and performance but presents a more comprehensive approach of the Triad's limited triangular view. Thus, RED-s addresses overall impaired physiological function, integrating factors such as metabolic rate, menstrual function, bone health, immune function, protein synthesis, cardiovascular and psychological health and likewise emphasizes performance issues (Mountjoy *et al.*, 2014).

The cause and effect between low EA and menstrual dysfunction was established by Loucks and colleagues through a series of observational and experimental studies in sedentary women and athletes (Loucks *et al.*, 2011). Long-term suppression of reproductive function through low EA can negatively impact musculoskeletal (De Souza *et al.*, 2014) and cardiovascular health (Rickenlund *et al.*, 2005). Ilhe and Loucks (2004) were able to show that low EA at <30kcal/kgFFM/d also leads to abrupt changes in markers of bone turnover and metabolic markers independent of estradiol. Due to the underlying aetiology of the Triad (i.e. low EA rather than DE or EDs), low EA is now recognized as the key link to both menstrual dysfunction and compromised bone mass (Nattiv *et al.*, 2007).

Osteoporosis presents a great risk for fragility fractures later in life. In older adults, osteoporosis develops over time through a gradual loss of bone mass. The World Health Organization (WHO) uses T-scores to diagnose osteoporosis in post-menopausal women (WHO, 1994), while the International Society for Clinical Densitometry (ISCD) and others (Mountjoy *et al.*, 2014; De Souza *et al.*, 2014) recommend using age-specific Z-scores to evaluate bone health in pre-meno-pausal women and young men, adolescents and children (Leib *et al.*, 2004; Leslie *et al.*, 2006).

Low EA is related to BMD Z-scores. Adolescent runners who consumed less energy than recommended (low EA) had low BMD Z-scores (Z-scores were < -1 at spine) compared with runners consuming more energy. They also had reduced bone turnover, lower body mass, lower BMI, lower 25 (OH) Vitamin D3, lower estradiol levels and reported fewer menstrual cycles in the past year (Barrack *et al.*, 2010).

Studies have also shown that female athletes with menstrual dysfunction have lower BMD than athletes with normal menstrual function. While initially thought a female problem, similar links between EDs/DE, suppression of sex steroid hormones and compromised BMD have recently been identified in male athletes (Hackney, 2008; Hind *et al.*, 2006; Castro *et al.*, 2002), especially endurance athletes (Stewart and Hannan, 2000), and this was also a decisive factor to expand the limited concept of the Female Athlete Triad to RED-s.

Not all athletes with reduced or low EA have an ED. When athletes suffer from low EA in the absence of an ED, they are thought to inadvertently under-eat, perhaps due to appetite suppression induced by high training intensity/volume, a high carbohydrate and fibre intake (Loucks *et al.*, 2011), or lack of time. Inadvertent low EA may occur in sports with high energy demands notorious for double workouts, long endurance sessions or high altitude training.

Low EA can also affect other systems beyond menstrual function and bone, including thyroid hormone, resulting in a decrease in resting metabolic rate. Low EA impairs muscle protein synthesis (Areta *et al.*, 2013), which particularly impacts a growing athlete regarding muscle protein accretion, recovery and training adaptation.

Finally, compromised energy and nutrient intakes affects growing athletes. Especially visible in gymnasts, growth retardation and delayed puberty is a side effect of high training volumes and inadequate nutrition (Weimann *et al.*, 2000). Catch-up growth after periods of weight reduction in young athletes (Roemmich and Sinning, 1997; Caine *et al.*, 2001) is possible; however, some bone loss may be irreversible (Drinkwater *et al.*, 1986). Some sports are also regulated in a manner that jeopardizes growth and development of young athletes into mature competitors, as Olympic qualification may depend on success in competitions that occurred nine months prior to the games. These athletes are at risk for energy and nutrient restriction because of their efforts to halt natural growth in order to compete in the same weight class (e.g. boxing).

Performance consequences of EDs and DE are multifold and acutely include glycogen depletion leading to reduction in mental and physical performance capacity. Athletes who lose weight rapidly over a short time (>5 per cent body mass) with little time to refuel post weigh-in will suffer from performance declines due to dehydration, glycogen depletion and low blood sugar levels with increased risk of injury, including heat illness (Brouns *et al.*, 1986; Tarnapolsky *et al.*, 1996; Viitasalo *et al.*, 1987). Chronically, low nutrient intakes compromise the immune system, increasing the susceptibility to illness and delaying recovery. In summary, consequences of EDs and DE on health and performance may be detrimental. Thus, it is important for athletes to be identified and treated if they are at risk.

Treatment of eating disorders in athletes

Screening, identification and diagnosis are the first steps before treatment for DE and EDs is initiated. The most valid and reliable screening approach is by clinical interview through a trained psychologist or during pre-participation examination through a physician. Short surveys or assessments can flag athletes for follow up in order to confirm risk of an ED or DE. Other health care professionals who work with athletes directly (e.g. athletic trainer, physical therapist, strength and conditioning coach) can act as eyes in the identification process. Once an athlete is identified, they need to be referred to the treatment team experienced in DE and EDs. It is important to determine whether DE and EDs occur transiently, associated with the specific demands of the sport (Sundgot-Borgen, 1996), or whether the symptoms are more consistent with an ED, as treatment will vary.

Reducing overall nutritional risk and clarifying myths through evidence-based education and hands-on training are critical to re-establish sound eating practices. Building a solid foundation of knowledge is important for the athlete to trust that increased food intake will lead to performance enhancement (perceived as positive) as opposed to weight gain (perceived as negative) and, often inaccurately, equated with a performance loss. Thus, a small-step approach is best (e.g. adding calories over time).

For athletes with low sex steroid hormones, increasing EA is the main goal. Studies have shown that female athletes can resume normal menstrual function within six months by adding dietary energy (Dueck *et al.*, 1996; Guebels *et al.*, 2011; Koppe Woodroffe *et al.*, 1999). These studies used a post-exercise carbohydrate and protein drink, adding an average 350 kcal per day.

Pharmacological treatment approaches (e.g. oral contraceptives) to regulate the menstrual cycle have not produced positive effects on bone mass and should be discouraged in young athletes. Bone is also regulated by nutritional means, and thus, failing to remedy nutritional deficits will likely affect bone mass independently from hypoestrogenism.

The treatment team also includes the sports medicine physician who should coordinate treatment after conducting a physical exam, including blood, urine, and bone parameters (Sundgot-Borgen and Torstveit, 2010). If a persistent ED exists the athlete needs psychological care (Beals, 2010), which may include the family, especially in young individuals (Lock, le Grange, Forsberg, and Hewell, 2006). Treatment guidelines are published in the Practice Guidelines for Treatment of Patients with Eating Disorders, third edition (APA, 2006).

Treatment approaches vary greatly. Whether an athlete is unfit to participate in training and competition should be determined on an individual basis among the treatment team members. The stop light system, published by the IOC Consensus Statement (Mountjoy *et al.*, 2014), is useful to assess risk of sport participation. Athletes with clinical EDs or practicing extreme weight loss methods should not be allowed to compete (RED), while those with various indicators (e.g. prolonged low percentage body fat, substantial weight loss of 5–10 per cent, attenuation of expected growth and development, menstrual dysfunction, abnormal hormone profile in men, reduced BMD, stress fractures, cardiovascular issues or lack of progress from treatment) are classified as YELLOW. These athletes should be carefully monitored. While treatment is necessary for athletes to return to play, prevention is the best treatment approach (Mountjoy *et al.*, 2014).

Prevention of eating disorders in athletes

Besides the policies and procedures to raise awareness and provide guidelines for identification and treatment of athletes with DE and EDs, sporting organizations should emphasize prevention through screening and education. Pre-participation physicals are the best opportunity to screen both male and female athletes (Nattiv *et al.*, 2007; Bonci *et al.*, 2008), allowing for early identification and secondary prevention and treatment.

Educational programmes should differentiate among audiences. Health care providers, including sports dietitians, need to be trained in the screening, identification, referral, and treatment approaches. Coaches, officials, parents and other support staff should understand which sports are at greatest risk and why. Education should also include trigger factors of DE and EDs in athletes.

Commenting on athletes' body weight and composition from coach, officials or parents should no longer be where weight pressures originate. Officials, coaches and parents should be educated about the potential impact their comments and actions may have on an athlete. Using role models of healthy athletes with normal body composition is a powerful message that winning does not relate to thinness but rather to fitness. In addition, coaches, officials and parents need to understand that athletes with DE and EDs are at risk for injuries and illness and that providing a supportive environment also promotes a safe and ethically just playing field.

Coaches and parents should be able to recognize the signs and symptoms of DE or ED and need a good understanding of short and long-term medical and performance complications. The misconception that a lower weight and body fat always lead to performance enhancement should be dispelled. Weight and body composition should be de-emphasized and performance should be the centre of attention (Beals *et al.*, 2010; Sundgot-Borgen and Torstveit, 2010). Highlighting the scientific evidence among topics of nutrition and fuelling, body weight and composition, and performance and health impacts can empower coaches with better understanding about sport and how nutrition relates to success. Weight and body composition assessment should be the task of trained professionals and the rationale for assessment communicated and methods chosen should be carefully considered (Meyer *et al.*, 2013). Weight classes for athletes in weight-category sports should be realistic with health prioritized.

Athlete education should focus on performance nutrition, including the importance of energy balance and availability as they relate to health, growth and performance. While many athletes are trying to meet body weight and composition goals, they should be trained to recognize both positive (e.g. slow, gradual weight/fat loss if indicated with enhanced energy levels) and negative effects (e.g. amenorrhea, fatigue, injuries, illness) of reduced EA. Education should target the extra need for calories when training intensity and duration are higher. If energy deficits are indicated dietary strategies should include increases in protein to preserve muscle mass (Mettler *et al.*, 2010) and ensure carbohydrate availability to support training and recovery (Burke *et al.*, 2011). Education should also target fuelling performance before, during and after exercise. While providing awareness of DE and EDs risk, signs and symptoms, and consequences, educational approaches should generally remain covert, positive and focus on performance nutrition using theoretical and practical, hands–on approaches.

Athletes should feel comfortable discussing concerns about body weight and composition with coaches, trainers and staff but this requires a de-stigmatization of DE and EDs. Athletes should no longer need to hide eating problems but feel trusting to discuss concerns with coaches. Coaches should refrain from approaching athletes with regard to changes in body weight and composition. In fact, these topics should be initiated by athletes, and coaching staff and/or health care providers should know the proper course of action for referral (Sundgot-Borgen and Torstveit, 2010; Sundgot-Borgen *et al.*, 2013).

Although preventing ED (as well as DE, the female athlete triad and The RED-S) among athletes has been recommended frequently (Beals, 2004; Bonci *et al.*, 2008 Drinkwater *et al.*, 2005; Mountjoy *et al.*, 2014; Nattiv *et al.*, 2007; Thompson and Sherman, 1993), only limited research exists aiming to prevent DE and ED among elite athletes.

Eating disorder prevention programmes

Prevention programmes on body dissatisfaction, dieting and DE have mainly been conducted in the general population (Shaw, Stice and Becker, 2009), while data in athletes are limited. ATHENA, a coach-led, peer-facilitated programme designed to reduce DE, smoking and substance abuse in female high school athletes, has shown promising effects on eating habits, self-efficacy in exercise, and substance abuse (Elliot *et al.*, 2004) and unhealthy weight loss behaviours (Ranby *et al.*, 2009). However, ATHENA has not been able to evoke a sustained effect on eating pathology (Elliot *et al.*, 2004). Body Sense, a three-month body image intervention in young female gymnasts, parents and coaches, resulted in a reduced perception by athletes in pressure to be thin from their sporting clubs. However, these changes in the sporting climate also had little effect on athletes' eating pathology (Buchholz *et al.*, 2008). The most recent intervention compared two types: a dissonance prevention and healthy weight intervention, previously used in non-athletes (Stice *et al.*, 2008) but modified for the use in athletes. Both interventions reduced thin idealization, dietary restraint, eating pathology, body shape and weight concerns. Interestingly, nutrition-based interventions, such as the healthy weight intervention may be preferred by athletes (Becker *et al.*, 2012). A covert approach to preventing DE and EDs may be more effective in athletes, and nutrition-based interventions are perfect to catch the athlete's attention due to the impact nutrition has on performance.

The most recent published study on ED prevention comes from Norway and included the total population of elite high school athletes and their coaches. This randomized control trial showed that a one-year, sport specific, school-based intervention programme can prevent new cases of ED and symptoms associated with EDs in adolescent female elite athletes (Martinsen *et al.*, 2014). Furthermore, an educational programme for coaches can be an effective addition to promoting long-term retention of information (at least nine months) on knowledge, weight-regulation and ED. The educational programme also demonstrated positive effects on the coaches' subjective evaluation of their ED knowledge (Martinsen *et al.*, 2014).

Due to the limited work on prevention of EDs in athletes, there is no consensus on best practice. However, focus on health-promoting factors has been highlighted as essential (Børresen and Rosenvinge, 2003). The Health, Body and Sports Performance Intervention (Martinsen *et al.*, 2014), previously discussed, was a sport-specific intervention built on the social-cognitive framework (Bandura, 1986) and the primary focus was to enhance self-esteem by strengthening the athletes' self-efficacy. It was also focused on systematic changes within the intervention schools and aimed at intervening at the social systems and individual level. The intervention was influenced by the elaboration–likelihood model (Petty and Cacioppo, 1986) and the cognitive-dissonance theory (Festinger, 1957). The study by Martinsen *et al.* (2013) provides an indication of the importance of including a long-term follow-up to fully characterise the effect of the prevention programme. Athletes (especially elite) constitute a unique population as they are under pressure to improve performance and conform to the requirements of sport, in addition to socio-cultural pressure. On the other hand, if the information indicates that healthy eating can increase the likelihood of good sport performance (e.g. by focusing on the relationship between body composition, health, nutrition and performance), the athletes would most likely pay more attention (Thompson and Sherman, 2010).

Although education is certainly an important aspect of ED prevention programmes, it is unlikely to be effective unless it is accompanied by preventive efforts designed to change the beliefs and behaviours of the participants (Beals, 2004). Interestingly, Nowicka, Eli, Ng, Apitzsch, and Sundgot-Borgen (2013) found, by interviewing eighteen Swedish elite coaches in high-risk sports, that those who did not have sufficient knowledge of ED symptoms easily questioned their own observations in the face of athletes' statement of denial. The researchers also found that knowledge of ED per se did not automatically entice the coaches to act. In fact, many of the coaches were uncomfortable and found it difficult to talk with their athletes when observing symptoms of ED (Nowicka *et al.*, 2013). Thus, health care professionals should continue to support efforts of ED prevention and recognize the need for coaches' education, even in the face of initial resistance.

While education can increase awareness and knowledge of the risks and consequences of DE and EDs in athletes, the culture of the sport may not allow for behaviour change. Thus, national and international sport governing bodies may seem to be the only other avenue by enforcing rules and regulation related to body mass and composition. As previously discussed, several sports have introduced such schemes, which have at least reduced the extremes of low body weight and composition and have provided a fairer playing field (Müller, 2009; Müller *et al.*, 2006; Oppliger *et al.*, 2006). Finally, experienced professionals may also break down cultural barriers and develop programmes to change the culture of the sport. This takes years of experience and a buy-in from the entire sporting organization.

Conclusion

This chapter provided an introduction into EDs and DE in young athletes, highlighting weight-sensitive sports in which athletes are perceived at increased risk. It is important to understand risks and triggers of EDs and DE, health and performance consequences and how to treat athletes diagnosed with an ED or DE. Prevention is the best treatment and should integrate education and screening for early identification. Sports with a high risk should develop policy and procedures that can be used on a national and local level, and education should target athletes, parents, volunteers, coaches, officials and health care providers.

References

Alderman, B., Landers, D.M., Carlson, J. and Scott, J.R. (2004). Factors related to rapid weight loss practices among international-style wrestlers. *Medicine and Science in Sports and Exercise*, 36(2): 249–52.

American Psychiatric Association Working Group on Eating Disorders. Practice Guideline for the treatment of patient with eating disorders. (2006). Third Edition. www.psych.org/MainMenu/PsychiatricPractice/PracticeGuidelines_1.aspx. Accessed, 1 May, 2011.

American Psychiatric Association. (2014). DSM-5 Development. Retrieved 15 May, 2014 from www.dsm5.org/Pages/Default.aspx.

American Psychiatric Association. (2013). Diagnostic and statistical manual of mental disorders, 5th edition (DSM-5). Washington, DC.

Areta, J.L., Burke, L.M., Ross, M.L. Camera, D.M., West, D.W., Broad, E.M., Jeacocke, N.A., Moore, D.R., Stellingwerff, T., Phillips, S.M., Hawley, J.A. and Coffey, V.G. (2013). Timing and distribution of protein ingestion during prolonged recovery from resistance exercise alters myofibrillar protein synthesis. *The Journal of Physiology*, 1;591(Pt 9): 2319–31.

Arthur-Cameselle, J.N. and Quatromoni, P.A. (2014). Eating disorders in collegiate female athletes:factors that assist recovery. *Eating Disorders*, 22(1): 50–61.

Artioli, G.G., Franchini, E., Nicastro, H., Sterkowicz, S., Solis, M.Y. and Lancha, Jr. A.H. (2010). The need of a weight management control programmes in judo: a proposal based on the successful H.case of wrestling. *Journal of the International Society of Sports Nutrition*, 4;7(1): 15.

Artioli, G.G., Gualano, B., Franchini, E., Scagliusi, F.B., Takesian, M., Fuchs, M. and Bandura, A. (1986). *Social foundations of thought and action – A social cognitive theory.* New Jersey: Prentice-Hall,

Barrack, M.T., Van Loan, M.D., Rauh, M.J. and Nichols, J.F. (2010). Body Mass, Training, Menses, and Bone in Adolescent Runners: A Three-Year Follow-up. *Medicine and Science in Sports and Exercise*, 43(6): 959–66.

Beals, K.A. *Disordered eating among athletes: a comprehensive guide for health professionals.* Champaign, III: Human Kinetics, 2004.

Beals, K.A. and Manore, M.M. (2002). Disorders of the female athlete triad among collegiate athletes. *International Journal of Sports Nutrition and Exercise Metabolism*, 12(3): 281–93.

Beals, K.A., Houtkooper, L. and Dalton, B. (2010). Disordered eating in athletes. In

Burke, L. and Deakin, V. 4th ed. *Clinical Sports Nutrition.* Sydney, Australia: Mc Graw Hill, pp. 171–190.

Becker, C., McDaniel, L., Bull, S., Powell, M. and Mcintyre, K. (2012). Can we reduce eating disorder risk factors in female college athletes? A randomized exploratory investigation of two peer-led interventions. *Body Image*, 2012. 9(1): 31–42.

Berkman, N.D., Lohr, K.N. and Bulik, C.M. (2007). Outcomes of eating disorders: a systematic review of the literature. *Int J Eat Disord* 40: 293–309.

Bonci, C.M., Bonci, L.J., Granger, L.R., Johnson, C.L., Malina, R.M., Milne, L.W., Ryan, R.R. and Vanderbunt, E.M. (2008). National athletic trainers' association position statement: preventing, detecting, and managing disordered eating in athletes. *Journal of Athletic Training*, 43(1): 80–108.

Børresen, R. and Rosenvinge, J.H. From Prevention to Health Promotion. Edited by Treasure, J., Schmidt, U. and van Furth, E. In: Handbook of Eating Disorders Chisester: Wiley, 2003. pp. 455–466.

Bratland-Sanda, S. and Sundgot-Borgen, J. (2013). Eating Disorders in athletes: overview of prevalence, risk factors and recommendations for prevention and treatment. *European Journal of Sports Science*, 13(5): 499–508.

Brouns, F., Saris, W.H. and Ten Hoor, F. (1986). Nutrition as a factor in the prevention of injuries in recreational and competitive downhill skiing. Considerations based on the literature. *The Journal of Sports Medicine and Physical Fitness*, 26(1): 85–91.

Brownell, K.D. and Rodin, J. (1992). Prevalence of eating disorders in athletes. In: Brownell K.D., Rodin, J. and Wilmore, J.H. (eds). *Eating, body weight and performance in athletes: disorders of a modern society.* Philadelphia: Lea and Febiger, pp. 128–45.

Buchholz, A., Mack, H., McVey, G., Feder, S. and Barrowman, N. (2008). BodySense: an evaluation of a positive body image intervention on sport climate for female athletes. *Eating Disorders*, 16(4): 308–21.

Burke, L.M., Hawley, J.A., Wong, S. and Jeukendrup, A.E. (2011). Carbohydrate for training and competition. *Journal of Sports Sciences*, 29 Suppl 1:S17–27.

Burke, L.M., Kiens, B. and Ivy, J.L. (2004). Carbohydrates and fat for training and recovery. *Journal of Sports Sciences*, 22(1): 15–30.

Byrne, S. and McLean, N. (2001). Eating disorders in athletes: a review of the literature. *Journal of Science and Medicine in Sport*, 4(2): 145–59

Byrne, S. and McLean, N. (2002). Elite athletes: effects of the pressure to be thin. *Journal of Science and Medicine in Sport*, 5(2): 80–94.

Caine, D., Lewis, R., O'Connor, P., Howe, W. and Bass, S. (2001). Does gymnastics training inhibit growth of females? *Clinical Journal of Sport Medicine*, 11(4): 260–70.

Carney, C.P. and Andersen, A.E. (1996). Eating disorders. Guide to medical evaluation and complications. *The Psychiatrics Clinics of North America*, 19(4): 657–79.

Castro, J., Toro, J., Lazaro, L., Pons, F. and Halperin, I. (2002). Bone mineral density in male adolescents with anorexia nervosa. *Journal of the American Academy of Child and Adolescent Psychiatry*, 41(5): 613–8.

Chatterton, J.M. and Petrie, T.A. (2013). Prevalence of disordered eating and pathogenic weight control behaviours among male collegiate athletes. *Eating Disorders*, 21(4): 328–41.

Chen, H. and Jackson, T. (2008). Prevalence and sociodemographic correlates of eating disorder endorsements among adolescents and young adults from China. *European Eating Disorders Review*, 16: 375–385.

De Souza Ferreira, J.E. and da Veiga, G.V. (2008). Eating disorder risk behaviour in Brazilian adolescents from low socio-economic level. *Appetite*, 51: 249–55.

De Souza, M.J., Nattiv, A., Joy, E., Misra, M., Williams, N.I., Mallinson, R.J., Gibbs, J.C., Olmsted, M., Goolsby, M. and Matheson, G. (2014). 2014 Female Athlete Triad Coalition Consensus Statement on Treatment and Return to Play of the Female Athlete Triad: 1st International Conference held in San Francisco, California, May 2012 and 2nd International Conference held in Indianapolis, Indiana, May 2013. *British Journal of Sports Medicine*, 48(4): 289.

Desbrow, B., McCormack, J., Burke, L.M., Cox, G.R. Fallon, K., Hislop, M., Logan, R., Marino, N., Swayer, S.M., Shaw, G., Vidgen, H. and Leveritt, M. (2014). Sports Dietitians Australia position statement: sports nutrition for the adolescent athlete. *International Journal of Sports Nutrition and Exercise Metabolism*, 24(5): 570–84.

Drinkwater, B.L., Nilson, K., Ott, S. and Chesnut, C.H. 3rd. (1986). Bone mineral density after resumption of menses in amenorrheic athletes. *Journal of the American Medical Association*, 256(3): 380–2.

Dueck, C.A., Matt, K.S., Manore, M.M. and Skinner, J.S. (1996). Treatment of athletic amenorrhea with a diet and training intervention programmes. *International Journal of Sport Nutrition*, 6(1): 24–40.

Elliot, D.L., Goldberg, L., Moe, E.L., Defrancesco, C.A., Durham, M.B. and Hix-Small, H. (2004). Preventing substance use and disordered eating: initial outcomes of the ATHENA (athletes targeting healthy exercise and nutrition alternatives) programmes. *Archives of Pediatrics and Adolescent Medicine*, 158(11): 1043–9.

Fairburn, C.G. and Harrison, P.J. (2003). Eating disorders. *Lancet*. 361(9355): 407–16.

Ferrand, C. and Brunet, E. (2004). Perfectionism and risk for disordered eating among young French male cyclists of high performance. *Perceptual and Motor Skills*, 99(3 Pt1): 959–67.

Festinger, L. (1957). *A theory of cognitive dissonance*. Stanford, Calif.: Stanford University.

Galli, N., Petrie, T.A., Greenleaf, C., Reel, J.J. and Carter, J.E. (2014). Personality and psychological correlated of eating disorder symptoms among male collegiate athletes. *Eating Behaviours*, 15(4): 615–8.

Guebels, C.P., Cialdella-Kam, L., Maddalozzo, G. and Manore, M.M. (2011). REMEDY: Menstrual status and energy availability in active women. *Medicine and Science in Sports and Exercise*, 43(5): S47.

Hackney, A.C. (2008). Effects of endurance exercise on the reproductive system of men: the "exercise-hypogonadal male condition". *Journal of Endocrinological Investigation*, 31(10): 932–8.

Hilton, L.K. and Loucks, A.B. (2000). Low energy availability, not exercise stress, suppresses the diurnal rhythm of leptin in healthy young women. *American Journal of Physiology. Endocrinology and Metabolism*, 278(1): E43–9.

Hind, K., Truscott, J.G. and Evans, J.A. (2006). Low lumbar spine bone mineral density in both male and female endurance runners. *Bone*, 39(4): 880–5.

Hudson, J.L. and Pope Jr, H.G. (2007). Genetic epidemiology of eating disorders and co-occurring conditions: the role of endophenotypes. *The International Journal of Eating Disorders*, 40 (suppl): S76–78.

Ihle, R. and Loucks, A.B. (2004). Dose-response relationships between energy availability and bone turnover in young exercising women. *Journal of Bone Mineral Research*, 19(8): 1231–40.

International Ski Federation. www.fis-ski.com. Retrieved, 15 January, 2015.

Jacobi, C., Haward, C., de Zwaan, M., Kraemer, H.C. and Agras, W.S. (2004). Coming to terms with risk factors for eating disorders: application of risk terminology and suggestions for a general taxonomy. *Psychological Bulletin*, 130: 1965.

Johnson, C., Powers, P.S. and Dick, R. (1999). Athletes and eating disorders: the National Collegiate Athletic Association study. *The International Journal of Eating Disorders*, 26(2): 179–88.

Jones, L., Meyer, N.L. and Gibson, J.C. (2014). Weight management practices of 2012 Olympians in combat sports. *International Journal of Wrestling Science*, 4(1): 56–64.

Kiningham, R.B. and Gorenflo, D.W. (2001). Weight loss methods of high school wrestlers. *Medicine and Science in Sports and Exercise*, 33(5): 8ten to3.

Kopp-Woodroffe, S.A., Manore, M.M., Dueck, C.A., Skinner, J.S. and Matt, K.S. (1999). Energy and nutrient status of amenorrheic athletes participating in a diet and exercise training intervention programmes. *International Journal of Sport Nutrition*, 9(1): 70–88.

Lancha, Jr. A.H. (2010). Prevalence, magnitude, and methods of rapid weight loss among judo competitors. *Medicine and Science in Sports and Exercise*, 42(3): 436–42.

Leib, E.S. Lewiecki, E.M. Binkley, N. and Hamdy, R.C. (2004). International Society for Clinical Densitometry. Official positions of the International Society for Clinical Densitometry. *Journal of Clinical Densitometry*, 7(1): 1–6.

Leon, G.R. (1991). Eating disorders in female athletes. *Sports Medicine*, 12(4): 219–27.

Leslie, W.D., Adler, R.A., El-Hajj Fuleihan, G., Hodsman, A.B., Kendler, D.L., McClung, M., Miller, P.D. and Watts, N.B. (2006). International Society for Clinical Densitometry. Application of the 1994 WHO classification to populations other than postmenopausal Caucasian women: the 2005 ISCD Official Positions. *Journal of Clinical Densitometry*, 9(1): 22–30.

Lock, J., le Grange, D., Forsberg, S. and Hewell, K. (2006). Is family therapy useful for treating children with anorexia nervosa? Results of a case series. *Journal of the American Academy of Child and Adolescent Psychiatry*. 45(11): 1323–8.

Loucks, A., Kiens, B. and Wright, H. (2011). Energy availability in athletes. *Journal of Sports Sciences*, 29 Suppl 1: S7–15.

Loucks, A.B. (1990). Effects of exercise training on the menstrual cycle: existence and mechanisms. *Medicine and Science in Sports and Exercise*, 22(3): 275–80.

Loucks, A.B. (2001). Physical health of the female athlete: observations, effects, and causes of reproductive disorders. *Canadian Journal of Applied Physiology*, 26 Suppl: S176–85.

Loucks, A.B. (2003). Energy availability, not body fatness, regulates reproductive function in women. *Exercise and Sport Science Reviews*, 31(3): 144–8.

Loucks, A.B. and Heath, E.M. (1994). Dietary restriction reduces luteinizing hormone (LH) pulse frequency during waking hours and increases LH pulse amplitude during sleep in young menstruating women. *The Journal of Clinical Endocrinology and Metabolism*, 78(4): 9ten to5.

Loucks, A.B. and Thuma, J.R. (2003). Luteinizing hormone pulsatility is disrupted at a threshold of energy availability in regularly menstruating women. *The Journal of Clinical Endocrinology Metabolism*, 88(1): 297–311.

Loucks, A.B. and Verdun, M. (1998). Slow restoration of LH pulsatility by refeeding in energetically disrupted women. *American Journal of Physiology*, 275(4 Pt 2): R1218–26.

Loucks, A.B., Laughlin, G.A., Mortola, J.F., Girton, L., Nelson, J.C. and Yen, S.S. (1992). Hypothalamic-pituitary-thyroidal function in eumenorrheic and amenorrheic athletes. *The Journal of Clinical Endocrinology and Metabolism*, 75(2): 514–8.

Loucks, A.B., Vaitukaitis, J., Cameron, J.L., Rogol, A.D., Skrinar, G., Warren, M.P., Kendrick, J. and Limacher, M.C. (1992). The reproductive system and exercise in women. *Medicine and Science in Sports and Exercise*, 24(6 Suppl): S288–93.

Loucks, A.B., Verdun, M. and Heath, E.M. (1998). Low energy availability, not stress of exercise, alters LH pulsatility in exercising women. *Journal of Applied Physiology*, 84(1): 37–46.

Manore, M.M., Meyer, N.L. and Thompson, J. (2009). Nutrition for the female athlete. In *Sport Nutrition for Health and Performance*. Champaign Illinois: Human Kinetics, pp. 449–476.

Martinsen, M., Bahr, R., Børresen, R., Holme, I., Pensgaard, A.M. and Sundgot-Borgen, J. (2014). Preventing eating disorders among young elite athletes: a randomized controlled trial. *Medicine and Science in Sports and Exercise*, 46(3): 435–47.

Martinsen, M., Bratland-Sanda, S., Eriksson, A.K. and Sundgot-Borgen, J. (2010). Dieting to win or to be thin? A study of dieting and disordered eating among adolescent elite athletes and non–athlete controls. *British Journal of Sports Medicine*, 44: 70–76.

Martinsen, M., Sherman, R.T., Thompson, R.A. and Sundgot-Borgen, J. (2014). Coaches' knowledge and management of eating disorders: a randomized controlled trial. *Medicine and Science in Sports and exercise*, in press.

Melin, A., Tornberg, A.B., Skounby, S., Møller, S.S., Sundgot-Borgen, J., Faber, J., Sidelmann, J.J., Aziz, M. and Sjödin, A. (2014). Energy availability and the female athlete triad in elite endurance athletes. *Scandinavian Journal of Medicine and Science in Sports*, in press.

Mettler, S. Mitchell, N. and Tipton, K.D. (2010). Increased protein intake reduces lean body mass loss during weight loss in athletes. *Medicine and Science in Sports and Exercise*, 42(2): 326–37.

Meyer, N.L., Sundgot-Borgen, J., Lohman, T.G., Ackland, T.R., Stewart, A.D., Maughan, R. and Muller, W. (2013). Body composition for health and performance: a survey of body composition assessment practice carried out by the Ad Hoc Research Working Group on Body Composition, Health and Performance under the auspices of the IOC Medical Commission. *British Journal of Sports Medicine*, 47(16): 1044–53.

Mountjoy, M., Sundgot-Borgen, J., Burke, L., Carter, S., Constantini, N., Lebrun, C., Meyer, N., Sherman, R., Steffen, K., Budgett, R. and Ljungqvist, A. (2014). The IOC consensus statement: beyond the Female Athlete Triad-Relative Energy Deficiency in Sport (RED- S). *British Journal of Sports Medicine*, 48(7): 491–7.

Müller, W. (2009). Towards research-based approaches for solving body composition problems in sports: ski jumping as a heuristic example. *British Journal of Sports Medicine*, 43(13): 1013–9.

Müller, W., Gröschl, W., Müller, R. and Sudi, S. (2006). Underweight in ski jumping: The solution of the problem. *International Journal of Sports Medicine*, 27(11): 926–34.

Nattiv, A., Loucks, A.B., Manore, M.M., Sanborn, C.F., Sundgot-Borgen, J. and Warren, M.P. (2007). American College of Sports Medicine. American College of Sports Medicine position stand. The female athlete triad. *Medicine and Science in Sports and Exercise*, 39(10): 1867–82.

Neumark-Sztainer, D. and Eisenberg, M.E. (2014). Body image concerns, muscle-enhancing behaviours, and eating disorders in males. *Journal of the American Medical Association*, 26;312(20): 2156–7.

Neumark-Sztainer, D. and Hannan, P.J. (2000). Weight-related behaviours among adolescent girls and boys: results from a national survey. *Archives of Pediatrics and Adolescent Medicine*, 154(6): 569–77.

Neumark-Sztainer, D., Wall, M., Larson, N.I., Eisenberg, M.E. and Loth, K. (2011). Dieting and Disordered Eating Behaviours from Adolescence to young adulthood: Findings from a 10-year longitudinal study. *Journal of the American Dietetic Association*. Jul; 111(7): 1004–11.

Nicely, T.A., Lane-Loney, S., Masciulli, E., Hollenbeak, C.S. and Ornstein, R.M. (2014).Prevalence and characteristics of avoidant/restrictive food intake disorder in a cohort of young patients in day treatment for eating disorders. *Journal of Eating Disorders*, 2;2(1): 21.

Nieman, DC (2008). Immunonutrition support for athletes. *Nutrition Reviews*, 66(6): 3–20.

Nowicka P., Eli, K., Ng, J., Apitzsch, E. and Sundgot-Borgen, J. (2013). Moving from Knowledge to Action: A Qualitative Study of Elite Coaches' Capacity for Early Intervention in Cases of Eating Disorders. *International Journal of Sports Science and Coaching*, 2013: 8: 343–355.

Oppliger, R.A., Case, H.S., Horswill, C.A., Landry, G.L. and Shelter, A.C. (1996). American college of sports medicine position stand. Weight loss in wrestlers. *Medicine and Science in Sports and Exercise*, 28(6): ix–xii.

Oppliger, R.A., Utter, A.C., Scott, J.R., Dick, R.W. and Klossner, D. (2006). NCAA rule change improves weight loss among national championship wrestlers. *Medicine and Science in Sports and Exercise*, 38(5): 963–70.

Otis, C.L., Drinkwater, B., Johnson, M., Loucks, A. and Wilmore, J. (1997). American College of Sports Medicine position stand. The Female Athlete Triad. *Medicine and Science in Sports and Exercise*, 29(5): i–ix.

Petty, R.E. and Cacioppo, J.T. (1986). Communication and persuasion: central and peripheralroutes to attitude change. New York: Springer-Verlag

Phillips, S.M. and Van Loon, L.J. (2011). Dietary protein for athetes: from requirements to optimum adaptation. *Journal of Sports Sciences*. 29 Suppl 1: S29–38.

Pomeroy, C. and Mitchell, J.E. (1992). Medical issues in the eating disorders. In: Brownell K.D. Rodin J. and Wilmore J.H. (eds) *Eating, body weight, and performance in athletes: disorders of modern society*. Philadelphia, PA: Lea and Febiger, pp. 202–221.

Ranby, K.W., Aiken, L.S., Mackinnon, D.P., Elliot, D.L., Moe, E.L., McGinnis, W. and Goldberg, L. (2009). A mediation analysis of the ATHENA intervention for female athletes: prevention of athletic-enhancing substance use and unhealthy weight loss behaviours. *Journal of Pediatric Psychology*, 34(10): 1069–83.

Rickenlund, A., Eriksson, M.J., Schenck-Gustafsson, K. and Hirschberg, A.L. (2005). *The Journal of Clinical endocrinology and metabolism*, 90(3): 1354–9.

Riebl, S.K., Subudhi, A.W., Broker, J.P., Schenck, K. and Berning, J.R. (2007). The prevalence of subclinical eating disorders among male cyclists. *Journal of the American Dietetic Association*, 107(7): 1214–7.

Roemmich, J.N. and Sinning, W.E. (1997). Weight loss and wrestling training: effects ongrowth-related hormones. *Journal of Applied Physiology*, 82(6): 1760–4.

Rosendahl, J., Bormann, B., Aschenbrenner, K., Aschenbrenner, F. and Strauss, B. (2009). Dieting and disordered eating in German high school athletes and non-athletes. *Scandinavian Journal of Medicine and Science in Sports*, 19(5): 731–9.

Shaw, H., Stice, E. and Becker, C.B. (2009). Preventing eating disorders. *Child and Adolescent Psychiatric Clinics of North America*, 18(1): 199–207.

Stellingwerff, T., Maughan, R.J. and Burke, L.M. (2011). Nutrition for power sports: Middle-distance running, track cycling, rowing, canoeing/kayaking and swimming. *Journal of Sports Sciences*, 29 Suppl 1: S79–89.

Stewart, A.D. and Hannan, J. (2000). Total and regional bone density in male runners, cyclists, and controls. *Medicine and Science in Sports and Exercise*, 32(8): 1373–7.

Stice, E., Marti, C.N., Spoor, S., Presnell, K. and Shaw, H. (2008). Dissonance and healthy weight eating disorder prevention programmes: long-term effects from a randomized efficacy trial. *Journal of Consulting and Clinical Psychology*, 76(2): 329–40.

Sundgot-Borgen, J,, Meyer, N.L., Lohman, T.G., Ackland, T.R., Maughan, R.J., Stewart, A.D. and Müller, W. (2013). How to minimise the health risks to athletes who compete in weight-sensitive sports review and position statement on behalf of the Ad Hoc Research Working Group on Body Composition, Health and Performance, under the auspices of the IOC Medical Commission. *British Journal of Sports Medicine*, 47: 1012–1068.

Sundgot-Borgen, J. (1993). Prevalence of eating disorders in elite female athletes. *International Journal of Sport Nutrition*, 3(1): 29–40.

Sundgot-Borgen, J. (1994). Risk and trigger factors for the development of eating disorders in female elite athletes. *Medicine and Science in Sports and Exercise*, 26(4): 414–9.

Sundgot-Borgen, J. (1996). Eating disorders, energy intake, training volume, and menstrual function in high-level modern rhythmic gymnasts. *International Journal of Sport Nutrition*, 6(2): 100–9.

Sundgot-Borgen, J. and Torstveit, M.K. (2004). Prevalence of eating disorders in elite athletes is higher than in the general population. *Clinical Journal of Sport Medicine*, 14(1): 25–32.

Sundgot-Borgen, J. and Torstveit, M.K. (2010). Aspects of disordered eating continuum in elite high-intensity sports. *Scandinavian Journal of Medicine and Science in Sports*, 20 Suppl 2: 112–21.

Tarnopolsky, M.A., Cipriano, N., Woodcroft, C., Pulkkinen, W.J., Robinson, D.C., Henderson, J.M. and MacDougall, J.D. (1996). Effects of rapid weight loss and wrestling on muscle glycogen concentration. *Clinical Journal of Sport Medicine*, 6(2): 78–84.

Thompson, R.A. and Sherman, R.T. *Eating disorders in sport.* New York: Routledge, 2010.

Torstveit, M.K. and Sundgot-Borgen, J. (2005). The female athlete triad: are elite athletes at increased risk? *Medicine and Science in Sports and Exercise*, 37(2): 184–193.

Treasure, J., Claudino, A.M. and Zucker, N. (2010). Eating disorders. *Lancet*, 13;375(9714): 583–93.

Viitasalo, J.T., Kyröläinen, H., Bosco, C. and Alen, M. (1987). Effects of rapid weight reduction on force production and vertical jumping height. *International Journal of Sports Medicine*, 8(4): 281–5.

Von Holle, A., Pinehiro, A.P. and Thornton, L.M. (2008). Temporal patterns of recovery across eating disorder subtypes. *Aust N Z J Psychiatry*, 42: 108–117.

Weimann, E., Witzel, C., Schwidergall, S. and Böhles, H.J. (2000). Peripubertal perturbations in elite gymnasts caused by sport specific training regimes and inadequate nutritional intake. *International Journal of Sports Medicine*, 21(3): 2ten to5.

World Health Organization (WHO). (1994). Assessment of fracture risk and its application to screening for postmenopausal osteoporosis: report of WHO study group technical report series 843. Geneva, Switzerland: WHO technical report series 843: 6.

Yeager, K.K., Agostini, R., Nattiv, A. and Drinkwater, B. (1993). The female athlete triad: disordered eating, amenorrhea, osteoporosis. *Medicine and Science in Sports and Exercise*, 25(7): 77.

39

EVERYDAY DISTORTIONS

Youth sport and body images

Michael Gard

I have hundreds, perhaps thousands of bodies. There is the body that confronts me at close quarters in the bathroom mirror first thing in the morning and, miraculously changed, last thing at night. There is the altogether more pleasing body that appears in softer lighting and at a slightly greater distance. My body appears to me as a different thing depending on whether it is dressed, half-dressed or naked and different again when clothed in each of the combinations that my wardrobe allows. All of the bodies I have been – thinner, fatter, younger, older, darker, more pale, sick, healthy – still live with me too. In fact, the memories of my body are utterly present in my life; in my mind, my photographs, the clothes that no longer fit. My body can change radically from moment to moment; pleasingly proportioned when I approach my reflection with deliberate forethought, unsettlingly unfamiliar when I catch a glimpse of it unexpectedly.

What do these bodies mean? Who are they? My body has been a sporting body for almost as long as I can remember being aware of it and it is partly on this premise that I propose in this chapter to explore some of the ways in which body images effect, govern and result from the involvement of young people in sport and physical activity. Although this has the potential to be a comfortingly theoretical and abstract exercise, there is another reason to think about body images: via a consideration of bodies *as images* we enrich our understanding of what they mean and who they are. In particular, my contention will be that the body images generated by and associated with sport and physical activity are now a dominant, perhaps pre-eminent, cultural economy through which young bodies are understood, experienced and consumed. In fact, by focusing on body images, sport and physical activity cease being what they are commonly assumed to be: health enhancing exercise, athletic competition or recreation.

Distorted images

It is now something of an academic orthodoxy to complain about the way psychologistic concerns with young women and eating disorders have monopolised 'body image' discourse (e.g., Probyn, 2009). While it is self-evident that there is more to the subject than the psychology of anorexia, the idea of the distorted body image is worth clarifying, if only for the comparisons it invites. According to Slade (1994), 'body image' first appeared as a significant subject of psychological inquiry in Paul Schilder's landmark work *The Image and Appearance of the Human Body*, first published in English in 1935. Drawing on neurophysiology, psychiatry, psychoanalysis and sociology, Schilder was concerned with a wide variety of somatic phenomena including apparent distortions in the way patients experienced and perceived the dimensions and appearance of their own body. Later, and with specific focus on anorexia, disordered eating and obesity, the American psychoanalyst Hilde Bruch laid much of the foundation for modern body image research by describing in great detail the personalities of patients. In her 1962 paper *Perceptual and conceptual disturbances in anorexia nervosa*, Bruch diagnosed twelve anorexia nervosa patients as manifesting both perceptual and conceptual disturbances; a delusionally distorted perception of their own bodily form and nutritional needs alongside what Bruch called 'an all-pervading sense of ineffectiveness' (p. 187) – an idea that would be translated into the language of 'low self-esteem' in following decades (see also Bruch, 1981, for a synopsis of her life's work in this area published shortly before her death in 1984).

In general terms, these lines of scholarship have filtered through to the present as a dual interest in the way bodies are perceived and evaluated, although a number of Bruch's conclusions have been questioned. For example, Slade (1994) pointed out that the propensity to overestimate one's body size is widespread among Western females and may not even be useful for diagnostic purposes. What this means, among other things, is that a distorted body image may actually be somewhat 'normal' and that severe or life-threatening eating disorders probably have a variety of proximate and ultimate causes, which may or may not include a distorted body image. If nothing else this allows us to see that bodies are not always, if ever, 'seen as they are'. As Slade (p. 502) writes: 'Body image is best viewed as a "loose mental representation of the body's shape, form and size", which is influenced by a variety of historical, cultural and social, individual and biological factors, which operate over varying timespans.'

Concern with the connections between sport, physical activity and young people on the one hand, and the psychology of disordered eating and distorted body images on the other, will be familiar enough to many readers. For example, a significant body of research has confirmed that young female ballet dancers appear to be more likely to dislike their body than young male ballet dancers or young people who are not dancers (Bettle *et al.*, 2001; Ravaldi *et al.*, 2006) and to misperceive the dimensions of their body (Pierce and Daleng, 1998).

Ballet is a particularly vexing and complex context for the study of body image. Perhaps more than any other codified movement form, practitioners are asked to pursue bodily ideals that have changed only slightly over preceding centuries. In a sense, the weight of history and tradition bears down on the way the dancers see, experience, evaluate and work on their bodies. For young females in particular, the idealised imagery of the sylph, the strictly defined gender roles and the ethos of perfectionism that pervades professional preparation, all invite a perpetual hostility to bodily imperfection especially in the form of body fat (for a detailed discussion see Novack, 1993). In turn, this implies that young female ballet dancers are more likely than their general population peers to develop overly restrictive or unhealthy food and eating practices, a proposition for which there is a significant body of supporting data (Abraham, 1996; Brickell, 1996; Ringham *et al.*, 2006). In fact, the assumed association between young female ballet dancers and disordered eating is so strong that a number of studies have directly compared the eating behaviours and body image distortion of dancers with anorexia patients (Meermann, 1983; Urdapilleta *et al.*, 2007).

Although comparisons are difficult, it is tempting to wonder whether ballet is perhaps only a more extreme example of a phenomenon that extends to competitive sports such as gymnastics and long distance running. In their study of eating disorders (EDs) among athletes, for example, Sundgot-Borgen and Torstveit (2004, p. 25) found: 'The prevalence of EDs is higher in athletes than in controls, higher in female athletes than in male athletes, and more common among those competing in leanness-dependent and weight-dependent sports than in other sports.' However, studies with young female gymnasts have tended not to report particularly high levels of body image distortion, body dissatisfaction or disordered eating (de Bruin, Oudejans and Bakker, 2007). Salbach *et al.* (2006) found only slightly elevated levels of disordered eating and body image distortion among teenage female rhythmic gymnasts.

Further afield the picture is predictably complex. Some research findings suggest that athletes in general feel *more* positively about their bodies that non-athletes (Hausenblas and Downs, 2001) while literature reviews tend to report only slightly elevated eating disorder prevalence and risk (which includes body image distortion) among female athletes from a range of sports (Byrne and McLean, 2001). At the same time, the literature is also sprinkled with findings that caution against underestimating the reach and impact of the image of the lean female body in competitive sports. For example, a relatively recent study found an eating disorder prevalence of 42 per cent among 138 U.S. Division 1 college level female equestrian riders and that: 'overall, participants perceived their body images as significantly larger than their actual physical sizes (self-reported BMI) and wanted to be significantly smaller in both normal clothing and competitive uniforms' (Torres-McGehee *et al.*, 2011, p. 431).

The purpose of the preceding discussion has not been to explain or estimate the prevalence of disordered eating, anorexia, body image distortion or particular psychological profiles among young female athletes. The research literature concerned with anorexia *per se*, for example, is voluminous and marked by divergent theoretical and empirical agendas. What we can say here, though, is that looking at sport and physical activity via the concept of body image unsettles straightforward assumptions about their 'healthiness'. In various ways, the moving female body comes to us pre-coded with meaning, expectation and bodily practices. In the case of ballet, a canon of barely distinguishable famous ballerinas inhabit the life-world of the aspiring dancer as much as the here-and-now practices – both healthy and unhealthy – intended to replicate ballet's cherished body images. It is true, of course, that ballet is its own kind of thing; both a specific and variable set of ideas and practices that more or less overlap with the ideas and practices of other codified movement traditions. The point, however, is that the *images* of bodies matter and exert a certain kind of agency on the lives of people who choose to participate in these traditions. Whether or not the force of these images leads to low self-esteem or disordered eating or anorexia is somewhat beside the point although there can surely be no doubt that the single-minded pursuit of bodies that look and perform in a particular way invites, if not demands, elaborate systems of internal and external surveillance. Because humans are variable, the effect of these systems of surveillance will also be variable and not always amenable to the vagaries of empirical study and parametric statistics. To go back to my introductory meditation on my own body, just because I feel good about the shape of my body today does not mean that I will feel the same way tomorrow. That an athlete or dancer circles a particular number on a psychological survey instrument rather than another number does not alter the near certainty that they all must continually encounter, evaluate and respond to the images of their own body and those of their peers, both living and dead.

The sporting body

Moving from a predominantly psychological register to the material practices of sport, I want now to develop the point I have just made, in passing, about the *agency* of sporting body images. It is self-evident that only certain kinds of bodies are welcome and can be successful in competitive sport. This is a matter with obvious equity implications. In the cases of the two South African runners Caster Semanya and Oscar Pistorius, the presence of genitally ambiguous (Semanya) and disabled (Pistorius) bodies appears to have presented mainstream elite sport with irresolvable questions. That is, which bodies are allowed to play and which are not? However, this is a related but separate matter from the kinds of bodies that sports produce and privilege.

To make this point more concrete, consider the work of the Australian researchers Tim Olds and Kevin Norton who analysed the anthropometric evolution of athletes in a range of sports during the twentieth century (Norton and Olds, 2001; Olds, 2001). Drawing on the available historical evidence, they describe how body size evolution among athletes in some sports far outstrips the secular trends recorded in the general populations and, in other sports, relative stasis. For example, in open sports like American football, rugby union and rugby league, the body mass of elite players became increasingly atypical as the twentieth century progressed. As more money came into these sports, the bodies of elite players grew heavier, more muscular and more unlike the populations from which they were drawn. In fact Olds (2001) presents data that suggest that in the latter part of the century the collective mass of international male rugby union teams correlated closely with their world ranking; the bigger, the better. There is, of course, a list of probable reasons for these changes including the globalisation of the talent pool, evolving training methods and the use of pharmacological substances that promote muscularity. Perhaps just as important, all three of these vigorous body contact sports have adopted rule changes – such as larger game-day squads, greater player interchanging and more compulsory stoppages in play – that were either deliberately or inadvertently favourable to larger players.

Olds and Norton (2001) report a similar phenomenon in elite male running, at least in the shorter events. Like football players, the bodies of male sprinters, both black and white, have grown heavier and more muscular. This is in complete contrast with runners in long distance events such as the 5000 metres, 10,000 metres and the marathon where the morphology of the most successful distance runners displays a particularly small amount of variation over time.

Although this kind of historical work has been relatively rare in the science of exercise and sports, Olds and Norton's work reflects a growing interest among researchers in the dimensions of the athletic body and its relationship to sports performance. Published in 1996, their textbook *Anthropometrica* (Norton and Olds, 1996) can be seen as the culmination of the twentieth century's increasing fascination with the measurement and production of sporting bodies. To put the point somewhat crudely, while particular kinds of bodies were previously seen as the *result* of sports participation, the sports and exercises sciences have gradually reversed the equation; sports performance now needs to be seen as dependent on selecting or producing particular kinds of bodies.

With respect to the sporting experiences of young people, it is absolutely clear that this new scientistic orientation to the shape and dimensions of sporting bodies has been consequential. The literature attests to both the breadth of sports in which the anthropometrical analysis of young athletes is seen to be worth knowing (for two examples from a large literature see Duncan, Woodfield and Al-Nakeeb, 2006; Ugarkovic *et al.*, 2002). Closer to the concerns of this chapter, the anthropometry literature includes many studies in which both the dimensions and composition of young athletes' bodies are presumed to be *predictive* of athletic success (Arrese and Ostáriz, 2006; Hoare, 2000). Once again, while there are dangers in glibly glossing the psychology of entire scientific fields, we can say that there is a pervasive view that the right kind of body is a prerequisite even for young athletes. Most obvious, the field of junior talent identification exists primarily because it is assumed that success in some sports – particularly (but not only) relatively 'closed' sports like rowing, swimming and track and field – is a matter of morphology as much it is of, say, skill or intrinsic interest in the sport.

It seems reasonable to assume that belief in the primacy of morphology will vary across the contexts in which junior athletes are selected and trained. Nonetheless, there is compelling evidence that young athletes are regularly subjected to questionable, misguided and damaging forms of bodily scrutiny and intervention. In their review article into the relationship between involvement in athletics and disordered eating, Thompson and Trattner Sherman (1999) concluded that many coaches of young athletes emphasise the reduction of body fat as a primary coaching goal. McMahon and her colleagues have produced a series of papers exploring the apparent preoccupation with body fat measurements among coaches of young elite Australian swimmers (McMahon and Dinan-Thompson, 2011; McMahon and Penney, 2013). In particular, this work highlights the agency of body images to demonise body fat, drive coaching practices and shape the identities and self-surveilling practices of young female swimmers and the women they will later become. Porter *et al.* (2013) have also described the detailed and highly self-critical ideas about body image used by a group 11–13-year-old female swimmers to talk about themselves and the 'look of success'. In a more biographical vein, Jones *et al.* (2005) in swimming and Zanker and Gard (2008) in long distance running have studied the stories of individual women and the apparent role played by coaches to feed a preoccupation with rigid bodily ideals.

At the other end of the morphological spectrum, some young athletes, notably sprinters, are confronted with bodily ideals that emphasise muscularity, a phenomenon that is probably being fed by the anthropometric evolution of sprinters' bodies described above. The young female college sprinters interviewed in Mosewich *et al.'s* (2009) study, for example, described the struggles associated with trying to live a healthy life while negotiating the competing expectations that they develop high levels of muscularity and low levels of body fat.

Of course, any discussion of muscularity and body image in sport leads inevitably to the subject of the widespread use of 'steroids' and other pharmacological body building agents, particularly among male athletes. While on a purely conceptual level we might think it important to make a distinction between doping that is intended to increase an athlete's chances of success and doping designed to produce a morphological goal or ideal, scholars have generally seen the two as interrelated. In their paper 'Doping among adolescent athletes', Yesalis and Bahrke (2000, p. 25) claim that 'the demand for performance-enhancing drugs [among adolescents] has been created by our societal fixation on winning and physical appearance'. The role of body images in this context is all the more intriguing given long standing questions over whether and to what extent substances such as anabolic steroids actually improve sports and exercise performance. Once again, the possibility emerges that changing ideas about what an athlete should look like, rather than what they can do, shape not only the experience of being a young athlete but the symbolic meaning and economic value of the sporting body image, matters to which we now turn.

The democratisation of distortion

In the context of Olds and Norton's work on the evolution of sporting bodies, it is interesting that less is known about the evolving morphology of players in the most globally popular of all the football codes, association football or soccer. One study has reported that professional soccer players may have generally grown heavier and taller, although it also found that tallness in soccer forwards is likely to be coupled with a more linear physique (Nevill *et al.*, 2009). Despite the relative scarcity of data, it is clear enough that because they do not have to endure the intense and repeated collisions found in other high profile football codes, elite soccer players exhibit comparatively lower body mass and muscularity. In fact, heavy muscularity would be a distinct disadvantage given that most players are expected to be mobile for long periods without the possibility of being rotated on and off the reserves bench. Nonetheless, with the world's major leagues now drawing in players from all over the world, particularly Africa, a chiselled muscular ideal has emerged. In an odd twist on the sauntering cat-walk model, players now regularly remove their shirt at the end of games for no apparent reason other than to parade in front of hungry cameras. The same happens in international athletics. In fact, in such a hurry are they, it is now commonplace for male sprinters to begin removing the top half of their running suits as soon as they cross the finishing line and well before they have even stopped running. The practice, which has spread to many other sports, seems to say a number of things: not simply *look at me* but *desire me* and *envy me*.

Changes in the morphology of some athletes have coincided – perhaps as part cause, part effect – with the increasing commodification and eroticisation of the sporting body (Rahman, 2011). In fact, we can say that the lean, muscular bodies of male and female athletes are an important part of the product range that highly commercialised sports like football and international athletics sell. From glossy wall calendars to celebrity gossip magazines and the advertisements for the sports themselves, we are invited to consume, perhaps even worship, the images and bodily exploits of athletes. When muscular athletes display their bodies to the world they are, among other things, advertising themselves. They know that their performances and their bodies are assets to be commercially exploited (Kane, LaVoi and Fink, 2013). But these bodies have also become discursive magnets, attracting and mashing together ideas about health, physical beauty and desirability. These are bodies that command authority *as images*. As images they can be used to do almost anything; sell products, launch public health campaigns, raise money for charity and symbolise both moral virtue and sexual power.

Little wonder then that the pursuit of an idealised muscular body shape has become one of the primary reasons why many young people participate in physical activity at all. Once again, it is the image that appears to sit at the heart of things. There is, for example, a growing body of research that documents the way young people – including school-age children – combine steroids and other doping agents with the exercise they do in pursuit of the body image they want for themselves (Faigenbaum *et al.*, 1998). In fact, writing in *The Lancet*, Sjöqvist *et al.* (2008) described steroid use among recreational exercisers and sportsmen and women as a serious public health concern. Needless to say, researchers have also explored body image distortion and disordered eating among recreational gymnasium users and body-builders (Ravaldi *et al.*, 2003).

The spread of the muscular ideal from professional sports to celebrity culture and the general public raises an interesting theoretical question that takes us back to the discussion of body image distortion that began this chapter: what should be our attitude be to people who vigorously pursue bodily transformation through exercise, perhaps to the detriment of some aspects of their health? Are they abnormal or suffering from a distorted body image? After all, the potential population of young people we might now be talking about is potentially very large. To take just one example, Jong (2015) has documented the remarkable popularity of online fitness communities in which young women appear to expend a great deal of time and energy exchanging information about exercise routines and diets. What is most striking about these communities is the role of images of very lean, muscular bodies. For example, participants generate and circulate thousands of images of their own often headless bodies on social media. The communities are also dominated by celebrity fitness gurus who use images of their ripped bodies to attract followers and generate markets for the diet and training advice that they sell. According to Jong, the popularity of diets and training programs in online fitness communities often *begins* with the image that is attached to them; body images, in other words, appear to be both the catalyst for and the currency of these communities. Should anyone be concerned about this activity? Is it unhealthy to desire an extreme body?

Likewise, *Boys and the buff culture* (ABC, 2012), an Australian Broadcasting Commission radio documentary, described the importance of body images in the body modification practices of young Australian men. Many of the young men interviewed described intensive weight lifting training, steroid use and tattooing as a way to give them more confidence when pursuing sexual partners. They also explicitly linked the popularity of tattooing to the images of heavily tattooed athletes. In fact, some young men clearly felt that women found the combination of muscles and tattoos irresistible and that this look had been mainstreamed primarily via the media images of football players. Similar to Jong's research into online fitness communities, the documentary highlighted the importance celebrity bodybuilders such as the Russian-born Australian Aziz Shavershian – better known as *Zyzz* – whose image appears to have been the cornerstone of his large internet fan base. For his part, Shavershian claimed to be an advocate for exercise and healthy living, despite lingering suspicions about his steroid use. Shavershian's subsequent death, aged just 22, created a heated debate about the healthiness or otherwise of the obsession with bodily perfection for which he became an icon.

Whatever else we might say about these behaviours, they are surely not inconsistent with Bordo's diagnosis of what she called anorectic Western culture (Bordo, 2003). That is, the differences between the seriously body conscious gym goer, the anorexic and the steroid user may only be of degree. On the other hand, presumably only a minority of the people, young and not so young, who participate in these sub-cultures is likely to be harmed, in the same way that we would not prevent a young woman becoming a ballet dancer simply because ballet dancers may be over-represented in the population of people suffering from disordered eating or anorexia.

At the very least, it is important to at least register the point that sport and physical activity are, for many young people, exercises in body image management. Certainly modern elite sport is nothing if not an exercise in the creation and curation of idealised bodies for public consumption. As such, sporting bodies participate in the body image economies that each of us is immersed in. For Weiss (1999; 2013), one of the enduring problems with body image research, including much of the research I have cited in this chapter, is its tendency to see body image 'as a cohesive, coherent phenomenon that operates in a fairly uniform way in our everyday existence' (2013, p. 1). In fact, in the psychological literature it is common to diagnose the sporting or dancing anorexic as somebody who lacks a clear and precise body image of themselves; because their body is in a state of constant flux they have struggled to arrive at a sense of what their body really looks like. In complete contrast, Weiss argues that we need to dispense with the idea of a person's body *image*, and instead think of 'a multiplicity of body images, body images that are copresent in any given individual, and which are themselves constructed through a series of corporeal exchanges that take place both within and outside of specific bodies' (2013, p. 2). In fact, Weiss claims that it is 'precisely the lack of *destabilization* in the anorexic's body image that is the source of its deadly destructiveness' (1999, p. 54, italics in original). To put this another way, Weiss thinks that each of us is engaged in a process of distortion whereby we see, construct, imagine, reject and desire different kinds of bodies for ourselves. Drawing on the psychoanalytic and poststructuralist theorising of Kristeva, Grosz and Butler, Weiss's point is that none of us could ever bear to live with an accurate image of our bodies as they are and that normal life involves the constant *othering* of the abject bodies that haunt us. For Weiss, the problem comes when the images we have of ourselves become excessively coherent and singular. She writes:

> For the nonpathological subject, I would argue, it is the very multiplicity of these body images that guarantees that we cannot invest too heavily in any one of them,

and these multiple body images themselves offer points of resistance to the development of too strong an identification with a singularly alienating specular (or even cultural) image. That is, these multiple body images serve to destabilize the hegemony of any particular body image ideal, and are precisely what allows us to maintain a sense of corporeal fluidity.

(Weiss, 1999, p. 54)

As the elite ends of competitive sports became more professional during the twentieth century, the bodies playing them became more specialised, more atypical and – within each particular sport – more uniform. At the same time as sporting labour was becoming more divided, scientists set themselves the task of discovering the ideal body for each sporting job. A similar thing happened, I would argue, in the world of professional dance; as each of its sub-fields (such as ballet, modern, jazz) matured as art forms, idiosyncratic bodies were chased from the stage. With more professionalism, more training institutions and more competition for paying jobs, employers were increasingly free to choose only those dancers whose bodies most closely matched the ideal. For aspiring young athletes and dancers, these changes have meant increasing pressure to specialise earlier in life, the physical and psychological dangers of which have been highlighted at some length (e.g., Baker *et al.*, 2009).

When scholars and other commentators talk about 'body image' and the darker sides of young people's involvement in sport, dance, gym culture and other physically demanding forms of physical activity, discussion tends to focus on the supposedly damaged psychology of the participant or particular 'unhealthy' practices within the specific field of activity. If the body image theorist Gail Weiss wrote about sport, which to my knowledge she does not, I think she would direct our attention instead to the kind of things professional (and increasingly recreational) forms of physical activity have been turned into body factories. It is not so much that a great deal of demanding work needs to go into producing these bodies, a fact that has its own risks and rewards. Rather, both by accident and design, the spectrum of acceptable bodies within and across fields of activity has been radically narrowed. Not only have we elevated the body image to a perplexing level of hyper-sexual, quasi-religious seriousness, we have done so with peculiarly twentieth century scientific precision.

Reclaiming a degree of playful fluidity about bodies will be all the more tricky given public health's escalating global war on obesity. Perhaps part of the solution here is to restore a degree of playfulness to physical activity itself, a development that would probably be financially negative for industrial physical activity like professional sports that rely on its consumers treating it with melodramatic earnestness. For the rest of us though, particularly young people, a little more psychic breathing space and bodily choice may at least be worth a try.

References

ABC (2012) Boys and buff culture. Radio documentary for the *Background Briefing* programme broadcast on ABC Radio National 1/1/2012.

Abraham, S. (1996). Eating and weight controlling behaviours of young ballet dancers. *Psychopathology*, *29*(4), 218–22.

Arrese, A. L. and Ostáriz, E. S. (2006). Skinfold thicknesses associated with distance running performance in highly trained runners. *Journal of Sports Sciences*, *24*(1), 69–76.

Baker, J., Cobley, S. and Fraser_Thomas, J. (2009). What do we know about early sport specialization? Not much! *High Ability Studies*, *20*(1), 77–89.

Bettle, N., Bettle, O., Neumarker, U. and Neumarker, K. J. (2001). Body image and self-esteem in adolescent ballet dancers. *Perceptual and Motor Skills*, *93*(1), 297–309.

Bordo, S. (2003). *Unbearable Weight: Feminism, Western Culture, and the Body*. University of California Press.

Brickell, T. (1996). Anorexia and bulimia: a ballet perspective. *The ACHPER Healthy Lifestyles Journal* 43(3): 17–22.

Bruch, H. (1962). Perceptual and conceptual disturbances in anorexia nervosa. *Psychosomatic Medicine*, 24(2), 187–194.

Bruch, H. (1981) Developmental considerations of anorexia nervosa and obesity. *The Canadian Journal of Psychiatry/La Revue Canadienne de Psychiatrie*, 26(4), 212–217.

Byrne, S. and McLean, N. (2001). Eating disorders in athletes: a review of the literature. *Journal of Science and Medicine in Sport*, 4(2), 145–159.

de Bruin, A. K., Oudejans, R. R. and Bakker, F. C. (2007). Dieting and body image in aesthetic sports: A comparison of Dutch female gymnasts and non-aesthetic sport participants. *Psychology of Sport and Exercise*, 8(4), 507–520.

Duncan, M. J., Woodfield, L. and Al-Nakeeb, Y. (2006). Anthropometric and physiological characteristics of junior elite volleyball players. *British Journal of Sports Medicine*, 40(7), 649–651.

Faigenbaum, A. D., Zaichkowsky, L. D., Gardner, D. E. and Micheli, L. J. (1998). Anabolic steroid use by male and female middle school students. *Pediatrics*, 101(5), e6–e6.

Hausenblas, H. A. and Downs, D. S. (2001). Comparison of body image between athletes and nonathletes: A meta-analytic review. *Journal of Applied Sport Psychology*, 13(3), 323–339.

Hoare, D. G. (2000). Predicting success in junior elite basketball players—the contribution of anthropometic and physiological attributes. *Journal of Science and Medicine in Sport*, 3(4), 391–405.

Jones, R. L. Glintmeyer, N. and McKenzie, A. (2005). Slim Bodies, Eating Disorders and the Coach-Athlete Relationship A Tale of Identity Creation and Disruption. *International Review for the Sociology of Sport*, 40(3), 377–391.

Jong. S. (2015). Online fitness communities and health literacies: Critical digital awareness. Paper presented at the ACHPER National Conference, 13–15 April 2015 Prince Alfred College, Adelaide, South Australia.

Kane, M. J., LaVoi, N. M. and Fink, J. S. (2013). Exploring elite female athletes' interpretations of sport media images: A window into the construction of social identity and 'selling sex' in women's sports. *Communication and Sport*, DOI: 10.1177/2167479512473585.

McMahon, J. and Dinan-Thompson, M. (2011). 'Body work—regulation of a swimmer body': an autoethnography from an Australian elite swimmer. *Sport, Education and Society*, 16(1), 35–50.

McMahon, J. A. and Penney, D. (2013). (Self-) surveillance and (self-) regulation: living by fat numbers within and beyond a sporting culture. *Qualitative Research in Sport, Exercise and Health*, 5(2), 157–178.

Meermann, R. (1983). Experimental investigation of disturbances in body image estimation in anorexia nervosa patients, and ballet and gymnastics pupils. *International Journal of Eating Disorders*, 2(4), 91–100.

Mosewich, A. D., Vangool, A. B., Kowalski, K. C. and McHugh, T. L. F. (2009). Exploring women track and field athletes' meanings of muscularity. *Journal of Applied Sport Psychology*, 21(1), 99–115.

Nevill, A., Holder, R. and Watts, A. (2009). The changing shape of "successful" professional footballers. *Journal of Sports Sciences*, 27(5), 419–426.

Norton, K. and Olds, T. (eds). (1996). *Anthropometrica: A Textbook of Body Measurement for Sports and Health Courses*. Sydney, UNSW Press.

Norton, K. and Olds, T. (2001). Morphological evolution of athletes over the twentieth century. *Sports Medicine*, 31(11), 763–783.

Novack, C. (1993). Ballet, gender and cultural power. *Dance, Gender and Culture*. H. Thomas. London, Macmillan: 34–48.

Olds, T. (2001). The evolution of physique in male rugby union players in the twentieth century. *Journal of Sports Sciences*, 19(4), 253–262.

Pierce, E. F. and Daleng, M. L. (1998). Distortion of body image among elite female dancers. *Perceptual and Motor Skills*, 87(3), 769–770.

Porter, R. R., Morrow, S. L. and Reel, J. J. (2013). Winning looks: body image among adolescent female competitive swimmers. *Qualitative Research in Sport, Exercise and Health*, 5(2), 179–195.

Probyn, E. (2009). Fat, feelings, bodies: a critical approach to obesity. *Critical Feminist Approaches to Eating Disorders*. H. Malson and M. Burns. London, Routledge: 113–123.

Ravaldi, C., Vannacci, A., Bolognesi, E., Mancini, S., Faravelli, C. and Ricca, V. (2006). Gender role, eating disorder symptoms, and body image concern in ballet dancers. *Journal of psychosomatic research*, 61(4), 529–535.

Ravaldi, C., Vannacci, A., Zucchi, T., Mannucci, E., Cabras, P., L., Boldrini, M., Murciano, L., Rotella, C. M. and Ricca, V. (2003). Eating disorders and body image disturbances among ballet dancers, gymnasium users and body builders. *Psychopathology*, 36(5), 247–254.

Rahman, M. (2011). The burdens of the flesh: star power and the queer dialectic in sports celebrity. *Celebrity Studies, 2*(2), 150–163.

Ringham, R., Klump, K., Kaye, W., Stone, D., Libman, S., Stowe, S. and Marcus, M. (2006). Eating disorder symptomatology among ballet dancers. *International Journal of Eating Disorders, 39*(6), 503–508.

Salbach, H., Klinkowski, N., Pfeiffer, E., Lehmkuhl, U. and Korte, A. (2006). Body image and attitudinal aspects of eating disorders in rhythmic gymnasts. *Psychopathology, 40*(6), 388–393.

Schilder, P. (1935). *The Image and appearance of the Human Body: Studies in the Constructive Energies of the Psyche*. London: Kegan Paul.

Slade, P. D. (1994). What is body image? *Behaviour Research and Therapy 32*(5): 497–502.

Sjöqvist, F., Garle, M. and Rane, A. (2008). Use of doping agents, particularly anabolic steroids, in sports and society. *The Lancet, 371*(9627), 1872–1882.

Sundgot-Borgen, J. and Torstveit, M. K. (2004). Prevalence of eating disorders in elite athletes is higher than in the general population. *Clinical Journal of Sport Medicine, 14*(1), 25–32.

Thompson, R. A. and Trattner Sherman, R. (1999). Athletes, athletic performance, and eating disorders: Healthier alternatives. *Journal of Social Issues, 55*(2), 317–337.

Torres-McGehee, T. M., Monsma, E. V., Gay, J. L., Minton, D. M. and Mady-Foster, A. N. (2011). Prevalence of eating disorder risk and body image distortion among National Collegiate Athletic Association Division I varsity equestrian athletes. *Journal of Athletic Training, 46*(4), 431–437.

Ugarkovic, D., Matavulj, D., Kukolj, M. and Jaric, S. (2002). Standard anthropometric, body composition, and strength variables as predictors of jumping performance in elite junior athletes. *The Journal of Strength and Conditioning Research, 16*(2), 227–230.

Urdapilleta, I., Cheneau, C., Masse, L. and Blanchet, A. (2007). Comparative study of body image among dancers and anorexic girls. *Eating and Weight Disorders-Studies on Anorexia, Bulimia and Obesity, 12*(3), 140–146.

Weiss, G. (1999). The abject borders of the body image. *Perspectives on Embodiment: The Intersections of Nature and Culture*. G. Weiss and H. F. Haber. New York, Routledge: 41–59.

Weiss, G. (2013). *Body Images: Embodiment as Intercorporeality*. New York, Routledge.

Yesalis, C. E. and Bahrke, M. S. (2000). Doping among adolescent athletes. *Best Practice and Research: Clinical Endocrinology and Metabolism, 14*(1), 25–35.

Zanker, C. and Gard, M. (2008). Fatness, fitness, and the moral universe of sport and physical activity. *Sociology of Sport Journal, 25*(1), 48.

40

YOUTH SPORT, CIGARETTES, ALCOHOL AND ILLICIT DRUGS

Patrick Peretti-Watel, Fabrice Lorenté and Laurent Grélot

Introduction

Does sport participation prevent young people using licit and illicit drugs? The answer is far from simple, as *sport participation* and *drug use* are vague notions referring to eminently heterogeneous behaviours. In the present chapter, our aim is to illustrate the complexity of the sports–drugs relationship during youth, the necessity to take into account the context and the characteristics of sports participation as well as youths' motives, and the variety of possible interpretations.

First, we will discuss the so-called deterrence hypothesis that gives an unreserved positive answer to the question above. Subsequent sections will illustrate how sports participation may either facilitate drug use, cause it or simply go with it. Regardless which type of sport is practised, sports participation is a social activity involving social control and socialisation issues that frame opportunities and motives to use drugs; orientation toward competition and success may also encourage drug use among young athletes; finally, sports participation and drug use may be driven by similar motives or values, such as impulses for sensation-seeking.

The deterrence hypothesis: a dubious myth?

For a long time, sport has been considered as a panacea for almost all youth problems. According to the so-called deterrence hypothesis, sports participation provides social and human capital that may reduce the likelihood of involvement in deviant and/or risky behaviours (Eitle *et al.*, 2003). For example, young people who practise a sport are supposed to socialise, to channel their violence and thus are not likely to participate in criminal activities (Carmichael, 2008), to enhance some crucial individual capabilities (such as self-esteem, self-efficacy, self-discipline, tenacity and the taste for effort, etc.), to learn some fundamental values (such as fairness, tolerance and solidarity) and even to improve their academic performances (Trudeau and Shephard, 2010).

Sport is also associated with many health benefits, including learning how to take care of one's body through proper nutrition, sleep and general self-care. Within this perspective, sport and drug use are incompatible, and the promotion of sports participation is considered as a way to foster healthy habits and to prevent alcohol, tobacco and illicit drug use among youth. Such alleged incompatibility can be illustrated in many different ways, referring to either biological, psychological or sociological mechanisms. For example, regular cigarette smoking reduces aerobic fitness thus compromising endurance performance. Furthermore, according to the American College of Sports Medicine, acute ingestion of alcohol can exert a deleterious effect upon a wide variety of psychomotor skills such as reaction time, hand-eye coordination, accuracy, balance, and complex coordination, and also may decrease strength, power, local muscular endurance, speed and cardiovascular endurance. Moreover, thanks to sport participation, young athletes may socialise with conformist peers instead of deviant ones, and young males may express their masculinity in legitimate ways instead of expressing it through deviant activities (Wichstrøm and Wichstrøm, 2009).

Thus, sport participation has been widely regarded as a means of encouraging teenagers to develop healthy habits while steering them away from tobacco, alcohol and other drugs. Nevertheless, the deterrence hypothesis is not supported by strong empirical evidence. The scientific literature on the drug–sport relationship expanded rapidly during the 1980s and the 1990s, with mixed results regarding this hypothesis. A study conducted in the early 1980s among American adolescents aged 17–18-years old found no statistical relationship between sports participation and alcohol use or illicit drug use, and a modest negative correlation between sports participation and cigarette smoking. The author concluded that the alleged relationship between sports and clean living was a 'useful myth': sports participation had a very little effect on drug use. Nevertheless, sports can still symbolize goodness, fun and fair play, notwithstanding what athletes really do (Rooney, 1984).

Regarding cigarette smoking, in several studies sports participation was found to be a protective factor for cigarette smoking among adolescents (Donato *et al.*, 1997; Escobedo *et al.*, 1993), especially among girls (Aaron *et al.*, 1995), but the effect of physical exercise on smoking cessation remained unclear (Nishi *et al.*, 1998). Regarding alcohol, some studies failed to find a unequivocal relationship between sports participation and alcohol use (Overman and Terry, 1991; Thorlindsson *et al.*, 1990); other studies found that teenagers involved in sports reported lower levels of use (Donato *et al.*, 1994; Thorlindsson, 1989), but the opposite result was also observed (Faulkner and Slattery, 1990), especially among boys (Aaron *et al.*, 1995; Eitle *et al.*, 2003). It was also suggested that the link between alcohol use and sporting activities may be curvilinear: on the average, athletes drink less alcohol than those who perform no physical activity, but teenagers who play sports intensively drink more than those who reported a moderate practice (Choquet and Hassler, 1997). Furthermore, regarding alcohol and tobacco use, a survey conducted among African-American female basketball players found that the protective effect of sport could be only seasonal: they reduced their drug use during the competitive season, but consumed just as much as other adolescents during the rest of the year (Bower and Martin 1999).

Concerning illicit drug use, most studies found that participation in sports was negatively correlated to such use, but some found a positive relationship (Green *et al.*, 2001; Rockafellow and Saules, 2006) or a relationship varying with sport and gender (Ford, 2007; Peretti-Watel *et al.*, 2002). Another study even found a curvilinear relationship for cannabis use among French adolescents (with highest prevalence at low levels and high levels of sports participation) (Aquatias *et al.*, 1999).

These contradictory results illustrate the fact that the deterrence hypothesis is much too general. The relationship between sports participation and drug use at adolescence may depend on many aspects related either to sports participation (informal practice with peers or under the supervision of a coach, recreational or competition-oriented practice, or team sport or individual sport, for example) or drug use (which substance, which level of use) (Lorenté, 2002; Peretti-Watel *et al.*, 2002). More recently, an exhaustive review of thirty-four peer-reviewed quantitative data-based studies investigating the relationship between sports involvement and drug use at adolescence was published in 2009. It concluded that sports participation is positively correlated with alcohol use, and negatively correlated with both cigarette smoking and illicit drug use, but the results displayed also varied according to the characteristics of sports participation and drug use (Lisha and Sussman, 2009).

Moreover, some other aspects of usage may be important. For example, these relationships may depend on age and gender, as well as on the timing of monitoring, as illustrated by the longitudinal analyses conducted by Wichstrøm and Wichstrøm (2009). In their study, alcohol intoxication and sports participation were negatively correlated at baseline, but sports participation at baseline was positively correlated with alcohol intoxication measured seven years later. These authors also found that the drug-sport link can mediate gateway effects: for example, initial sports participation reduced later tobacco use via lower levels of cannabis initiation.

Let's consider now how sports participation, and which type of sports participation, may either facilitate, induce or go with different kinds of drug use.

Sports participation, social control and socialisation

In some cases, sports participation can be a contextual protecting factor for drug use, as it is a time-consuming activity frequently involving age and gender segregation (instead of socialising with older adolescents, which may increase the risk of drug use) and adult supervision (Wichstrøm and Wichstrøm, 2009). Sporting practice can be either formal (registration in a club, practice supervised by adult coaches in specific facilities), informal (playing sports alone or with friends, especially in public space such as streets and parks) or both formal and informal (Lorenté, 2002). Practising sports alone or with friends in public space can make it easier to use substances because it takes adolescents away from adults' control, whereas practice in a club under a well educated coach's supervision extends the social control usually performed by school or family). This opportunity effect induced by a loosening of social control is a well-known result in the sociology of deviance (Becker, 1963; Cloward and Ohlin 1960; Osgood *et al.*, 1996). Lay people also know about this potential effect. According to a Canadian study published in 1995, many parents were keeping their children out of sport precisely because of the issue of drugs in sport (Lorenté, 2002). Among French adolescents aged 18, for example, outings and other peer-oriented activities, including informal sport practice, were positively and strongly correlated with cannabis use, while formal sport practice was negatively correlated with such use, and these relationships also depended on which levels of use were considered (Peretti-Watel and Lorenté, 2004). Indeed, occasional use of cannabis was more common among respondents who participated in many different outdoor activities, while regular use was associated with a more selective lifestyle, focusing on music-oriented outings and time spent at a friend's home in the evening. In other words, drug experimentation and occasional use may depend on opportunities provided by one's lifestyle, including sports participation, but reciprocally regular users may select specific activities chosen for their convenience to cannabis use. Similarly, adolescents practising sport in a club reported less frequent tobacco use than those who were not, but after adjustment on various confounding factors this relationship remained significant for daily smoking, not heavy smoking (smoking at least ten cigarettes per day) (Peretti-Watel *et al.*, 2002).

Moreover, as a social activity, sports participation may boost socialisation among teammate peers (Thombs and Hamilton, 2002), especially regarding team sports (such as the famous third half in rugby). Among university sportspeople, team cohesion was found to be a significant predictor of alcohol consumption (Zhou *et al.*, 2014), and several studies also found that high-school and university students involved in team sports were more likely to report recent alcohol use or drunkenness (Lorenté *et al.*, 2004; Martha *et al.*, 2009; Peretti-Watel *et al.*, 2002). This relationship persists during early adult years (Wichstrøm and Wichstrøm, 2009), and it was also observed among elite student-athletes trained in specialized public centres (Peretti-Watel *et al.*, 2003). In this case, the sociability induced by sports participation may be more important than what sport is being played, but the cultural meaning of some team sports (such as soccer, rugby, hockey or American football) and their association with masculine values is also an important factor (Dunning, 1986). Regarding cigarette smoking, another study used specific statistical tools designed to capture network effects among a sample of American adolescents aged 10–13 (Fujimoto, Unger and Valente, 2012). It found that smoking initiation was more frequent among adolescents exposed to teammates who smoke through participation in school-based organized sports activities.

Finally, beyond young athletes' socialization, there are also issues related to later de-socialization. Indeed, adolescents strongly involved in competitive sports are constantly supervised by coaches, their training and competition schedule shape their daily lives, but their world may suddenly collapse if they are no longer competitive or seriously injured. Such brutal desocialization may expose them to drug use, as suggested by the relatively high prevalence of drug abuse among former high-level athletes (Lowenstein *et al.*, 2000).

Orientation toward success and drug use

Orientation toward competition and success may also encourage drug use among young athletes. Of course, alcohol, cigarettes and illicit drugs are usually not considered as doping agents, but even so-called 'recreational drugs' could be used to enhance sportive performance. For example, at the beginning of the twentieth century, road racing cyclists used to drink a sip of champagne to boost their performance before downhill sections (Laure, 2004). During the last decade, in France, positive tests for cannabinoids steadily ranged between 20 and 30 per cent of all positive doping tests.

According to a survey conducted among French university sport students (aged 18–24), 13 per cent of them had already used cannabis to enhance their sporting performance, and the risk of such use was twice higher among those involved in national or international competitions (Lorenté *et al.*, 2005). Similarly, in France, among young elite athletes trained in specialized public centres, girls competing at international level were more likely to smoke cigarettes and cannabis than those competing at lower levels, suggesting that tobacco and cannabis can be used to alleviate competitive stress and anxiety, which are frequent among young athletes (Peretti-Watel *et al.*, 2003). The same interpretation has been already proposed regarding alcohol drinking among young athletes (Lisha and Sussman, 2009).

Such drug use reflects a general contemporary trend toward the integrative use of so-called recreational drugs that can be used to increase efficiency or manage stress. Of course, this phenomenon is not confined to sports. For example, cannabis could be used for managing anxiety and increasing efficiency before a competition but also before another stressing event, such as an examination or a combat situation (Grélot, 2011). Drug use in the US Army, for example, reached levels far greater than in civilian society (Riker-Coleman, 1996). In the study quoted above, 36 per cent of university sports students reported that they had already used cannabis to enhance academic performance, and both kinds of enhancing-substance use (for sportive and non-sportive performances) fuelled each other (Lorenté, Peretti-Watel and Grélot, 2005).

Moreover, among young elite student-athletes, those who consider doping as a dangerous but necessary adjunct to both sporting and non-sporting achievements (for example, to earn money and to experience new sensations) were also more prone to report alcohol or cannabis use (Peretti-Watel *et al.*, 2004).

More generally, human existence is increasingly medicalized nowadays, especially in sports (Waddington, 2000). Elite athletes become accustomed to taking a lot of nutritional supplements and medication to avoid tiredness and speed-up recovery, to treat injuries or to obtain a competitive edge (Alaranta *et al.*, 2008; Leroux, 2002). Socialization into competitive sport may, therefore, teach teenagers to use various kinds of psychoactive substances to cope with everyday life, including using so-called 'recreational' drugs for 'non-recreational' purposes.

Motives and values expressed through sports and drug use

Sports participation and drug use may also be impelled by similar motives or values. For example, according to psychologists, sensation seeking is a trait of personality expressed through many behaviours, including X-treme sports (which are often sliding sports) and drug use (Zuckerman, 1994). Some studies echoed this statement as they found that practicing a sliding sport (either windsurfing, skiing, snowboarding, surfing or sailing) was positively associated with alcohol and cannabis use. For example, in France young elite student-athletes aged 16–24 and trained in specialized public centres were less likely to report cigarette, alcohol or cannabis use than other adolescents and young adults, but among them practising a sliding sport increased both the risk of recent alcohol use among boys and the risk of recent cannabis use among girls (Peretti-Watel *et al.*, 2003). Similarly, among sport science students aged 18–24, those who practised a sliding sport strongly were more likely to report having already use cannabis to enhance sportive or non-sportive performances (Lorenté *et al.*, 2005). In this case, both sliding sports participation and drug use may be impelled by sensation-seeking: to search for exhilaration, thrill, vertigo or *flow* (Caillois, 1967; Lyng, 1990; Stranger, 2009, 2011). Both behaviours can also appear as complementary features of the same subculture, as social practices that give access to authenticity of selfhood by confronting the barriers of social conventions. Furthermore, psychoactive substances could be used as an adjunct to sensation-seeking during sliding sport practice.

Sport is frequently seen as one of the last strongholds for masculine values such as confrontation, physical strength and endurance (Dunning, 1986). Drunkenness provides another way to express commitment to such virile values: when male teammates challenge each other to show that they can hold their liquor, it can turn a binge drinking session into a true test of stamina. This may explain why sport science students drink less frequently but report more episodes of intoxication than their counterparts in the general population (Lorenté *et al.*, 2003), why young athletes are much more likely to engage in binge drinking and consistently consume larger quantities than non-athletes (Martens *et al.*, 2006), or why team leaders (and especially male team leaders) tend to consume more alcohol and to binge more often than other team members (Leichliter *et al.*, 1998).

Finally, some recent evidence showed that body image is an increasingly important issue for adolescent boys. Around two-thirds of them are dissatisfied with their bodies, and this is equally split between those who desire weight loss and those who want to gain muscle. Adolescent boys with increased body dissatisfaction exhibited positive attitudes towards drug use in sport (Yager and O'Dea, 2014). Thus, body dissatisfaction is becoming a new concern with adolescent health as the use of protein powders and supplements predicts the use of anabolic steroids (Backhouse *et al.*, 2013).

Conclusion

Does sports participation prevent young people to use licit and illicit drugs? The existing scientific literature provides some insight regarding our introductory question. From a very general point of view, sports participation tends to be positively correlated with alcohol use, but negatively correlated with cigarette smoking and illicit drug use. Nevertheless, such statement should be strongly qualified. First, it depends on the kind of use considered: what is true for smoking initiation or binge drinking may not be true for daily smoking or occasional drinking. Second, it also depends on the characteristics of sports participation: there are many different kinds of sports; sporting practice can be either formal or informal; competition-oriented or recreational; and so forth. Third, some results may be gender-specific, or observed only for university students and not for younger people. This variety of results demonstrates the complexity of the relationship between sports participation and drug use at adolescence. In some cases, sporting practice induces a structural change in opportunities to experiment various substances and/or to use them occasionally as part of a socialisation process. In other cases, young athletes may decide to use recreational drugs for enhancing their sportive performances, or for alleviating competitive stress and anxiety, and such use may be extended to non-sportive activities. Furthermore, sporting practice and drug use may express the same impulses for specific motives and values, such as sensation-seeking. These examples illustrate the necessity to take into account the fact that both sports participation and drug use are social practices, associated to and supported by specific meanings and motives. Moreover, these aspects are shared with and learned from peers, and they may change across socio-historical contexts.

References

Aaron, D. J., Dearwater, S. R. Anderson, R., Olsen, T., Kriska, A. M. and Laporte, R. E. (1995). Physical activity and the initiation of high-risk health behaviours in adolescents, *Medicine and Science in Sports and Exercise, 27*, 1639–1645.

Alaranta, A., Alaranta, H. and Helenius, I. (2008). Use of prescription drugs in athletes, *Sports Medicine, 38 (6)*, 449–463.

Aquatias, S., Desrues, I., Leroux, M., Stettinger, V. and Valette-Viallard C. (1999). *Activités sportives, pratiques à risque, usages de substances dopantes et psychoactives: recherche sur la pratique moderne du sport.* Paris, Ministère de la jeunesse et des sports, RESSCOM.

Backhouse, S., Whitaker, L. and Petroczi, A: (2013). Gateway to doping? Supplement use in the context of preferred competitive situations, doping attitude, beliefs, and norms, *Scandinavian Journal of Medicine and Science in Sports, 23*, 244–252.

Becker, H. S. (1963). *Outsiders.* New York: The Free Press.

Bower, B.L. *and* Martin, M. *(1999)* African American female basketball players: an examination of alcohol and drug behaviors, Journal of American College Health, *48*, 129–133.

Caillois, R. (1967). *Les jeux et les hommes. Le masque et le vertige* [Man, Play and Games]. Paris: Gallimard.

Carmichael, D. (1996). *Youth Sport vs. Youth Crime.* Brockville: Active Heathy Links Inc. 2008. www.lin.ca/Files/12569/YouthSportvsYouthCrime2008[2].pdf

Choquet, M. and Hassler, C. (1997). Sports and alcohol consumption during adolescence. Alcoologie and Addictologie, *19*, 21–27.

Cloward, R. and Ohlin, L. (1960). *Delinquency and Opportunity.* New York: The Free Press.

Donato, F., Assanelli, D., Marconi, M., Corsini, C., Rosa, G. and Monarca, S. (1994). Alcohol consumption among high school students and young athletes in North Italy, *Revue Epidémiologique et Santé Publique, 42*, 198–206.

Donato, F., Assanelli, D., Chiesa, R., Poeta, M. L., Tomasoni, M. and Turla, C. (1997). Cigarette smoking and sports participation in adolescents: a cross-sectional survey among high school students in Italy, *Substance Use and Misuse, 32*, 1555–1572.

Dunning, E. (1986). Sport as a male preserve: notes on the social sources of masculinity and its transformations. In N. Elias and E. Dunning (eds) *Quest for excitement: sport and leisure in the civilizing process* (pp. 267–307). Oxford: Basil Blackwell.

Eitle, D., Turner, R.J. and Eitle, T.M. (2003). The Deterrence Hypothesis Reexamined: Sports Participation and Substance Use among Young Adults, *Journal of Drug Issues, 33 (1)*, 193–221.

Escobedo, L.G., Marcus, S.E., Holtzman, D. and Giovino, G.A. (1993). Sports participation, age at smoking initiation, and the risk of smoking among US high school students, *Journal of the American Medical Association, 269*, 1391–1395.

Faulkner, R.A. and Slattery, C.M. (1990). The relationship of physical activity to alcohol consumption in youth, 15–16 years of age, *Canadian Journal of Public Health, 81 (2)*, 168–169.

Ford, J.A. (2007). Substance use among college athletes: A comparison based on sport/team affiliation, *Journal of American College Health, 55*, 367–373.

Fujimoto, K., Unger, J.B. and Valente, T.W. (2012). A network method of measuring affiliation-based peer influence: assessing the influences of teammates' smoking on adolescent smoking, *Child Development, 83 (2)*, 442–51.

Green, G.A., Uryasz, F.D., Petr, T.A. and Bray, C.D. (2001). NCAA study of substance use and abuse habits of college student-athletes, *Clinical Journal of Sport Medicine, 11*, 51–56.

Grélot, L. (2011). Le dopage mental est-il possible? [Is mental doping possible?]. In F. Xavier-Alario (ed.) *Toutes les questions que vous vous posez sur votre cerveau* (pp. 176–179). Paris: Odile Jacob.

Laure, P. (2004). *Histoire du dopage et des conduites dopantes.* [History of doping behaviours] Paris: Vuibert.

Leichliter, J.S., Meilman, P.W., Presley, C.A. and Cashin, J.R. (1998). Alcohol Use and Related Consequences Among Students With Varying Levels of Involvement in College Athletics, *Journal of American College Health, 46 (6)*, 257–262.

Leroux, M. (2002). Consommations intégrées et sport de haut-niveau [integrated drug use among top athletes]. In C. Faugeron and M. Kokoreff (eds) *Sociétés avec drogues: enjeux et limites* (pp. 79–98). Ramonville Saint-Agne: Erès.

Lisha, N.E. and Sussman, S. (2010). Relationship of high school and college sports participation with alcohol, tobacco, and illicit drug use: a review, *Addictive Behaviors, 35 (5)*, 399–407.

Lorenté, F.O. (2002). Sports involvement can be both formal and informal at the same time: a comment on Peretti-Watel *et al.*, *Addiction, 97*, 1609.

Lorenté, F.O., Souville, M., Griffet, J. and Grélot, L. (2004). Participation in sports and alcohol consumption among French adolescents, *Addictive Behaviors, 29 (5)*, 941–946.

Lorenté, F.O., Peretti-Watel, P., Griffet, J. and Grélot L. (2003). Alcohol use and intoxication in sport university students. *Alcohol and Alcoholism, 38 (5)*, 427–430.

Lorenté, F.O., Peretti-Watel, P. and Grélot, L. (2005). Cannabis use to enhance sportive and non-sportive performances among French sport students, *Addictive Behaviors, 30 (7)*, 1382–1391.

Lowenstein, W., Arvers, P., Gourarier, L., Porche, A.S., Cohen, J.M., Nordmann, F., Prévot, B., Carrier, C. and Sanchez M. (2000). Activités physiques et sportives dans les antécédents des personnes prises en charge pour addictions [history of sports participation and physical exercise among patients receiving addiction treatment], *Annales de Médecine Interne, 151 (suppl. A)*, A18–A26.

Lyng, S. (1990). Edgework: A Social Psychological Analysis of Voluntary Risk Taking, *American Journal of Sociology, 95*, 851–866.

Martens, M.P., Dams-O'Connor, K. and Beck, N.C. (2006). A systematic review of college student-athlete drinking: Prevalence rates, sport-related factors, and interventions, *Journal of Substance Abuse Treatment, 31*, 305–316.

Martha, C., Grélot, L. and Peretti-Watel, P. (2009). Participants' sports characteristics related to heavy episodic drinking among French students, *International Journal of Drug Policy, 20 (2)*, 152–160.

Nishi, N., Jenicek, M. and Tatara, K. (1998). A meta-analytic review of the effect of exercise on smoking cessation, Journal of Epidemiology, *8*, 79–84.

Osgood, D.W., Wilson, J.K., O'Malley, P.M., Bachman, J.G. and Johnston, L.D. (1996) Routines activities and individual deviant behaviour, *American Sociological Review, 61*, 635–655.

Overman, S.J. and Toni Terry, B.S. (1991). Alcohol use and attitudes: a comparison of college athletes and nonathletes, *Journal of Drug Education, 21 (2)*, 107–117.

Peretti-Watel, P., Beck, F. and Legleye, S. (2002). Beyond the U-curve: the relationship between sport and alcohol, cigarette and cannabis use, *Addiction, 97 (6)*, 707–716.

Peretti-Watel, P., Guagliardo, V., Verger, P., Pruvost, J., Mignon, P. and Obadia, Y. (2003). Sporting activity and drug use: alcohol, cigarette and cannabis use among elite-student-athletes, *Addiction, 98*, 1249–1256.

Peretti-Watel, P. and Lorenté, F.O. (2004). Cannabis use, sport practice and other leisure activities at the end of adolescence, *Drug and Alcohol Dependence, 73 (3)*, 251–257.

Peretti-Watel, P., Guagliardo, V., Verger, P., Mignon, P., Pruvost, J. and Obadia, Y. (2004). Attitudes toward doping and recreational drug use among French elite student-athletes, *Sociology of Sport Journal, 21 (4)*, 1–17.

Riker-Coleman, E. (1996). *Reaping the Whirlwind. Systemic failure of leadership in the US Army, 1969–1971.* www.unc.edu/~chaos1/whirlwind.pdf

Rockafellow, B.D. and Saules, K.K. (2007) Substance use by college students: The role of intrinsic versus extrinsic motivation for athletic involvement, *Psychology of Addictive Behavior, 20*, 279–287.

Rooney, J.F. (1984). Sports and clean living: a useful myth?, *Drug and alcohol Dependence, 13 (1)*, 75–87.

Stranger, M. (1999). The aesthetics of risk: a study of surfing, *International Review for the Sociology of Sport, 34*, 265–276.

Stranger, M. (2011). *Surfing Life. Surface, Substructure and the Commodification of the Sublime.* Burlington: Ashgate Publishing Company.

Thombs, D. and Hamilton, M. (2002). Effects of a Social Norms Feedback Campaign on the Drinking Behavior of Division I Student-Athletes, *Journal of Drug Education, 32 (3)*, 227–244.

Thorlindsson, T. (1989). Sport participation, smoking, and drug and alcohol use among Icelandic youth, *Sociology of Sport Journal, 6*, 136–143.

Thorlindsson, T., Vilhjalmsson, R. and Valgeirsson G. (1990). Sport participation and perceived health status: a study of adolescents, *Social Science and Medicine, 31 (5)*, 551–556.

Trudeau, F. and Shephard, R.J. (2010). Relationships of physical activity to brain health and the academic performance of schoolchildren. *American Journal of Lifestyle Medicine, 4 (2)*, 138–150.

Waddington, I. (2000). *Sport, health and drugs. A sociological perspective.* London: EandFN Spon.

Wichstrøm, T. and Wichstrøm, L. (2009). Does sports participation during adolescence prevent later alcohol, tobacco and drug use? *Addiction, 104 (1)*, 138–149.

Yager, Z. and O'Dea, J.A. (2014). Relationships between body image, nutritional supplement use, and attitudes towards doping in sport among adolescent boys: implications for prevention programs, *Journal of the International Society of Sports Nutrition, 11 (1)*, 13.

Zhou, J., O'Brien, K.S. and Heim, D. (2014). Alcohol consumption in sportspeople: The role of social cohesion, identity and happiness, *International Review for the Sociology of Sport, 49 (3–4)*, 278–293.

Zuckerman, M. (1994). *Behavioural Expressions and Biosocial Bases of Sensation Seeking.* Cambridge: Cambridge University Press.

SECTION 7

Elite youth sport

41

INTRODUCTION

Andy Smith

It is now well established that since the 1970s, in particular, elite sport has become an increasingly central and perhaps defining feature of the sport policy priorities of many countries across the world. As Houlihan and Green (2008: 2) have noted, the almost irresistible obsession among a diverse range of governments with pursuing elite sport success has most often been underpinned by a concern for international prestige and diplomatic recognition, ideological competition and a belief that 'international sporting success generates domestic political benefits ranging from the rather nebulous "feel good factor" to more concrete economic impacts associated with the hosting of elite competitions.'

Such is the perceived value of sport, and especially elite sport, as a 'high-visibility, low-cost and extremely malleable resource which can be adapted to achieve, or at least give the impression to the public/electorate of achieving, a wide variety of domestic and international goals' (Houlihan and Green, 2008: 3), there are now few governments who fail to make a publicly claimed commitment to the promotion of elite sport and competition – if they possess the necessary resources to do so. Even in times of global recession and austerity, it is not uncommon for many governments to retain elite sport as a core policy priority albeit under more pressured economic conditions. In the UK, for example, despite the significant economic recession that beset the home countries at the time, it was reported in 2012 that £125 million of Exchequer and National Lottery money would be given annually to UK Sport to distribute to Olympic and Paralympic sports to assist in the preparation of athletes intending to compete at the Rio 2016 Olympic and Paralympic Games. The monies were to be spent as part of UK Sport's broader no-compromise approach to medal-based funding, which as a consequence does not benefit sports and individual athletes uniformly but was symbolic of the retained commitment to elite sport by the then Coalition government.

The prioritization of elite sport at the heart of much sport policy, and the funding used in the pursuit of elite sports success, has increasingly constrained countries to engage in a variety of practices that maximize their chances of succeeding on the global stage. As the first two chapters in Section 7 make clear, among these practices are the systematic talent development and talent identification processes used by many sports organizations that seek to recruit young athletes into their elite performance environments and structures. In *The elements of talent development in youth sport*, Matthew Vierimaa, Karl Erickson and Jean Côté outline one of the more dominant approaches taken to talent development by many countries, namely, the Long-

Term Athlete Development (LTAD) model (Balyi and Hamilton, 2004). Following the work of others (e.g. Bailey *et al.*, 2010; Ford *et al.*, 2011), Vierimaa *et al.* argue that despite its attractive simplicity the LTAD model is 'primarily uni-dimensional and lacking in scientific rigour in terms of supporting empirical evidence'. In contrast, they suggest that the Developmental Model of Sport Participation (DMSP) is a more adequate 'conceptual framework that integrates the developing person in its environment with objective processes and outcomes that can be measured and tested', and proceed to discuss the concepts of specialization and sampling in youth sport and the learning environments that have been associated with talent development during the first stage of involvement in sport. Having reviewed the various ways in which young athletes learn and develop in sporting contexts, Vierimaa *et al.* conclude that given 'the equivocal evidence surrounding the optimal prescriptive approach for talent development, young athletes should be given the opportunity to engage in and learn from activities that are both adult and youth-led and are intrinsically and extrinsically valued'.

Various models of development and their application to talent development approaches in youth sport are also the subject of Steve Cobley's chapter, *Talent identification and development in youth sport*. Considering what he calls 'the developmental model view of talent', Cobley argues that youthful sporting talent can be conceptualized as comprising the presence or absence of a set, or combination, of particular skills and qualities that are grounded in the complex interaction between individual-level characteristics, specific sport tasks, the social environment as well as the policy priorities which underpin elite sport. Acknowledging the rapid growth of talent identification and development systems in youth sport, Cobley then outlines the key debates associated with these systems which can be identified in the existing literature. These debates he divides into three broad categories:

1   Immediate competitive success in junior and youth sport;
2   Early sport specialization accompanied by intensified, highly structured and specific training; and
3   Adherence to the performance social ecology.

An appreciation of the processes involved in each of these stages of talent identification and development, it is held, is vital for understanding the likely efficacy of elite youth sport talent practices in a diverse range of sports.

In their chapter, *Health, well-being and the 'logic' of elite youth sports work*, Chris Platts and Andy Smith move beyond the more dominant performance-oriented approaches to elite youth sport (such as that which is often evident in discussions of talent identification and development) and explain why the trend toward earlier and more intensive involvement in elite sport by many young people has not been an unalloyed blessing. Drawing upon ideas most widely developed in analyses of risk, pain and injury in sport, Platts and Smith outline how in elite youth sport there is an institutionalized expectation that athletes will take serious risks with their health within the cultures of risk which characterize their workplaces. These risks, they suggest, often emerge out of many athletes' commitment to the norms and values of what Hughes and Coakley (1991) refer to as the 'sport ethic' that frequently constrains athletes to engage in often health-compromising behaviours, and which characterizes aspects of the relational constraints to which young athletes are subject.

Following a consideration of the subcultural meanings that are often associated with various processes that constitute the cultures of risk in youth sport, Platts and Smith examine some of the structural features and realities of the work situations of young elite sports workers. To that end, they suggest that young elite athletes are constrained from an early age to internalize the logic of sports work and the values of the sports worlds they inhabit. These values, it is held, include the routine punishment of mistakes, the close and regular surveillance of performance (including weight) that may result in a variety of publically enforced punishments, and constant social comparisons between oneself and others which often encourages young athletes to ensure they live up to (and preferably exceed) expectations. The costs to young athletes' health of the strategies they adopt in relation to the management of emotions, their interpersonal relations in the workplace, and the difficulties they may face in managing the often blurred boundaries between their public and private lives concludes the chapter.

In the final chapter of Section 7, Melanie Lang, Mike Hartill and Bettina Rulofs provide a review of international research and prevention policy on child abuse in sport. Building upon the earlier work of Brackenridge (2001), Lang *et al.* note that while children and young people have for many years engaged in sport at a variety of levels, only relatively recently has there been a recognition of the potential for maltreatment of children and young people in sport. The increased interest in children's rights and the prevention of child maltreatment, they suggest, is closely associated with the introduction in 1989 of the United Nations Convention on the Rights of the Child (United Nations General Assembly, 1989) and the emergence in several countries of high-profile cases of abuse in sport. In their chapter, Lang *et al.* review evidence of the physical, emotional and sexual abuse in sport but add that much of the available literature in this regard 'has predominantly emanated from high-income countries and has focused on the sexual abuse of athletes, particularly of able-bodied athletes'. To illustrate some of the ways in which sports organizations have responded to concerns of child abuse, the chapter concludes with a case study of child protection in sport in Germany, which demonstrates some of the difficulties, as well as the potential benefits, of implementing policy intended to tackle child abuse in sport.

References

Bailey, R., Collins, D., Ford, P., MacNamara, A., Pearce, G. and Toms, M. (2010). *Participant development in sport: an academic literature review*. Commissioned report for Sports Coach UK. Leeds: Sports Coach UK.

Balyi, I. and Hamilton, A. (2004). *Long-term athlete development: trainability in children and adolescents. Windows of opportunity, optimal trainability*. Victoria, BC: National Coaching Institute British Columbia and Advanced Training and Performance, Ltd.

Brackenridge, C. H. (2001) *Spoilsports: Understanding and Preventing Sexual Exploitation in Sport*. London, Routledge.

Ford, P., De Ste Croix, M., Lloyd, R., Meyers, R., Moosavi, M., Oliver, J. and Williams, C. (2011). The long-term athlete development model: physiological evidence and application. *Journal of Sports Sciences*, 29(4), 389–402.

Houlihan, B. and Green, M. (2008). Comparative elite sport development. In B. Houlihan and M. Green (eds). *Comparative elite sport development: systems, structures and public policy*. Oxford: Butterworth-Heinemann.

Hughes, R. and Coakley, J. (1991). Positive deviance among athletes: the implications of overconformity to the sport ethic. *Sociology of Sport Journal*, 8(4), 307–25.

United Nations General Assembly (1989). *Convention on the Rights of the Child*. Available online at: www.unhcr.org/refworld/docid/3ae6b38f0.html

42

THE ELEMENTS OF TALENT DEVELOPMENT IN YOUTH SPORT

Matthew Vierimaa, Karl Erickson and Jean Côté

Introduction

The development of talent in young athletes is often regarded as the fundamental goal of youth sport programmes. Indeed, countries around the world spend countless dollars designing and implementing athlete development programmes aimed at fostering athletic talent in youngsters to allow them to compete at elite levels of sport. One such approach to talent development that has been adopted by multiple countries is the Long-Term Athlete Development model (LTAD; Balyi and Hamilton, 2004). The LTAD model has been well-received and implemented by national sporting organizations in countries such as Canada, the United Kingdom and Australia (Bailey *et al.*, 2010). For example, in Canada, a general LTAD model has been published by Canada Sport for Life (2008), which has since been adapted and implemented by over fifty unique Canadian sport organizations.

Given the widespread implementation of the LTAD by sport organizations and the corresponding required financial investments, it would be reasonable to assume that these organizations would have thoroughly reviewed the model to ensure that it is relevant and empirically based and tested. However, it seems that the LTAD model relies upon approachability and simplicity for the average coach or parent as a primary strength. All of the resources related to the LTAD are well-illustrated and clearly indicative of a professional product. This, paired with a straightforward prescriptive approach to youth sport, clearly appeals to the general public and average parents and coaches. However, it has been suggested that therein lie the limitations of the LTAD in that it is primarily uni-dimensional and lacking in scientific rigour in terms of supporting empirical evidence (Bailey *et al.*, 2010; Ford *et al.*, 2011). Despite its advertised holistic approach to athlete development (Canadian Sport for Life, 2008), it is evident that the LTAD was developed largely on principles of physiology and motor development (Ford *et al.*, 2011). This is not inherently problematic, but it has further been noted that the creators of the LTAD have occasionally made questionable assumptions and gone beyond the literature in their integration of existing research in the development of the model (Bailey *et al.*, 2010; Ford *et al.*, 2011). More transparency in this regard would be advantageous so that the general public is aware of which sections of the model are empirically supported and which are not; a shift in perspective is necessary so that the LTAD is viewed as a working model rather than a finished product (Ford *et al.*, 2011). The strong emphasis on physiological and motor development can be viewed as a strength of the LTAD, but it is also a weakness in its goal of promoting holistic athlete development. Only brief passing references are made to research from other pertinent areas of the literature; in particular, a growing body of research on athlete development from the psychology domain could be utilized to help strengthen the validity and overall applicability of the LTAD model (Bailey *et al.*, 2010).

To this end, the Developmental Model of Sport Participation (DMSP) is a conceptual framework that integrates the developing person in its environment with objective processes and outcomes that can be measured and tested (Côté *et al.*, 2009). The DMSP addresses how changes in athlete development can be tracked over time and make specific hypotheses about the range of activities in youth sport that lead to long-term participation and talent development. The DMSP and its seven postulates have the ability to quantitatively chronicle the transitions of athletes along the talent development pathway by contrasting approaches to sport programming that are based on diversification before specialization and play before practice (Côté and Abernethy, 2012).

The DMSP has three sport participation trajectories:

1   recreational participation through early diversity and deliberate play;
2   elite performance through early diversity and deliberate play;
3   elite performance through early specialization and deliberate practice.

Pathways one and two have the same foundation and include an initial stage of sport involvement (approximately ages 6–12) labelled the sampling years. The sampling years are characterized by a diversity of sport experiences, both across and within sports, with participation primarily concerned with fun and enjoyment. Within pathway two toward elite performance, participants then build on this early diversity by beginning to specialize in their chosen sport and gradually incorporating more targeted practice activities (approximately ages 13–15), before investing heavily in the chosen sport at a high performance level at approximately age 16. Conversely, pathway three is an alternative pathway to sport expertise that is classified as an early specialization trajectory. Early specialization is defined as involvement in one sport and intense investment in sport-specific practice in particular during the early years of participation in sport. The different stages within and between trajectories are thus based on the type of developmental activities that dominates a specific sport and changes in the amount of involvement in different sports.

The sampling years of the DMSP infer that the passion to pursue elite performance in sport emerges from the positive environment that comprises a diversified and play-oriented environment in youth sport. The sampling years of the DMSP focus on the youth sport participants' immediate needs and assets instead of focusing on skill acquisition and the long-term outcomes of sport. Contrary to commercially available models of talent development in sport such as the LTAD, the DMSP provides a flexible structure for sport involvement by focusing on activities that are most appropriate for the developing athlete. In other words, talent development is not the primary focus of sport involvement during the sampling years of the DMSP, but rather the emergent by-product of successful and healthy personal development in supportive youth sport environments.

The purpose of this chapter is first to briefly describe the concepts of specialization and sampling in youth sport and second to provide an overview of the learning environments that have been associated with talent development during the first stage of involvement in sport.

Early specialization versus early sampling

Early specialization

Early specialization implies a focus on elite performance in youth sport and increased training during childhood. An early specialization pathway in youth sport mainly focuses on the short-term performance outcome of a selected number of youth, often reducing the overall and positive long-term impact that youth sport can have on children. The application of an early specialization approach may be effective for the development of talent in sports with a large base of participants (such as soccer in England, baseball and basketball in the United States, or ice hockey in Canada). However, it excludes a large number of children that are interested in recreational sport or that do not currently perform at a comparatively high level and therefore may not be selected as a child but could still develop into elite level athletes. In other words, it artificially reduces the pool of interested and committed athletes from an early age (Fraser-Thomas and Côté, 2009).

There is evidence that early specialization can lead to elite performance in adult sport (e.g. Ward *et al.*, 2004). However, the personal development and long-term participation costs of early specialization when implemented widely can be devastating for a large number of youth. It is clear, for instance, that early specialization leads to less enjoyment in sport and more dropout, burnout and injuries (Fraser-Thomas *et al.*, 2008a, 2008b Strachan *et al.*, 2009; Wall and Côté, 2007).

Early sampling

The underpinning principle of sampling different sports and/or different activities and participation contexts within a particular sport during childhood is to provide playing and training opportunities for a large number of children across various sports (and different positions or participation contexts within sports) as a mechanism to promote sport participation among a large pool of motivated youth (Côté *et al.*, 2009). The most important aspects for providing a sampling environment during childhood sport is to attract children to sport and motivate them to stay involved so that they can intentionally choose a recreational or elite pathway during adolescence (Côté and Abernethy, 2012). Diversity and play in the sampling years allow youth to experience a range of opportunities and provides young athletes with a breadth of experiences and variety of skills that help them make clear choices about their future involvement in sport.

A sampling approach to children's sport programming is consistent with a developmental perspective that emphasizes long-term participation, personal development and performance as important considerations of youth sport involvement. Considering the difficulty of measuring and predicting sport talent during childhood, it is important that youth sport programmes offer balanced opportunities in sport that benefit a large number of children. The benefits of participating in different sports (Côté *et al.*, 2009) and combining play and practice activities during childhood (Côté *et al.*, 2013) have been highlighted as positively impacting personal development and continued participation as well as developing sport expertise in adulthood (Côté and Abernethy, 2012). Several DMSP studies have supported the concept of diversity before specialization and a mixture of play and practice activities with more play during childhood and increasing practice time during adolescence as important elements of youth sport that lays the foundation for talent development in one sport (e.g. Baker *et al.*, 2003; Baker *et al.*, 2005; Barreiros *et al.*, 2014; Berry *et al.*, 2008; Bridge and Toms, 2013; Gulbin and Gagné, 2010; Leite and Sampaio, 2012; Lidor and Layvan, 2002; Robertson-Wilson and Côté, 2003; Soberlak and Côté, 2003).

Learning environments associated with a sampling approach to talent development in youth sport

Over the years, there have been a number of different lines of research examining the type of activities and environments that are important at different stages of development to maintain participation and develop talent in sport. Côté *et al.* (2013) recently suggested that four principal types of learning environments exist in youth sport, which differ according to the personal values and the social structure that characterize the main developmental activities of each unique learning environment. The personal values and social structure of each learning environment are, in turn, influenced by the social relationships that transpire within sport, along with the setting in which each activity takes place. Personal values and social structure come together along two axes to form a taxonomy that describes four main types of learning environments in youth sport (Figure 42.1). Personal values can range from extrinsic (e.g. involved in activity to improve performance) to intrinsic (e.g. involved in activity because it is enjoyable). The social structure axis refers to the social agents (i.e. adults or youth) who organize and direct the activity. On one end of the axis are sport environments, which are entirely organized and supervised by adults (e.g. coaches), while at the other end are environments in which youth play an active role and adult involvement is minimal. The resultant matrix formed by these two axes describes four main learning environments: rational, emotional, informal and creative. The intersection of these learning environments is the organized competitive setting of youth sport that can be described as 'applied learning'. Each of these learning environments, illustrated in Figure 42.1, occupies a unique position along these axes and creates contexts for distinct developmental activities that are beneficial to the healthy development of youth athletes.

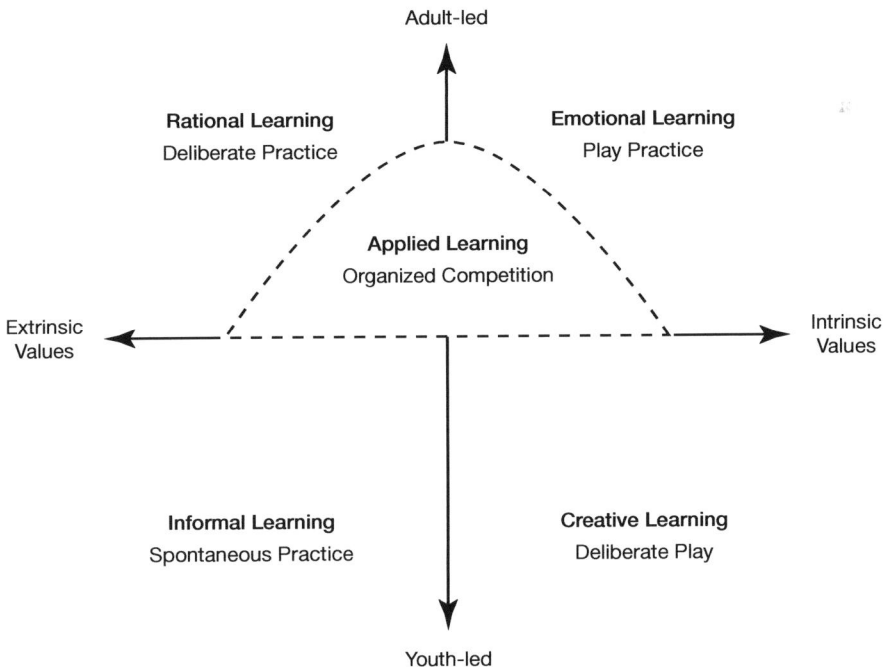

Figure 42.1 A taxonomy of learning environments and developmental activities in youth sport (adapted from Côté et al., 2013)

Rational learning

Rational learning is systematic and logical in nature, and activities utilizing this type of learning are prescribed or led by an adult to improve youth's specific sport skills. The constraints of the activity are initially determined and controlled by an adult, predicated on the transmission of knowledge and skills to the learner by a more capable other (i.e. the coach). The design of these activities are therefore focused on the most efficient means of transmitting relevant information and providing the learner with maximal opportunities to implement and correct the use of this information towards a predetermined 'ideal' performance pattern. Key concerns within this process are breaking performance down into its primary component elements and minimizing irrelevant contextual stimuli – both of which require extensive knowledge of the sport by the adult in charge of designing the training environment.

Deliberate practice

A prototypical example of a developmental activity incorporating rational learning is deliberate practice (Ericsson *et al.*, 1993). According to Ericsson and colleagues (1993), engagement in deliberate practice requires effort, generates no immediate rewards and is motivated by the goal of improving performance rather than its inherent enjoyment. Within Côté and colleagues' (2013) taxonomy, deliberate practice represents the prototype activity of the quadrant defined by high adult involvement and extrinsic values. Ericsson *et al.* (1993) suggested that to achieve expert performance, deliberate practice must be sustained over a period of at least ten years. Based on this and other findings, as well as the intuitive appeal of highly structured environments for talent development, singular participation in deliberate practice activities from an early age has typically composed the foundation of early specialization approaches.

Studies that assess sport-specific practice (i.e. deliberate practice) patterns throughout development generally indicate that expert athletes accumulate more hours of practice over the course of their development; however, the differences between elite and less elite athletes do not occur until adolescence for sports in which peak performance is achieved after puberty (Côté *et al.*, 2007). On the other hand, the overly structured, competitive and adult-driven aspect of organized sport and deliberate practice during childhood can lead to negative outcomes such as early exclusion of late-maturing athletes and the increased prevalence of overuse injuries and dropout, all of which can potentially limit the talent development pool for certain sports (Côté and Abernethy, 2012). Highly structured, adult-driven approaches to skill learning through deliberate practice may also result in an over-dependence on explicit forms of skill learning and, with this, limits on the extent to which skill performance can remain robust under various psychological and physiological stressors (Masters and Maxwell, 2004).

Creative learning

A creative learning context removes most of the external constraints imposed by adults and minimizes the emphasized outcome of performance. The child-directed nature of activities within this environment contributes to the creative aspect of learning through two key characteristics:

1   a high degree of novelty and unpredictability
2   flexibility in structure and form.

While the rational learning context of adult-driven deliberate practice seeks to limit unpredictability in the name of conditioning set responses to specific situations, youth-led play inherently emphasizes physical, social and emotional unpredictability to which the participating children must adapt. With control of the structure and form of the activity, children's self-guided adaptation to these novel physical, social and emotional experiences creates a flexible participation trajectory. Without the actual or perceived pressure from controlling adults to produce a specific performance outcome, the ramifications of failure or unsuccessful attempts are drastically reduced; thus, in combination with adaptation to unpredictability and flexibility, is free experimentation necessary for creative learning.

Deliberate play

Deliberate play is a child-led activity that offers unique characteristics when compared to the adult-led activities of organized sport. Côté (1999) first suggested the term deliberate play to describe a fun and playful activity, which is often the way in which athletes first experience sport. In contrast with Ericsson and colleagues' (1993) notion of deliberate practice, deliberate play is inherently designed to maximize fun, enjoyment and intrinsic motivation. Deliberate play activities, such as playing basketball in a driveway with peers, are regulated by rules adapted from standardized sport rules. These activities are set up and monitored by the children involved in the activity. As such, deliberate play represents the prototype activity for the quadrant within the youth sport activity taxonomy defined by low adult involvement (i.e. child-directed) and high intrinsic value. The unique environment of deliberate play provides motivational and learning advantages that have been associated with long-term sport participation, personal development, and the achievement of expertise (e.g. performance; Côté *et al.*, 2013).

Even though deliberate play activities are designed to maximize enjoyment, there is also research to suggest that play is also important in the development of sport expertise in young athletes, particularly during childhood. Deliberate play is widely regarded as a foundational activity for the well-rounded development of young athletes. Indeed, multiple studies have found that elite level athletes engage in relatively high levels of deliberate play during their childhood (e.g. Berry *et al.*, 2008 Carlson, 1988; Côté, 1999; Soberlak and Côté, 2003; Wall and Côté, 2007) Even though elite athletes in sports such as tennis and swimming sometimes specialize in their chosen sport at a young age, research has shown that these athletes often engaged in high amounts of fun, playful activities (e.g. Bloom, 1985; Carlson, 1988).

Sports for which peak performance is achieved before adulthood often require early specialization and higher amount of deliberate practice during childhood to allow young athletes to acquire the necessary technical skills during adolescence. This is particularly true in sports where athletes reach their peak level of performance at a young age, such as gymnastics and figure skating (Law *et al.*, 2007; Starkes *et al.*, 1996). However, the lack of exposure to child-directed and intrinsically valued deliberate play activities may also have negative implications for both long-term talent and psychosocial development (Côté *et al.*, 2009).

Emotional learning

Adults can create an emotional learning environment by trying to integrate fun into skill development practice by integrating playful activities during structured training sessions. This environment prioritizes affective outcomes and is generally structured to provide opportunities for full participation and success for all participants within a game-like structure. Theoretically, emotional learning inverts traditional deliberate practice-based training by positing that enjoyment and engagement with the sport in game form is both the primary goal of participation and the foundation for technical/tactical skill development (Griffin and Butler, 2005), rather than the reverse. Rather than performance objectives in and of themselves, technical/tactical skill development is conceptualized as merely a tool for more full enjoyment and engagement with playing the game.

Play practice

Activities that cannot be defined as either deliberate practice or deliberate play are the specific pedagogical games/play designed by adults to prioritize affective outcomes over performance. While this general class of activities have been also described as game sense (Light, 2006), and teaching games for understanding (Griffin and Butler, 2005), we argue that Launder's (2001) term 'play practice' is the most appropriate label for this developmental activity. Play practice activities are led or prescribed by adults and emphasized fun and games. With these characteristics, play practice is the prototype activity for the taxonomy quadrant defined by high adult involvement and high intrinsic value. An important aspect of play practice activities is to keep youth motivated by designing learning activities that are enjoyable and typically represent the games that are played by youth.

Studies on non-specific sport training, which approximates many of the tenets of play practice, suggest that this type of developmental activity holds substantial promise in the development of innovation and talent among young athletes (Memmert et al., 2010; Memmert and Roth, 2007). Indeed, a recent review of the literature suggests that game-based approaches to coaching utilizing emotional learning principles are effective in the development of technical and tactical sport skills (Jarrett and Harvey, 2013).

Informal learning

An informal learning environment occurs outside of formal institutions or programmes (e.g. organized sports; Livingstone, 2002), and maintains the low external pressure atmosphere of deliberate play but is directed towards specific skill development. From a nonlinear pedagogy perspective, variability, flexibility and adaptability in motor skill performance is key to talent development and successful athletic performance. Chow and colleagues (2013) argued that the child-directedness characterizing these informal learning environments provides optimal conditions for the encouragement of variability in motor skill practice. Without adults directing or prescribing practice drills toward a specific motor pattern, children are free to attempt a diversity of strategies to solve any skill-based problem.

Spontaneous practice

The term spontaneous practice differs from deliberate play in that it is structured by athletes with the overall goal of improving their sport skills (e.g. extrinsic value). However, unlike the adult-directed nature of deliberate practice, in spontaneous practice children lead and coordinate the activities themselves, and do not necessarily follow a plan previously specified by an adult, or work on the skills most essential to their sport performance. Rather, spontaneous practice is more sporadic as it is planned and coordinated entirely by young athletes themselves. Thus, spontaneous practice is the prototype activity representing the taxonomy quadrant defined by low adult involvement (i.e. child-directed) and extrinsic value. Spontaneous practice activities provide a setting in sport where youth can experiment with new behaviors in a safe but stimulating environment (Balish and Côté, 2013). This setting allows youth to make errors without being criticized, be creative without being judged, try a new skill without being told 'how to do it', and do sport without an explicit focus on the technical aspect of performing.

Applied learning

Applied learning describes a learning environment that, in the adult world, could be described as 'workplace learning' (Malloch *et al.*, 2010). It is a form of learning that is at the intersection of the different types of learning environments described above (i.e. rational, creative, informal and emotional), as it includes a mix of intrinsic and extrinsic motivational conditions, and is monitored by adults. This particular learning environment is unique in that it allows young athletes to apply the varied skills that they have developed in all other learning environments. In this sense, it affords individuals the opportunities to access direct support from adults (coaches, parents, referees) and being evaluated in terms of performance outcomes. These applied learning situations in sport will usually happen in competitive activities that are structured and organized and will stimulate the young athletes to reflect on their performance, skills and learning.

Organized competition

Participation in organized competition is an activity led by adults, which requires concentration and effort but could vary greatly in terms of enjoyment or extrinsic value. Thus, the structure and adult-directed nature of organized competition situates it in a unique location relative to the developmental activities that occur in the other learning environments. Among elite athletes, organized competition has been considered one of the most helpful types of training for developing physical fitness, skill execution and decision-making (Baker, Côté and Abernethy, 2003). Organized competition supervised by adults has personal properties that resemble deliberate play, deliberate practice, spontaneous practice and play practice.

In sum, although youth sport is often perceived as being solely adult-led and focused on performance, the sampling years of the DMSP suggest that youth-led activities and enjoyment should also be integrated into youth sport programmes. The different learning environments and developmental activities of Figure 7.2.1 have been shown to uniquely contribute to long-term talent development in sport and concurrently the personal development of young athletes. The following section outlines the contribution of each environment to overall athlete development outcomes and highlights the need for integrated balance of developmental activities in youth sport.

Learning environments and outcomes of sport

Côté and Gilbert (2009) posited that four constructs termed the 4 Cs – competence, confidence, connection and character – collectively make a group of athlete outcomes that include measures of performance (competence), along with other important psychosocial factors related to talent development in sport such as self-confidence, positive social relationships and moral development. Improving in each of these four areas results in positive youth development (PYD), which can ultimately lead to long-term improvements in sport performance, participation and personal development (Fraser-Thomas *et al.*, 2005). Just as each learning environment and prototype activity can provide a unique context for talent development, the same can be suggested in consideration of the broader framework of the 4 Cs and PYD. We argue that the most comprehensive development of young peoples' talent potential in sport necessarily requires the integration of all 4 Cs, and not simply sport skill or ability (i.e. competence).

Inherent to a rational learning environment or deliberate practice is a clear emphasis on skill development, which should ideally improve athletes' competence in those discrete skills. In turn, if athletes improve their competence through rational learning, they are also likely to be more confident in their overall ability in a given sport. Furthermore, the adult-directed nature of this social context provides structured opportunities for athletes to engage in meaningful interactions with coaches, ultimately helping to facilitate adaptive coach-athlete relationships.

In addition, creative learning environments may influence the development of the 4 Cs in different ways. While rational learning and deliberate practice emphasize skill development as a primary outcome, increased competence may result as an indirect by-product of participating in a creative learning environment. In these youth-led social contexts, young athletes have more freedom and flexibility to be creative in sport and try out different skills, strategies and positions. This experimentation can lead to improved competence and confidence by helping youth develop more varied skill sets that they can later utilize in a rational learning environment. The lack of adult direction and supervision can also have significant implications on young athletes' peer relationships. Young athletes in a creative learning context need to engage in constructive peer interactions and effectively resolve conflicts in order to facilitate a positive experience. Through this process, youth have the potential to improve their social connections with peers and character as they navigate the occasional conflicts that can arise in this less structured environment.

Emotional learning represents a social context that shares similarities with both rational and creative learning environments. Play practice is adult-led, but emphasizes fun and enjoyment as opposed to skill development. This environment may therefore be beneficial to developing athletes' competence under the watchful eye of the coach, but through participation in activities that may be enjoyable to a broader range of young athletes given the focus on fun and enjoyment. Coaches that design game situations that allow all athletes to experience success on a regular basis will also have a significant impact on athletes' confidence and connection with others. The adult-led game situations can also help coaches to control certain scenarios that offer teachable moments for the development of athletes' character.

An informal learning environment is characterized by spontaneous practice activities where youth engage in structured drills, but do so voluntarily outside of an organized sport context. Thus, this type of environment may be conducive to the development of competence and confidence in young athletes, since they are able to practice previously learned skills and drills in a self-regulated manner without the added stress and watchful eye of a coach. Depending on the number of young people involved and the dynamic of the setting, informal environments can also potentially contribute to athletes' connection and character.

Finally, applied learning environments have the potential to develop competence and confidence in young athletes by allowing opportunities to integrate their learning from the different learning environments into competitive performance contexts. However, another aspect of learning that occur in youth competitive environments such as organized games is the use of real-time situations to transmit values related to positive relationships (connection) and character. The many ups and downs afforded by competition allow young athletes to develop personal bonds with their teammates and, if supported appropriately, strong moral character. When games are structured such that external rewards are de-emphasized, healthy competition becomes a source of enjoyment and effort, which sets a foundation that allows young athletes to truly excel in sport (Shields and Bredemeier, 2009).

Learning environments: a summary

Rational, creative, emotional, informal and applied learning are not intended to form a complete list of all youth sport environments. Together, however, they represent a handful of the varied social contexts that young athletes may be exposed to. Each learning environment is comprised of unique contextual characteristics, which can be further described by the prototype activities suggested by Côté and colleagues (2013): Deliberate practice, deliberate play, play practice, spontaneous practice and organized competition. This collection of activities and their unique characteristics are representative of the diverse sport involvement that is typical of the sampling years. Thus, through participation in each of these activities, young athletes are likely to have a much broader range of sport experiences than would be likely if they were only exposed to a smaller subset of learning environments and activities.

Deliberate practice, play practice, spontaneous practice, deliberate play and organized competition all vary according to the social structure and personal values of the learning environment. However, each activity plays an important role in maintaining youths' motivation to participate in sport and ultimately develop new skills and talent. Indeed, previous studies have demonstrated that as children, elite-level athletes appeared to engage in a wide range of activities that could be generally classified as deliberate practice, deliberate play, play practice, spontaneous practice and organized competition (e.g. Baker *et al.*, 2003; Berry, Abernethy and Côté, 2008; Ford *et al.*, 2009). Thus it appears that the different learning environments of these varied activities facilitated the development of different personal and social skills, which in turn helped to promote their continued sport participation. The intrinsically motivating and self-directed nature of more play-oriented activities contrasts with the outcome-oriented and often adult-driven nature of more practice-oriented activities. The nurturing of talent through the sampling of different learning environments without a sole focus on a rational (or adult-led) type of learning will result in more positive outcomes and less negative consequences for all children involved in sport, while still facilitating development toward expertise.

The complementary nature of these different learning environments and developmental activities suggests that youth sport programmes should include a variety of these activities to optimize the personal and talent development of young athletes. The characteristics of each specific context provide unique opportunities to facilitate the development of important outcomes exemplified by the 4 Cs. The sampling years of the DMSP thus refers to a balance of learning environments and activity types. Youth's relative participation in these different sport activities then sets the foundation for their long-term talent development trajectories. Unfortunately, many organized youth sport programmes primarily focus on rational learning, and while these programmes might sometimes be considered effective in developing talented young athletes, youth are at the same time prevented from reaping the additional benefits that would have been afforded to them in more varied learning environments. A limited view of the breadth of activities pertinent to the acquisition of sport expertise fails to acknowledge the crucial developmental assets that influence athlete development throughout childhood (Côté *et al.*, 2007). Structured models of athlete development such as the LTAD would be well-served to begin to integrate the evidence supporting the benefits of varied developmental activities and learning environments for developing talented young athletes. Given the equivocal evidence surrounding the optimal prescriptive approach for talent development, young athletes should be given the opportunity to engage in and learn from activities that are both adult and youth-led and are intrinsically and extrinsically valued.

References

Bailey, R. P. and Toms, M. (2010). *Participant Development in Sport: An Academic Literature Review*. Commissioned report for Sports Coach UK. Leeds: Sports Coach UK.

Baker, J. and Abernethy, B. (2003). Learning from the experts: Practice activities of expert decision makers in sport. *Research Quarterly for Exercise and Sport*, 74: 342–347.

Baker, J. and Deakin, J. (2005). Expertise in ultra-endurance triathletes: Early sport involvement, training structure, and the theory of deliberate practice. *Journal of Applied Sport Psychology*, 17: 64–78

Balish, S. and Côté, J. (2013). The influence of community on athletic development: an integrated case study, *Qualitative Research in Sport, Exercise and Health*, DOI:10.1080/2159676X.2013.766815

Balyi, I. and Hamilton, A. (2004). *Long-Term Athlete Development: Trainability in Children and Adolescents. Windows of Opportunity, Optimal Trainability*. Victoria, BC: National Coaching Institute British Columbia and Advanced Training and Performance, Ltd.

Barreiros, A. and Fonseca, A.M. (2014). From early to adult sport success: Analyzing athletes' progression in national squads. *European Journal of Sport Science*, 14(sup1): S178–S182.

Berry, J. and Côté, J. (2008). The contribution of structured practice and deliberate play to the development of expert perceptual and decision-making skill. *Journal of Sport and Exercise Psychology*, 30: 685–708.

Bloom, B.S. (1985). *Developing Talent in Young People*. New York: Ballantine.

Bridge, M. W. and Toms, M. R. (2013). The specialising or sampling debate: a retrospective analysis of adolescent sports participation in the UK. *Journal of Sports Sciences*, 31(1): 87–96.

Canadian Sport for Life (2008). Long term athlete development resource paper v2. Vancouver, BC: Canadian Sport Centres. Retrieved from http://canadiansportforlife.ca/sites/default/files/resources/CS4Lper cent20Resource per cent20Paper.pdf

Carlson, R. (1988). The socialization of elite tennis players in Sweden: An analysis of the players' backgrounds and development. *Sociology of Sport Journal*, 5(2): 241–256.

Chow, J. Y. and Button, C. (2013). The acquisition of movement skill in children through nonlinear pedagogy. In J. Côté and R. Lidor (eds), *Conditions of Children's Talent Development in Sport* (pp. 41–60). Morgantown, WV: Fitness Information Technology.

Côté, J. (1999). The influence of the family in the development of talent in sports. *The Sport Psychologist*, 13: 395–417.

Côté, J. and Abernethy, B. (2012). A developmental approach to sport expertise. In S. Murphy (ed), *The Oxford Handbook of Sport and Performance Psychology* (pp. 435–447). New York: Oxford University Press.

Côté, J. and Abernethy, B. (2007). Practice and play in the development of sport expertise. In R. Eklund and G. Tenenbaum (eds), *Handbook of Sport Psychology* (3rd edition,pp. 184–202). Hoboken, NJ: Wiley.

Côté, J. and Abernethy, B. (2013). Practice and play in sport development. In J. Côté and R. Lidor (eds), *Condition of Children's Talent Development in Sport* (pp. 9–20). Morgantown, WV: Fitness Information Technology.

Côté, J. and Wilkes, S. (2009). The benefits of sampling sports during childhood. *Physical and Health Education Journal*, 74(4): 6–11.

Côté, J. and Fraser-Thomas, J. (2007). Youth involvement in sport. In P. Crocker (ed), *Sport Psychology: A Canadian Perspective* (pp. 270–298). Toronto, ON: Pearson.

Côté, J. and Gilbert, W. (2009). An integrative definition of coaching effectiveness and expertise. *International Journal of Sports Science and Coaching*, 4: 307–323.

Côté, J. and Hackfort, D. (2009). To sample or to specialize? Seven postulates about youth sport activities that lead to continued participation and elite performance. *International Journal of Sport and Exercise Psychology*, 9: 7–17.

Ericsson, K. A. and Tesch-Römer, C. (1993). The role of deliberate practice in the acquisition of expert performance. *Psychological Review*, 100: 363–406.

Ford, P. and Williams, C. (2011). The long-term athlete development model: Physiological evidence and application. *Journal of Sports Sciences*, 29(4): 389–402.

Fraser-Thomas, J. and Côté, J. (2009). Understanding adolescents' positive and negative developmental experiences in sport. *The Sport Psychologist*, 23: 3–23.

Fraser-Thomas, J. and Deakin, J. (2005). Youth sport programmes: An avenue to foster positive youth development. *Physical Education and Sport Pedagogy*, 10: 49–70.

Fraser-Thomas, J. and Deakin, J. (2008a). Examining adolescent sport dropout and prolonged engagement from a developmental perspective. *Journal of Applied Sport Psychology*, 20: 318–333.

Fraser-Thomas, J. and Deakin, J. (2008b). Understanding dropout and prolonged engagement in adolescent competitive sport. *Psychology of Sport and Exercise*, 9: 645–662.

Griffin, L. L. and Butler, J. I. (2005). *Teaching Games for Understanding: Theory, Research, and Practice.* Champaign, Illinois: Human Kinetics.

Gulbin, J. P. and Gagné, F. (2010). A look through the rear view mirror: Developmental experiences and insights of high performance athletes. *Talent Development and Excellence,* 2(2): 149–164.

Jarrett, K. and Harvey, S. (2013). Recent trends in research literature on game-based approaches to teaching and coaching games. In R. Light, S. Harvey, O. Quay, and A. Mooney (eds) *Contemporary Developments in Games Teaching* (pp. 87–98). London: Routledge.

Launder, A. G. (2001). *Play Practice: The Games Approach to Teaching and Coaching Sports.* Champaign, Illinois: Human Kinetics.

Law, M. and Ericsson, K. A. (2007). Characteristics of expert development in rhythmic gymnastics: A retrospective study. *International Journal of Sport and Exercise Psychology,* 5: 82–103.

Leite, N. M. and Sampaio, J. E. (2012). Long-term athletic development across different age groups and gender from Portuguese basketball players. *International Journal of Sports Science and Coaching,* 7(2): 285–300.

Light, R. (2006). Game sense: Innovation or just good coaching? *Journal of Physical Education New Zealand,* 39(1): 8–19.

Livingstone, D. W. (2002). *Mapping the iceberg.* Retrieved from www.nall.ca/res/54DavidLivingstone.pdf

Malloch, M. and O'Connor, B. N. (eds). (2010). *The SAGE Handbook of Workplace Learning.* London: SAGE.

Masters, R. S. W. and Maxwell, J. P. (2004). Implicit motor learning, reinvestment and movement disruption: What you don't know won't hurt you? In A. M. Williams and N. J. Hodges (eds), *Skill Acquisition in Sport: Research, Theory and Practice* (pp. 207–228). London: Routledge.

Memmert, D. and Bertsch, C. (2010). Play and practice in the development of sport_specific creativity in team ball sports. *High Ability Studies,* 21(1): 3–18.

Memmert, D. and Roth, K. (2007). The effects of non-specific and specific concepts on tactical creativity in team ball sports. *Journal of Sports Sciences,* 25(12): 1423–1432.

Robertson–Wilson, J. and Côté, J. (2003). Childhood sport involvement in active and inactive adult females. *AVANTE,* 9: 1–8.

Shields, D. L. and Bredemeier, B. L. (2009). *True Competition: A Guide to Pursuing Excellence in Sport and Society.* Champaign, Illinois: Human Kinetics.

Soberlak, P. and Côté, J. (2003). The developmental activities of professional ice hockey players. *Journal of Applied Sport Psychology,* 15: 41–49.

Starkes, J. L. and Hayes. and *Games* (pp. 81–106). Mahwah, NJ: Erlbaum.

Strachan, L. and Deakin, J. (2009). "Specializers" versus "samplers" in youth sport: Comparing experiences and outcomes. *The Sport Psychologist,* 23: 77–92.

Wall, M. and Côté, J. (2007). Developmental activities that lead to drop out and investment in sport. *Physical Education and Sport Pedagogy,* 12: 77–87.

Ward, P. and Starkes, J. L. (2004). Deliberate practice and expert performance: Defining the path to excellence. In. A. M. Williams and N. J. Hodges (eds), *Skill Acquisition in Sport: Research Theory and Practice* (pp. 231–258). New York: Routledge.

43

TALENT IDENTIFICATION AND DEVELOPMENT IN YOUTH SPORT

Steve Cobley

Developmental science and models of development

Developmental science attempts to describe, explain and optimize the intra and inter-individual biological, psychological, social and behavioural changes that occur across the life span, including childhood and youth (Damon, 2004; Lerner, Fisher and Weinberg, 2000). This field emerged, in part, to address the limitations, dualistic tensions and the impasse arising from the nature and nurture perspectives put forward to account for development. These limitations include an inability to adequately explain the diversity of individual differences, such as psychological resilience versus frailty (Feldman *et al.*, 2004) as well as other existential outcomes and experiences that occur across the life-course, and which can result from inappropriate development, such as compromised health (Gottlieb *et al.*, 2006; Overton, 2006). Other limitations stem from the use of reductionist as opposed to multi-disciplinary research paradigms.

To overcome these perspectives and better explain human complexity and experiences, developmental science increasingly considers that change and development in youth occurs via both functional and dysfunctional relationships between the individual and the potential multiple levels of the ecological context (Bronfenbrenner, 1979, 2005; Lerner, 1995). In other words, the integration or fusion of all factors within and between the individual and the environment at all levels (Tobach and Greenberg, 1984); often represented as 'individual context' relations (Lerner, 1991).

Contemporary developmental system models (e.g. Ford and Lerner, 1992) emphasize that there are potentially multiple reciprocal effects and influences shaping youth development. These include factors associated with the individual, social others (e.g. family, peers, and coaches) and context (e.g. school and sports system) with their range relating to intra-individual genes and cell physiology, individual mental and behavioural functioning, local community (e.g. quality of school provision), broader institutions of society, culture and its history (temporality) as well as the designed (i.e. built) and natural environments (see Figure 1 in Lerner and Castellino, 2002). The potential inherent interactions, whether simple, such as positive affection between two individuals, or complex (e.g. parental work commitments limiting evening social-interaction) regulates, facilitates, inhibits, accelerates and/or actively constrains youth development. When

476

these relations between the individual and context are mutually beneficial, they provide a highly adaptive fit, often referred to as 'relative plasticity' (Baltes, 1987; Lerner, 1998). Importantly, as adaptation takes place, it also deflects the likelihood for development to move in negative directions, which might include school failure and dropout, violence, drug and alcohol abuse and/or non-participation in physical activity, sport and social clubs.

The developmental model view of talent

From a developmental model viewpoint, youthful sporting talent could be construed as reflecting the presence or absence of a set, or combination, of particular individual skills (e.g. intrinsic motivation, self-regulation and social confidence) and qualities (e.g. gene allele adaptability, biological growth, height, low body-fat and training history). These may emanate from multiple causal pathways, and influential relationships between the individual, specific sport tasks, social environment, as well as wider social policy (e.g. age-group provision) and culture (e.g. history of attainment at local club and state investment in infrastructure). Not all potential individual-context relations would need to be present or functionally active at any one time point to underpin talent. Further, these relations and processes may also be diverse and different for athletes in their particular developmental ecologies. Overall though, some level of plasticity is required to evidence development. When this occurs, it can underpin a valued set of physical, psychological, technical and tactical attributes necessary within a given sport context.

While multiple individual-context relations seem possible, it also appears logical that the nature of the sport task itself could also be influential. We might consider, for instance, the beneficial factors in rowing versus field-hockey. Rowing has relatively fewer requisite components that constitute the task, which suggests a more narrow and specific set of individual-context relations (see Figure 43.3 and supporting explanation in Vaeyens *et al.*, 2008). Performance here may be more predicated on both genetically inherited and trained anthropometric and physical individual characteristics such as height, $VO_{2\,max}$, low body mass as well as endurance training exposure in childhood and beyond (e.g. Ingham *et al.*; Lawton *et al.*, 2012). Many of these factors are constrained by biological growth and development and endurance training exposure rather than potential influences in the wider ecology, such as access to coaching expertise and exposure to water-based rowing per se.

By comparison, field-hockey not only has anthropometric and physiological requisites, but also contains continuously adaptive perceptual-cognitive/motor and technical components that have to be acquired and applied in the game (e.g. see Keogh *et al.*, 2003; Elferink-Gemser *et al.*, 2004). These requisites may require more time to initiate and complete their developmental trajectories (e.g. neural development in executive and motor brain areas). Importantly, they may be more highly dependent on ecological contexts that stimulate their development. For example, development may hinge on access to equipment and space, and opportunities to play the game and learn from peers, parents, players and knowledgeable coaches. Such diversity and their potential interactions suggest that a complex set of pathways are possible, and many are yet to be identified within research. It also highlights that across and within sports uneven and different profiles of development may occur, each contributing potentially uniquely to the emergence of talent and to which underlies further onward long-term development.

If identifying the functional requisites and individual-context factors underpinning sport talent is not challenging enough, proceeding to optimally develop the multiple skills and physiological competencies within changing ecologies adds to that challenge. Developmental models assume that the progression of time leads to potential change within youth, their social environments, and their relations. For instance, each individual will follow a distinctive pattern of biological growth and maturation, alongside the evolution of their social interactions and relationships. Additionally, there are planned and often inevitable transitions, such as changing school/ college alongside unplanned gradual and abrupt changes, such as loss of a loved one or trauma from an injury or accident, that can impact the life-course of youth. Changes also occur within the sport context itself (e.g. selection or non-selection for a team) and in other life contexts (e.g. parent/teacher/coach relationships).

Taken together, sporting talent can be said to develop through a favourable alignment of individual-context characteristics and conditions, which add or provide multiplicative benefits (Simonton, 1999) for the completion of a task or activity. Another perspective is that some of these characteristics predict onward acceleration in cognitive learning and physical performance into adulthood. Contrary to popular perceptions, individual-context dynamics expressed over time highlight the likelihood that talent is not predominantly a fixed set of individual traits and characteristics that are usually on display at an early age. Instead, talent is better understood as a temporary state from which there are:

1   multiple non-linear paths and trajectories and
2   where talent can emerge late, regress, surge and be lost across ages and stage of sporting development, due to multiple individual-context mechanisms within the ecological system
(Abbott et al., 2005; Simonton, 2001)

Talent identification and development systems (TIDS) in sport

Reflecting the desire to systematically manufacture exceptional adult athletes, the installation and deployment of national and local child/youth based TIDS has grown markedly in the last 15–30 years. While the fundamental purpose has remained consistent, the intensity of the experience of being enrolled in such a programme has intensified in recent years. Two features characterise this intensification:

1   the identification of precocious young athletes earlier and earlier in their lives (Williams and Reilly, 2000) and
2   attempts to accelerate the youngsters' performance through provision of supposedly more optimal training conditions and environments (Abbott and Collins, 2004).

For instance, alongside the commercial growth, media and popular interest in sport, there has been a wave of government investment and policy promoting sporting competition in schools within the UK (Green, 2006). This has been justified by claims that sport can be an avenue for individual and social health, community and urban development (e.g. Coalter, 2007). Similarly, there has been a marked attempt to identify athletic talent through national search programmes such as Sporting Giants (UK Sport 2007), and strategically funding developing athletes in preparation for an impending home Olympics (UK Sport, 2008). In parallel, independent sport governing bodies and local professional sports clubs have adopted or adapted (inappropriately, in some cases) TID models. For example, many sports clubs adapted one-dimensional *stage* or linear step-like practical models, such as Long-Term Athlete Development (LTAD) (Arellano, 2010; Balyi and Hamilton, 2004) from other sporting contexts. Whether accepted as part of policy implementation or absorbed via external influences and values, TIDS have become increasingly popular. This popularity has gone hand-in-hand with the perception that earlier selection into TIDS optimises progression into elite sport and subsequent achievements. Such notions are reinforced by research revealing how skill and performance benefits accrue from long-term and intensive training, as highlighted by the deliberate practice framework (Ericsson *et al.*, 1993). Overall, the UK case exemplifies how a social-cultural ecology and climate can begin to exert influence, shaping junior/youth sporting experiences.

Structurally, TIDS invariably adopt a pyramid structure of participation (Güllich and Emrich, 2012, p. 245), with local junior age-group bands and recreational participation often constituting the so-called 'broad base'. Competitive performance and assessment at set ages and time point milestones usually determines onward selection into higher tiers of local-national representation, depending on performance and skill level. Tiers of representation across the pyramid highlight the path and transfer between linear stages. At every representative stage, the pool of athletes reduces until a small, elite sample is reached (Cobley *et al.*, 2012, p. 6). Typically, throughout adolescence, programmes offer age-group bands ending at youth or adult/senior ages (e.g. 18–21 years). Ultimately, the structure means that most recruits (perhaps up to 99 per cent of participants) will experience de-selection, withdrawal and dropout in childhood and youth, and it is rare that substantial numbers of athletes transfer across TID contexts.

Across the research literature (e.g. Rongen *et al.*, 2015) and athlete/practitioner experience, several intertwined features of current sport-based youth TIDS have been identified and debated. Considerable energy has been devoted to evaluating the potential – both positive and negative – of TIDS to influence youth athletes. These debates often focus on the emphasis and value of:

1   immediate competitive success in junior and youth sport;
2   early sport specialization accompanied by intensified, highly structured and specific training; and
3   adherence to a performance social ecology model.

From a developmental science perspective, many of these features appear contradictory to, or misaligned with, current developmental models and highlight a discrepancy between system-athlete needs. Accordingly, this raises questions about the functionality of programme components and whether practices and social ecologies within TIDS are, in fact, optimally developmental. Sport TIDS have received criticism for their role in compromised developmental health consequences. But even when avoiding these pitfalls, TIDS often appear fixed, rigid and inconsiderate towards actual developmental changes, diverse trajectories, and the developmental needs of youth.

Immediate competitive success in junior and youth sport

A core concern of critics tends to be the focus on competitive performance. They recognise that many TIDS have, to date, followed a heuristic approach toward athlete development based on backward extrapolation, starting with adult sport models; that is to say, the best way to prepare 'up and coming' athletes is to replicate and mimic the nature and content of adult elite sport competition. Thus, intensive frequent local-international competition is often a key feature of TIDS involvement. Such a focus places a premium on identifying and selecting athletes who can deliver immediate success, which is then used to justify continuing in this way. This can result in a myopic and narrow conception of talent, suggesting that universal, one-dimensional performance indicators can be used to identify and evaluate athletic talent. To complicate matters, sport TIDS themselves can promote such a view insofar as they employ and evaluate their delivery staff (e.g. coaches and youth development coordinators) on the basis of short-term competitive performance successes as opposed to longer-term developmental processes.

There are at least three limitations confronting proponents of TIDS that focus on performance. First, predictive factors for performance success in youth will change at each age and stage until the elite level (Cobley *et al.*, 2012). So a singular approach is unlikely to fit all. Second, biological growth and development (e.g. Meylan *et al.*, 2010; Pearson *et al.*, 2006) proceeds discontinuously and episodically, making it difficult to identify athletic talent. Third, important attributes and skills that appear to provide the scaffold for both immediate and long-term successes (e.g. psychological self-regulation skills; Cleary and Zimmerman, 2001; Jonker *et al.*, 2010) take time to develop. In terms of biological growth, increases in anthropometric height, weight, fat tissue and organ size occur as an individual ages across youth (Malina *et al.*, 2004; Tanner, 1962). But then to complicate matters, maturation – associated with the final growth spurt (Malina, 1994) – is characterised by variable timing and tempo upon onset during adolescence (i.e. 12–15 years of age for males; 11–14 for females), changing many structural and functional features in the body, such as converting cartilage to bone in the skeleton and the appearance of secondary sexual characteristics.

Although less consistently related to skill or technical competencies, such as soccer ball control and dribbling (Votteler and Höner, 2014), growth is highly predictive of physical capacities such as aerobic power, muscular strength, endurance, and speed (e.g. Viru *et al.*, 1998; 1999; Vandenendriessche *et al.*, 2012). These characteristics also underlie, or partly constitute, many athletic contexts and provide physical performance advantages for older children/youth – whether the characteristics are determined chronologically (i.e. between age groups) or relatively (i.e. within age groups; Malina *et al.*, 2007; Musch and Grondin, 2001). To exacerbate anthropometric and physiological characteristic differences, older children/youth – however categorised or considered – are more likely to enter maturation earlier and with unpredictable tempos. All this adds to the physical performance variability that exists between individuals. When stabilisation finally occurs, at 15–16 years of age or beyond, differences that previously existed reduce in magnitude, especially for anthropometric and physiological variables (e.g. Baxter-Jones *et al.*, 2005). However, before this point, the mismatch within a single age group can exceed the equivalent of two biological years (Cobley and Till, in press; Malina *et al.*, 2004). Crucially, these events coincide with the time when many team sport TIDS are implementing their programmes from school level.

The result of biological growth processes is that the earlier maturing and relatively older are more likely to be selected as talented and be participating in TID age-group structures (e.g. Sherar *et al.*, 2007; Simmons and Paull, 2001). For example, in a sample of young Rugby League players (aged 13–16 years; N = 683), Till *et al.* (2010a) compared growth status against aged-matched UK reference percentiles (Freeman *et al.*, 1995). For height, 92.4 per cent of selected players were taller than the fiftieth percentile, and 33.3 per cent were above the ninety-seventh percentile. For weight, 96.0 per cent and 30.3 per cent were above the fiftieth and ninety-seventh percentiles respectively. When one considers that the average age of peak height velocity in maturation for European boys occurs between 13.8–14.2 years (Malina *et al.*, 2004), these young UK rugby league players were maturing earlier (i.e. peak height velocity = 13.61 ±0.58 years; Mirwald *et al.*, 2002). Studies in other team sports replicate these observations (e.g. soccer – Phillippaerts *et al.*, 2006; handball – Mohammed *et al.*, 2009; ice-hockey – Sherar *et al.*, 2007).

Relative Age Effects (RAEs) in TIDS also reflect the link between a performance emphasis and biological growth. Referring to an interaction between an athletes' birth-date, and the dates used for chronological [bi]annual age grouping (such as under 14–16s) within a TID system (Wattie *et al.*, 2008), a relatively older athlete (i.e. born in the initial months after an age group cut-off date, e.g. 1 January) is more mature than a relatively younger athlete (i.e. born in the last few months of the age-group). And relatively older athletes are also more likely to be selected onto a TIDS, due to the benefit of up to potentially 364 days additional growth and maturation per year. Studies, particularly in male team sport contexts (e.g. ice-hockey, soccer, rugby union and league) reveal that RAEs magnify progressively in youth ages (i.e. 14–18 years of age), and across TID stages. Ratios between relatively older and younger athletes have been found to range from 3:2 to 9:1 at the local to national stages respectively (Cobley *et al.*, 2009; Till *et al.*, 2010b). So although relatively younger athletes are present in TIDS, they often need to be earlier maturing (Carling *et al.*, 2009; Till *et al.*, 2010b).

The interaction between biological growth and TIDS, characterised by early age entry point restrictions and a step-like linear structure, has profound effects. It increases the likelihood of later age, later maturing, and later emerging talent being either excluded, denied developmental opportunities, de-selected or simply being missed by the system. In the long term, incorrect or missed TID results in fewer – actually skilfully talented – athletes successfully transitioning into elite sport, outcomes which are counterproductive and paradoxical for TIDS. To illustrate, Till *et al.* (2014) recently tracked eighty-one junior Rugby League players, aged 13–15, within a TIDS. Their data demonstrated not only that early-maturing players were more likely to be present, possessing more preferable anthropometric (e.g. height) and fitness characteristics (e.g. VO_2 max), but also that a later maturing group improved their height, upper body strength and lower body power (e.g. sprint times) proportionately more across the same two-year tracking period. Players in the prop position, characterised by superior height, strength and body mass – advantageous to competitive success at the under 13–14s stage – became the worst performing on fitness tests among under 15s. They were also more likely to retain body fat, a factor likely to impede performance later in the TID, where game speed and intensity increases. Props were subsequently less likely to be involved in higher TIDS ages and stages, and less likely to reach the professional game.

At their final stages, TIDS bridge into the group of adult professional athletes. Deaner *et al.* (2013) examined 2,736 Canadian outfield ice-hockey players who entered the professional NHL ice-hockey draft, 1980–2012, and their subsequent NHL career productivity profiles. On draft

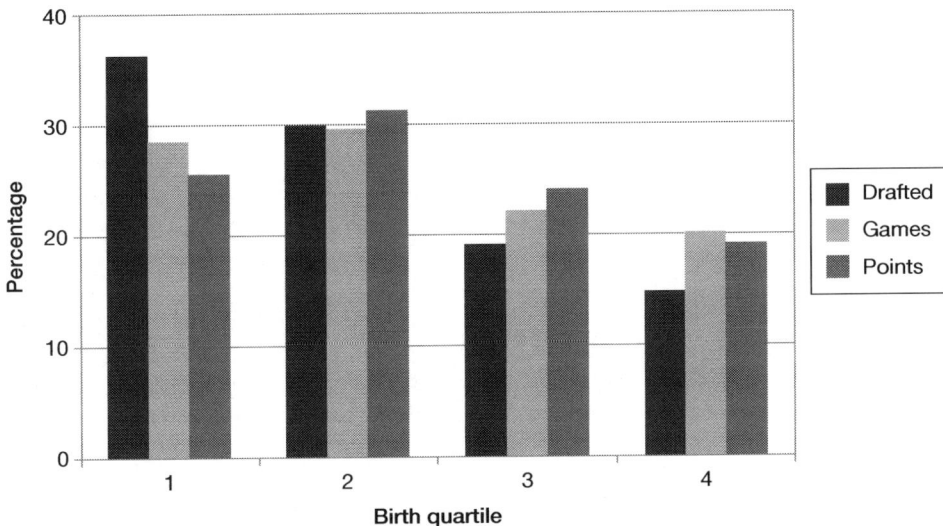

Figure 43.1 Percentage of NHL draftees (spanning 1980–2012), games played, and points scored according to relative age (or birth quartile)

entry at ages 18–20, 36 per cent were relatively older (i.e. quartile 1) with only 14.5 per cent relatively younger (i.e. quartile 4) athletes (Figure 43.1). Yet, 45 per cent of this draft sample never played in a single NHL game; and when controlling for other factors, the relatively younger actually went on to play in 20 per cent of NHL games, contributing 19 per cent of total points scored. In addition, the relatively younger were twice as likely to attain career benchmarks (i.e. 400–600+ games played). By contrast, the relatively older were less likely to play a single game, and underperformed given their overrepresentation, suggesting that they were overvalued at the draft stage. This may reflect a legacy of RAE mechanisms that prevailed in youth, and valuing early physical capacities for producing competitive success. The professional-level success of relatively younger players was related to a combination of

1 late emerging maturation and/or performance,
2 adaptive development in an adverse youth TID climate, including heightened technical skill proficiency, and
3 social escalation processes, such as being able to contribute unique skills.

Early sport specialization and intensive training

Early specialisation is typified by sole participation and intensive training in one sport context on a year-round basis from an early age (American Academy of Paediatrics, 2000; Baker *et al.*, 2009). It is favoured in sports like gymnastics where peak performance occurs at approximately 15–16, compared to others (e.g. soccer) where peak performance happens between ages 24–30. Nonetheless, even within late specialisation sports, TIDS are promoting and stipulating earlier specialization. Linked to broader socio-cultural movements (e.g. national sport and education policy in the UK), this has involved *inter alia* implementing more selection and participation tiers within national-local TID models. The approach is based on the unfounded assumption that 'more training and competition is better' and that earlier capture and involvement will realise 'athletic promise' at younger ages. Another feature, the imposed behaviour regulation on athletes (such as non-participation in other sports) is proposed as a benign approach to reducing risk of non-sport specific injury (e.g. Green, 2009).

The effects of earlier specialization are hypothesized as being diverse and far-reaching across individual and broader sport ecologies. Broadly, TID growth is actively changing when the participation pyramid narrows, due to differentiation and selection; and resources are concentrated on fewer talented athletes at an earlier age (Figure 43.2). Competition and performance success is increasingly valued, prioritised, and transmitted throughout the sport system, supported by youth institutions and members (e.g. schools and sport clubs) at lower levels of the sport participation pyramid. As a consequence, few models of contemporary youth are prioritising social inclusion, physical activity and/or health promotion, over performance success (Collins *et al.*, 2012). Inevitably, these priorities colour the experiences, perceptions, and values that young people then link to sport, even after initial exposures. Before having opportunities to experience intrinsic developmental outcomes – such as experiences of fun, enjoyment, satisfaction; perceptions of self-competence, affiliation; and being able to build social relationships – youth are being shaped to match-up and/or accept as 'part of the game' the intensified striving and increasingly discriminating system.

Yet carefully balanced and managed TIDS – for the included and selected – permit focused opportunities for the positive development of psychological (e.g. self-esteem, social connectedness) and physiological capacities (e.g. VO_2 max, power; Malina, 2010), fundamental movement skills, sport-specific motor skills, as well as healthier anthropometry (e.g. lower body

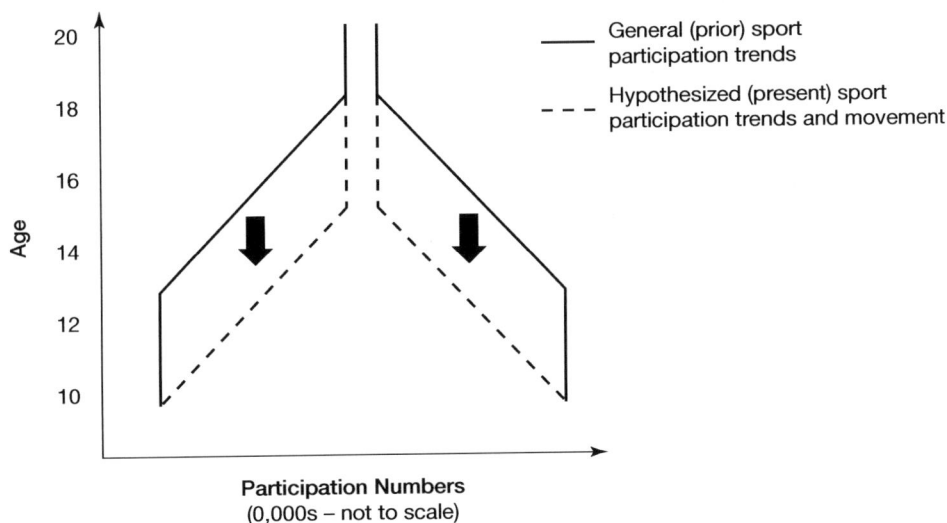

Figure 43.2 Illustration highlighting the changing sport participation pyramid due to a growing emphasis on athlete TID in sport

mass index) and cardiovascular profiles. These outcomes are clearly beneficial for long-term cognitive and physical health (Armstrong and Oomen-Early, also 2009; Bailey, *et al.*, 1999; Ford *et al.*, 2009). Nevertheless, early TID involvement continues to be associated with high volume, intense and repetitive sport-specific training over an extended period of the year (Baxter-Jones and Helms, 1996; Lang, 2010), running the risk of over-reaching into negative consequences, such as unbalanced fundamental movement skills (e.g. Branta, 2010), pre-disposure to injury (e.g. repetitive strain injuries; e.g. Brenner, 2007) as well as compromised psychosocial and physical health. These risks appear to interrelate with decreased motivation and enjoyment, social isolation (Coakley, 2010), heightened perceptions of stress and poor physical health (Boyd and Yin, 1996; Law *et al.*, 2007) as well as overtraining and burnout (e.g. Wiersma, 2000; Matos and Winsley, 2007). If prolonged and severe, these experiences are most likely to disaffection and overall withdrawal from sport (e.g. Fraser-Thomas *et al.*, 2008).

The justification for early specialization in later peak-age sports has also been questioned, following review of retrospective data from elite athletes. Significantly, this suggests that an 'early diversified, later specializing' approach is more conducive to long-term (performance) development. Voluntary sampling across childhood sports, with little emphasis on training and a high emphasis on play prior to investment later in youth, are deemed at least equally beneficial in facilitating progression toward elite sport, while also better facilitating physical and psychosocial health (e.g. Baker *et al.*, 2003; Côté *et al.*, 2009). A diversified approach, so the logic goes, fosters intrinsic interest and self-determined behaviour via the playful nature of pick-up-and-go adaptive games, created and led by children. To a greater or lesser extent, these activities resemble sport contexts from the child's perspective. But involvement in multiple games/activities, with their diverse physical and motor requirements, help stimulate generic perceptual-cognitive skills, and provide a strong physical foundation for more specific and intense training in later youth (Baker and Côté, 2006).

In exploring the benefits of diversification, Moesch, Elbe, Hauge and Wikman (2011) recently examined the participation trajectories of 148 elite (i.e. top 10 finish at a European/World championship or Olympics) and 95 near–elite Danish athletes across sports such as cycling, rowing, swimming, sailing, track and field. The results revealed that elite success, compared to near-elites, was associated with less training in childhood, less specific accumulated training up to 15 years of age, a later age of specialization, accelerated training in youth (specifically, 18–21 years) and a shorter amount of time on junior TID stages (i.e. national teams). Findings that resonate with observations in other sport contexts (e.g. Carlson, 1988; Lidor and Lavyan, 2002). It seems that early specialization is positively correlated with immediate, junior success, but negatively associated with adult level attainment (Vaeyens *et al.*, 2009) and the likelihood of continued sport participation in adulthood (Russell and Limle, 2013). Early sampling and later specialization is associated with increased physical capacity and motor skill base (e.g. Bailey *et al.*, 2010), a better ability to transfer motor and psychological skills to other sports (e.g. Fransen *et al.*, 2012), increased motivation, confidence and self-direction (e.g. Côté and Fraser-Thomas, 2008) and a longer likelihood of involvement on national teams (e.g. Barynina and Vaitsekhovskii, 1992).

Adherence to a performance social ecology

Some TIDS can promote social values and micro-systems that also emulate the adult sport ecology. That is, encouraging and reinforcing distinctive behaviours, narratives and focused identities (Carless and Douglas, 2009; Douglas and Carless, 2006). Recognised and reinforced by those with vested interests in competition success (e.g. selectors, governing bodies, financial investors and media), the strength of these discourses is such that they consistently favour athletes who resolutely offer personnel commitment and contribution from early ages and stages, including playing when injured and 'putting the body on the line'. Those athletes are then held up as personified exemplars of 'real-athletes' (e.g. McGillivray, Fearn and McIntosh, 2005), especially when they link to performance domination, achieved through physical strength and aggression. These narratives are powerful and compelling. They generate expectancies and support the adoption of specific behaviours that then become part and parcel of an athletic identity. For those unfamiliar and unexposed, such psychological conditions can be perceived as pressurising to conform, ego-based, anxiety inducing and stressful (e.g. Pensgaard, and Roberts, 2000).

Acceptance and compliance to any social ecology centred on performance explicitly moulds and shapes 'athletic identity' (e.g. Christensen and Sorensen, 2009; Lamont-Mills and Christensen, 2006). In the most visible examples, this is characterised by a single-mindedness and a strong association of the self and personal mission with athletic behaviours (Brewer *et al.*, 1993). Of course, an athletic identity can benefit psychological health (e.g. increased self-esteem and positive body image) and enhance performance. But conversely, problems can occur through early athletic identities or 'identity foreclosure' (Murphy *et al.*, 1996) at a time when exploring and developing a multi-faceted identity in divergent contexts often occurs (Adams and Marshall, 1996). In sport contexts where specific body characteristics predict performance, rapid weight loss/gain strategies, using performance enhancing substances and adopting disordered eating patterns can all indicate over-commitment, often more frequently in those with strong athletic identities (e.g. Pipe, 2001; Sundgot-Borgen and Torstveit, 2010). The strong athletic identities may also experience psychological difficulties when coping with performance setbacks that can accompany involvement in TIDS, including being de-selected (Brown and Potrac, 2009), or when forced to make transitions (e.g. out of sport – Wylleman, and Lavallee, 2004), leading to mental health problems such as social isolation (Horton and Mack, 2000), depression and identity loss (Douglas and Carless, 2006, 2009).

Implicitly, performance social ecologies can also engender forms of 'elitism' (Tännsjö and Tamburrini, 2000). In contrast to a sense of belonging, athletic elitism can involve: physical domination and distancing; psychological self-valuing, narcissism and a sense of 'betterness'; as well as social processes that typically symbolize and construct forms of separation, difference(s) and distinctiveness. Since TIDS invoke separation (via selection) and exclusivity on performance meritocratic grounds from an early age/stage, moral, ethical and behavioural side effects may accrue toward non-members, such as demeaning and disparaging behaviours. Again, these processes are at odds with developmental models, which favour development of individual-context relationships that promote positive self and social development.

Realigning developmental and TID system needs

With particular reference to 'later-age peak performance' sports, the previous sections highlight how the structure and content of sporting TIDS have progressively maligned system and youth developmental needs. The urgencies of competition exaggerate the role of performance as an indicator of athletic talent, overlooking the multitude of interacting temporal factors that play out as talent emerges and regresses. Selection continues to favour biologically advanced youngsters, rarely addressing the discontinuities and variations that affect growth trajectories. Equally, early specialization risks compromising psychological and physical development and appears to reduce the likelihood of becoming an adult elite athlete. Within some TIDS, social ecologies promote adherence to narrow identities and behaviours at the expense of youth controlling, exploring, and developing their own behaviours and identities prior to adulthood. These ecologies are also likely to produce unwanted psychological challenges and detrimental outcomes.

If it is accepted that these TID processes are less effective than their counterparts, how can these trends be realigned? From a pragmatic stance, researchers, clinicians and parents need to press for greater matching of TID practices with the developmental and health needs of young people. At the same time, deliverers of TIDS will probably be more motivated to respond to data continuing to show both lost or missed talent, combined with less than optimal perform-ance attainment at junior/youth/national competition. Done well, TIDS can handle each set of priorities. Development models, existing reviews (e.g. Jayanthi et al., 2013) and position state-ments (e.g. DiFiori et al., 2014) all now recommend changing convention, and highlight potential macro–micro levels of intervention. Table 43.1 draws on models of development and provides a summary of some possible implicated strategies on the basis of the content in this chapter. These strategies are not tried and tested. Rather they are intended to generate discussion and help improve the structure, function and effectiveness of TIDS.

Sport TIDS will continue to have an important role in developing individual skill and performance alongside biological, psychological, social and other broader health assets. But beyond athleticism, TIDS are also well placed to help address wider concerns affecting youth and society, such as pre-youth physical inactivity and obesity (Collins et al., 2012). TIDS represent contexts, often available locally, making them important accessible community assets for developing human resources. By marrying closer attention to youth individuality and diversity, temporal developmental changes and broader societal concerns, TIDS have the potential to foster mutually beneficial outcomes of positive and healthy development. Table 43.1 considers the possibility of coordinating inclusive multi-sport activity programmes in the junior years. With-holding competition aims to foster greater initial participation, intrinsic interest and diversified engagement. At the same time, this could contribute in reducing physical inactivity and helping with obesity prevention. Overall, this structure arguably facilitates long-term development and

Table 43.1 Illustration of possible strategies to improve athlete development and TID effectiveness in 'later peak age sports'

TIDS Feature	Present TID Trends	Developmental Preference
TID Macro–System: Policy	Early mandated talent ID and selection. Early specialized and intensive training and TID related competition.	Mandated no talent ID and selection in/exclusion prior to maturation. Delayed talent ID and specialization until post maturation (16 years +). Low–progressive training increment over time. No TID related competition. Post 16 structuring into skill/attribute and performance stages.
TID policy and programme integration	Active competition for junior/athlete participation in one-sport TID. Control on athlete behaviour.	No cross-TID competition for athlete recruitment pre 16. Coordination of multi-sport activity programmes to foster participation and diversification. No control on participant behaviour.
TID model or framework	Tiers of fixed/rigid age and performance stages progression steps within and across a performance model.	No progression stages on the basis of performance prior to 16. Fluid/open approach to talent emergence. Emphasis on assessment and development of multi-disciplinary skill/attributes, i.e., assets.
TID Aim	Immediate and adult competitive performance success	Skill/attribute development Long-term (adult) performance preparation.
Meso–System: Process	High frequency, repetitive, highly structured training and competition in sport context from an early age. Emphasis on learning how to win now/next; Learning via stress exposure.	Lower frequency, less-repetitive, low structure (non-specific games in junior years, transitioning later into mini/adapted games structures similar to sport context.

Learning skills, movement, and progressive training. Emphasis on self and group skill learning and asset building as well as sport-specific knowledge. |
Competition Function	High competition participation at junior/youth local-international tournaments.	Low (if any) competition participation and emphasis at junior/youth local-international tournaments. Become integral at 16 and beyond.
Outcomes desired	Performance and competition success.	Human development, i.e., physical, psychological, social, i.e., to underpin later adult performance.
Practitioner/Coach employment	Performance focused often short-term.	Skill/attribute development focused and longer-term.
Micro–System: Social ecology	Celebrated and reinforced performance narratives; focused athletic identity. Implicit athletic elitism.	Emphasis on developmental narratives. Support for multi-faceted identity exploration/development. Alternative activity and social group participation. Avoidance of athletic elitism. Social/community inclusion/participation and contribution.
Coaching climate	Performance focused; Competitive and ego-orientated. Individual focus. Relationships short-term and unstable.	Fun, enjoyment, satisfaction emphasis progressing to learning/training skill/attribute development. Personal and group development focus, Task-orientated, stable and longer-term relationships.

a better health trajectory prior to a performance emphasis, reducing the presence of factors known to be associated with detrimental outcomes. Likewise, it may better contribute in attaining what developmental models hypothesise as the achievement of 'optimal functional plasticity' in one or several contexts, specifically the maximal creation and exposure to a multitude of positive individual–context human interactions and relations.

References

Abbott, A. and Collins, D. (2004). Eliminating the dichotomy between theory and practice in talent identification and development: considering the role of psychology. *Journal of Sports Sciences*, 22(5): 395–408.

Abbott, A. and Collins, D. (2005). Unnatural selection: talent identification and development in sport. *Nonlinear Dynamics, Psychology, and Life Sciences*, 9(1): 61–88.

Adams, G. R. and Marshall, S. K. (1996). A developmental social psychology of identity: Understanding the person-in-context. *Journal of Adolescence*, 19(5): 429–442.

American Academy of Pediatrics Committee on Sports Medicine and Fitness. (2000). Intensive training and sports specialization in young athletes. *Pediatrics*, 106(1), 154–157.

Arellano, R. (2010). Interpreting and implementing the long term athlete development model: English swimming coaches' views on the (swimming) LTAD in practice – A commentary. *International Journal of Sports Science and Coaching*, 5: 413–419.

Armstrong, S. and Oomen-Early, J. (2009). Social connectedness, self-esteem, and depression symptomatology among collegiate athletes versus nonathletes. *Journal of American College Health*, 57(5): 521–526.

Bailey, R. and Pearce, G. (2010). *Participant Development in Sport: An Academic Review*. Leeds: Sports Coach UK. Commissioned report for Sports Coach UK.

Bailey, D. A. and Faulkner, R. A. (1999). A six-year longitudinal study of the relationship of physical activity to bone mineral accrual in growing children: The university of Saskatchewan bone mineral accrual study. *Journal of Bone and Mineral Research*, 14(10): 1672–1679.

Baker, J. and Côté, J. (2006). Shifting training requirements during athlete development: Deliberate practice, deliberate play and other sport involvement in the acquisition of sport expertise. In D. Hackfort and G. Tenenbaum (eds), *Essential Processes for Attaining Peak Performance* (pp. 92–109). Oxford: Meyer and Meyer Sport.

Baker, J. and Abernethy, B. (2003). Learning from the experts: Practice activities of expert decision makers in sport. *Research Quarterly for Exercise and Sport*, 74: 342–347.

Baker, J. and Fraser-Thomas, J. (2009). What do we know about early sport specialization? Not much! *High Ability Studies*, 20(1): 77–89.

Baltes, P. B. (1987). Theoretical propositions of life-span developmental psychology: On the dynamics between growth and decline. *Developmental Psychology*, 23: 611–626.

Balyi, I. and Hamilton, A. (2004). *Long-term athlete development: Trainability in childhood and adolescence. Windows of opportunity and optimal trainability*. Victoria: National Coaching Institute British Columbia and Advanced Training and Performance Ltd.

Barynina, I. I. and Vaitsekhovskii, S. M. (1992). The aftermath of early sports specialization for highly qualified swimmers. *Fitness and Sport Review International*, 27(4): 132–133.

Baxter-Jones, A. D. G. and Helms, P. J. (1996). Effects of training at a young age: a review of the Training of Young Athletes (TOYA) study. *Pediatric Exercise Science*, 8: 310–327.

Baxter-Jones, A. and Sherar, L. (2005). Controlling for maturation in pediatric exercise science. *Pediatric Exercise Science*, 17(1): 18–30.

Boyd, M. P. and Yin, Z. (1996). Cognitive–affective sources of sport enjoyment in adolescent sport participants. *Adolescence*, 31: 383–395.

Branta, C. (2010). Sport specialization: Development and learning issues. *Journal of Physical Education, Recreation, and Dance*, 81: 19–28.

Brenner, J. S. (2007). Overuse injuries, overtraining, and burnout in child and adolescent athletes. *Pediatrics*, 119(6): 1242–1245.

Brewer, B. W. and Linder, D. E. (1993). Athletic identity: Hercules' muscles or Achilles heel? *International Journal of Sport Psychology*, 24(2): 237–254.

Brown, G. and Potrac, P. (2009). 'You've not made the grade, son': De-selection and identity disruption in elite level youth football. *Soccer and Society, 10*(2): 143–159.

Brewer, B. W. and Linder, D. E. (1993). Athletic Identity: Hercules' muscles or Achilles heel? *International Journal of Sport Psychology, 24*: 237–254.

Bronfenbrenner, U. (1979). *The ecology of human development: Experiments by nature and design.* Cambridge, MA: Harvard University Press.

Bronfenbrenner, U. (2005). *Making human beings human: Bioecological Perspectives on Human Development.* Thousand Oaks, CA: Sage.

Carless, D. and Douglas, K. (2009). "We haven't got a seat on the bus for you" or "All the seats are mine": Narratives and career transition in professional golf. *Qualitative Research in Sport and Exercise, 1*(1): 51–66.

Carling, C. and Williams, A. M. (2009). Do anthropometric and fitness characteristics vary according to birth date distribution in elite youth academy soccer players? *Scandinavian Journal of Medicine and Science in Sports, 19*(1): 3–9.

Carlson, R. C. (1988). The socialization of elite tennis players in Sweden: An analysis of the players' backgrounds and development. *Sociology of Sport Journal, 5*, 241–256.

Christensen, M. K. and Sorensen, J. K. (2009). Sport of School? Dreams and dilemmas for talented young Danish football players. *European Physical Education Review, 15*(1): 115–133.

Cleary, T. J. and Zimmerman, B. J. (2001). Self-regulation differences during athletic practice by experts, non-experts, and novices. *Journal of Applied Sport Psychology, 13*(2): 185–206.

Coakley, J. (2010). The "logic" of specialization: Using children for adult purposes. *Journal of Physical Education, Recreation and Dance, 81*(8): 16–25.

Coalter, F. (2007). *A Wider Social Role for Sport: Who's Keeping the Score?* London: Routledge.

Cobley, S. and Till, K. (2015). Talent identification, development, and the young rugby player. In P. Worsfold and C. Twist, (eds) *The Science of Rugby* (pp. 237–52). London: Routledge.

Cobley, S. and Schorer, J. (2012). Identification and development of sport talent: A brief introduction to a growing field of research and practice. In J. Baker, S. Cobley and J. Schorer (eds), *Talent Identification and Development in Sport: International Perspectives* (pp. 1–10). London: Routledge.

Cobley, S. and McKenna, J. (2009). Annual age-grouping and athlete development: A meta-analytical review of relative age effects in sport. *Sports Medicine, 39*(3): 235–256.

Collins, D. and Pearce, G. (2012). Three Worlds: New directions in participant development in sport and physical activity. *Sport, Education and Society, 17*(2): 225–243.

Côté, J. and Fraser-Thomas, J. (2008). Play, practice and athlete development. In D. Farrow, J. Baker, C. MacMahon (eds), *Developing Elite Sport Performance: Lessons From Theory and Practice* (pp. 17–28). New York: Routledge.

Côté, J. and Hackfort, D. (2009). ISSP Position Stand: To sample or to specialize? Seven postulates about youth sport activities that lead to continued participation and elite performance. *International Journal of Sport and Exercise Psychology, 7*(1): 7–17.

Damon, W. (2004). What is positive youth development? *Annals of the American Academy of Political and Social Science, 591*: 13–24.

Deaner, R. O. and Cobley, S. (2013). Born at the wrong time: Selection bias in the NHL Draft. *PLoS One, 8*(2): 1–7.

DiFiori, J. P. Benjamin, H. J., Brenner, J. S., Gregory, A., Jayanthi, N., Landry, G. L. and Luke, A. (2014). Overuse injuries and burnout in youth sports: a position statement from the American Medical Society for Sports Medicine. *Clinical Journal of Sports Medicine, 24*(1): 3–20.

Douglas, K. and Carless, D. (2006). Performance, discovery, and relational narratives among women professional tournament golfers. *Women in Sport and Physical Activity Journal, 15*(2): 14–27.

Douglas, K. and Carless, D. (2011). A narrative perspective: Identity, well-being, and trauma in professional sport. In D. Gilbourne and M. Andersen (eds), *Critical essays in applied sport psychology* (pp. 3–22). Champaign, Illinois: Human Kinetics.

Elferink-Gemser, M. and Mulder, T. (2004). Relation between multidimensional performance characteristics and level of performance in talented youth field hockey players. *Journal of Sports Sciences, 22*(11–12): 1053–1063.

Ericsson, K. A. and Tesch-Römer, C. (1993). The role of deliberate practice in the acquisition of expert performance. *Psychological Review, 100*: 363–406.

Feldman, B. J. and Burzette, R. G. (2004). Traumatic events, psychiatric disorders, and pathways of risk and resilience during the transition to adulthood. *Research in Human Development, 1*(4): 259–290.

Fransen, J. Pion, J., Vandendriessche, J., Vandorpe, B., Vayens, R., Lenoir, M. and Philippaerts, R. M. (2012). Differences in physical fitness and gross motor coordination in boys aged 6–twelve years specializing in one versus sampling more than one sport. *Journal of Sport Sciences*, *30*(4): 379–386.

Fraser-Thomas, J. and Deakin, J. (2008). Understanding dropout and prolonged engagement in adolescent competitive sport. *Psychology of Sport and Exercise*, *9*(5): 645–662.

Freeman, J. and Preece, M. (1995). Cross sectional stature and weight reference curves for the UK, 1990. *Archives of Disease in Childhood*, *73*(1): 17–24.

Ford, D. L. and Lerner, R. M. (1992). *Developmental systems theory: An integrative approach*. Newbury Park, CA: Sage.

Ford, P. R. and Williams, A. M. (2009). The role of deliberate practice and play in career progression in sport: the early engagement hypothesis. *High Ability Studies*, *20*(1): 65–75.

Gottlieb, G. and Lickliter, R. (2006). The significance of biology for human development: A developmental psychobiological systems view. In W. Damon and R. M. Lerner (eds). *Handbook of child psychology: Theoretical models of human development* (6th edn). Hoboken, NJ: Wiley. Vol 1.

Green, C. (2009). *Every Boy's Dream. English Football Future on the Line*. London: A&C Publishers.

Green, M. (2006) From 'Sport for All' to not about 'Sport' at all? *European Sport Management Quarterly*, *6*: 217–238.

Güllich, A. and Emrich, E. (2012). Individualistic and collectivistic approach in athlete support programmes in the German high-performance sport system. *European Journal of Sport and Society*, *9*(4): 243–268.

Horton, R. S. and Mack, D. E. (2000). Athletic identity in marathon runners: Functional focus or dysfunctional commitment? *Journal of Sport Behavior*, *23*(2): 101–119.

Ingham, S. and Nevill, A. (2002). Determinants of 2,000 m rowing ergometer performance in elite rowers. *European Journal of Applied Physiology*, *88*(3): 243–246.

Jayanthi, N. and LaBella, C. (2013). Sports specialization in young athletes evidence-based recommendations. *Sports Health: A Multidisciplinary Approach*, *5*(3): 251–257.

Jonker, L. and Visscher, C. (2010). Differences in self-regulatory skills among talented athletes: The significance of competitive level and type of sport. *Journal of Sports Sciences*, *28*(8): 901–908.

Keogh, J. W. and Dalton, C. T. (2003). Evaluation of anthropometric, physiological, and skill-related tests for talent identification in female field hockey. *Canadian Journal of Applied Physiology*, *28*(3): 397–409.

Lamont-Mills, A. and Christensen, S. A. (2006). Athletic identity and its relationship to sport participation levels. *Journal of Science and Medicine in Sport*, *9*: 472–478.

Lang, M. (2010). Intensive training in youth sport: A new abuse of power? In: Lang, M. and Vanhoutte, K. P. (eds) *Bullying and the Abuse of Power: From the Playground to International Relations* (pp. 57–64). Oxford: Freeland Inter-Disciplinary Press.

Law, M. and Ericsson, K. A. (2007). Characteristics of expert development in rhythmic gymnastics: A retrospective study. *International Journal of Exercise and Sport Psychology*, *5*: 82–103.

Lawton, T. W. and McGuigan, M. R. (2012). Anthropometry, strength and benchmarks for development: A basis for junior rowers' selection? *Journal of Sports Sciences*, *30*(10): 995–1001.

Lerner, R. M. (1991). Changing organism-context relations as the basic process of development: A developmental contextual perspective. *Developmental Psychology*, *27*: 27–32.

Lerner, R. M. (1995). *America's Youth in Crisis: Challenges and Options for Programs and Policies*. Thousand Oaks, CA: Sage.

Lerner, R. M. (1998). Theories of human development: Contemporary perspectives. In W. Damon and R. M. Lerner (eds) *Handbook of Child Psychology: Theoretical Models of Human Development* (5th edn). New York: Wiley, Vol. 1 (pp. 1–24).

Lerner, R. M. and Castellino, D. R. (2002). Contemporary developmental theory and adolescence: Developmental systems and applied developmental science. *Journal of Adolescent Health*, *31*(6): 122–135.

Lerner, R. M. and Weinberg, R. A. (2000). Toward a science for and of the people: Promoting civil society through the application of developmental science. *Child Development*, *71*(1): 11–20.

Lidor R, Lavyan Z. (2002). A retrospective picture of early sport experiences among elite and near-elite Israeli athletes: developmental and psychological perspectives. *International Journal of Sport Psychology*, *33*: 269–289.

Malina, R. M. (1994). Physical growth and biological maturation of young athletes. *Exercise and Sport Sciences Reviews*, *22*(1): 280–284.

Malina, R. M. (2010). Early sport specialization: Roots, effectiveness, risks. *Current Sports Medicine Reports*, *9*: 364–371.

Malina, R. M. and Bar-Or, O. (2004). *Growth, Maturation, and Physical Activity*. Champaign, Illinois.: Human Kinetics Publishers.

Malina, R. M. and Cumming, S. P. (2007). Characteristics of youth soccer players aged 13–15 years classified by skill level. *British Journal of Sports Medicine, 41*(5): 290–295.

Matos, N. and Winsley, R. J. (2007). Trainability of young athletes and overtraining. *Journal of Sports Science and Medicine, 6*(3): 353–367.

McGillivray, D. and McIntosh, A. (2005). Caught up in and by the beautiful game: A case study of Scottish professional footballers. *Journal of Sport and Social Issues, 29*(1): 102–123.

Meylan, C. and Hughes, M. (2010). Talent identification in soccer: The role of maturity status on physical, physiological and technical characteristics. *International Journal of Sports Science and Coaching, 5*(4): 571–592.

Mirwald, R. L. and Beunen, G. P. (2002). An assessment of maturity from anthropometric measurements. *Medicine and Science in Sports and Exercise, 34*(4): 689–694.

Moesch, K. and Wikman, J. M. (2011). Late specialization: the key to success in centimeters, grams, or seconds (cgs) sports. *Scandinavian Journal of Medicine and Science in Sports, 21*(6): e282-e290.

Mohamed, H. and Philippaerts, R. (2009). Anthropometric and performance measures for the development of a talent detection and identification model in youth handball. *Journal of Sports Sciences, 27*(3): 257–266.

Murphy, G. M. and Brewer, B. W. (1996). Identity foreclosure, athletic identity, and career maturity in intercollegiate athletes. *The Sport Psychologist, 10*(3), 239–246.

Musch, J. and Grondin, S. (2001). Unequal competition as an impediment to personal development: A review of the relative age effect in sport. *Developmental Review, 21*(2): 147–167.

Overton, W. F. (2006). Developmental psychology: Philosophy, concepts, methodology. In W. Damon and R. M. Lerner (eds). *Handbook of Child Psychology: Theoretical Models of Human Development* (6th ed). Hoboken, NJ: Wiley. Vol 1.

Pearson, D. and Torode, M. (2006). Predictability of physiological testing and the role of maturation in talent identification for adolescent team sports. *Journal of Science and Medicine in Sport, 9*(4): 277–287.

Pensgaard, A. M. and Roberts, G. C. (2000). The relationship between motivational climate, perceived ability and sources of distress among elite athletes. *Journal of Sports Sciences, 18*(3): 191–200.

Philippaerts, R. M. and Malina, R. M. (2006). The relationship between peak height velocity and physical performance in youth soccer players. *Journal of Sports Sciences, 24*(3): 221–230.

Pipe, A. (2001). The adverse effects of elite competition on health and well-being. *Canadian Journal of Applied Physiology, 26*(S1), S192-S201.

Rongen, F. Cobley, S., McKenna, J. and Till, K. (2015). Talent identification and development: The impact on athlete health? In J. Baker, P. Safai and J. Fraser-Thomas (eds), *Health and Elite Sport: Is High Performance Sport a Healthy Pursuit?* Abingdon, UK: Routledge.

Russell, W. D. and Limle, A. N. (2013). The relationship between youth sport specialization and involvement in sport and physical activity in young adulthood. *Journal of Sport Behavior, 36*: 82–98.

Sherar, L. B. and Russell, K. W. (2007). Do physical maturity and birth date predict talent in male youth ice hockey players? *Journal of Sports Sciences, 25*(8): 879–886.

Simmons, C. and Paull, G. C. (2001). Season-of-birth bias in association football. *Journal of Sports Sciences, 19*(9): 677–686.

Simonton, D. K. (1999). Talent and its development: An emergenic and epigenetic model. *Psychological Review, 106*(3): 435–457.

Simonton, D. K. (2001). Talent development as a multidimensional, multiplicative, and dynamic process. *Current Directions in Psychological Science, 10*(2): 39–43.

Sundgot-Borgen, J. and Torstveit, M. K. (2010). Aspects of disordered eating continuum in elite high-intensity sports. *Scandinavian Journal of Medicine and Science in Sports, 20*(s2): 112–121.

Tanner, J. (1962). *Growth at adolescence*. Oxford: Blackwell Scientific Publications.

Tännsjö, T. and Tamburrini, C. (2000). *Values in Sport: Elitism, Nationalism, Gender Equality and the Scientific Manufacture of Winners*. London: E. and FN Spon Ltd.

Till, K. and Cooke, C. (2010a). Anthropometric, physiological and selection characteristics in high performance UK Junior Rugby League players. *Talent Development and Excellence, 2*: 193–207.

Till, K., Cobley, S., O'Hara, J., Cooke, C. and Chapman, C. (2014). Considering maturation status and relative age in the longitudinal evaluation of junior rugby league players. *Scandinavian Journal of Medicine and Science in Sports. 24*(3), 569–576.

Till, K. and Chapman, C. (2010b). The prevalence, influential factors and mechanisms of relative age effects in UK Rugby League. *Scandinavian Journal of Medicine and Science in Sports, 20*(2): 320–329.

Tobach, E. and Greenberg, G. (1984). The significance of T. C. Schneirla's contribution to the concept of levels of integration. In G. Greenberg and E. Tobach (eds) *Behavioral Evolution and Integration Levels.* Erlbaum, Hillsdale, NJ (pp. 1–7).

UK Sport (2007). Sporting Giants. Retrieved on 3 January, 2014 from www.uksport.gov.uk/pages/sportinggiants/

UK Sport (2008). 'No Compromise' funding strategy. Retrieved on 10 January, 2014 from www.uksport.gov.uk/pages/london-2012/

Vaeyens, R. and Philippaerts, R. (2009). Talent identification and promotion programmes of Olympic athletes. *Journal of Sports Sciences, 27*(13): 1367–1380.

Vaeyens, R. Lenoir, M. Williams, A. M., and Philippaerts, R. M. (2008). Talent identification and development programmes in sport. *Sports Medicine, 38*(9): 703–714.

Vandendriessche, J. B. andorpe, B. and Philippaerts, R. M. (2012). Biological maturation, morphology, fitness, and motor coordination as part of a selection strategy in the search for international youth soccer players (age 15–16 years). *Journal of Sports Sciences, 30*(15): 1695–1703.

Viru, A. and Viru, M. (1999). Critical periods in the development of performance capacity during childhood and adolescence. *European Journal of Physical Education, 4*(1): 75–119.

Viru, A. and Viru, M. (1998). Age periods of accelerated improvement of muscle strength, power, speed and endurance in the age interval 6–18 years. *Biology of Sport, 15*(4): 211–227.

Votteler, A. and Höner, O. (2014). The relative age effect in the German Football TID Programme: Biases in motor performance diagnostics and effects on single motor abilities and skills in groups of selected players. *European Journal of Sport Science, 14*(5), 433–442.

Wattie, N. and Baker, J. (2008). Towards a unified understanding of relative age effects. *Journal of Sports Sciences, 26*(13): 1403–1409.

Wiersma, L. (2000). Risks and benefits of youth sport specialization: Perspectives and recommendations. *Pediatric Exercise Science, 12*: 13–22.

Williams, A. and Reilly, T. (2000). Talent identification and development in soccer. *Journal of Sports Sciences, 18*: 657–667.

Wylleman, P. and Lavallee, D. (2004). A developmental perspective on transitions faced by athletes. In M. R. Weiss (ed), *Developmental Sport and Exercise Psychology: A Lifespan Perspective* (pp. 503–523). Morgantown, W. Virginia: Fitness Information Technology.

44

HEALTH, WELL-BEING AND THE 'LOGIC' OF ELITE YOUTH SPORTS WORK

Chris Platts and Andy Smith

Introduction

Writing over two decades ago, Donnelly (1993) drew attention to some of the central problems that he associated with the involvement of young people in elite or high performance sport settings. Based on findings from a sample of forty-five recently retired Canadian high performance sport athletes, he identified not only the positive experiences of elite sport recalled by athletes, but also many more negative experiences, among which the following were regarded as being of central importance: relationship difficulties with family, friends and coaches; educational problems; physical and psychological problems; dietary and body image problems; the use of performance enhancing drugs; internal politics of sports teams and organizations; and retirement (Donnelly, 1993). Many of these problems, Donnelly added, were experienced when athletes were young and were likely to be exacerbated by the earlier and more intensive involvement of children and young people in elite sport settings which he observed at the time. In particular, he noted that:

> As children encounter opportunities for increasingly lucrative careers as professional athletes, parents are tempted to encourage their children to become heavily involved in professional sports at early ages. As evidenced by increasing demands for international success in sport as a justification for government and corporate spending on elite participation, and by a variety of attempts to establish schemes for the early identification athletic talent, there is an obvious trend toward earlier and more intensive athletic involvement for younger and younger children.
>
> *(Donnelly, 1993: 96)*

There is little reason to think that the situation described by Donnelly has improved significantly since; indeed, in 2005, David (2005: 55) claimed that 'unless a child starts training at a very early age, it is almost impossible to reach the top in many sports', while almost a decade later DiFiori *et al.* (2014: 5) concluded that 'the increasing highly competitive nature of youth sports has fuelled trends of extensive training, sport specialization, and participation in large numbers of competitive events at young ages'. They added that: the 'emphasis on competitive success has become widespread, resulting in increased pressure to begin high-intensity training at young ages' (DiFiori *et al.*, 2014: 6).

Although it is clear that some athletes have undoubtedly positive experiences of their careers, working in elite sports environments is not without its 'costs', perhaps especially so during the youth life-stage when many young athletes often work intensely to seek entry into the apparently lucrative world of elite sport. Indeed, the trend towards earlier and more intensive involvement in elite sport by many young people is not an unalloyed blessing for, as the evidence reviewed in this chapter indicates, this is often associated with significant health costs that may or may not have been anticipated. This is not altogether surprising since studies of athletes whose health – physical, mental and social – has been compromised while working in elite sport are almost innumerable, and it is clear that in many sports there is an institutionalized expectation that athletes (including elite youth athletes) will take serious risks with their health within the 'cultures of risk' that characterize their workplaces.

These introductory remarks represent the starting point for this chapter, the central objective of which is to consider some of the workplace pressures to which young athletes are subject in elite sport and their impact on athletes' welfare. More specifically, the chapter examines:

1   the norms and values of what Hughes and Coakley (1991) refer to as the 'sport ethic', which frequently constrains athletes to engage in often health-compromising behaviours;
2   the cultures of risk in which young athletes are bound up and that frequently compromise their health and well-being, including through the normalization and acceptance of pain, injury and 'playing hurt'; and
3   the key structural features of the workplace which must be understood if we are to develop a more adequate understanding of the realities of young elite sports workers' lives.

The sport ethic and elite youth sport

Hughes and Coakley (1991) have argued that in elite sport, the attitudes and behaviours of many athletes, coaches and other sports workers are often guided by what they refer to as the *sport ethic*. The sport ethic, it is held, is what many elite sports workers use to define what it means to be a real athlete, and is formed around four norms (Hughes and Coakley, 1991). These norms, which are strengthened through the socialization of workers in elite sports cultures, are:

* athletes must be dedicated to their sport above everything else;
* athletes should always strive for distinction and perfection;
* athletes should accept risk and play through pain and injury as part of the culture of risk which exists in sport; and
* athletes should accept no obstacles in the pursuit of possibilities throughout their careers
(Coakley and Pike, 2014; Hughes and Coakley, 1991)

These norms, Coakley and Pike (2014: 160) suggest, are 'accepted uncritically, without question or qualification, and often followed without recognizing limits or thinking about the boundaries that separate normal from deviant'. This is thought to be particularly true of many young athletes who, especially during the early stages of their working lives, are constrained to accept the values of the sport ethic from important gatekeepers who to a large extent control access to the world of elite sport (Brackenridge, 2001; Roderick, 2006a). That is, from a young age, elite sports workers are socialized into accepting the dominant values, ideologies and practices of their sport and are required to demonstrate their commitment to the sport, and significant others, by engaging in deviant over-conformity (Hughes and Coakley, 1991), such as playing with injury, engaging in self-injurious behaviours, and adopting unhealthy dietary and weight control practices.

Deviant over-conformity, or positive deviance (Hughes and Coakley, 1991), is common in elite sport and while such behaviour is likely to vary between different historical periods, and from one sport to another and from one country to another, many athletes do not perceive their over-conformity to the sport ethic as deviant. Instead, despite the obvious health risks involved, a significant proportion of athletes often regard their actions as necessary occupational hazards. These hazards are frequently rationalized as necessary sacrifices that need to be made should they wish to become an elite sports worker, and if they are to be accepted by others (such as coaches, managers and performance directors) who regularly encourage over-conformity. In contrast, many young athletes seek to avoid engaging in deviant under-conformity (or negative deviance) where they are often perceived as failing to accept the norms of the sport ethic (e.g. by refusing to play with pain, or follow instructions), and where others question their commitment (Hughes and Coakley, 1991); in such cases, athletes are also routinely subject to a variety of stigmatizing processes which threaten their sense of self, self identity, and feelings of authenticity which compromise their mental as well as physical and social well-being (Roderick, 2013; Roderick and Gibbons, 2015).

We shall return to these issues later, but it is worth noting that while the sport ethic is a useful framework for making sense of the workings of elite sport, Hughes and Coakley (1991) do not explain why athletes engage in both types of deviance. It is also unlikely that all young athletes are equally accepting of the sport ethic, and their commitment to the norms and values of the sport ethic is likely to vary throughout their careers. These matters are of empirical and theoretical importance since more needs to be known about how and why young athletes in elite sport negotiate decisions about engaging in positive and negative deviance, and what the health (and other) costs are. One appropriate starting point for such an analysis is the network of relationships involved in elite sport, and particularly those associated with the culture of risk that characterizes that workplace.

Cultures of risk and working in elite youth sport

According to Nixon (1992, 1993, 1994), there exists in sport (especially elite sport) a culture of risk in which athletes are exposed to what he calls a 'conspiratorial alliance' of coaches, administrators and sports physicians who collectively comprise 'sportsnets', by which Nixon refers to as webs of interaction that directly or indirectly link members of social networks in a particular sport-related setting. These sportsnets, Nixon argues, foster the acceptance by athletes of pain and injury and insulates them from, and inhibits them from seeking, medical care and other forms of support from outside sport (Nixon, 1992, 1993, 1994). Sportsnets and associated cultures of risk are likely to vary in significant respects between sports and between different levels of sport, and between different societies in which sport is played. In the elite sport context, however, Nixon (1992: 132) argues that sportsnets are 'relatively more likely to entrap athletes in the culture of risk and foster a self-abusive pattern of pain and injury' when these networks of relationships are larger, denser, more centralized, more closed, more homogeneous and more stable, and where athletes are more accessible to others in greater positions of power, control and authority within the sporting world (Nixon, 1992). In such contexts, athletes are also more likely to receive 'biased messages of "support" that reinforce the culture of risk more than they contribute to the welfare of the athletes' (Nixon, 1993: 190). Where sportsnets are smaller, less dense, less centralized, less closed and less stable then they are, in Nixon's terms, less likely to 'entrap' athletes and less likely to constrain them towards engaging in various forms of 'self-abusive addiction' (Nixon, 1993: 189).

Although focused on risk, pain and injury in sport, Nixon's work provides a useful framework for understanding key aspects of the workplace conditions in which various elite sports workers (Roderick, 2006b; Waddington, 2012), including young athletes, find themselves and how their work situations may compromise health and well-being. This is because Nixon's work, and especially the concept of sportsnets, places particular emphasis upon understanding the complex and contradictory relational constraints to which young athletes are subject in the workplace, how these are negotiated and managed and how they also enable athletes to pursue their careers successfully. In elite youth sport, it is adults who frequently dominate the sportsnets into which young people are socialized and subsequently work, and these adults are often in greater positions of power to make decisions which may compromise, as well as safeguard and enhance, the welfare of young elite athletes (Brackenridge, 2001; Brackenridge *et al.*, 2007; David, 2005). David (2005: 35), for example, has argued that elite youth sport often 'exists largely to satisfy adults. Even more than their peers, children involved in competitive sports grow up in a world dominated by adults with little space for freedom, self-initiative and creativity. Adults – parents, coaches and trainers, officials, managers and agents, journalists and sponsors – control competitive sport at all levels.'

Thus, for David (2005), a central characteristic of the work situations in which young elite athletes find themselves is an often tightly integrated set of adult-dominated relationships where vested interests are played out by, among other groups, parents, coaches, managers and support staff, sometimes at the expense of the interests of the young athletes with whom they work. In this regard, elite sport represents a working context in which very unequal power ratios often exist between adults and young people, and which are frequently tilted in favour of adults, one consequence of which is that young athletes' welfare may be more likely to be compromised. This is perhaps increasingly common when young athletes gradually spend more and more time in the company of adults as their elite careers unfold, and as their training and competition schedules become more intense and regular (Brackenridge, 2001; David, 2005). In other words, as young elite athletes become increasingly integrated into adult-dominated sportsnets – which, in Nixon's terms, are large, dense, centralized, closed, and largely homogeneous and stable – they routinely work within a closed social world where they 'usually create strong emotional and dependency bonds with the adults in charge of them' (David, 2005: 58).

Since 'discipline and obedience are also key elements' (David, 2005: 58) of adult-dominated relationships in elite youth sport, so young athletes may find it increasingly difficult to question and disobey the instructions they receive from adults who are entrusted with their care, and on whom they may be heavily dependent for future success, including being selected for international squads, being offered professional contracts, and receiving a favourable recommendation to other teams in the elite sports environment (Brackenridge, 2001; Roderick, 2006a; Roderick *et al.*, 2000). It is thus important in any study of the workplace conditions of elite youth sport, and the associated impacts on athletes' health and well-being, that young athletes are located within their various networks of relationships and how these influence their experiences of elite sports work. In the remaining sections of this chapter, we shall briefly review some of these experiences and reflect upon how these are connected to the 'logic' of workplace practices in elite sport.

Violence, abuse and elite youth sport

As David (2005: 58) has noted, it is 'increasingly recognized that young athletes are potentially vulnerable to serious abuses of trust and power, which may lead to severe forms of violence', much of which is often socially sanctioned and accepted as one of the key organizing principles and attractions of elite sport (Young, 2012). The findings of numerous studies have now indeed indicated that, in many sports, athletes are socialized from a relatively young age into accepting that abuse, intimidation and threat or real use of physical violence is a central element of workplace cultures and practices (Brackenridge *et al.*, 2007; Kelly and Waddington, 2006; Parker, 1996; Roderick, 2006a; Roderick *et al.*, 2000). For example, in Kelly and Waddington's (2006: 152) study, one professional footballer commented on his experiences of the use by his manager of physical violence as a means of intimidating and imposing discipline on young players at an English Premier League club as follows:

> I remember [the manager] smacked us all in the head with a cricket bat once. We had training and I remember I was a youth team player at the time, and we used to get kitted in the morning and then get changed, put on fresh kit, go up [for food] but we were meant to put the old kit in the wash bags for the wash man to wash, but I think [the manager] walked by and saw the kit on the ground, went up to his office and got the cricket bat out. He lined us all up, turned the cricket bat to one side . . . and smacked us all on the head. Yeah, and it was a good hard smack as well.
> *(Kelly and Waddington, 2006: 152)*

In his ethnographic study that explored the way young athletes learn to normalize the norms and values that underpin workplace practices in sports such as professional football, Parker (1996) also drew attention to the ways in which the well-being of young players was routinely challenged by the prevailing 'shop floor culture' (Willis, 2009 [1978]) that exists within the game. One feature of the work situations occupied by young players included 'the stylized adoption of a sexually explicit and often derogatory vocabulary which was ideally characterized by a sharp-pointed form of delivery' (Parker, 1996: 223). Often described as 'banter' (Collinson, 1988; Parker, 1996; Platts, 2012; Roderick, 2006a), Parker (1996: 224) argued that this culture revolved around 'administering verbal "wind-ups" to the point where the young athletes failed to cope with the pressures in hand and ultimately "snapped"' having been so exposed to the authoritarianism, ruthlessness and hyper-masculine practices of the workplace (Parker, 1996). A more recent study of education and welfare provisions in professional football academies in England and Wales also revealed that the verbal abuse of young players aged 16–18 (n=303), often intended to illicit a 'response' from them by being administered publicly in front of teammates, was a common technique deployed by coaches and managers frequently with little regard for player welfare. The comments of a group of players from a Premier League club are particularly illustrative of the experiences recalled by other players in the study (Platts, 2012: 154):

Tim: If you do something he'll just go 'That was shit'.
Jack: You'll have the game of your life, and like you'll have played well, but he'll still point out
Tim: [Interrupts] Something bad you've done.
Jack: 'Oh but you done this, just work on that' . . .
Tim: It's in front of everybody.
Jack: Yeah it is, he'll go round.
Ash: He'll go through the whole team and say 'You did this, you did that'.
Matt: He did it today. Everyone was standing there and he went though everyone.
Jack: Make an absolute show of someone . . .
Ash: Once he went to me 'Listen bollocks' . . . I thought 'Fuckin' hell, that's a bit harsh innit?'

Other players in the study explained that the use by coaches of verbal abuse was part of the broader strategies they used to encourage young players to show them respect, and as part of post-match interactions. Players frequently referred to the ways in which derogatory language was used by coaches to humiliate and isolate them and to emphasize the view that players had not tried hard enough, as the following extract taken from a discussion held with players from a Championship club indicates:

Andy: We get 'shit bags' a lot.
Kieran: Or 'shit house' . . .
James: Like tearing you apart . . .
Ste: Total humiliation . . .
Kieran: Sometimes he [coach] singles you out.
Fabian: Sometimes it can be like character building or, you know, what I mean, dealing wi' abuse . . .
Ste: It's not if you lose, it's the fact on how you play, so if you play shit and don't show any determination, or desire to wanna play for the team, you just get fucked.

(Platts, 2012: 136)

The verbal abuse and criticism to which players were subject were seen as important parts of the steep learning curve they were constrained to undertake while preparing for a career in professional football. Indeed, 'despite being couched in humorous and seemingly harmless terms' (Roderick, 2006a: 72) and often described by coaches as 'banter', the mocking of players and their performances was perceived as part-and-parcel of everyday life within professional football (Roderick, 2006a), and players often rationalized this as a necessary part of their football education and socialization into the workplace culture of the game.

In football, as in many other sports, the willingness of young athletes to accept without question instances of verbal abuse is often part of the broader pressures on them to convey a 'good attitude', which is commonly regarded as a central characteristic of the 'good professional' (Roderick, 2006a; Roderick *et al.*, 2000). Although verbal abuse and hyper-aggressivity are often characteristics needed to convey a good attitude in the working environments inhabited by male athletes (Kelly and Waddington, 2006; Young, 2012), they have also been shown to be common in sports involving women. The findings of a study that investigated the workplace practices of elite female ice-skating, for example, found that possessing a good attitude invariably meant accepting various dressing downs from coaches and engaging in long and demanding training sessions (Grenfell and Rinehart, 2003). As Grenfell and Rinehart (2003: 82; emphases in the original) have noted:

"Dressing downs" are relatively common; they are certainly . . . for the girls' "own good". Not only are coaches to teach the *skills* of figure skating, they are to teach the *attitude* of figure skating.

Demonstrating a good attitude also meant that the young ice skaters were prepared to make the sacrifices necessary to pursue and maintain a career at the elite level, and to show adult coaches and parents that they were totally committed to the norms and values of the sport. Accordingly, the uncritical acceptance by athletes as well as other members of their networks of the sport ethic which underpinned the sub-cultural world of ice skating meant 'parents and coaches may not even be aware of the negative effects that highly competitive programs have on the child's development and happiness. The parent/child/coach coalition becomes so focused on the shared idea that the child *has the talent* and has *made the commitment* that this seems to justify any amount of work and sacrifice to attain a competitive-related goal' (Grenfell and Rinehart, 2003: 80; emphases in the original)

The pressures to which young ice skaters were subject thus led Grenfell and Rinehart (2003: 79) to describe the workplace conditions these athletes often inhabited as being comparable to 'the working conditions for children which led to the passage of child labor laws early in the twentieth century'.

Pain and injury in elite youth sport

An additional way in which elite young athletes seek to demonstrate a good attitude in the workplace is by competing with pain and injury, which has now been shown unequivocally to be a feature of the experiences of older professional and non-elite athletes competing in many sports, including gymnastics (e.g. Pike and Scott, 2015), ballet (e.g. Turner and Wainwright, 2003; Wainwright and Turner, 2006), rugby union (e.g. Malcolm and Sheard, 2002), football (e.g. Roderick, 2006a; Roderick *et al.*, 2000) and rowing (e.g. Pike, 2005).

Although it is difficult to estimate accurately the scale of youth sports injuries, the findings of several studies have indicated that sport is a – if not *the* – major cause of injury among young people (e.g. Hastmann-Walch and Caine, 2015; James *et al.*, this volume; Maffulli *et al.*, 2010; Maffulli *et al.*, 2011). As James *et al.* (this volume) make clear, the heightened risk to young people of participating in sport (particularly at higher intensities and frequencies) often occurs at a time of major physiological as well as psychological and social change. In the United States, between 2001 and 2009, an estimated 2,651,581 under 19-year-olds were treated annually for sports and recreation related injuries, of which 6.5 per cent were non-fatal concussions treated in emergency departments (Gilchrist *et al.*, 2011). A recent systematic review of injuries among rugby union and league players under 21-years old also revealed that just under three in ten (28 per cent) of players involved in a rugby match playing season are likely to sustain an injury (Freitag *et al.*, 2015). Approximately 12 per cent of players were also identified as being likely to sustain an injury severe enough to require at least seven days absence from play, with the most frequently reported types of injury being sprains, strains and soft tissue injuries; more severe injuries, including concussion and bone fractures, were also commonly reported by young players (Freitag *et al.*, 2015).

The prevalence and seriousness of injury among young rugby players was also identified in a prospective cohort study of injuries among 470 Scottish secondary school pupils between January and April 2009. Thirty-seven injuries were reported by all rugby-playing pupils, of which 70 per cent were inflicted during matches and 30 per cent during training (Nicol *et al.*, 2011). The incidence for all reported competitive match injuries was 10.8 injuries per 1,000 player-hours (Nicol *et al.*, 2011), and over one-half of all injuries in the study were treated at an accident and emergency department, including serious injuries such as shoulder dislocations and concussions (Nicol *et al.*, 2011). In addition, just over one-third of all injuries (35 per cent) left players unable to compete for up to two weeks, 46 per cent were unable to play for 3–6 weeks, and 19 per cent were unable to return to play for seven weeks or more (Nicol *et al.*, 2011).

The risk of injury to young people from participating in sport is clear, but there is by comparison to studies of recreational sport 'a paucity of information on injury risk related to the young athlete competing in elite, high-level sport' (Hastmann-Walch and Caine, 2015: 66). This is particularly significant for, as Safai *et al.* (2015: 2) have argued, the tolerance of pain and injury by athletes and other sports workers (e.g. coaches, medical personnel) is 'part-and-parcel of the high performance sport experience', and there is thus a need to explore whether the 'routine normalization and romanticizing of the pain and injury involved in the high performance sport process' (Safai et al., 2015: 2) is true also of the working lives of young elite athletes. One study that has examined experiences of pain and injury among this population is Platts's (2012) study of young elite academy footballers referred to earlier. As in studies of their professional counterparts (e.g. Roderick, 2006a; Roderick et al., 2000), almost all players in the study explained that they regularly concealed injuries from their peers and above all their coaches, often because of performance-related concerns and a desire to get game time that was thought necessary to maximize the possibility of securing a full-time professional contract. One group of players from a Championship club discussed their experiences thus:

Scott:	I try and not say 'I'm injured', I wouldn't want to risk that . . .
Leo:	Obviously it is such a big year.
Chris:	[Interrupts] Unless it is really, really bad.
Leo:	I just want to play as many games as I can to like show I am good enough really . . .
Scott:	Oh, yeah, I have been playing with a bad ankle for about two weeks but I don't want to say . . . 'I'm injured'.
Joe:	Like my knee . . .
Scott:	Obviously I'm getting it strapped up and that, and it's painful when I play and train, but it's one of them, I'm just gonna have to get through it.
Joe:	My knee's been hurting for like two weeks, then on Saturday it swelled up for no reason, but I'm still training. I can't afford to stop.

(Platts, 2012: 256)

In this regard, the players appeared locked into an occupational trap in which they had been socialized into accepting that 'their work setting is largely intolerant to injury' (Young, 2012: 104), and this often led them to engage in the kinds of 'self-abusive addiction' that Nixon (1993) claims is common among members of sportsnets in the context of elite sport. Although the concealment of injury was among players' most pressing occupational concerns that at times defined their everyday working lives, they were simultaneously encouraged to engage in overt displays of deviant over-conformity (that is, playing with pain and injury) by their coaches. As the following comments of another group of players at a Championship club indicate, this was because it enabled them to demonstrate character and commitment that were regarded as central elements of a professional attitude:

Dave:	They [the coaches] said it shows character, and that's what they like to see or something like that.
Kenny:	That's just fuckin' stupid.
Interviewer:	They like to see character by playing injured?
Greg:	So you are risking your health.
Jimmy:	It shows you care for your team.
Dave:	They think you are being tough . . .
Dean:	But it's like the professional attitude again, like we said about the old managers . . . Tradition they say, 'Oh yeah, broken arm, play through it, you're alright' sort of thing.

If players failed to play when in pain or when injured, or were unavailable for selection because of injury, then coaches often ignored them and questioned whether they were really injured (Roderick, 2006a, 2013; Roderick *et al.*, 2000). When asked about the process of being ignored by coaches at their Premier League club, one group of players described their experiences as follows:

Paul:	The coaches, they ignore you.
Iain:	They palm you off.
Paul:	Like they don't say a word to you. They pretend you are not even there.
Justin:	They won't talk to you, only the physios will deal with you . . .
Iain:	Sometimes they just think you are on a jolly up.
3.	Sometimes they think 'He ain't really injured, he just don't want to train'.
Nick:	Some of the coaches . . . think that they should just be like soldiers and carry on and play through it.

(Platts, 2012: 262)

In this respect, the experiences players recalled provided clear evidence of the cultures of risk that must be negotiated and managed, often in the context of very public relationships with others, during their everyday working lives in elite football academies. The avoidance of stigma, of being ignored and labelled as a non-producer, and of meeting the high (sometimes unrealistic) expectations of coaches were uppermost in the minds of players whose work situations constrained them to make a number of personal sacrifices, often in the form of significant physical and mental health costs. While the physical and emotional costs of players' attempts to meet the exacting standards of coaches were in part observable to others, many of the emotional costs remained hidden and were instead internalized, kept private and managed away from the workplace. We shall briefly consider such privatization of emotion and fear of stigma and shame as an aspect of the 'logic' of elite sports work next.

The 'logic' of elite (youth) sports work

As Roderick and Gibbons (2015) have noted, accounts of the everyday realities of working in elite sport are all too often absent from many portrayals of athletes' lives. However, in contrast to the often one-sided, overly romanticized and glorified media-led presentations of elite sport, there is a small but growing body of academic research that indicates that, for many elite sports workers, their lives are frequently 'celebrated, sensationalized, mortified, dehumanized, and commodified' (Roderick and Gibbons, 2015: 153; see also Hoberman, 1992; Roderick, 2006a, 2013). The conditions of work for many elite athletes are structured by a series of performance-oriented practices intended to maximize the likelihood of success, and which emerge out of the dominant norms and values that inform the sports ethic. Central among these practices, it is claimed, is the constant observation, regulation and modification of working bodies, and the regular monitoring and development of talent (Roderick, 2013; Roderick and Gibbons, 2015), as well as an apparently 'permanent and obsessive search for perfection which leads to perpetual improvement of results' (David, 2005: 67).

For reasons explained earlier, elite athletes are constrained from an early age to internalize this logic of sports work and the values of their respective sports worlds (Nixon, 1992, 1993; Roderick and Gibbons, 2015), perhaps especially during the early years of their careers when seeking entry to the workplace of elite sport often dominates many other concerns. These are often work environments, it should be noted, in which mistakes are often published and are to be avoided, where the close and regular surveillance of performance (including weight) may result in a variety of publically enforced punishments, and where constant social comparisons between one's teammates and fellow workers often encourages young athletes to ensure they live up to (and preferably exceed) expectations. In this regard, young athletes may become centrally concerned with projecting 'a sense of infallibility and not show weakness or self-doubt' (Flett *et al.*, 2014: 168), often by presenting a particular, preferred self image (Goffman, 1959), hiding distress through significant investments in publicly-staged emotional labour (Hochschild, 1983), and avoiding help-seeking in the sporting context (Roderick, 2006a, 2013). Just as many athletes are expected (and willing) to accept the normative values and behaviours that underpin the sport ethic, so too are these processes 'rationalized and justified as fundamental features of the logic of sports work' (Roderick and Gibbons, 2015: 153). As Roderick and Gibbons (2015: 153–4) have noted, this is a logic that 'espouses the twin ideas that athletes must always strive to win and be successful, and that they must love their work and treat it as a privilege; they must realize, and not squander, their God-given talents. The effects of the power of this discourse – one which has no meaningful rival – are to camouflage often chronic underlying (mental) health issues and stifle athletes' genuine motives for seeking help.'

Indeed, the 'relentless self-identity constraints and performance scrutiny that characterise sports work' (Roderick and Gibbons, 2015: 150) that athletes encounter are not without their costs; at all stages of their career, athletes often pay a heavy physical and emotional cost for their working lives. Many of these costs are often paid away from the purview of athletes' public (in some cases, celebrity) lives. It is often in the more privatized spheres of social life where many athletes bear many of the health costs of their publicly-oriented reputations and working selves, and where they can be who they really are; that is to say, where they can be their more authentic selves rather than who they need to be at work (see Douglas and Carless, 2015; Roderick, 2013; Roderick and Gibbons, 2015).

One consequence of the privatization of emotion and avoidance of help-seeking is the constraint on athletes to manage their experiences of mental illness, and other health conditions, away from the workplace often out of shame and fear of being stigmatized. Little academic attention has so far been given to understanding the complex relationships that exists between the working lives of elite athletes and the development and experience of mental illness, and more is currently known about this dimension of athletes' lives once their careers have ended rather than throughout periods of their sporting careers (Roderick and Gibbons, 2015). What is clear, however, is that elite athletes are not immune to mental illness (Mummery, 2005) and that conditions including depression, anxiety, self-harm and forms of addiction are commonly experienced during and at the end of athletes' sporting careers. A recent study of 301 current and former professional footballers by the World Players' Union, FIFPro, reported that symptoms associated with depression and anxiety 'are highly prevalent among professional footballers', especially among former recently retired players who reported more mental health problems than current players (FIFPro, 2014). The study found that of the 121 former players in the sample, 39 per cent reported experiencing depression or anxiety, 32 per cent reported adverse alcohol behaviour and 18 per cent were found to be in distress. Among the 180 current players, one-quarter (26 per cent) reported experiencing depression or anxiety, 19 per cent reported adverse alcohol behaviour and 10 per cent were found to be in distress (FIFPro, 2014). The study concluded that while there remains an 'acute lack of scientific data about mental illness among professional footballers', the findings suggest that 'mental illness in football is widespread, and higher than normal among former professional players compared to other studied populations' (FIFPro, 2014).

Such health problems are not confined to older players, for it is also clear that mental illness is common among young players. In 2015, the charity XPRO, that supports former professional players in the United Kingdom and Ireland, was said to be supporting around sixty players under 20-years old who had depression and a further 250 players who were currently in young offenders' institutions having been released from their clubs without a professional contract (Ducker, 2015). Another study by Dr David Blakelock at Teeside University revealed that 55 per cent of almost 100 15–18-year-olds had mental illnesses such as depression and anxiety, or engaged in legal and illegal drug use that contributed to impaired everyday functioning, within one month of being released from their football clubs (cited in Ducker, 2015). For young and older footballers, like many other athletes, experiences of mental illness and the structural conditions of the workplace may contribute (directly or indirectly) to the incidence of suicide which now attracts greater media attention, but which is not yet very well understood. While many more people with mental illness do not die by suicide than those who do, one risk factor for suicide is known to be the 'tendency for perfectionists to engage in perfectionistic self-presentation and to be characterized by self-concealment behaviors that enable them to hide their sense of shame, self-loathing, and hopelessness behind a mask of apparent invulnerability' (Flett *et al.*, 2014: 156). Not all elite athletes – young or old – may be regarded as perfectionists, but that so many feel constrained to manage and conceal their emotions in the workplace, and to hide their real selves in public behind masks of apparent invulnerability and self-confidence, should at least encourage us to better understand and take seriously the potential risks of such behaviour for athletes' health and well-being.

Conclusion

In this chapter we have been centrally concerned with exploring some of the workplace pressures to which young athletes are subject in elite sport, the impact of these pressures on health and well-being, and how these collectively contribute to the 'logic' of sports work for young people. As we have emphasized, these are matters that are not very well understood and much more academic attention needs to be given to the ways in which many young athletes' over-conformity to the sport ethic and immersion within the cultures of risk in which they are bound up during their careers, however short or long, comes to impact on their health and well-being. Part of this enterprise, as Roderick and Gibbons (2015: 160) have noted, involves recognizing that the 'all-encompassing nature of sports work on athletes' sense of self breeds a lack of autonomy and freedom of expression. A key sociological problem however for all who have an interest in this unusual work is overcoming the value-laden idea that it is hard to understand such well-being issues for athletes gifted with talent, who stereotypically live celebrated and privileged careers.'

It is also essential that we seek to better understand the comingling of young athletes' public and private lives, how their work situations are experienced in complex ways with the broader changes in their lives as they pass through the transitional youth life-stage, and how all these are managed and negotiated within the interdependent networks that they inhabit with others. This is not only an intellectually important exercise, but one that is of real practical value and which should be undertaken with the well-being of young people in mind.

References

Brackenridge, C. (2001). *Spoilsports*. London: Routledge.

Brackenridge, C., Pitchford, A., Russell, K. and Nutt, G. (2007). *Child welfare in football: an exploration of children's welfare in the modern game*. London: Routledge.

Coakley, J. and Pike, E. (2014). *Sports in society: issues and controversies*. (2nd ed). Berkshire: McGraw Hill.

Collinson, D. (1988). 'Engineering humour': masculinity, joking and conflict in shop-floor relations. *Organization Studies*, 9(2), 181–99.

David, P. (2005). *Human rights in youth sport*. London: Routledge.

DiFiori, J., Benjamin, H., Brenner, J., Gregory, A., Jayanthi, N., Landry, G. and Luke, A. (2014). Overuse injuries and burnout in youth sports: a position statement from the American Medical Society for Sports Medicine. *Clinical Journal of Sports Medicine*, 24(1), 3–20.

Donnelly, P. (1993) Problems associated with youth involvement in high-performance sport. In B. Cahill and A. Pearl (eds) *Intensive participation in children's sports*. Champaign, Illinois: Human Kinetics.

Douglas, K. and Carless, D. (2015). *Life story research in sport: understanding the experiences of elite and professional athletes through narrative*. London: Routledge.

Ducker, J. (2015). From superstars to scrapheap: meet the game's lost generation. *The Times*, 15 January, pp. 68–69.

FIFPro (2014). *Depression highly prevalent in footballers*. Available at: www.fifpro.org/en/news/depression-highly-prevalent-in-footballers [Accessed 2 April 2014].

Flett, G., Hewitt, P. and Heisel, M. (2014). The destructiveness of perfectionism revisited: implications for the assessment of suicide risk and the prevention of suicide. *Review of General Psychology*, 18(3), 156–72.

Freitag, A., Kirkwood, G., Scharer, S., Ofori-Asenso, R. and Pollock, A. (2015). Systematic review of rugby injuries in children and adolescents under 21 years. *British Journal of Sports Medicine*, 49, 511–19.

Gilchrist, J., Thomas, K., Xu, L., McGuire, L. and Corondo, V. (2011). Nonfatal traumatic brain injuries related to sports and recreational activities among persons aged ≤ 19 years – United States, 2001–2009. *Centers for Disease Control and Prevention, Morbidity and Mortality Weekly Report* 60: 1337–42.

Goffman, E. (1959). *The presentation of self in everyday life*. London: Penguin.

Grenfell, C. and Rinehart, R. (2003). Skating on thin ice. Human rights in youth figure skating. *International Review for the Sociology of Sport*, 38(1), 79–97.

Hastmann-Walch, T. and Caine, D. (2015). Injury risk and long-term effects of injury in elite youth sports. In J. Baker, P. Safai and J. Fraser-Thomas (eds) *Health and elite sport: is high performance sport a healthy pursuit?* London: Routledge.

Hoberman, J. (1992). *Mortal engines: the science of performance and the dehumanization of sport*. New York: Free Press.

Hochschild, A. (1983). *The managed heart: commercialization of human feeling*. Berkerley, CA: University of California Press.

Hughes, R. and Coakley, J. (1991). Positive deviance among athletes: the implications of overconformity to the sport ethic. *Sociology of Sport Journal*, 8(4), 307–25.

James, E., Bahr, R. and LaPrade, R. (2016). Youth sport, health and physical activity. In K. Green and A. Smith (eds) *The Routledge handbook of youth sport*. London: Routledge.

Kelly, S. and Waddington, I. (2006). Abuse, intimidation and violence as aspects of managerial control in professional soccer in Britain and Ireland. *International Review for the Sociology of Sport*, 41(2), 147–64.

Maffulli, N., Longon, U., Gougoulias, N., Loppini, M. and Denaro, V. (2010). Long-term health outcomes of youth sports injuries. *British Journal of Sports Medicine*, 44(1), 21–5.

Maffulli, N., Longon, U., Spiezia, F. and Denaro, V. (2011). Aetiology and prevention of injuries in elite youth athletes. In. N. Armstrong and A. McManus (eds). *The elite young athlete*. Basel: Karger.

Malcolm, D. and Sheard, K. (2002). "Pain in the assets": the effects of the commercialization and professionalization on the management of injury in English rugby union. *Sociology of Sport Journal*, 19(2), 149–69.

Mummery, K. (2005). Essay: depression in sport. *The Lancet*, 366, S36–S37.

Nicol, A., Pollock, A., Kirkwood, G., Parekh, N. and Robson, J. (2011). Rugby union injuries in Scottish schools. *Journal of Public Health*, 33(2), 256–61.

Nixon, H.L. II (1992). A social network analysis of influences on athletes to play with pain and injuries. *Journal of Sport and Social Issues*, 16(2), 127–35.

Nixon, H.L. II (1993). Accepting the risks of pain and injury in sport: mediated cultural influences on playing hurt. *Sociology of Sport Journal*, 10(2), 183–96.

Nixon, H.L. II (1994). Coaches' views of risk, pain, and injury in sport, with special reference to gender differences. *Sociology of Sport Journal*, 11(1), 79–87.

Parker, A. (1996). *Chasing the 'big-time': football apprenticeship in the 1990s*. Unpublished PhD Thesis. Warwick: University of Warwick.

Pike, E. (2005). 'Doctors just say "rest and take Ibuprofen"'. A critical examination of the role of non-orthodox health care in women's sport. *International Review for the Sociology of Sport*, 40(2), 201–219.

Pike, E. and Scott, A. (2015). Safeguarding, injuries and athlete choice. In M. Lang and M. Hartill (eds) *Safeguarding, child protection and abuse in sport*. London: Routledge.

Platts, C. (2012). *Education and welfare in professional football academies and centres of excellence: a sociological study*. Unpublished PhD Thesis. Chester: University of Chester.

Roderick, M. (2006a). *The work of professional football. A labour of love?* London: Routledge.

Roderick, M. (2006b). The sociology of pain and injury in sport: main perspectives and problems. In S. Loland, B. Skirstad and I. Waddington (eds). *Pain and injury in sport: social and ethical analysis*. London: Routledge.

Roderick, M. (2013). From identification to dis-identification: case studies of job loss in professional football. *Qualitative Research in Sport, Exercise and Health*, 6(2), 143–60.

Roderick, M. and Gibbons, B. (2015). 'To thine own self be true': sports work, mental illness and the problem of authenticity. In J. Baker, P. Safai and J. Fraser-Thomas (eds) *Health and elite sport: is high performance sport a healthy pursuit?* London: Routledge.

Roderick, M., Waddington I. and Parker, G. (2000). Playing hurt: managing injuries in English professional football. *International Review for the Sociology of Sport*, 35(2), 165–80.

Safai, P., Fraser-Thomas, J. and Baker, J. (2015). Sport and health of the high performance athlete: an introduction to the text. In J. Baker, P. Safai and J. Fraser-Thomas (eds) *Health and elite sport: is high performance sport a healthy pursuit?* London: Routledge.

Turner, B. and Wainwright, S. (2003). Corps de Ballet: the case of the injured ballet dancer. *Sociology of Health and Illness*, 25(4), 269–88.

Waddington, I. (2012). Sports medicine, client control and the limits of professional autonomy. In D. Malcolm and P. Safai (eds) *The social organization of sports medicine: critical socio-cultural perspectives*. London: Routledge.

Wainwright, S. and Turner, B. (2006). 'Just crumbling to bits'? An exploration of the body, ageing, injury and career in classical ballet dancers. *Sociology*, 40(2), 237–55.

Willis, P. (2009) [1978] *Learning to labour: how working class kids get working class jobs*. Farnham: Ashgate.

Young, K. (2012). *Sport, violence and society*. London: Routledge.

45

CHILD ABUSE IN SPORT

From research to policy and protection

Melanie Lang, Mike Hartill and Bettina Rulofs

Introduction

Children's participation in sport is generally regarded as beneficial, a component of a healthy childhood and a long, healthy adulthood (United Nations Children's Fund [UNICEF], 2004). UNICEF (2004: 1) states that sport has the potential to 'promote the spirit of friendship, solidarity and fair play, teach teamwork, self-discipline, trust, respect for others.' Governments worldwide have sought to harness these benefits, and non-governmental organizations are increasingly using sport and physical activity as tools to achieve international health, social and educational goals (Darnell, 2010).

However, in recent years child maltreatment in sport has been recognised as a significant problem (Brackenridge *et al.*, 2010). A growing interest in preventing child maltreatment has primarily been driven by high-profile cases of sexual abuse in sport across several countries during the 1990s (Lang and Hartill, 2015). Protecting children from maltreatment is a key strand in the children's rights agenda and stakeholders in sport, such as coaches, are named as key individuals 'with clear, recognized legal, professional-ethical and/or cultural responsibility for the safety, health, development and wellbeing of the child' (Committee on the Rights of the Child, 2011: para. 33).

Maltreatment and the context of sport: what do we know?

The World Health Organization (WHO) (1999: 15) defines child maltreatment as:

> the abuse and neglect that occurs to children under 18 years of age. All forms of physical and/or emotional ill-treatment, sexual abuse, neglect or negligent treatment or commercial or other exploitation, resulting in actual or potential harm to the child's health, survival, development or dignity in the context of a relationship of responsibility, trust or power.

Three forms of abuse are identified here: physical abuse, emotional abuse and sexual abuse. This chapter focuses on these and we direct readers to David (2005) and Lang and Hartill (2015) for information on other forms of exploitation in youth sport.

It is important to note, however, that the figures presented in this chapter should be treated with some caution as all forms of child abuse are significantly underreported and under prosecuted (Finkelhor, 2008; Gilbert *et al.*, 2009). In addition, research in this area to date has predominantly emanated from high-income countries and has focused on the sexual abuse of athletes, particularly of able-bodied athletes; more research is needed from low- and middle-income countries and on other forms of maltreatment, including among disabled groups.

Physical abuse

Physical abuse is defined as either a single or repeated behaviour that 'results in actual or potential physical harm from an interaction or lack of an interaction, which is reasonably within the control of a parent or person in a position of responsibility, power or trust' (WHO, 1999: 15).

The Child Protection in Sport Unit (CPSU) in England – the only state-backed agency with responsibility for safeguarding and child protection in sport – provides examples of behaviours that constitute physical abuse in sport, such as: 'when a child is forced into training and competition that exceeds the capacity of his or her immature and growing body, or where the child is given drugs to enhance performance or delay puberty' (CPSU, 2012).

Research on physical abuse in sport is limited, possibly because of the widespread acceptance of the 'no pain, no gain' mentality that links developing physical toughness with achieving sporting success (McKay *et al.*, 2000) and because a grey area exists between determining what constitutes a challenging but tolerable part of competitive preparation and what constitutes physical abuse (Brackenridge *et al.*, 2007).

Anecdotal cases of physical abuse in sport occasionally appear in the media. Large-scale prevalence studies of physical abuse in sport are, nevertheless, rare. In one of the only such studies – a retrospective of 1,430 youth athletes in the United Kingdom (UK) – 24 per cent of respondents reported experiencing at least one behaviour categorized as causing physical harm, such as being hit, shaken or forced to train when injured or exhausted (Alexander *et al.*, 2011). Figures were slightly higher for males than females (26 per cent and 23 per cent, respectively). Meanwhile, a study of former and current British and Irish professional footballers revealed that managers used verbal and physical abuse to intimidate young players and induce fear (Kelly and Waddington, 2006).

Coaches are the most common perpetrators of physical abuse and reported (to the relevant authorities) incidences of physical abuse increase the higher the athlete goes up the performance spectrum. For example, in the Alexander, Stafford and Lewis (2011) study from the UK, 83 per cent of international-level athletes reported experiencing physically harmful behaviour from their coach, compared to 60 per cent of national-level athletes, 43 per cent of district-level athletes and 25 per cent of recreational-level athletes.

Meanwhile, some authors have drawn attention to the manner in which elite player development models – that over-emphasize high volumes of training for children (Lang and Light, 2010), alongside pressure on coaches to create successful athletes – effectively encourage developmentally inappropriate training loads for children (Lang, 2010a). This highlights the fine line between appropriate training and practices that might, under the CPSU's definition of physical abuse (CPSU, 2012), constitute physical abuse. Scholars have also identified the practice of coaches setting punishments, such as additional training loads, on athletes who perform below expectations or who fail to conform to strict standards (Alexander *et al.*, 2011; Hong, 2004).

To highlight this issue, Kerr (2010) coined the term 'forced physical exertion' and growing awareness of this practice has prompted some sport organizations, including the Australian Sports Commission (2000), to outlaw the practice.

Emotional abuse

The emotional abuse of youth athletes has also been side-lined from critical debate until recently. Emotional abuse is defined as:

> acts towards the child that cause, or have a high probability of causing, harm to the child's health or physical, mental, spiritual, moral or social development . . . including restriction of movement, patterns of belittling, denigrating, scapegoating, threatening, scaring, discriminating, ridiculing or other non-physical forms of hostile or rejecting treatment.
>
> *(WHO, 1999: 15)*

In addition to these behaviours, putting children under consistent pressure to perform in sport to unrealistically high standards can also be deemed emotional abuse (CPSU, 2012).

As with physical abuse, the dearth of empirical research on emotional abuse in sport may be a legacy of such behaviours being part of a sports culture that normalizes practices that would be considered abusive in other social settings (Brackenridge, 2001). In addition, there is considerable debate over the definition and measurement of emotional abuse, including whether it should be defined in terms of specific behaviours perpetrated by someone with 'a significant influence over an individual's sense of safety, trust and fulfilment of needs' (Stirling and Kerr, 2013: 87) – an athlete's coach, for example – or in terms of the impact the behaviour has on an individual, as is the case with many definitions of bullying.

Increasingly, however, attention is being paid to emotional abuse in sport, albeit at the elite level primarily. As a result, the widespread nature of emotional abuse within sport at all competitive and age levels is beginning to be understood as a 'habitual coaching tool used by coaches of elite child athletes' (Gervis and Dunn, 2004: 220). A UK study of children's experiences in sport (Alexander *et al.*, 2011) supports this. It found that emotional harm was the most common form of maltreatment experienced by youth athletes, afflicting 75 per cent of respondents. Of these, 79 per cent reported being criticized about their performance, 77 per cent being embarrassed or humiliated about something in a sports context and 51 percent being shouted or sworn at in sport.

Lang (2010b) argues that adherence to common coaching practices, underpinned by understandings of coaches as experts and athletes as novices, encourages athletes to conform to normative behaviours in sport, leading them to submit to various abusive practices. Mindful of this, sports organizations are increasingly including emotional abuse in their policies. Indeed, a spate of cases of high-profile coaches being fired or suspended over allegations of emotionally abusing athletes (Stirling and Kerr, 2015) suggests sports organizations may at last be addressing this issue.

Sexual abuse

Research into the sexual abuse of child athletes has received more attention in academic circles to date than physical or emotional abuse, despite a lack of consensus on its definition (Brackenridge, 2001). The WHO provides the following broad definition:

Child sexual abuse is the involvement of a child in sexual activity that he or she does not fully comprehend, is unable to give informed consent to, or for which the child is not developmentally prepared and cannot give consent, or that violate the laws or social taboos of society . . . This may include but is not limited to: the inducement or coercion of a child to engage in any unlawful sexual activity; the exploitative use of a child in prostitution or other unlawful sexual practices; the exploitative use of children in pornographic performances and materials.

(WHO, 1999: 15–6)

The most robust study of the prevalence of sexual abuse in sport to date comes from Australia, where researchers used a legal definition of sexual abuse to question 370 elite- and recreational-level athletes about their experiences in sport (Leahy *et al.*, 2002). They found that 31 per cent of females and 21 per cent of males reported experiencing sexual abuse. Among females who had experienced sexual abuse, 41 per cent said this was perpetrated by a member of the sports personnel, compared to 29 per cent for males. Meanwhile, a national-level study of elite and recently retired elite athletes in Canada found that 22 per cent of the 266 respondents reported having sexual intercourse with someone in a position of authority in sport, including 9 per cent who said this was forced (Kirby and Greaves, 1996). In a UK study, 3 per cent of respondents reported experiencing what the researchers called sexual harm, which included behaviours such as 'being forced to kiss someone,' 'being touched sexually against your will,' 'being forced to have penetrative sex' (Alexander *et al.*, 2011). Meanwhile, a study of athletes in Norway found 42 per cent of those aged over 23 and 17 per cent of those aged between 15–18 reported experiencing sexual harassment and abuse in sport (Fasting *et al.*, 2003).

Further empirical evidence of the prevalence and incidence of child sexual abuse in sport is necessary in order to establish the extent of the problem. Brackenridge and Kirby (1997) argue that young athletes are most vulnerable to sexual abuse when they are on the cusp of the elite level – what is called the 'Stage of Imminent Achievement' – because that is when an athlete's dependency on their coach peaks. Girls, particularly those with older coaches, are most at risk of sexual abuse (Brackenridge, 2001), although Hartill (2009, 2014) and Parent and Bannon (2012) have drawn attention to the sexually abused male child in sport.

Furthermore the culture of sport, particularly its heterosexist masculine character and the relationship of dependency often present between coaches and athletes, disempowers athletes and facilitates abuse and harassment (Klein and Palzkill, 1998; Lang, 2010b). Writing for a UNICEF publication on violence to children in sport, Brackenridge and colleagues (2010: 13) identified 'the acceptance of psychologically abusive coaching practices and the often–unregulated power of authority figures to isolate young athletes' as key risk factors for abuse in sport, particularly sexual abuse.

International policy developments

In recent years the world's most influential sports organization, the International Olympic Committee (IOC), has committed itself to protecting children from abuse in sport: for example, by adopting consensus statements on sexual harassment and abuse in sport (IOC, 2007), on training the elite child athlete (IOC, 2005), on evaluating the health of elite athletes (IOC, 2009), and on the health and fitness of young people through physical activity and sport (Micheli *et al.*, 2011). In 2012, the IOC also published online education resources to raise awareness of child welfare issues in sport. Meanwhile in 2012, UNICEF initiated the creation of the International Safeguarding Children in Sport Working Group to draft a set of child safeguarding standards that all sports organizations should have in place to protect children (Paramasivan, 2012). These so-called International Standards were piloted in several sports organizations worldwide in 2013–14 prior to being introduced globally.

On a European level, the Lanzarote Convention (Council of Europe, 2007) provides a framework for EU countries to meet their obligations to safeguard and protect children. The guidelines, known formerly as the Council of Europe Convention on the Protection of Children against Sexual Exploitation and Sexual Abuse, came into force in 2010. While they focus on preventing the *sexual* exploitation of children, the guidelines are underpinned by a children's rights discourse that foregrounds the best interests of the child and have, therefore, the potential to impact on all forms of child maltreatment in sport. However, while such developments should be viewed positively, their influence on sports practice remains unknown.

Thus, while there have been great strides in recent years in the development of policies aimed at protecting children from abuse in sport, the focus has predominantly been on preventing *sexual* abuse. In this regard, it has been suggested that the driver for change in some cases has been concern among sports organizations about potential litigation in conjunction with pre-empting reputational damage, rather than a desire to safeguard child athletes per se see (Independent Football Commission, 2005). Nevertheless, given that measures to protect children from maltreatment in sport are relatively recent additions to the international sport policy agenda, such developments are to be welcomed, and it is hoped that the influence of leading international organizations such as the IOC and UNICEF will prompt national agencies to take these issues seriously and act to protect their millions of child members.

The remainder of the chapter presents a case study of child protection in sport in Germany, focusing on how sports organizations became aware of child abuse in their ranks and how they have responded to these concerns.

Child protection developments in German sport

Ethical issues in children's elite sport have been a long-standing concern in German academic discourse (e.g. Meinberg, 1984). Yet the term *child protection* was neglected in German sport for a long time. Rather, studies tended to focus on developmental issues such as the risks and opportunities within elite sport for adolescents or questions around doping prevention (e.g. Bette *et al.*, 2002; Frei *et al.*, 2000). In recent years, however, the term *child protection* has emerged on the sport-political agenda, although it is strongly connected to activities concerning the prevention of sexual harassment and abuse and has not, so far, included discourses on emotional and physical abuse.

Concerns about child abuse in sport first entered German public discourse in 1995 when the media reported that Karel Faifr, an internationally acclaimed figure skating coach, was found guilty of eleven cases of sexual abuse and two cases of bodily harm against elite female youth athletes.[1] Faifr received a two-year suspended sentence and a fine and was banned from coaching for three years (Hettrich, 1995). In response to Faifr's sentence, a pilot study on violence against women and girls in German sport was conducted (Klein and Palzkill, 1998). The study included qualitative interviews with victims of sexual harassment and abuse and with key stakeholders in sport. On the basis of the study, it was argued that the structure of sport – for example gender hierarchies, relationships of dependency, and the intense focus on the body and success in sport – facilitates sexual harassment and abuse.

In reaction to the study, a handful of sport organizations developed campaigns on preventing sexual harassment and abuse in sport. Others, however, including the national umbrella organization for sport, did nothing, and some sports organizations even opposed public dissemination of the findings, due to concern that they could damage their reputations. In the years that followed Klein and Palzkill's (1998) study, several cases of sexual harassment and abuse in sport were made public. In 2009, for example, a national athletics coach known in the media by the anonymous pseudonym Ewald K. was sentenced to eight years imprisonment for sexually abusing young male athletes over several years (Spiegel Online, 18 August 2009). However, it was not until 2010 that sport stakeholders finally accepted that the prevention of sexual harassment and abuse in German sport required a sustained prevention campaign. Public outcry over reports of sexual abuse in the Church and in boarding schools prompted the German federal government to act. In May 2010, it introduced a national helpline for people affected by harassment and abuse. Some fifteen months later, a systematic review of the helpline's data revealed that it had received 1,094 calls from people alleging sexual abuse in institutions (e.g. schools, churches, clubs and children's homes). These figures included sixty-four instances in which callers pinpointed 'clubs' as locations of sexual abuse, with twenty-six of these specifically referring to sports clubs (Fegert et al., 2012). However, while the figures from the helpline indicate that sport is indeed a site where abuse takes place, the prevalence of child abuse in German sport remains unknown.

The results of a recent general large-scale survey of elite German athletes (n=1,154) (Breuer and Hallmann, 2013) also underlines the need for a broad and sustainable strategy on providing a safe environment for young people in sport – 11 per cent of respondents admitted to suffering from burnout; 9 per cent complained of depression; and 41 per cent admitted to knowingly risking their health in pursuit of their sporting career. Yet despite this, the German approach to child protection in sport continues to focus on the prevention of sexual abuse, neglecting other forms of abuse and exploitation. While sexual abuse in and beyond sport remains a serious issue, in light of the issues raised in Breuer and Hallmann's (2013) study, consideration also needs to be paid to the broader issues that impact on athletes' welfare.

Child protection and prevention policies in German sport

Since 2010, the German federal government has required all youth organizations in the country, including the German Olympic Sports Confederation (Deutscher Olympischer Sportbund or DOSB), to develop their own child protection, prevention and intervention policies. The first major step towards removing the taboo surrounding sexual harassment and abuse in German sport was the adoption of the so-called *Munich Declaration* at the 2010 DOSB general assembly, where the DOSB and its subsidiary bodies committed to preventing sexual harassment and abuse (DOSB, 2010a). This goal was further solidified in a DOSB position paper from 2010 (DOSB, 2010b). In connection with this, the organization German Sport Youth (Deutsche Sportjugend or DSJ) assembled a working group of experts to advise its executive committee on a child protection, prevention, and intervention strategy. Since then, the DSJ and its expert panel have driven the development and implementation of numerous national-level policies. These have included the launch of an internet platform on child protection in sport, the publication of guidelines on child protection for sports clubs (cp. Rulofs et al., 2011), and the creation of a training package on preventing sexual harassment and abuse in sport and a code of conduct for coaches. In addition, the DSJ requires each of its ninety-eight member organizations to appoint a designated child protection officer and holds annual symposia for them to exchange ideas.

These developments mark a significant advance in the protection of children in sport in Germany. However, not all sports organizations agree about the extent to which sport should be required to address child protection. One issue surrounds whether volunteers and temporary employees at sports clubs should be required to produce a certificate of good conduct to, for example, serve as a coach or youth leader. National child protection laws require full-time employees who work with children to provide a certificate of good conduct, and beyond the sport sector these and other mandatory measures relating to child protection (such as police record background checks) are well established. However, with much of German sport run by volunteers – at the last count, there were 8.8 million volunteers in sports clubs (cp. DOSB 2013) – some sports organizations have expressed concern that applying this standard to sport will discourage volunteers (cp. Rulofs and Emberger, 2011). Meanwhile, researchers argue that background checks on staff with contact with children are crucial for effective child protection (Brackenridge 2001). Nevertheless, this and other mandatory regulations effecting adults working in youth sport are highly contested and evoke strong feelings in Germany.

In sum, there have been significant changes in relation to child protection in and beyond sport in recent years in Germany, including a long-overdue end to the silence surrounding sexual harassment and abuse. There are several reasons for this. First, the media has been crucial as critical and sustained reporting of cases of abuse were the catalyst behind the emerging societal expectation that youth organizations take responsibility for child protection. Equally important was the German federal government's decision to prompt youth organizations, including those in sport, to tackle child abuse. Of central importance in the future is sustaining a strategy that is broad enough to prevent various forms of child abuse in sport and effective enough to create a safe environment for children in each of the 91,000 German sport clubs.

Conclusion

While the policy response to child abuse in sport emerged in industrialized countries in the mid-1990s, acknowledgment of the problem within global sports governance remains far from uniform (Lang and Hartill, 2015). Indeed, there is some way to go before responsibility for children's protection and welfare could be said to be embedded within sports governance and practice. Furthermore, developments to date have largely excluded the perspectives of children, who tend to remain some distance from the decision-making process within sport. In addition, limited robust evaluation research has been conducted in this field (Hartill and O'Gorman, 2015). To be most effective, research needs to become embedded within the safeguarding and child protection policy development *process* rather than being viewed as a convenient tool to justify policy decisions in hindsight.

Note

1   The case is still causing trouble in German sport: in 2014, Fajfr wanted to coach a prominent German figure skating pair during the Winter Olympics in Sochi. The German Association for Figure Skating supported Fajfr, but the German Olympic Sport Confederation decided not to nominate him for the Olympic team due to ethical reasons (Spiegel Online 23 January 2014).

References

Alexander, K., Stafford, A. and Lewis, R. (2011). *The Experiences of Children Participating in Organized Sport in the UK*. Edinburgh: University of Edinburgh/NSPCC.

Australian Sport Commission (2010). *Australian Sport Commission: Ethics in Sport*. Online. Available HTTP: <secure.ausport.gov.au/__data/assets/pdf_file/0003/417117/ASC_Ethics_report.pdf> (accessed 28 August 2010).

Bette, K.-H., Schimank, U. Wahlig, D. and Weber, U. (2002). *Biographical Dynamics in Competitive Sports: Possibilities of Doping Prevention in Adolescence*. Cologne: Sport and Buch Strauß.

Brackenridge, C. H. (2001). *Spoilsports: Understanding and Preventing Sexual Exploitation in Sport*. London: Routledge.

Brackenridge, C. H. and Kirby, S. (1997). Playing safe? Assessing the risk of sexual abuse to elite child athletes. *International Review of the Sociology of Sport, 32*: 407–18.

Brackenridge, C. H., Fasting, K., Kirby, S. and Leahy, T. (2010). *Protecting Children from Violence in Sport: A Review with a Focus on Industrialized Countries*. Florence: UNICEF Innocenti Research Centre.

Brackenridge, C. H., Pitchford, A., Russell, K. and Nutt, G. (2007). *Child Welfare in Football: An Exploration of Children's Welfare in the Modern Game*. London: Routledge.

Breuer, C. and Hallmann, K. (2013). *Dysfunctions of Elite Sport: Doping, Match-fixing and Health Risks as Seen from the Perspective of Population and Athletes*. Bonn: Federal Institute for Sport Science.

CPSU (2012). *Defining Child Abuse*. Online. Available HTTP: <www.nspcc.org.uk/Inform/cpsu/helpand advice/organisations/defining/definingchildabuse_wda60692.html> (accessed 17 September 2012).

Committee on the Rights of the Child (2011). *Convention on the Rights of the Child: General Comment No. 13*. Online. Available HTTP: <www.unicef-irc.org/portfolios/general_comments/CRC.C.GC. 13_en.doc.html> (accessed 27 February 2014).

Council of Europe (2007). *Council of Europe Convention on the Protection of Children against Sexual Exploitation and Sexual Abuse, CETS No.: 201*. Online. Available HTTP: <http://conventions.coe.int/Treaty/ Commun/QueVoulezVous.asp?NT=201andCM=8andDF=andCL=ENG> (accessed 27 May 2013).

Darnell, S. C. (2010). Power, politics and 'sport for development and peace': Investigating the utility of sport for international development, *Sociology of Sport Journal, 27* (1): 54–75.

David, P. (2005). *Human Rights in Youth Sport: A Critical Review of Children's Rights in Competitive Sports*. New York: Routledge.

DOSB (2010a). *Protection from Sexual Violence in Sport*. Online. Available HTTP: <www.dosb.de/ fileadmin/fm-dosb/downloads/Sexualisierte_Gewalt/Sexualisierte_Gewalt_Schutz_Praevention_DOSB_ Erklaerung.pdf> (accessed 27 February 2014).

DOSB (2010b). *Position Paper: Preventing and Combating Sexual Violence and Abuse of Children and Young People in Sport*. Online. Available HTTP: <www.dsj.de/fileadmin/user_upload/Dokumente/Handlungs felder/Praevention/sexualisierte_Gewalt/Positionspapier_DOSB-Praesidium_2010_php.pdf> (accessed 27 February 2014).

DOSB (2013). *Short Profile of the German Olympic Sports Confederation*. Online. Available HTTP: <www. dosb.de/de/organisation/philosophie/kurzportraet-des-dosb/> (accessed 27 May 2013).

Fasting, K. Brackenridge, C. H. and Sungot-Borgen, J. (2003). Experiences of sexual harassment and abuse among Norwegian elite female athletes and non-athletes. *Research Quarterly for Exercise and Sport. 74*(1): 84–97.

Fegert, J. M., Rassenhofer, M., Schneider T., Seitz, A., König, L. and Spröber, N. (2012). Listening to victims: results of the scientific research on the helpline of the independent commissioner for the clearing of child sexual abuse and the discussion of a research agenda. In S. Andresen and W. Heitmeyer (eds) *Destructive Processes: Disrespect and Sexual Violence Against Children and Adolescents in Institutions*. (pp. 111–129). Basel: Beltz Juventa.

Finkelhor, D. (2008). *Childhood Victimization: Violence, Crime and Abuse in the Lives of Young People*. Oxford: Oxford University Press.

Frei, P., Lüsebrink, I., Rottländer, D. and Thiele, J. (2000). *Pressures and Risks in Female Gymnastics: Part 2: Insider Views, Educational Perspectives and Consequences*. Schorndorf: Hofmann.

Gervis, M. and Dunn, N. (2004). The emotional abuse of elite child athletes by their coaches. *Child Abuse Review, 13*: 215–23.

Gilbert, R., Kemp, A., Thoburn, J., Sidebotham, P., Radford, L., Glaser, D. and MacMillan, H. L. (2009). Recognising and responding to child maltreatment. *The Lancet, 373*: 167–80.

Hartill, M. (2009). The sexual abuse of boys in organized male sports. *Men and Masculinities, 12*(2): 225–49.

Hartill, M. (2014). Suffering in gratitude: Sport and the sexually abused male child. In J. Hargreaves and E. Anderson (eds) *Routledge Handbook of Sport, Gender and Sexuality*. (pp. 426–34). London: Routledge.

Hartill, M. and O'Gorman, J. (2015). Evaluation in safeguarding and child protection in sport. In M. Lang and M. Hartill (eds) *Safeguarding, Child Protection and Abuse in Sport: International Perspectives in Research, Policy and Practice*. (pp. 181–91). London: Routledge.

Hettrich, A. (1995). *Faijfr Guilty: Figure Skating Coach Received Two Years Suspended Sentence*. Online. Available HTTP: <www.welt.de/print-welt/article664514/Fajfr-schuldig-gesprochen.html> (accessed 24 July 2013).

Hong, F. (2004). Innocence lost: Child athletes in China. *Sport in Society: Cultures, Commerce, Media and Politics. 7*: 338–54.

Independent Football Commission (2005). *Report on Child Protection in Football*. Stockton-on-Tees: Independent Football Commission.

IOC (2005). *Consensus Statement on Training the Elite Child Athlete*. Online. Available HTTP: <www.olympic.org/content/news/media-resources/manual-news/1999-2009/2005/11/14/consensus-statement-adopted-on-training-the-elite-child-athlete/> (accessed 21 February 2014).

IOC (2007). *IOC Consensus Statement on Sexual Harassment and Abuse in Sport*. Online. Available HTTP: <www.olympic.org/Documents/Reports/EN/en_report_1125.pdf> (accessed 15 November 2013).

IOC (2009). *IOC Consensus Statement on Periodic Health Evaluation of Elite Athletes*. Online. Available HTTP: <www.olympic.org/Documents/Reports/EN/en_report_1448.pdf> (accessed 15 November 2013).

Kelly, S. and Waddington, I. (2006). Abuse, intimidation and violence as aspects of managerial control in professional soccer in Britain and Ireland. *International Review for the Sociology of Sport*. 41(2):147–64.

Kerr, G. (2010). Physical and Emotional Abuse of Elite Child Athletes: the case of forced physical exertion. In C. H. Brackenridge and D. Rhind (eds) *Elite Child Athlete Welfare: International Perspectives*. London: Brunel University.

Kirby, S. and Greaves, L. (1996). *Foul Play: Sexual Harassment and Abuse in Sport*. Paper presented to the Pre-Olympic Scientific Congress, Dallas, USA, July 11–14.

Klein, M. and Palzkill, B. (1998). *Violence Against Girls and Women in Sport*. Dusseldorf: Ministry of Women, Youth, Family and Health: North Rhine-Westphalia.

Leahy, T. Pretty, G. and Tenenbaum, G. (2002). Prevalence of sexual abuse in sport in Australia. *Journal of Sexual Aggression*, 2: 16–36.

Lang, M. (2010a). Intensive training in youth sports: A new abuse of power? In K. P. Vanhoutte and M. Lang (eds) *Bullying and the Abuse of Power: From the Playground to International Relations*. (pp. 57–64). Freeland: Inter-Disciplinary Press.

Lang, M. (2010b). Surveillance and conformity in competitive youth swimming. *Sport, Education and Society*, 12: 19–37.

Lang, M. and Hartill, M. (eds) (2015). *Safeguarding, Child Protection and Abuse in Sport: International Perspectives in Research, Policy and Practice*. London: Routledge.

Lang, M. and Light, R. (2010). Interpreting and implementing the Long Term Athlete Development Model: English swimming coaches' views on the (swimming) LTAD in practice. *International Journal of Sports Science and Coaching*, 5 (3): 389–402.

Meinberg, E. (1984). *Children's High-Performance Sport: Heteronomy or Self-development – Educational, Anthropological and Ethical Orientation*. Cologne: Strauß.

McKay, J. Messner, M. and Sabo, D. (2000). *Masculinities, Gender Relations and Sport*. Thousand Oaks, Sage.

Micheli, L., Mountjoy, M. and Engebretsen, L. *et al.* (2011). International Olympic Committee consensus statement on the health and fitness of young people through physical activity and sport. *British Journal of Sport Medicine*, 45: 839–48.

Paramasivan, M. (2012). *UNICEF Takes Safeguarding Procedures Beyond Paper*. Online. Available HTTP: <www.sportanddev.org/?4769/UNICEF-takes-safeguarding-procedures-beyond-paper> (accessed 31 January 2014).

Parent, S. and Bannon, J. (2012) Sexual abuse in sport: What about boys? *Children and Youth Services Review*, 34(2): 354–59.

Rulofs, B. With Brandi, H., Busch, G., Gramkow, K., Hunz, J., Korn, M., Rittgasser, N., Sahle, D. and Witte, K. (2011). *Against Sexual Violence in Sport: Annotated Guidelines for Sports Clubs to Protect Children and Adolescents*. Frankfurt: German Sport Youth and the German Olympic Sports Confederation.

Rulofs, B. and Emberger, D. (2011). *Prevention of Sexual Violence in Sport: Between Voluntarism and Commitment? Analysis of the Perception and Acceptance of Specific Prevention Measures of the Sports Federation in North Rhine-Westphalia from the Perspective of Functionaries in Sport*. Unpublished report to the Ministry for Sport North Rhine-Westphalia.

Spiegel Online (18 August 2009). *Bavaria: German National Coach Confesses to Hundredfold Child Abuse*. Online. Available HTTP: <www.spiegel.de/panorama/justiz/bayern-bundestrainer-gesteht-hundert fachen-kindesmissbrauch-a-643530.html> (accessed 1 April 2012).

Spiegel Online (23 January 2014.) *Contested Coach: Figure Skating Coach Fajfr is Not Allowed to go to Sochi*. Online. Avalable HTTP: <www.spiegel.de/sport/wintersport/eiskunstlauf-trainer-fajfr-darf-nicht-mit-nach-sotschi-a-945138.html> (accessed 23 March 2014).

Stirling, A. and Kerr, G. (2013). The perceived effects of elite athletes' experiences of emotional abuse in the coach–athlete relationship. *International Journal of Sport and Exercise Psychology*, 11(1): 87–100.

Stirling, A. E. and Kerr, G. A. (2015). Safeguarding athletes from emotional abuse. In: M. Lang and M. Hartill (eds) *Safeguarding, Child Protection and Abuse in Sport: International Perspectives in Research, Policy and Practice*. (pp. 143–52). London: Routledge.

UNICEF (2004). *Sport, Recreation and Play*. Geneva: UNICEF.

United Nations General Assembly (1989). *Convention on the Rights of the Child*. Online. Available HTTP: <www.unhcr.org/refworld/docid/3ae6b38f0.html> (accessed 15 March 2013).

WHO (1999). *Report of the Consultation on Child Abuse Prevention*. Geneva: WHO.

SECTION 8

Politics and policy in youth sport

46

INTRODUCTION

Andy Smith

In the final section of the Handbook, the authors explore some key aspects of the politics and policy of youth sport. Each of the contributions address the central issues that have been examined in the preceding sections of this Handbook, and collectively they indicate how youth sport constitutes a 'crowded policy space' (Houlihan, 2000) in which young people are in much demand by policy makers and those responsible for programme delivery. As in other areas of social and welfare policy, the chapters in Section 8 reveal how youth sport remains a setting in which policy 'is introduced into a context where differing and often competing interests will view young people variously as future or potential workers and citizens, health sector clients, elite athletes, consumers of leisure services, etc' (Houlihan, 2000: 181). Many of these sectoral interests in young people are represented in the four chapters which address elite youth sport policy (De Bosscher *et al.*), youth sport development in small states (Sam), youth-focused sport-for-change programmes (Coalter), and community sport for young people (Ives *et al.*).

Before briefly reviewing each of the chapters in turn, it is worth noting that 'the pervasive and nearly unshakable belief in the inherent purity and goodness of sport' (Coakley, 2015: 403) continues to inform the assumptions, priorities and direction of much youth sport policy in many countries. Since the roots of these assumptions, which view sport as an unambiguously positive and wholesome activity, can be traced back to the nineteenth century, it seems almost unnecessary to draw attention to the existence of what Coakley (2015: 403) calls the 'great sport myth'. This myth, he argues, is almost universally accepted by those predisposed to view sport in this way and who 'already know the truth about sport and their faith in that truth is much like religious faith – isolated from empirical reality and regularly expressed through unquestioned support of policies and programs in which sport is the focus' (Coakley, 2015: 403). Despite an abundance of international evidence, which seriously brings into question the 'great sport myth', it nevertheless remains a persuasive and powerful one which proves attractive to politicians, policy makers, funders of sports programmes and many people who participate in sport whether directly or indirectly. This appears particularly true for those with an interest in youth sport who regularly relate beliefs underpinning the 'great sport myth' with two others:

1   the purity and goodness of sport is transmitted to those who participate in or consume it; and
2   sport inevitably leads to individual and community development.

(Coakley, 2015: 403)

As readers will see, these beliefs frequently provide the context within which the contributors to this section of the Handbook variously locate their work.

In their chapter, *Elite youth sport policy and dual career support services in fifteen countries*, Veerle De Bosscher, Camilla Brockett and Hans Westerbeek revisit some of the key themes which underpinned the contributions presented in Section 7, namely, talent identification and development, talent recognition scouting, and the selection of young athletes for national and international competitions. These features of elite sport policy are discussed in light of the emergence of state-sponsored, elite sport development 'systems' that over the last fifty years have become an increasingly prominent feature of sport policy in many countries throughout the world (Bloyce and Smith, 2010; Green and Houlihan, 2005; Oakley and Green, 2001; Sotiriadou and De Bosscher, 2013). Among other things, this process has been associated with the growing social significance of sport internationally and the tendency for many governments, and sports organisations such as national governing bodies of sport, to prioritize investment in sports and athletes most likely to result in elite sports success.

As De Bosscher *et al.* note in their chapter, the constraints experienced by sports organizations within this highly competitive and pressurised elite sport policy environment has often involved the earlier, intense and more systematic identification of athletes at a very young age. To help address the lack of research on the support needed during the talent development of young athletes, De Bosscher and colleagues present data from fifteen countries involved in the *Sports Policy Factors Leading to International Sporting Success* (known as SPLISS 2.0) study between 2009 and 2014 (De Bosscher *et al.*, 2015). In particular, the authors examine strategies deployed in national elite sport policy intended to develop young talented athletes, and to assist in the management of their engagement in elite sport and academic study commitments that are regarded as important for their well-being. The findings of the study revealed that there exists significant variation between the fifteen nations in relation to the level of national coordination of talent identification and development systems. In general terms, the coordination of talent identification and development in larger countries (defined in terms of land size and population) such as Canada was more complex and expensive to organize, while comparatively smaller-sized countries such as Flanders, Switzerland and the Netherlands were said to have capitalized on their 'small size' to operate more effectively and competitively in relation to talent identification and talent development. More particularly, smaller nations were identified as adopting a more comprehensive approach to planning for youth talent identification and development, with significant age-related and level-appropriate support for young athletes being provided by sport scientists. These countries were also said to provide young athletes with nationally coordinated support services, which better enabled them to combine their participation in elite sport with academic study, while in other countries there existed a complex network of centralized and decentralized systems to assist the sporting and education participation of young elite athletes.

The findings reported by De Bosscher *et al.* raise important questions about the degree to which the talent development and talent identification processes involved in elite youth sport are increasingly becoming part of the 'global sporting arms race' which characterizes the broader elite sport policy context (De Bosscher *et al.*, 2008; Oakley and Green, 2001). They should also encourage further reflection upon the degree to which elite youth sport, as part of broader elite sports development systems, is characterized by processes of diminishing contrasts and increasing varieties (Bloyce and Smith, 2010), which not only have consequences for the success of nations, but also the well-being of elite youth athletes.

The next two chapters by Michael Sam and Fred Coalter explore additional features of young people's development and sport participation in other policy contexts, and consider some of the issues addressed in the various contributions on youth sport around the world (Section 2), socialization (Section 4) and social dynamics (Section 5). In *Youth sport policy in small states*, Sam addresses some of the issues associated with the organization and provision of youth sport in so-called small nations such as New Zealand, Singapore and the Nordic states. He argues that, in (youth) sport, 'size matters' though how and why it matters is said to depend on the complex interdependence between population size, geography and political economy. Sam explains how there exists immense variation among and between small states, and concludes that 'it is probable that internationalized youth sport would yield distinctive responses compared to global superpowers', not least because of the often 'limited human and financial resources, close personal ties, and frameworks of legitimacy' which exist in small states. However, in an echo of the arguments surrounding processes of diminishing contrasts and increasing varieties which underpins analyses of elite sport policy (such as that offered by De Bosscher et al., in the preceding chapter), Sam also draws attention to the ways in which sport policy in small states such as Trinidad and Tobago has been modelled on Australian sport policy, while in New Zealand comparisons have been made with the sport policy priorities of Australia and the UK. This having been said, Sam rightly argues that the ways in which 'small states enact such modelling or mimicking must necessarily take place in an environment marked by each state's responses to global pressures, by the domestic realities of having limited resources, and by its close-knit networks of accountability', each of which need to lie at the heart of future youth sport research.

Fred Coalter's chapter *Youth and sport-for-change programmes: what can you expect?* builds upon his longstanding concern with better understanding sports programmes intended to contribute to 'development' and promote among young people a variety of pro-social behaviours (e.g. Coalter, 2007, 2011). In his present contribution, Coalter reports the findings of research based on an evaluation of six sport-based projects in various parts of the UK, which were funded by Comic Relief over a five-year period. These projects were targeted towards at-risk youth (often perceived to lack aspiration and ambition) in areas of deprivation and sought to reduce conflict between young people which was based on territoriality, gang culture, and racist and sectarian attitudes. Having reviewed the evidence of these projects – many of which were *sport plus* and *plus sport* programmes (Coalter, 2007) – Coalter proceeds to outline a framework for developing programme theories that help identify 'the processes, relationships and experiences which *might* achieve the desired impacts and, perhaps, outcomes' of sport-for-change programmes. In this regard, Coalter draws upon the work of Weiss and Pawson, among others, to emphasize the importance of understanding the middle range mechanisms – the processes, experiences and relationships – which might help programme workers to achieve more of their desired impacts on young people's behaviour. 'The identification of the possible communalities of such mechanisms across a variety of interventions', Coalter suggests, 'can assist in the development of, or linking with, broader theoretical and analytical frameworks, providing a more robust and potentially generalisable version of what works, in what circumstances, for whom and why'. A central dimension of this analysis, and a theme that runs throughout Coalter's contribution to this Handbook, involves recognizing that while sport might provide the context for positive experiences among young people, it is the social *process* of participation which is essential for understanding what happens on programmes intended to affect desired behavioural change. Much more attention needs to be given to this significant – but often overlooked – process-oriented approach to understanding the workings of sports-based programmes, and much remains to be learned about the mechanisms that are associated with the experiences participants have of such programmes.

The importance of context and process in youth sport programmes is a theme picked up in *Enacting youth sport policy: towards a micro-political and emotional understanding of community sports coaching work*, by Ben Ives, Laura Gale, Lee Nelson and Paul Potrac. In this chapter, Ives *et al.*, outline the beginnings of an important topic that has so far been a much neglected feature of youth sport research: the everyday realities of working life for community sports coaches who are charged with the responsibility of enacting youth sport policy in the UK. This is an important development for, if young people's involvement in sport and physical activity is to be adequately understood, then it is clearly important to understand something of the experiences of the significant others to whom their care is entrusted, including sports coaches, youth mentors and other (often adult) figures who assist in the organization of programmes. The workplace conditions that characterized the lives of two community sports coaches – Greg and James – are explored to illuminate the everyday demands and dilemmas that they experience, and the ways in which this comes to impact on the degree to which they can achieve desired policy goals. As well as delivering various sports and physical activities, the stories of Greg and James are ones in which attention is also drawn to other tasks (e.g. administration of attendance registers), cultures of payment-by-results, and pressures to meet participation targets that were played out in the context of sometimes strained and intense employer-employee relations. As Ives *et al.*, make clear, there were significant costs to coaches' well-being of working in this highly uncertain and pressurised policy context, and the significant investment by coaches of emotional labour in the enactment of youth sport policy is clearly a much under-acknowledged area of policy analysis. As Ives *et al.*, themselves note, future research on community sports coaches' work, lives and careers will have much to offer in analyses of youth sport and especially 'the design, delivery, monitoring and evaluation of various programmes and interventions'.

References

Bloyce, D. and Smith, A. (2010). *Sport policy and development: an introduction.* London: Routledge.

Coakley, J. (2015). Assessing the sociology of sport: on cultural sensibilities and the great sport myth. *International Review for the Sociology of Sport*, 50(4–5), 402–06.

Coalter, F. (2007). *A wider social role for sport. Who's keeping score?*, London: Routledge.

Coalter, F. (2011). *Sport, conflict and youth development.* London: Comic Relief.

De Bosscher, V., Bingham, J., Shibli, S., van Bottenburg, M. and De Knop, P. (2008). *The global sporting arms race: an international comparative study on sports policy factors leading to international sporting success.* Aachen: Meyer and Meyer.

De Bosscher, V., Shibli, S., Westerbeek, H. and van Bottenburg, M. (2015). *Successful elite sport policies. An international comparison of the sports policy factors leading to international sporting success (SPLISS 2.0).* Aachen: Meyer and Meyer.

Green, M. and Houlihan, B. (2005). *Elite sport development.* London: Routledge.

Houlihan, B. (2000). Sporting excellence, schools and sports development: the politics of crowded policy spaces. *European Physical Education Review*, 6(2), 171–93.

Oakley, B. and Green, M. (2001). Elite sport development systems and playing to win: uniformity and diversity in international approaches. *Leisure Studies*, 20(4), 247–67.

Sotiriadou, P. and De Bosscher, V. (eds) (2013). *Managing high performance sport.* London: Routledge.

47

ELITE YOUTH SPORT POLICY AND DUAL CAREER SUPPORT SERVICES IN FIFTEEN COUNTRIES

Veerle De Bosscher, Camilla Brockett and Hans Westerbeek

Introduction

For every Olympic gold medal athlete, there have been thousands of aspiring and talented children training hard to achieve their dreams of elite sporting success. The '10-year rule', first applied to the game of chess (Simon and Chase, 1973) and later to other areas, such as sport, is often used to express what it takes to develop talent towards success. At least 10,000 hours of deliberate practice in a period of ten years is a minimum requirement to reach the level of being an expert (Ericsson, 2003). Recent research has found that in sport this timeframe has increased as athletes are younger when they first enter their sport (2.3 years younger) and their elite sport career takes on average 3.7 years longer than about fifteen years ago (De Bosscher and De Croock, 2010; van Bottenburg, 2009). Furthermore, athletes train longer and more national and international championships are organized for young athletes (Gullich et al., 2004). Responding to this increasing performance pressure for athletes, several countries have established programmes to support talent identification and talent development over the past decades. Without support services during talent development, athletes are unlikely to reach their full performance potential (De Bosscher et al., 2015).

A plethora of studies has attempted to understand what determines success for talented youth at the micro-level (individual athlete) perspective (such as physical, genetics, physiology, perceptual motor, psychological applications) (e.g. Elferink-Gemser et al., 2004; Vaeyens et al., 2008; Wylleman et al., 2008). Several talent development models have been developed on that basis (e.g. Balyi and Hamilton, 2004; Bloom, 1985; Côté, 1999; Côté and Fraser-Thomas, 2007; Wylleman and Lavallee, 2004). Since 2000, an emerging body of literature has emerged that has paid attention to meso-level factors (organisation) – especially in national level of sport policy – that can contribute to international sporting success (e.g. Andersen and Ronglan, 2012; Bergsgard et al., 2007; De Bosscher, et al., 2006 and 2008; Digel, Burk and Fahrner, 2006; Green and Houlihan, 2005; Houlihan and Green, 2008; Gulbin, 2011; Oakley and Green, 2001). These studies focus on the systems and programmes developed by sport organisations and governments to support athletic careers. Research on the support needed during talent development of young athletes has been largely ignored, and the European Union has also recognized the need to focus on young athletes' dual careers in which their sport participation is combined with study and work (European Commission, 2007). Drawing on data collected from fifteen countries (as part of the SPLISS study), this chapter examines strategies at the national level of sport policies intended to develop young talented athletes and how this is facilitated, particularly those intended to help young people combine their engagement in elite sport with academic study.

Elite youth sport policy: data from SPLISS 2.0

The results presented in this chapter are based on a large-scale international project that took place between 2009 and 2014 and compared Sports Policy factors Leading to International Sporting Success (SPLISS), known as SPLISS 2.0 (De Bosscher *et al.*, 2015). SPLISS identifies nine Pillars at the national policy level that can influence international sporting success, and specifies thirty-one sub-dimensions that include ninety-six Critical Success Factors (CSFs) and 750 sub-factors as key elements that are necessary to improve the elite sport success of a nation. These Pillars have been compared in fifteen nations: Australia, Belgium (separated by Flanders and Wallonia), Brazil, Canada, Denmark, Estonia, France, Finland, Japan, South-Korea, the Netherlands, Northern Ireland (as part of the United Kingdom), Portugal, Spain and Switzerland. The focus of the SPLISS model is on the relationship between policies and international sporting success, and provides insights into the factors that shape elite sport policies that in turn influence the pathways to success in different nations. The project is characterized by the use of mixed-methods research, including the development of a scoring system to measure the competitive position of nations in elite sport for each Pillar of the theoretical model. This scoring system is – in addition to qualitative data – a supportive and tangible way of understanding elite sport policies more broadly, in relation to sporting success. In this respect the SPLISS–study is complementary to, both in methodological and theoretical terms, existing knowledge on elite sport policies, that is descriptive in nature. One key point in the methodology is the involvement of the main stakeholders (3142 athletes, 1376 coaches and 241 performance directors) in the evaluation process. This way, in addition to measuring quantifiable variables, such as inputs (money) and outputs (medals), the project also seeks to understand the *black box* of throughput or processes of elite sport policies. The collaborative project is a collaboration of fifty-eight researchers (who funded their own research contribution or collaborated voluntarily) and thirty-three policy partners across the world (De Bosscher *et al.*, in press; De Bosscher *et al.*, 2006; De Bosscher *et al.*, 2010).

The fourth Pillar of the SPLISS model deals with 'talent identification and development systems', which is the focus of this chapter. This Pillar is composed of twelve CSFs including 169 sub-factors. These are presented in the next section together with the summarized average results of the sample relative to five sub-dimensions. The chapter will then focus, in particular, on the so-called dual careers of young athletes, and how countries provide support to facilitate the combination of high performance training with educational support for athletes.

Critical success factors of national talent identification and development policies (Pillar 4)

Pillar 4 of the SPLISS model consists of two main elements: talent identification and talent development. The talent identification process starts when a talented athlete is identified and special attention is provided to this athlete. In order to detect talent, monitoring systems to scan talent characteristics and minimize drop out are required, underpinned by well-organized scouting systems (Rowe, 1994). Talent identification is concerned with different phases of talent recognition (i.e. monitoring systems based on criteria that recognize young talent), talent scouting (i.e. the processes undertaken to recruit young athletes) and selection processes (the process of selecting young athletes for specific purposes (e.g. training activities, competitions). The majority of talent identification issues need to be analysed on a sport-specific basis as young talented athletes are usually recruited from within one sport. At the national level of Pillar 4, policy is mainly related to planning and national coordination and these processes were evaluated by six CSFs, grouped under one sub-dimension, as shown below (De Bosscher *et al.*, 2009):

I. There is an effective system for the identification of young talented athletes, so that the maximum number of potential top level athletes are reached at the right time (age)

CSF 4.1	There is a systematic talent selection process to identify potential elite athletes from outside a sport's participant base or by talent transfer.
CSF 4.2	NGBs [national governing bodies; that is to say, national sports federations] can receive funding for the identification (recognition and scouting) of young talented athletes in their sport.
CSF 4.3	There is comprehensive planning for talent identification: NGBs are encouraged to have (and have) detailed long-term policy plans describing how talents in their sport are recognised, identified and selected in order to receive funding
CSF 4.4	NGBs receive sport specific support to develop a testing system (tests for the recognition of young talents) and monitoring system with clear criteria for the identification of young talents in each sport.
CSF 4.5	The talent identification system is informed and covered by scientific research (including the socio-psychological development of children and the development of a stage-specific, individualized and balanced approach).
CSF 4.6	There is a national framework on how the talent identification and selection process has to look like (or different frameworks as guidelines for different sports).

During the talent development phase, athletes become highly committed to their sport, train more and for longer and become more specialized. They have usually made the transition from the local sports club to formal competitive sport with a view to improving performance. As they progress along the talent development pathway, these pre-elite athletes are regularly evaluated to confirm their performance potential. At the point when they are selected for a significant benchmark event, such as a regional or national (youth) championships, this is often the time when talented/pre-elite athletes start to receive special attention and extra benefits from their sport club (or personal coach), governing bodies and/or governments. Since the 1990s, many countries have developed programmes to provide athletes with a balanced and flexible approach to academic and sporting commitments (De Knop *et al.*, 1999). The talent development system was measured by six CSFs in the SPLISS project, grouped under four sub-dimensions:

II. There is nationally coordinated planning for NGBs in order to develop an effective system for the development of young talents in their sports

CSF 4.8	NGBs have a coordinated long-term and short-term planning for talent development (how talents in their sport are developed from club level to regional level to national level in order to receive funding) that is covered by scientific research.

CSF 4.7   NGBs and/or sports clubs can receive funding specifically for talent development and receive information, knowledge and support services (other than financial) in order to develop their talent development programmes.

III. Young talents receive multidimensional support services that are needed to develop them as young athletes at the highest level

CSF 4.9   Young talents receive age/level appropriate multidimensional support services at different levels, including training and competition support, medical/ paramedical support and lifestyle support.

IV. Young talents receive nationally coordinated support for the combination of sports development and academic study during secondary education (12–16/18 years) and where relevant primary education (for early specialisation sports where such a system is required)

CSF 4.10   There is a legal framework (whereby young talents have their elite sport status recognised contractually by the sports and education ministries at an age appropriate to their sport) and governments/NSA recognise the cost involved with elite sport and study in secondary education

CSF4.11   There is a nationally coordinated system that facilitates the combination of elite sport and studies during secondary and primary education.

V. Young talents receive nationally coordinated support for the combination of sports development and academic study during higher education (university/college level)

CSF4.12   There is a nationally coordinated system that facilitates the combination of elite sport and academic studies in higher education and governments/NSA recognise the cost involved with it.

Data on these CSFs have been collected by two different research instruments:

1   An overall elite sport policy inventory, a comprehensive research instrument in its own right, was used to collect mainly qualitative data on all Pillars. It was completed by the researchers in each country through interviews with policy agencies and analysis of existing secondary sources such as policy documents.
2   As noted earlier, a survey completed by 3,142 athletes, 1,376 coaches and 241 performance directors (of national governing bodies) across the fifteen sample nations, which examined the elite sport climate both objectively and subjectively.

Overall, one-third of the CSFs were identified through the elite sport climate survey and two-thirds through the overall sport policy inventory.

The data analysis reflected findings from economic studies that measure competitiveness in market research using composite indicators (De Pelsmacker and Van Kenhove, 1999). In addition to descriptive content analysis, SPLISS used a scoring system for two reasons: first, to objectify comparison in nine Pillars and to recognize patterns of well-developed elite sport policies and, second, to find possible relationships between elite sport policies (independent variables) and sporting success (dependent variable) (Sandelowski *et al.*, 2009). Nations received a score for each CSF, which were then aggregated into one percentage score for the sub-dimensions and then for the total Pillar (De Bosscher *et al.*, 2010; 2015).

Global evaluation of national talent identification (TID) and development (TD) policies

There appears to be a degree of ambivalence towards talent identification and development in many nations (Figure 47.1). Pillar 4 scores vary markedly between countries and the presence of a nationally coordinated talent identification and development system does not correlate high with success ($r_{s(summer)}$ = -.148 [p=0.629] and $r_{s(winter)}$ = .237 [p=0.435]). It appears that mainly smaller nations, both in terms of land size and to a lesser extent population, score better on Pillar 4. The scores are generally low. The best level of development was found in Flanders, Switzerland and the Netherlands. These countries adopt a comprehensive approach to planning in relation to talent identification and development. Much of this relates to support provided by sport scientists, multidimensional support services specific to the age and level of development of young athletes, and nationally coordinated support to combine elite sport with academic study.

As Figure 47.1 indicates, the average score on talent identification across six CSFs (sub-dimension I) is just 35 per cent. Switzerland and Japan are the most advanced nations. According to the high performance directors, the general planning of talent identification by the NGBs is still limited, and particularly with respect to having an integrated talent identification strategy from club, to regional, to national level. Furthermore, less than 40 per cent of the performance directors from NGBs (n=187) reported that their TID systems are based on scientific knowledge of the sport. One possible explanation for these low scores may be that the majority of countries do not offer scientific personnel or research funds to develop sport-specific talent identification systems. Talent identification is increasingly seen as a specialist area within elite sport development systems, and the problem consistently reported by nations in the sample is that there is a lack of, and access to, suitably qualified professionals in this field (i.e. talent coaches and scientists). Switzerland's Prognostic Integrative Systematic Trainer Evaluation (PISTE) system can be considered the most advanced and detailed talent selection system. It provides assessment criteria for selecting young athletes based on coaching science. Criteria include: competition results, performance tests, performance development, athlete motivation, athlete biography and biological development assessment. Talent cards and subsequent funding by the Swiss Olympic Association (SOA) are allocated based on the PISTE criteria and ranking provided by each sport.

The highest score across the five sub-dimensions is reached in the multidimensional support services that young talented athletes receive (sub-dimension III), measured by only one CSF, but by forty-four different objective and subjective criteria that have been evaluated retrospectively by athletes, and confirmed by coaches and performance directors. In summary, the support services that young athletes had received, including extra training opportunities, training schedules, access to international competitions, equipment, reimbursement of expenses, medical support services, mental coaching (psychological support), nutritional advice and biomechanical analysis, were deemed of reasonable quality across the nations, with 47 per cent of all athletes, on average, receiving these kind of services. However, only 27 per cent of the coaches (n=1144) and 39 per cent of the athletes (n=2932) rated the support they received as an emerging talent from their NGB as sufficient (De Bosscher *et al.*, 2015). There were no differences between top 16 athletes and others. A maximum score was reported in the Netherlands and the lowest level of development was found in Canada. The low score in Canada is related to the lack of national coordination of support, and dissatisfaction about this among Canadian elite athletes and coaches. Coaches are more critical of the provision of talent identification and development than athletes. This may be because coaches are more experienced and have greater knowledge

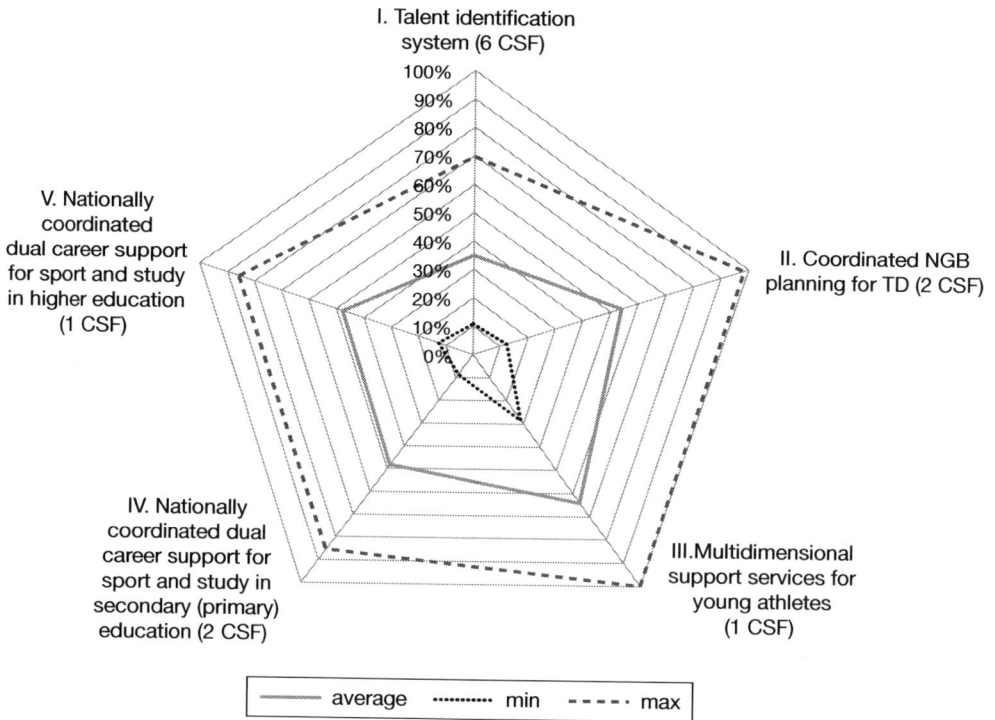

Figure 47.1 Average scores (and min/max) on five sub–dimensions of talent identification and development systems (pillar 4) among 15 nations in the SPLISS sample

of what is recognized as best practice globally, and because coaches are often in a stronger position to make informed judgements and comparisons than athletes (De Bosscher *et al.*, 2015).

Sub-dimensions IV and V are concerned with the programme support offered for career and education. Considering the special attention these programmes have received over the last decade in many countries, the next section will explore young athletes' dual career provision in more depth.

Dual career support: combining education and sport in secondary education

The increasing demands of elite sport careers make it difficult for young athletes to balance attending school and practicing sport at the elite level. It can be argued that the most time and resource intensive talent development phase in sport coincides with attending secondary and tertiary education. It is almost impossible for athletes to combine an average of 20–30 hours training per week with regular schooling without having to prioritize one over the other, which is often associated with high dropout from elite sport. As most countries have compulsory education laws up until the age of 16 or 17, many athletes will face the challenge of balancing their academic and athletic development (De Knop, *et al.*, 1999). Some athletes choose to invest fully in their sport often at the expense of education and, in less commercialized sports, their financial future. But many (especially European) athletes eventually prioritize education over their participation in sport. This is partly explained by the fact that – especially in Europe –

there is no elite sport pathway through high school or intercollegiate sports comparable to that which exists in North America. Accordingly, elite sport and study programmes have been developed in many countries since the 1990s to provide athletes with a balanced and flexible approach to academic and sporting commitments (De Knop *et al.*, 1999). The European Union has also expressed a concern about the dual careers of young athletes and works to protect young athletes in terms of, among other matters, young athletes educational rights and their ability to integrate academic study into their working lives in sport. Both at secondary and higher education levels, several initiatives have been taken to provide young talents with all kinds of support services. in relation to academic study, these include reduced school attendance requirements, flexibility in examination scheduling, absence from school/university (for international competitions), individualized study schedules, alternative access to delivery of courses (distance learning), individual or small group tutoring, study coordinators and career coaching/planning and scholarships. In relation to sport, services comprise extra training during school time, coaching support, medical and psychological support, sport science support, training facilities at school, apparel and sporting equipment, participation in international competitions and boarding (Aquilina and Henry, 2010; De Bosscher *et al.*, 2008; Radtke and Coalter, 2007).

In secondary education (which typically encompasses ages 11/12–18/19-years old), some countries have set up specific schools and/or programmes for talented young athletes that enable them to train during the day, participate in international competitions, have distance learning guided by a study coordinator, and receive other tailored support. Overall, 61 per cent of all athletes in the fifteen nations reported that their educational establishment offered them special treatments in recognition of their status as an elite athlete; this was highest in Finland and Flanders and lowest in Brazil and Northern Ireland (see Figure 47.2).

Nine countries (Australia, Denmark, Finland, Flanders, France, Japan, Switzerland, the Netherlands and Wallonia) operate some kind of nationally coordinated systems for the flexible combination of elite sport activities and secondary education. There are various methods for integrating academic and sporting careers ranging from highly centralized state (i.e. national government) controlled systems to much more informal laisez-faire approaches (De Bosscher *et al.*, in press). There is seemingly no single best approach, as will be explained further.

The discussion on centralization can also be seen in the light of early specialization versus early diversification; whether athletes need to limit their childhood sport participation to a single sport, with a deliberate focus on training and development in that sport or the opposite perspective

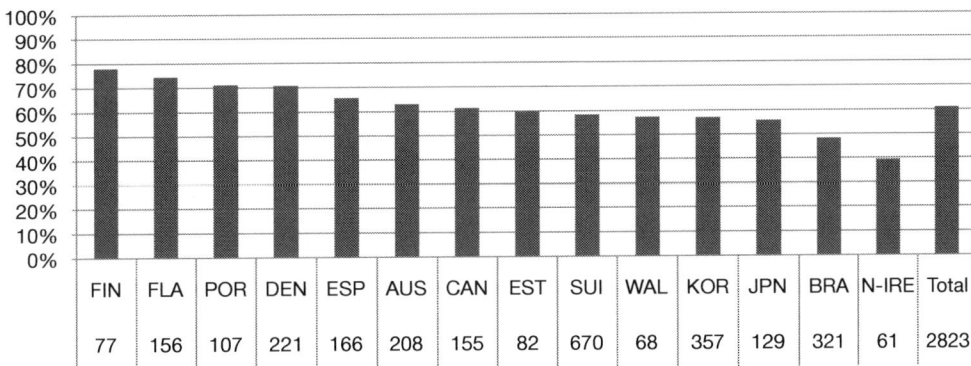

Figure 47.2 Percentage of athletes indicating that their educational establishment offered them any special treatment in recognition of their status as an elite athlete during secondary education (n = 2,823)

that favours a focus on involvement in a number of different sports through which an athlete develops multilateral physical, social and psychological skills, before specializing in later stages of development (Côté *et al.*, 2007; Wiersma, 2000; Baker, 2003). The answer to what is the best system seems to lie in how a central and decentralized approach can be combined. For example while there is a nationally coordinated and centralized training centre (including national agreements with local schools) in Australia, France, and Spain, the system of educating elite athletes is considered to take place away from the central governing body. Similar combined systems also exist in the Netherlands. The survey results also revealed that 68 per cent of the athletes (n = 2603) are satisfied with the support they have received during their secondary education. There seems to be no great desire by athletes to be supported centrally in that regard, a decentralized system based on local agreements seems to work fine for many athletes.

Another matter of debate seems to be the degree of national coordination, the level of state/National Sports Agency (NSA) intervention ranging from a strong hands-on approach to virtual laissez-faire. Since secondary (and primary) education is compulsory in most countries, a national statute can ensure that flexible educational arrangements for athletes do not depend on individual initiatives from athletes, coaches, clubs or NGBs. Aquilina and Henry (2010) provided a typology of four approaches for higher education, which we have applied to secondary education to classify elite sport and study in secondary education in the SPLISS nations. The four levels are:

- In a *state/NSA-centric regulation*, there is a directive towards the schools, to provide flexible opportunities for student-athletes typically via legislation, statutory requirement or government regulation (usually in collaboration with the NSA). For example Flanders and the Netherlands have a national law/covenant in partnership with both the ministry of education and the ministry of sports, and both ministries contribute financially to the system. Entry requirements, curriculum, location, adapted programs are all nationally determined.
- State/NSA as *a sponsor/facilitator* is an approach where by the state promotes formal agreements to ensure that student-athletes' needs are being met, for example through permissive legislation (rather than statutory requirement). The state or NSA plays a less direct interventionist role, enabling rather than regulating responses to the specific needs of the student-athlete (e.g. with regard to entry requirements, flexible timetables, distance learning and scholarships). Denmark, Finland, Portugal, Wallonia, Australia, Switzerland, Spain and France have all been classified under this category.
- *NGBs/institutes as intermediary* is an approach in which there is an established system of recognized channels for sporting advocates (usually NGBs) to act on behalf of the student to negotiate flexible educational provision with schools and where staff may advise and act on behalf of the student-athlete. In this approach, there are no state/NSA regulations and athletes are dependent on their NGBs as a facilitator. Although there exists national funding for elite sport and study in Japan, there is no national regulation, for example, with regard to absence from school.
- In the *Laissez-Faire* approach, there are no formal structures in place and arrangements rely on individually negotiated agreements. Brazil, Northern Ireland and Canada are typical examples of this. In Canada, the educational system is run by the Provincial ministries/departments of Education and directed by the district school boards who decide what flexibilities they provide. There are some individual initiatives, for instance, the National Sport School in Calgary (provincial level), and the Edge School (a private school, with relatively high tuition fees).

State/NSA-centric		NED	FLA
State/NSA as facilitator	DEN, FIN, POR, WAL, SUI	AUS*, ESP*, FRA*	
NGB as intermediary (no state/NSA involvement)		JPN	
Laissez Faire (no formal structures)	BRA, N-IRL, CAN		
	(low)	Centralization	.... (high)

(low) coordination (high)

Note: * the systems in these countries are generally decentralized except from the national training centres

Figure 47.3 Typology of state co-ordination (Aquilina & Henry, 2010) and centralization of elite sport and study systems in secondary education in the SPLISS nations (Adapted from De Bosscher et al., 2015)

The key feature of central coordination concerns the fact that young athletes do not depend on the individual decisions and (lack of) flexibility of their educational institutes to receive support services. This degree of coordination is cross-tabulated against the level of centralization of these elite sport and study systems in Figure 47.3. A high level of centralization is present when young athletes train, live and go to school at one place and when there are a limited number of elite sport schools. A high degree of decentralization is present when young athletes mainly train in their home environment. It seems that countries with a long tradition in having national training centres, such as Australia (The Australian Institute of Sport, AIS) and France (the National Institute of Sport and Physical Education, INSEP), have moved on from centralized provision to a combined centralized and decentralized talent development support system.

Figure 47.4 reveals that most of the countries with a high level of national coordination (state centric/as a facilitator) apply a decentralized approach to the development of elite youth sport and academic study, or a mixed centralized/decentralized approach, which means that central coordination is combined with high flexibility for local negotiation and implementation. Accordingly, these elite sport schools are regionally spread (sports-orientated schools) or normal schools can agree to provide flexible study (status benefits) patterns for young elite athletes who attend them.

Dual career support: combining education and sport in higher (tertiary) education

Since higher (tertiary) education is not compulsory, support at the national level does not require legislation that allows athletes to train during the day. Flexibility to combine sport and study for students-athletes (aged 18 and above) therefore means that the NSA or the state act

	State/NSA-centric	Spain**, Portugal*
(low) coordination (high)	State/NSA as facilitator	France*, Australia*, Denmark*, Finland*, Flanders and Wallonia
	NGB as intermediary	In the countries with *, the NGB makes the arrangements with educational institutions
	Laissez Faire (no formal structures)	Brazil, Canada, Netherlands, Japan, Northern Ireland, Switzerland and countries with **

Figure 47.4 Typology of state/NSA coordination (Aquilina & Henry, 2010) in higher education in the SPLISS nations (Adapted from DeBosscher *et al.*, 2015)

as facilitators to ensure athletes are not dependent on decisions made by individual educational institutes. Individual athletes, their coaches, clubs and preferably NGBs can negotiate on an athlete's behalf. Compared to secondary education, national coordination working towards flexible arrangement has not been a priority and is still in an early stage of development in most countries. The NSA or the state acts as a facilitator in six SPLISS countries (France, Australia, Denmark, Finland, Flanders and Wallonia). Portugal and Spain provide athletes with legal elite athlete status which has associated benefits when studying at universities such as placement quotas for elite athletes (who meet entry criteria), timetable flexibility, permitted absence and access to study mentors. In most nations, the NGBs are the intermediary to organize elite youth sport and study. Many countries reported that the systems for supporting young athletes attending higher education institutions were still based on a laissez faire approach (Brazil, Canada, Japan, the Netherlands, Northern Ireland, Switzerland). In the Netherlands, NOC★NSF provides a list of the services and facilities that universities/high schools offer, but there is no national coordination, legislation or regulation, nor finance to facilitate this. A summary overview from the fifteen SPLISS nations is shown in Figure 47.4.

Conclusion

This chapter examined national level elite youth policies regarding talent development based on the results of the SPLISS 2.0 study involving fifteen nations (De Bosscher *et al.*, 2015). A significant degree of variation was found between the sample nations in relation to the level of national coordination of talent identification and development systems, though higher scores were notable in smaller countries. This may have derived from the fact that in larger countries the coordination of talent identification and development was more complex and expensive to organize. Smaller sized countries have capitalized on their small size competitive advantage in this Pillar over other countries. In relation to elite youth sport and study systems in secondary education, mixed centralized and decentralized systems were observed, which offered nationally centralized training opportunities by adopting an individual approach to the needs of young talents within different sports. In higher education, national coordination is typically less refined in most countries compared to coordination in secondary education, which may lead to a higher than otherwise drop-out rate of student-athletes in higher education. The advantages of centralized and decentralized systems are presented in Table 47.1.

Talent identification and development requires analysis at a sport-specific level as young talented athletes are usually recruited from within the existing participation base of a sport. Once young people have chosen to participate in a sport on a regular basis, NGBs play an important role in ensuring that young talents can be identified and developed. Some recent studies have explored elite sport policies within specific sports (e.g. Andersen and Ronglan, 2012; Böhlke and Robinson, 2009; Brouwers *et al.*, in press; Robinson and Minikin, 2011; Sotiriadou *et al.*, 2013; Truyens *et al.*, 2013). From a sport policy point of view, increased financial pressures within sport organisations and pressure to perform have driven sports teams and organizations to attempt and identify future stars at a very young age. However, the predictive accuracy of early talent detection models would appear inversely related to the length of time over which the prediction is intended to span (Vaeyens *et al.*, 2008). How successful talent can be identified also depends on the type of sport. Sports where one or two variables have a high predictive value for success (e.g. running, sprint) can better apply talent identification systems than multi-skill sports such as tennis or volleyball. Furthermore, the prediction of success is likely to be easier in closed (e.g. throwing a javelin or shooting at a target) rather than open sports (e.g. team sports, tennis) because in closed sports are less affected by the environment and fewer components are likely to impact on performance (Vaeyens *et al.*, 2008). This most likely explains why national federations have invested more resources in closed sport TID models (e.g. rowing, cycling, athletics, canoeing and weightlifting) and are now recruiting potential medal winners at later ages, for example through talent transfer (Bullock *et al.*, 2009) or by identifying sporting giants, such as in the UK. The principles of early specialization (e.g. Côté, Fraser and Thomas, 2007) versus diversification (also known as late specialization) (Wiersma (2000), and deliberate practice (Ericsson *et al.*, 1993) need to be thought about carefully before being written into elite sport policy and high performance sport management. A too narrow approach to elite youth sport development and the pitfalls of identifying talent too early may lead to increased drop-out among young elite athletes. In this regard, some researchers have emphasized the

Table 47.1 Advantages of centralised versus decentralised systems for training and study (De Bosscher & De Croock, 2010)

Advantages of decentralised systems	Advantages of centralised systems
• Athletes sleep in their home environment, train with club coach • Avoid early drop out and burnout • Investment in a broader talent development pyramid with potential for more athletes • More individual approach to athletes' development • Motivation of sports clubs to be involved in athletic performance development; room for local implementation and approach of sport development	• Athletes live, study and train in one place • Cheaper cost per athlete; efficient inputs • Allows more 'all inclusive' services • Time efficiency (e.g., less travelling time) • 'better athletes make athletes better': higher training level • Centralisation of expertise: best coaches, sport science and sport medicine support • Quality services for talent development in sport clubs are often under developed

importance of deliberate play (maximizing fun, intrinsic motivation and enjoyment) and adapting sport rules to accommodate this. This will contribute to decreasing drop-out (from sport in general and from young talents in particular), reduce injuries and improve sustainable sport participation, personal development and learning (e.g. Baker and Cobley, 2013; Côté, 1999; Vaeyens *et al.*, 2008; Wiersma, 2008). While this new sport science continues to evolve and gain momentum with elite sport coaches, there is a paucity of information in elite sport policy and talent programme literature. Programmes sometimes over-emphasize immediate performance, often because of key performance indicators set by funding agencies (such as government) that fail to consider sufficiently the longer-term effects of performance on athletic development within a sport. While our research shows there is no evidence for talent development as a prerequisite for success in elite sport, two issues are brought to light. First, it could be assumed that for short-term goals Pillar 4 is not a priority Pillar in terms of effectiveness, but in the longer term it may provide a competitive advantage by delivering more athletes on the podium more frequently and consistently. Second, as mainly smaller nations have better scores on Pillar 4, this is an area for development and future increased competitiveness in larger nations. To that end it can be argued that Pillar 4 (talent identification and development) offers great scope for development across most nations. Nations that invest strategically may work towards (short- or maybe even long-term) competitive advantage, which maximizes the future success of all athletes.

References

Andersen, S. S. and Ronglan, L. T. (2012). *Nordic Elite Sport: Same Ambitions, Different Tracks*: Copenhagen Business School Press.

Aquilina, D. and Henry, I. (2010). Elite athletes and university education in Europe: A review of policy and practice in higher education in the European Union Member States. *International Journal of Sport Policy*, 2(1), 25–47.

Augestad, P. and Bergsgard, N. A. (2008). Chapter 8 – Norway. In B. Houlihan and M. Green (eds), *Comparative Elite Sport Development* (pp. 194–217). Oxford: Butterworth-Heinemann.

Baker, J. (2003). Early specialization in youth sport: A requirement for adult expertise? *High Ability Studies*, 14(1), 85–94.

Baker, J. and Cobley, S. (2013). Outliers, talent codes, and myths: play and practice in developing the expert athlete. In D. Farrow, J. Baker and C. MacMahon (eds), *Developing sport exercise: Researchers and coaches put theory into practice*. New York: Routledge.

Balyi, I. and Hamilton, A. (2004). *Long term athlete development: Trainability in childhood and adolescence*. Victoria: National Coaching Institute British Columbia and Advanced Training and Performance ltd.

Bloom, B. (1985). *Developing talent in young people*. New York: Ballantine

Böhlke, N. and Robinson, L. (2009). Benchmarking of élite sport systems. *Management Decision*, 47(1), 67–84.

Brouwers, Sotiriadou, De Bosscher (in press). Sport specific policies and factors that influence international success: The case of tennis. *Sport Management Review* (accepted).

Bullock, N. Gulbin, J.P., Martin, D.T, Ross, A., Holland, T. and Marino, F. (2009). Talent identification and deliberate programming in skeleton: Ice novice to Winter Olympian in 14 months, *Journal of Sports Sciences*, 27(4), 397–404.

Côté, J. (1999). The influence of the family in the development of talent in sport. *Sport Psychologist*, 13(4), 395.

Côté, J. and Fraser-Thomas, J. (2007). Play, practice, and athlete development. In D. Farrow, J. Baker and C. MacMahon (eds), *Developing sport exercise: Researchers and coaches put theory into practice*. New York: Routledge.

De Bosscher, V. and De Croock, S. (2010). *Effectiviteit van de Topsportscholen in Vlaanderen [Effectiveness of the elite sport schools in Flanders]*. Research report for the department CJSM, Flemish government. Brussel: Vrije Universiteit Brussel.

De Bosscher, V., De Knop, P. and van Bottenburg, M. (2009). An analysis of homogeneity and heterogeneity of elite sports systems in six nations. *International journal of sports marketing and sponsorship*, *10*(2), 111–131.

De Bosscher, V., De Knop, P., van Bottenburg, M. and Shibli, S. (2006). A Conceptual Framework for Analysing Sports Policy Factors Leading to International Sporting Success. *European Sport Management Quarterly*, *6*(2), 185–215.

De Bosscher, D., Shibli, S., Westerbeek, H. and van Bottenburg, M. (2015). *Successful elite sport policies. An international comparison of the Sports Policy factors Leading to International Sporting Success (SPLISS 2.0).* Aachen: Meyer and Meyer.

De Knop, P., Wylleman, P., Van Hoecke, J. and Bollaert, L. (1999). Sports management – A European approach to the management of the combination of academics and elite-level sport. In S. Bailey (ed), *Perspectives – The interdisciplinary series of physical education and sport science. Vol. 1 School sport and competition* (pp. 49–62). Oxford: Meyer and Meyer Sport.

De Pelsmacker, P. and Van Kenhove, P. (1999). *Marktonderzoek: methoden en toepassingen [Market research: methods and applications]* (3rd edition). Leuven Apeldoorn, BE: Garant.

Digel, H., Burk, V. and Fahrner, M. (2006). *High-performance sport. An international comparison* (Vol. 9). Weilheim/Teck, Tubingen: Bräuer.

Elferink-Gemser, M. Visscher, C., Lemmink, K. and Mulder, T. (2004). Relation between multi-dimensional performance characteristics and level of performance in talented youth field hockey players. *Journal of Sports Sciences*, *22*(11–12), 1053–1063.

Ericsson, K. A. (2003). Development of elite performance and deliberate practice: An update from the perspective of the expert performance approach. In K. Starkes and K. A. Ericsson (eds), *Expert performance in sports: Advances in research on sport expertise* (pp. 49–85). Champaign, Illinois: Human Kinetics.

European Commission. (2007). *White Paper: White Paper on Sport.* Brussels: European Commission Retrieved from www.publications.parliament.uk/pa/cm200708/cmselect/cmcumeds/347/347.pdf.

Green, M. and Houlihan, B. (2005). *Elite Sport Development. Policy learning and political priorities.* New York: Routledge.

Gulbin, J.P. (2011). Applying talent identification programs at a system wide level: the evolution of Australia's national program. In Baker, J., Cobley, S. and Schorer, J. (eds), *Talent Identification and Development in Sport: International Perspectives* (pp 147–165), London, Routledge.

Gullich, A., Emrich, E., Espwall, S., Olyslager, M., Parker, R. and Rus, V. (2004). *Cooperation between elite sport and education in Europe.* Brussels: European Commission.

Houlihan, B. and Green, M. (2008). *Comparative Elite Sport Development. Systems, structures and public policy.* London, UK: Elsevier.

Oakley, B. and Green, M. (2001). The production of Olympic champions: International perspectives on elite sport development system. *European Journal for Sport Management*, *8*, 83–105.

Radtke, S. and Coalter, F. (Producer). (2007, 28/11/2010). Sports schools: An international review. Retrieved from www.dualcareer.eu/media/ccpages/2012/11/12/Elite_Sports_Schools_by_Dr._Sabine_Radtke.pdf

Rowe (1994). *Talentdetectie in basketbal [Talent detection in basketball].* Unpublished doctoral dissertation, Catholic University of Leuven, BE.Ericsson, K., Krampe, R. and Tesch-Römer, C. (1993). The role of deliberate practice in the acquisition of espert performance. *Psychological Review*, 100, 363–406.

Sandelowski, M., Voils, C. and Knafl, G. (2009). On quantitizing. *Journal of Mixed Method Research*, *3*, 208–222.

Simon, H. and Chase, W. (1973). Skill in chess. *American Scientist*, *61*, 394–403.

Sotiriadou, P., Gowthorp, L. and De Bosscher, V. (2013). Elite sport culture and policy interrelationships: the case of Sprint Canoe in Australia. *Leisure Studies*, *33*(6), 598–617.

Truyens, J. De Bosscher, V., Heyndels, B. and Westerbeek, H. (2013). A resource-based perspective on countries' competitive advantage in elite athletics. *International Journal of Sport Policy and Politics*, *6*(3), 459–489.

Vaeyens, R., Lenoir, M., Williams, A. M. and Philippaerts, R. (2008). Talent identification and development programmes in sport: Current models and future directions. *Sports Medicine*, *38*(9), 703–714.

van Bottenburg, M. (2009). *Op jacht naar goud. Het topsportklimaat in Nederland, 1998–2008. [the hunt for gold. The elite sport climate in the Netherlands, 1998–2008].* Niewegein, Netherlands: Arko Sports Media.

Wiersma, L. D. (2000). Risks and benefits of youth sport specialization: perspectives and recommendations. *Pediatric exercise science*, *12(1)*, 13–22.

Wylleman, P. and Lavallee, D. (2004). A developmental perspective on transitions faced by athletes. In M. Weiss (ed), *Developmental sport and exercise psychology: A lifespan perspective* (pp. 507–527). Morgantown, WV: Fitness Information Technology.

Wylleman, P., Alfermann, D. and Lavallee, D. (2004). Career transitions in sport: European perspectives. *Psychology of Sport and Exercise*, *5*(1), 7–20.

48

YOUTH SPORT POLICY IN SMALL NATIONS

Michael Sam

Introduction

To begin, it is worth putting the concept of 'small nations' in perspective. For example, according to recent estimates, China has 400 million basketball participants (Sport in China, 2014). Even if this is an overestimation, it provides a significant contrast to observations that 60 per cent of the world's nations have populations of less than 10 million and 48 per cent of nations have less than 5 million inhabitants. When it comes to sport, size matters, hence differences in scale have been a frequent independent variable in studies examining elite sport success (De Bosscher *et al.*, 2008). Generating explanations regarding how and why size matters for elite youth sport raises questions regarding the possible differences, challenges and opportunities of being a small nation.

In this chapter, I want to demonstrate the importance of scale in the development of policies and programmes around youth sport. I first outline the case for studying small states and consider the key characteristics that might distinguish small states from large ones, focusing in particular on the conceptual dimensions of vulnerability and resilience. I follow this with a reading of what these characteristics mean for youth sport development. In particular, I discuss whether the development of international sport for youth might have a proportionately larger impact on small states' sport systems. At the same time, it is suggested that youth in small states may have wider opportunities for international competition and its benefits (travel, cultural exchange, etc.). Following a review of relevant sport studies, the chapter concludes by suggesting that the importance of these works lies with the distinctive 'ecologies' of small states.

What is a small nation?

The identification of small states is problematic given the myriad of ways size can be expressed (Thorhallsson and Wivel, 2006). Size is contested in theory and practice but for comparative purposes, three dimensions are relevant. The first is population and as one might expect there are a number of proposed cut-off points, ranging from 1 million to 20 million (Tõnurist, 2010). In studies of Commonwealth countries, the threshold for small is set at under 1.5 million, a figure also generally accepted as the approximate cut-off for what are referred to as micro states. The threshold for smallness thus generally depends on the interest of the academic field itself

(Tõnurist, 2010). In some European studies, for example, smallness as a function of population has been arbitrarily set in relation to the Netherlands (i.e. approximately 16 million) because of the wide gap between it and the next largest nation, Poland (pop. 38 million) (Thorhallsson, 2006). Sam and Jackson's (forthcoming) collection on 'sport policy in small nations' uses an arbitrary population of under 10 million, a relatively high threshold in part because of the dearth of research scholarship on sport in states under 5 million. A second related dimension is geographical size, where small states are generally understood to have small land areas. Island states like Fiji and Samoa in the South Pacific, or Mauritius and Malta would fit this description. Here again, however, the size of a nation is relative; some states such as Mongolia (pop. 2.8 million) or Namibia (pop. 2.3 million) can have large land areas and therefore very low population densities. Ultimately, in light of the imprecise nature of definitions and thresholds, it has become accepted that smallness is best viewed as lying upon a continuum (Sutton, 2011; Tõnurist, 2010).

A third, more commonly used dimension in relation to small state studies is the size of a nation's economy. This dimension is usually with reference to a state's Gross Domestic Product (GDP), narrow base for trade (e.g. agriculture or tourism), small domestic market, comparative expenditures on defence, health, etc. Economic scale could be said to affect many facets of youth sport. A smaller tax base means less revenue that can be used for the provision of sport and recreation facilities. A narrower economic base also translates into a fewer number of large companies that can limit the pool of potential corporate sponsors. Furthermore, given their limited economic power and lack of influence, small states are 'price takers' (Tõnurist, 2010) and this fact has great relevance in the world of international professional sport. Larger markets typically command larger athlete salaries, pressuring small states to either meet expectations in their own domestic competitions and/or institute a range of policies discouraging player migration. The New Zealand Rugby Union, for example, has tried to discourage outward migration by negating a player's eligibility to play for the national team should they take up contracts in other leagues. For its part however, NZ welcomes the migration of Samoan, Tongan and Fijian rugby players into its national ranks, contributing to the depletion of human capital in those comparatively smaller Pacific nations (Grainger, 2009; Kanemasu and Molnar, 2013).

Insofar as broadcasting revenue depends on the size of audiences, small states arguably have less control over the makeup of leagues or the timing of major events (e.g., Kanemasu and Molnar, 2013). More significantly perhaps is that with the exception of Qatar and the United Emirates, small nations are susceptible to the inflationary financial pressures around the hosting of events, rendering these beyond reach or causing the governments of small states to engage in a race to the bottom (i.e. making commitments that can be ill-afforded in order to win the bid).

Taken together, a country's vulnerability is what sets small nations apart. For reasons of geography and economy they are prone to economic shocks, and heavily constrained in their development by global forces beyond their control (Neumann and Gstöhl, 2004). Globalization is therefore an important theoretical dimension in relation to small states, as one of its key themes surrounds the vulnerability of the local in relation to the global. The fall of oil prices in the 1980s for instance resulted in a sharp economic downturn for Trinidad and Tobago, resulting in delayed social programmes (including sport) that would not be revisited until the late 1990s when commodity prices began to rise again (McCree, 2009). Perhaps one the most direct pressures in relation to this handbook comes from the emergence of a global youth sport agenda, associated with the growth of age-group International Federation competitions (Under 18s, Under 16s) and the Youth Olympic Games (YOG).

The impact of the YOG on small states should not be underestimated for the simple reason that the policies and strategies enabling the preparation of youth at that level may have profound effects at subsequent levels. Certainly the increased financial investment required to broaden elite sport support to youth is the most obvious implication. But the increasing importance accorded to elite sport could also arguably translate into an attendant demand for earlier specialization. Indeed central agencies, national sport federations and regional bodies all support junior development programmes in earnest as proof of their adherence to whole-of-sport planning and talent identification pathways (Bloyce and Smith, 2010). More practices/trainings per week and longer seasons (owing to off-season development camps) may have significant flow-on effects in small nations. If sports require a growing commitment from youth, it may translate into them playing a fewer number of different sports. With their already small economies of scale, small states thus face the prospect of organizations trying to recruit at younger and younger age groups in order to capture their markets. The view that it may be too late to take up a new sport at the age of say, 12-years old, may become more common as a result, doing little to encourage adolescent sport-for-all objectives.

Another likely scenario is that the performances of youth athletes will become closely monitored by existing government sport agencies, effectively becoming markers of a sustainable system. The tendency for markers (or indicators) to become the targets over time (Bevan and Hood, 2006), means that the YOG will potentially generate a new elite sport political economy focused on youth. While speculative, these scenarios point to two important considerations in small state research. The first is with respect to the ways in which small states cope with vulnerability while the second is in relation to the persistent tensions that command attention in a small state.

Small states and resilience

Where vulnerability emerged as the bridging concept in identifying small nations, scholars sought to move away from pessimistic views of 'small as weak' that typified international relations literature. *Resilience* has since become an important part of the lexicon in small state studies. Katzenstein's (1985) proposition in this regard is that through their experience of vulnerability at particular historical junctures (e.g. Great Depression, World War I), small states have developed political capacities to respond successfully. The adaptive effects of smallness thus include:

1   the establishment of corporatist institutions (i.e. government partnership with selected interest groups);
2   the development of policies aimed at social integration (e.g. language policy);
3   the coordination of responses to public problems.

Echoing these ideas, others point out that the resilience of small nations lies with their capacities for social partnership, cooperation and sacrifice (Campbell and Hall, 2009; Lowenthal, 1987).

In reflecting on his own seminal book *Small States in World Markets* (1985), Peter Katzenstein (2003: 11) remarked that the most 'important explanatory variable' 20 years later was that:

> Small size was a code for something more important . . . What really mattered politically was the perception of vulnerability, economic and otherwise. Perceived vulnerability generated an ideology of social partnership that had acted like glue for the corporatist politics of the small European states.
>
> *(Peter Katzenstein, 2003: 11)*

The possibility of closer personal ties is thus what sets small nations apart. More trusting relationships and repeated interactions act as a means to supplant stricter principal–agent relations.

Put another way, the development of social capital serves to remove the distrust in impersonal contacts. Indeed, it would be difficult to challenge the notion that small nations are also small societies (Benedict, 1967) with highly personalised role relationships (Farrugia, 1993) that can provide a capacity for resilience. And in light of the above, it is not surprising that small states should pursue sport as a means of inducing social integration and national unity.

In one of the few comparative studies focusing on small states, Girginov *et al.* (2006) explored the cultural orientations of sport managers in Malta, Cyprus, Iceland, Luxembourg, San Marino, Monaco and Liechtenstein. While the sample of individuals was small (n=fifteen managers), the research acknowledged the cultural differences in how administrators deal with dilemmas. Germane to the present subject is the observation that these managers considered it normal to reconcile tensions and conflicts, as against the general tendency of western sport management to want to seek more definitive resolutions.

One explanation is that people in small states are accustomed to compromise, reflecting Lowenthal's (1987: 39) thesis of a 'managed intimacy', where:

> Small-state inhabitants learn to get along, like it or not, with folk they will know in myriad contexts over their whole lives. To enable the social mechanism to function without undue stress, they minimise or mitigate overt conflict. They become expert at muting hostility, deferring their own views, containing disagreement, avoiding dispute, in the interest of stability and compromise.

This is not to suggest that the sport sectors of small states would lack detractors but rather that small size perhaps necessitates 'sophisticated modes of accommodation' (Lowenthal, 1987: 39).

Cases, contradictions and tensions

If fewer 'degrees of separation' and close ties provide a source of resilience, a significant counter-balance has been the transformation of small states to align with neoliberal institutions. Indeed one important source of transformation for small states has been the role of international or supra-national organisations such as the International Monetary Fund (IMF), World Bank and European Union. Given the legitimacy of these agencies and the interest they have in small states, it is not surprising that their prescriptions should influence domestic policies including those related to sport (e.g., Girginov and Sandanski, 2008; McCree, 2009).

One prescription or strategy concerns the need for small states to specialise, to consolidate and target specific industries (Bray, 1991; Sarapuu, 2010). Smallness and the comparative resource scarcity that goes with it, thus invites consolidation, the narrowing of objectives, targeting and rationing. Hence in their wider economies, small states may choose to focus their investments in technology, agriculture or tourism (Browning, 2006). Contemporary investment in sport falls under similar logic. The tendency to consolidate efforts around particular sports appears to be evident in both small and large nations – China, for example, has identified nine superior sports (about the same number as New Zealand's targeted or priority sports). However it is doubtful that the narrowing of priorities in a large country distorts their sporting systems to the same degree.

In states like Singapore (pop. 5.4 million), New Zealand (pop. 4.3 million) and Finland (pop. 5.3 million), the doctrines of New Public Management (NPM) have been pursued with substantive effects on the organization of sport. The governments of these countries have sought to achieve greater alignment between sport and business practices, while demonstrating a preference for using contracts and their associated targets, benchmarks and performance-based budgeting (cf. Collins, 2011; Sam, 2012; Teo, 2011). Insofar as these strategies are largely premised on distrust, small nations may struggle to reconcile the ideals of social partnerships with the contemporary emphasis on accountability. Neoliberal doctrines thus present small nations with a paradox: scale invites consolidation, targeting and rationing, while also invoking strategies to break the very communal bonds that provide them with the fertile conditions for growth and competitive advantage.

This paradox is certainly not a trajectory that states are compelled to follow. While New Zealand's standing as the model neoliberal reformer has encouraged the development of a centralised system for elite sport (Sam, forthcoming), Nordic countries have by design maintained the autonomy of their sport organizations. Indeed, according to Koski (forthcoming), Finland has eschewed the targeting of particular sports. Norway's system has maintained a similar outlook, owing to the legitimacy of its traditional grassroots system and the representative structures of its umbrella organization, the Norwegian Sports Federation (Ronglan, forthcoming). Clearly, then, the paradox between neoliberal reforms and small societies does not play out the same way, but it remains a recognisable tension and one in need of further analysis.

Common themes in small state sports research

Perhaps the most common theme around small state sport is in regards to how sport is portrayed in the national psyche. Bairner's (1996) analysis of Sweden, Scotland and the Republic of Ireland is instructive in this regard, suggesting that the construction of 'sporting nationalisms' is shaped by dimensions of homogeneity and by the relative historical significance of national identity. In the Finnish context, Koski (forthcoming) maintains that sport strengthened national pride during that country's path to independence. Likewise, rugby's importance to the development of national identity is well documented in New Zealand (Scherer and Jackson, 2010) as well as Fiji (Kanemasu and Molnar, 2013). The contemporary use of sport as a means of projecting national identity is also an emerging theme, particularly in relation to the pursuit of events hosting by small (but economically successful) nations such as Singapore (Fry and McNeill, 2011) and Arab nations Bahrain, Qatar and United Emirates.

Another common theme in the narratives of small nation sport relates to issues around migration. Two broad storylines appear in this regard. The first tells of the tendency for athletes (especially young athletes) to leave their small home nations in search of more lucrative opportunities, producing a kind of brawn drain. McGovern (2000), for example, documents the departure of Irish footballers to English Premier League clubs, suggesting that this contributes to football's underdevelopment in the Republic. The second storyline surrounds the initiatives of small states to develop their sporting capacities by effectively purchasing talent from abroad. Qatar has been the most forthright in this practice, having for instance purchased an entire weightlifting team from Bulgaria in the late 1990s (Girginov and Sandanski, 2008) and nationalising a Kenyan steeplechase runner in 2003 to boost the country's standing in athletics (Hunter, 2003). To the extent that other nations (e.g. New Zealand) encourage this kind of re-settlement through special immigration categories (Chang et al., forthcoming), we see that sporting talent is an increasingly valued skillset and one that small states may be keen to attract. However, against the migratory patterns of elite athletes, coaches and technical directors, it is nevertheless possible that youth sport may become an area of activity that is increasingly nationalistic. Home-grown talent may become more valued than imported talent or talent principally nurtured and developed in larger overseas hot houses (e.g. U.S. colleges).

Yet another important theme is with respect to how small states attempt to coordinate the competing demands around sport. The tension between sport-for-all and elite sport is ubiquitous but it is notably more muted in Nordic countries characterised by strong member associations, links with workers' organizations and a longstanding public perception of sport as a social movement (Ronglan, forthcoming). However, the lack of a critical mass of athletes to provide high-level competition also features as problematic in small nations. Reflecting this concern, a common issue raised in small state research relates to the coordination between the education and sport sectors. In the context of Barbuda and Antigua, for example, Darko and Mackintosh (2014) point to the persistent compartmentalization between physical education and sport, between levels of education and between layers of government. Paradoxically and speaking to the hegemony of sport, the authors observe that despite the unimportance accorded to physical education, the nation still has a national sport policy. In Sweden, the sport movement has begun to influence physical education in schools not simply by advancing sport's importance and status, but by becoming a primary supplier, offering coaches and programmes in the curriculum (Ferry *et al.*, 2013). The growing tendency for outsourcing physical education to sport specialists is a trend in Singapore and New Zealand as well (Fry and McNeill, 2011; Pope, 2002) with the emergence of sport-specific boarding schools and academies in those countries further reflecting sport's importance in the market reforms of education sectors. Taken together, the tensions and coordination challenges between education and sport sectors (even in small states) point to the possibility that the schism is not easily reconciled.

If the combination of scale and neoliberalism potentially results in unwanted distortions, it is important to acknowledge that, at an individual level, there may be advantages for young athletes in small states. One advantage is that it is perhaps more likely that they will have the opportunity to compete internationally. In some cases this may be through intentional government design; Namibia's Ministry of Youth, for example, has actively pursued international junior programmes in a number of sports (Chappell, 2005). But even anecdotally, one could speculate that there is something significant in being the big fish in a small pond. In a developed state like New Zealand, there are national representatives in many sports, from the major sports (such as cricket, rugby, netball and football) to comparatively minor sports (such as ice hockey and volleyball) and everything in between. Insofar as a country such as this maintains a wide gamut of sports, the chances of rising to the top would seem to be proportionately greater than they would be otherwise. While it would be difficult to determine the statistical chances of being a national representative, the intuitive assumption is a dimension worth exploring. Indeed, is the wider range of possibilities to be a big fish a help or hindrance with respect to participation patterns? What is the impact on youth sport when role models are so accessible and characterized by only two degrees of separation?

Conclusion

Though what defines a small state is fairly fluid, it is generally agreed that scale matters. How and why it matters, however, depends on the interplay between population size, geography, political economy and the subject area under analysis. Indeed, a small state's sources of vulnerability and resilience in relation to sport are as context-specific as they might be in relation to agriculture or international security. Though there is immense variation among and between small states, it is probable that internationalized youth sport would yield distinctive responses compared to global superpowers, owing to the former's limited human and financial resources, close personal ties and frameworks of legitimacy.

In contrast to this view are predictions around isomorphism, stipulating the pressure/tendency for organizations to resemble one another over time (Powell and DiMaggio, 2012). One proposition in this regard is that small states would tend to mimic larger states because they are perceived to be successful. McCree's (2009) study of sport policy in the Caribbean, for example, notes that that Trinidad and Tobago's policy was formulated using the Australian sport policy as a model, while Sam (2003; forthcoming) documented similar discourses in New Zealand's comparisons with Australia and the United Kingdom. Yet, the ways in which small states enact such modelling or mimicking must necessarily take place in an environment marked by each state's responses to global pressures, by the domestic realities of having limited resources, and by its close-knit networks of accountability. In this light, an attention towards small states may help scholars and policy makers to better understand the significance of having fewer degrees of separation and the implications this has for youth sport.

Acknowledgment

I would like to acknowledge Professor Steven J. Jackson for his useful insight into an earlier draft of this chapter and for his contribution as co-editor for the special issue on which this chapter is based.

References

Bairner, A. (1996). Sportive nationalism and nationalist politics: A comparative analysis of Scotland, the Republic of Ireland, and Sweden. *Journal of Sport and Social Issues*, *20*(3), 314–334.

Benedict, B. (1967). Sociological aspects of smallness. In B. Benedict (ed), *Problems of smaller territories* (pp. 45–55). London: University of London/Athlone Press.

Bevan, G. and Hood, C. (2006). What's measured is what matters: Targets and gaming in the English public health care system. *Public Administration*, *84*(3), 517–538.

Bloyce, D. and Smith, A. (2010). *Sport policy and development: An introduction*. London: Routledge.

Bray, M. (1991). *Making small practical: the organisation and management of ministries of eduction in small states*. London: Commonwealth Secretariat.

Briguglio, L., Cordina, G., Farrugia, N. and Vella, S. (2009). Economic vulnerability and resilience: concepts and measurements. *Oxford Development Studies*, *37*(3), 229–247.

Bromber, K. and Krawietz, B. (2013). The United Emirates, Qatar, and Bahrain as a modern sport hub. In K. Bromber, B. Krawietz and J. Maguire (eds), *Sport across Asia: Politics, cultures and identities* (pp. 189–212). New York: Routledge.

Browning, C. S. (2006). Small, smart and salient? Rethinking identity in the small states literature. *Cambridge Review of International Affairs*, *19*(4), 669–684.

Campbell, J. L. and Hall, J. A. (2009). National identity and the political economy of small states. *Review of International Political Economy*, *16*(4), 547–572.

Chappell, R. (2005). Sport in Namibia: conflicts, negotiations and struggles since independence. *International Review for the Sociology of Sport*, *40*(2), 241–254.

Collins, S. (2011). Finland. In M. Nicholson, R. Hoye and B. Houlihan (eds), *Participation in sport: International perspectives* (pp. 109–125). New York: Routledge.

Darko, N. and Mackintosh, C. (2014). Challenges and constraints in developing and implementing sports policy and provision in Antigua and Barbuda: which way now for a small island state? *International Journal of Sport Policy and Politics*, DOI:10.1080/19406940.2014.925955.

De Bosscher, V., Bingham, J., Shibli, S., van Bottenburg, M. and De Knop, P. (2008). *The global sporting arms race: An international comparative study on sports policy factors leading to international sporting success*. Aachen: Meyer and Meyer Verlag.

Farrugia, C. (1993). The special working environment of senior administrators in small states. *World Development*, *21*(2), 221–226.

Ferry, M., Meckbach, J. and Larsson, H. (2013). School sport in Sweden: what is it, and how did it come to be? *Sport in Society*, *16*(6), 805–818.

Fry, J. M. and McNeill, M. C. (2011). 'In the Nation's good': Physical education and school sport in Singapore. *European Physical Education Review, 17*(3), 287–300.

Girginov, V., Papadimitriou, D. and López De D'Amico, R. (2006). Cultural orientations of sport managers. *European Sport Management Quarterly, 6*(1), 35–66.

Girginov, V. and Sandanski, I. (2008). Understanding the changing nature of sports organisations in transforming societies. *Sport Management Review, 11*(1), 21–50.

Grainger, A. (2009). Rugby, Pacific peoples, and the cultural politics of national identity in New Zealand. *The International Journal of the History of Sport, 26*(16), 2335–2357.

Henry, I. P., Amara, M. and Al-Tauqi, M. (2003). Sport, arab nationalism and the Pan-Arab games. *International Review for the Sociology of Sport, 38*(3), 295–310.

Hunter, J. (2003). Flying the flag: Identities, the nation, and sport. *Identities: Global Studies in Culture and Power, 10*(4), 409–425.

Kanemasu, Y. and Molnar, G. (2013). Collective identity and contested allegiance: a case of migrant professional Fijian rugby players. *Sport in Society, 16*(7), 863–882.

Katzenstein, P. J. (1985). *Small states in world markets: Industrial policy in Europe*: Cornell University Press.

Katzenstein, P. J. (2003). Small states and small states revisited. *New Political Economy, 8*(1), 9–30.

Koski, P. (forthcoming). A David in the global Goliath's sporting arena: Finland as a small sports nation. *International Journal of Sport Policy and Politics*.

Lowenthal, D. (1987). Social features. In C. Clarke and T. Payne (eds), *Politics, security and development in small states* (pp. 26–49). London: Allen and Unwin.

McCree, R. (2009). Sport Policy and the New Public Management in the Caribbean: Convergence or resurgence? *Public Management Review, 11*(4), 461–476.

McGovern, P. (2000). The Irish brawn drain: English League clubs and Irish footballers, 1946–19951. *The British Journal of Sociology, 51*(3), 401–418.

Neumann, I. B. and Gstöhl, S. (2004). *Lilliputians in Gulliver's world? Small states in international relations*: University of Iceland.

Pope, C. C. (2002). Plato makes the team: the arrival of secondary school sport academies. *Waikato Journal of Education, 8*, 89–100.

Powell, W. W. and DiMaggio, P. J. (2012). *The new institutionalism in organizational analysis*: University of Chicago Press.

Ronglan, L-T. (forthcoming). Elite sport in Scandinavian welfare states: Legitimacy under pressure? *International Journal of Sport Policy and Politics*.

Sam, M. P. (2003). What's the big idea? Reading the rhetoric of a national sport policy process. *Sociology of Sport Journal, 20*(3), 189–213.

Sam, M. P. (2012). Targeted investments in elite sport funding: Wiser, more innovative and strategic? *Managing Leisure, 17*(2), 206–219.

Sam, M. P. (forthcoming). Small state vulnerability and resilience: The case of New Zealand sport. *International Journal of Sport Policy and Politics*.

Sarapuu, K. (2010). Comparative Analysis of State Administrations: The size of State as an independent variable. *Administrative Culture*(11–1), 30–43.

Scherer, J. and Jackson, S. J. (2010). *Globalization, sport and corporate nationalism: The new cultural economy of the New Zealand All Blacks*. Oxford: Peter Lang.

Sport in China. (2014). Retrieved 3 November, 2014, from http://en.wikipedia.org/wiki/Sport_in_China

Sutton, P. (2011). The concept of small states in the international political economy. *The Round Table, 100*(413), 141–153.

Teo, L. (2011). Singapore. In M. Nicholson, R. Hoye and B. Houlihan (eds), *Participation in sport: International perspectives* (pp. 183–208). New York: Routledge.

Thorhallsson, B. (2006). The size of states in the European Union: Theoretical and conceptual perspectives. *European Integration, 28*(1), 7–31.

Thorhallsson, B. and Wivel, A. (2006). Small states in the European Union: what do we know and what would we like to know? *Cambridge Review of International Affairs, 19*(4), 651–668.

Tõnurist, P. (2010). What is a "small state" in a globalizing economy. *Halduskultuur – Administrative Culture, 11*(1), 8–29.

49

YOUTH AND SPORT-FOR-CHANGE PROGRAMMES

What can you expect?

Fred Coalter

Introduction

This chapter examines the effectiveness of sports-based interventions that address issues of gang membership, racism, at-risk youth and a rather ill-defined notion of conflict. The chapter illustrates the varying centrality of sport in such programmes, and explores participants' experiences and perceptions of the programme elements that had the greatest impact on their values, attitudes and behaviour. The chapter draws on theories of change about how such programmes might work and emphasises the centrality of social relationships between leaders and participants and the development of respect, trust and reciprocity as a basis for potential changes in values, attitudes and behaviour.

Sufficient conditions and their commonality

The most consistent rationales underpinning public investment in sport have been based on the supposed ability of sport to teach lessons for life, to contribute to character building and to develop self-discipline and positive moral reasoning (President's Council on Physical Fitness and Sports, 2006). Sport has also consistently been promoted as having potential to contribute to crime prevention, to promote social inclusion and contribute to development (Coalter, 2007; Collins and Kay, 2014; Nichols, 2007).

However, there are several unresolved issues with interventions that are premised on these supposed benefits of sport participation. First, evidence of their effectiveness is limited – either because robust and comparable monitoring and evaluation has not been undertaken consistently (Coalter, 2007; Coakley, 2011; West and Crompton, 2001) or there are major methodological difficulties in measuring the impact of programmes on participants (Coalter, 2007; Hartmann and Kwauk, 2011; Nichols, 2007; Nichols and Crow, 2004; Taylor, 1999). Second, sport is a summative term that conceals more than it reveals. For example, the President's Council on Physical Fitness and Sports (2006) referred to the unhelpful nature of generalisations about 'sports' because of varying rule structures, different types of social interaction, different developmental stimuli, varying subcultures and implicit moral norms and the possibility that the experience of participants in the same programme varies substantially.

Third is the distinction between necessary and *sufficient* conditions and it is this issue that is the focus of this chapter. Clearly, participation is a necessary condition to obtain any of the benefits supposedly associated with sport. However, because such potential impacts are only a possibility (Svoboda, 1994) there is a need to consider *sufficient conditions*, that is, the conditions under which the potential impacts might be achieved (Patriksson, 1995). This is reflected is an emerging body of literature which takes Coakley's (1998: 2) lead in viewing 'sports as *sites* for socialisation experiences, not *causes* of socialisation outcomes'. Further, Hartmann (2003: 134) argues that 'the success of any sports-based social intervention program is largely determined by the strength of its non-sport components'.

Such comments indicate that, while sport might provide the context for positive experiences, the social *process* of participation is the key to understanding what is happening. For example, Fox (2000) emphasises the importance of 'attractiveness' factors in encouraging individuals to remain in programmes – for example, the qualities of the leader, the exercise setting and relationships with other participants – and these cannot be separated from the physical components of programmes in promoting self-esteem. Sandford *et al.* (2006: 262), in a review of research on the role of physical education programmes in re-engaging 'disaffected youth', note that 'it has been argued that the social relationships experienced during involvement in physical activity programmes are the most significant factor in effecting behavioural change'. Crabbe (2008: 35), on the basis of his evaluations of the United Kingdom (UK) Positive Futures programme, emphasises the need to obtain 'a deeper understanding of the complexities of participants' interactions and the often contradictory and fluid impact of initiatives'.

Such emphases on context, social and learning relationships and active cognition have similarities with social learning theory (Bandura, 1994; Pajares 2002) and its emphasis on participants as active and interpreting agents. Likewise, the realist evaluation approach of Pawson and Tilley (2004) emphasises that social interventions work by enabling participants to make different choices, which reflect their previous experiences, beliefs and attitudes and access to various types of resources. The making and sustaining of different choices requires a change in participants' reasoning (values, beliefs, attitudes, or the logic they apply to a particular situation) and/or the resources (e.g. information, skills, material resources, support) available to them. This combination of 'reasoning and resources' – the programme 'mechanism' – is what enables programme to work. This means that we have to shift analysis and understanding from families of programmes (i.e. sport) to *families of mechanisms* – the processes, experiences and relationships that might achieve desired impacts (Coalter, 2007, 2011). Therefore we need to understand the middle-range mechanisms that programme providers either assume, or try to build into their programmes. The identification of the possible commonalities of such mechanisms across a variety of interventions can assist in the development of, or linking with, broader theoretical and analytical frameworks, providing a more robust and potentially generalisable version of what works, in what circumstances, for whom and why.

From programmes to mechanisms

Tacon (2007) asserts that many sport-for-change projects have much in common with social work practice and the key mechanisms in generic youth work programmes for at-risk youth has been addressed by several researchers (e.g. Gambone and Arbreton, 1997; MacCallum and Beltman, 2002). Witt and Crompton's (1997) widely quoted analysis of the 'protective factors' essential to sports programmes for at-risk youth is derived from this literature. It is based on an examination of the factors in the lives of resilient youth that enable them to avoid the negative consequences of multiple risk environments. The protective factors approach shifts the focus from the risks to which young people are exposed to a concern that 'developing protective factors is central to promoting positive youth development in risk environments' (Witt and Crompton, 1997: 3).

There is broad agreement about the required elements: safe and supportive environments; adult caring role models; the development of a sense of belonging; challenging and interesting activities; opportunities to develop leadership and decision-making skills; and opportunities for volunteering. Further, there is a general agreement that such programmes work via strong relationships between participants and *relevant* role models/mentors (Bandura, 1994; Lyle, 2006), with the most effective programmes being those which develop long-term, supportive and reinforcing relationships. We can also draw on Pawson's (2006) conclusions from a realist review of published research on youth mentoring programmes for at-risk youth. He identifies four broad stages through which the mentor/mentee relationship proceeds:

- Befriending. Creating bonds of trust.
- Direction-setting. Promoting self-reflection and the reconsideration of values, loyalties and ambitions.
- Coaching. Coaxing and cajoling mentees into acquiring the skills, assets, credentials required to enter the mainstream.
- Sponsoring. Advocating and networking on behalf of the mentee to gain requisite contacts and opportunities.

These various stages, in which linear progression is not guaranteed, are based on movement from emotional and cognitive gains to social and vocational skills and career gains. Given the self-selecting nature of many programmes, it is important to note that Pawson (2006) suggests that progression is more likely for those who arrive with resilience and aspiration to move away from their present status.

This generic literature was drawn on to provide a broad theoretical framework for the in-depth interviews reported in this chapter and for the analysis of the data.

Methods

The research reported here is based on an evaluation of six sport-based projects in various parts of the UK, which were funded by Comic Relief over a five-year period. The funded organisations had broad and often ill-defined objectives. Their general targets were at-risk youth in areas of deprivation and the programmes sought to reduce conflict based variously on territoriality, gangs, racist and sectarian attitudes. They also sought to address issues relating to perceived lack of aspiration and ambition. Although work from all of the projects informs the analysis, the projects that are drawn on directly for this analysis are:

- A soccer-based programme in a deprived inner city area in Liverpool (in north-west England) which has a long history of gang-related violence and high levels of unemployment. Recreational and competitive football programmes were provided to address broad issues relating to at-risk youth and gang membership.
- A basketball-based project in several deprived areas of Glasgow in Scotland aimed at at-risk youth and immigrants and asylum-seekers. Recreational and competitive programmes were provided, with a close link with a professional basketball team.
- A programme based in the east end of London using football (and other activities) to address issues of gang-membership among Bengali youth.

- A sport-oriented project in Glasgow addressing issues of territoriality, gang-membership and substance abuse. Recreational football was combined with other sporting activities such as go-karting.

The programme personnel were asked to select a variety of participants who were over 14 years of age and preferably had been in the programme for at least three years. Individual in-depth interviews were conducted with thirty-seven male participants between 14 and 21 years of age. While it is not possible to comment on their representativeness, they included those who were only at risk via peer group membership, some who had been core gang members, some were recovering drug addicts and at least one who had recently served time in a young offenders institute for assault. The semi-structured interviews explored behaviour prior to joining the programmes, reasons for joining the programmes, reasons for staying with the programmes, the most significant aspects of the programmes from the participants' perspective and the impact that they perceived that it had had on them.

The relative role of sport

Although all were funded as sports-based projects, the relative centrality of sport varied.

- Sports programmes in which young people played both recreational and competitive football and basketball. It was hoped that the collective act of participation would break down barriers and lead to changed values, attitudes and behaviours.
- 'Sport-plus' (Coalter, 2007) in which sport was viewed as an important context for changing values, attitudes and behaviour, but this was not left to chance. For example, some used a 'red card' approach in which on-field unacceptable behaviour was addressed immediately, or workshops were used to discuss a range of issues (e.g. anger management, territoriality, drug use, sectarianism, violence).
- 'Plus-sport' (Coalter, 2007) youth-work organisations in which free access to sport was used as *fly paper* to attract young people.

Recruiting participants

Like most sport-for-development projects, these programmes had vague ideas of a 'target group' – usually some type of supposedly 'at risk' youth – and different ways of recruiting them. We can identify three broad types:

1   Open access, sports-only programmes in deprived areas open to all young people. Because such programmes deal with *self-selecting participants*, it is possible that the key target groups will not be attracted (if they actually exist). Such programmes work with an implicit *deficit model* based on a form of *environmental determinism* – all young people from areas designated as high crime, or recording racist attacks, will themselves be at-risk, or will have racist attitudes, low self-confidence, weak self-esteem or low aspirations. Such assumptions are essential rationales and form the basis for funding applications, although the evidence is that little systematic analysis of prior values, attitudes and behaviour is undertaken. There is a paradoxical danger of well-meaning projects being based on negative stereotypes of all young people from particular areas, with the attendant danger of misconceived provision and inappropriate performance indicators.

2   Relatively open access plus a targeting outreach approach to attract young people who were more obviously at risk. Some programmes regarded it as essential to recruit more widely in order not to stigmatise vulnerable young people and also to introduce them to ordinary kids as part of broader socialisation objectives.

3   Versions of outreach youth work, in which young people were befriended and recruited to programmes aimed almost wholly at them. These programmes included an opportunity to take part in sport, but as a social context for youth work and as an incentive to stay with the programme (e.g. free go-karting). However, even in such focused programmes, it was felt necessary for participants to participate in supervised activity sessions with other young people from different areas.

A further distinction is between once or twice a week programmes – mostly open-access – and more open-ended programmes with a 'base' where participants had on-going, 'drop-in' contact with staff. Such variations mean that participants were involved in a variety of social relationships and experiences, in which sport had a varied importance. All interviewees quoted below are from types (2) and (3) above.

The role of sport

Witt and Crompton (1997) suggest that participants should be provided with the opportunity to take part in an activity that they like and for which they have a perceived competence. Gambone and Arbreton (1997) also suggest that young people should be provided with challenging and interesting activities. It is clear that this is the presumed role that sport plays in some of these programmes. Despite this, football and basketball rarely featured in discussions about influences on claimed changes in values, attitudes and behaviour. Although in the basketball programme some saw sport as more central, this could reflect the programme's choice of interviewees, who were mostly skilled competitive players, some of whom had aspirations for basketball-related scholarships. For some refugees/immigrants, the team environment facilitated a degree of social connection and the development of language skills. However, for most participants, the key aspects of the programme related to general issues about the social climate and social relationships.

The social climate: 'there is loads of relationships there'

Witt and Crompton (1997) list two key protective factors – interested and caring adults, and a sense of acceptance and belonging. Similarly, Gambone and Arbreton (1997) refer to settings that help youth to develop a sense of safety and belonging, plus social support from adults. Pawson (2006: 124) identifies the basic stage of development as one in which the mentor's role is established via *befriending*, 'creating the bonds of trust and the sharing of new experiences so that the mentee recognises the legitimacy of other people and other perspectives'. Others, influenced by social learning theory, have referred to the importance of a lack of perceived social distance in such relationships (Bandura, 1994).

Although sport was an attraction and an important shared interest, the relationships established went beyond that of player and coach. The relative lack of social distance was part of the attraction:

> And he's great. He's like a mate to me. He's just like one of the lads. He's that close with us. He's just dead laid back.

Another referred to the coach as a trusted 'role model: He's like my best friend'. An interviewee who had played elsewhere, commented on a 'different approach to coaching':

> they wanted to know about you, they wanted to know what you wanted to achieve and they were there to help. Whereas with the other team I was with, were just really, 'you're good, we'll take you', ignore everybody else sorta thing.

Other comments indicate that diversion and rehabilitation work needs to 'go beyond the touchline'. The level of intimacy is often reinforced by a high level of access to staff, which interviewees found impressive: 'they give you a lotta time, know what I mean?'

> if you get yourself into trouble, like you can always come here and try and sort it out and talk to them and explain what's going on and see their point of view of what they're doing and get some advice what they would say. So yeah, it's just not football.

For others, the staff were regarded as family (or at least compensating for dysfunctional family relationships):

> It wasn't just [the programme which kept me out of trouble] but it helped. It helped a lot, especially, you see where you were talking about the friendship side of it . . . that helped big time 'cos I actually fell out with my mother, so, and I turned to [. . .] more, I turned to them more than I did my dad. I couldn't talk to my dad.

Respect, trust and reciprocity: the key mechanism

These various aspects – closeness, support, accessibility – combine to underpin the most significant aspect of the programmes: the development of the closely inter-dependent processes of respect, trust and reciprocity. This has a wider influence on both behaviour and aspiration – 'We like not to disappoint them like . . . we don't want to let them down'. In a competitively-oriented programme, this friendship relationship was based on a respect for the coach:

> They give you a lot of respect and they always, they always say to you, if I give you respect, you need to give me respect back . . . They demand respect from you 'cos they're gonna give you respect.

Initial respect for the leader/coach and the fact that they 'give so much of their time' and treated them 'like adults', leads to the development of a relative closeness and trust which many did not have with other adults in their lives. This then underpins the ability of the leaders to influence values, attitudes and behaviour. This was aided by the growing sense of *reciprocity* in which various individuals wanted to give something back and not disappoint the leader/coach and consequently began to change their attitudes and behaviour. For example, when asked how behaviour is controlled within the programmes one respondent stated:

> They'll stop really 'cos everyone respects him, so everyone gets on together. It doesn't mess, it's like he says behave, everyone'll behave.

What if . . . ?

Witt and Crompton (1997) list three protective factors relating to the understanding of consequences and changing behaviour: models for conventional behaviour; high controls against deviant behaviour; and ability to work out conflicts. In Pawson's (2006) second phase of 'direction-setting', self-reflection is promoted via the discussion of alternatives to enable participants to consider their loyalties, values and ambitions.

In addition to the strong moral influences on behaviour, some programmes addressed such issues directly and systematically. They stressed the need to be aware of the consequences of actions and to develop an ability to make mature choices – the need to move away from arbitrary risk-taking behaviour. Some interviewees referred to the phrase *what if*, which was used by staff to encourage them to think about the consequences if misbehaviour occurred in a less safe and supportive context. Respondents stated that 'the words kinda stick in your head':

> like if I do something stupid, like to [. . .] or something, like arsing about, it's like what if that goes wrong and what are the consequences that could happen. Like just stuff like that.

Some programmes used incidents during games to reinforce the need for self-control and the possible wider consequences of failing to do so. One incident in which the respondent lost his temper and left the pitch illustrates this:

> When I walked away, it was the coach who came up and spoke to us and he said 'if you're gonna do this at a job interview, if you're gonna do this when times get hard . . . you're not gonna have very much success in life'. So it makes you think . . . See the point when he tells you, you think, oh fuck, know what I mean, fuck you, fuck off . . . I did walk away a few times but then when you go home and you're sitting on your bed at night, you think about it a lot more, you think about the way you're trying to make of your life, if you are gonna do that in life, know what I mean? It doesn't just affect you on the court, it affects you when you go home as well. You don't want to be that same arsehole that you were two years ago.

'Go for your goal an' that!'

Witt and Crompton (1997) emphasise the need to place a high value on achievement and to promote positive attitudes to the future. Pawson's (2006) second stage of 'direction-setting' also includes the development of aspirations and his third 'coaching' stage involves participants being cajoled into acquiring the skills and assets required to enter the mainstream.

Issues of aspiration and goal setting were addressed via a mixture of support and exhortation. For one respondent the general message was 'don't let anyone put ye af it! . . . Go for your goal an' that!'. The impact is expressed succinctly: 'When I met . . . I actually started realising that I could do something with my life'. To reinforce and support such ambitions, some organisations provided access to free coaching awards and First Aid courses. However, there was also a proactive approach to helping to find employment: 'if you use . . . to its full strength, they really can like help you a lot, like CVs, help you write CVs out, getting your CVs around, getting you job interviews'.

Some also offered assistance similar to Pawson's (2006) final stage of 'sponsoring', in which the mentor networks assist the mentee to gain contacts and opportunities – a form of bridging social capital (Putnam, 2000). For example, one respondent appreciated the general assistance for job hunting:

> I'm not rich or nothing. So I've not got nothing and they helped me out by letting me use the computers in the office, letting me research some of the . . . to get my job and that, and let me prepare for my meetings and stuff. So then they also helped me get a job as well. Know what I mean? I could research . . . so if they asked me questions when I went to the meeting, I could answer them straight off. I knew what I was talking about.

As part of Pawson's (2006) 'direction-setting' phase, self-reflection is promoted via the discussion of alternatives to enable participants to consider their loyalties, values and ambitions. A key feature of the supportive, achievement-oriented environments was the opportunity to develop different values, attitudes and aspirations and change relationships with their previous peers. For example:

> I kept going along, just started from there, just kept playing and playing, then I started becoming further away from my friends. Just became further apart from them 'cos I was going and playing basketball more, it kept me away from all the trouble. So then, you know, if you don't speak to people, then you know, you're not friends anymore. I've kinda broke away from it 'cos I was playing basketball so much.

Volunteering and 'a sense of being needed'

Witt and Crompton (1997) suggest that a key programme component should be the development of the ability to work with others and Gambone and Arbreton (1997) propose that programmes should provide opportunities to develop leadership roles and opportunities to undertake volunteer and community service activities.

Confidence and self-worth

In one programme, the development of employment-related skills via Level 1 coaching was reinforced by the opportunity to coach on the programme: 'it gave me the sort of sense of importance I suppose, 'cos you're important to what they're doing. So it gave me that sense of being needed'. For others, it was not simply the experience of overcoming fear and developing self-confidence, but also passing on their experiences and helping younger ones to develop sporting skills – *'giving something back'*:

> Q: Which is the proudest bit? Playing or coaching the kids?
> A: I'd probably say coaching. See to help somebody else or pass on what I've learned from other guys, it's a big, big, big difference. See when you see some of the wee kids and you help them out with what he's doing or whatever, you take him aside and talk to him and he's back on and he seems happy, it's a big, big, big thing, because I tell you it changes your life.

For some the experience of volunteering and addressing their fears contributed to a growing maturity:

I think it's made me more mature really like because I think we just needed to grow up at the time but now that I've done like loads of voluntary work I can like talk to the younger groups and things like that . . . and like tell them how you shouldn't be like going, not tell them but advising them.

Growing up safely

For many participants, the organisations provided a safe, supportive, achievement-oriented environment in which they could mature. Many acknowledged their debt to the programmes and, especially, their close relationships with the staff and the way this *assisted* their growing maturity. Some believed that they would inevitably have matured over the time that they had been with the programme (reflecting a wider pattern of a decline in anti-social behaviour in later adolescence), but one acknowledged that the programme had quickened his maturity:

I think I probably would have matured later . . . and I would have kept doing that for a lot longer if basketball hadn't stopped me, you know . . . the basketball stopped me in my tracks, it stopped me from going that far . . . That's where it helped me personally, 'cos I was going down a really slippery slope but then basketball came in and it kinda cut me off from that.

Two steps forward . . .

Although we have identified a series of positive impacts associated with the programmes, we do not have data to enable us to assess the *relative* effectiveness of such programmes – for example, we have no interviews with those who dropped out. Further, Pawson (2006) illustrates that mentees' progress is often halting and non-linear. He argues that many disadvantaged young people have frequent and repetitive battles with authority, bust-ups with family and brushes with the law and that the mentee/mentor relationship is characterised by a persistent element of 'firefighting'. This is confirmed by our data, and it was clear that dealing with such individuals can be a long-term and emotionally intense work. Some continued to struggle with behavioural issues and lived in environments with constant pressures and temptations. In such circumstances changes in values, attitudes and behaviours were part of a process. Part of the key to the relative effectiveness of the organisations was that the staff continued to support those who erred. For example, one interviewee valued the support provided:

He helped me in court . . . Gave me a reference and that and, eh, stood up and said stuff and, you know, said I was going to [a foreign trip] with them and I've been doing, eh, loadsa voluntary and things like that . . . So he helped [me] in court really from going to jail.

Such actions reflected and reinforced the relationship based on respect, trust and reciprocity at the heart of the *sport plus* and *plus sport* programmes (Coalter, 2007, 2013). However, they also raise issues about how the effectiveness of such organisations should be assessed and the extent to which they can compensate for wider economic, social and cultural influences on young people's attitudes and behaviour (Spaaij, 2011). Some of the issues at stake are illustrated by Taylor *et al*'s (1999: 50) evaluation of programmes using sport to reduce recidivism when they state that although personal and social development 'may, sooner or later, improve offending behaviour, their impact is unpredictable in scale and timing. To expect anything more tangible is unrealistic'.

This is why a theory of behaviour change – a programme theory – cannot be assumed to be unilinear in terms of its impacts (values, attitudes) or outcomes (behaviour). As Pawson and Tilley (2004) argue, the programmes work by offering participants a series of resources and choices, but choice-making is always constrained by participants' previous experiences, beliefs and attitudes, opportunities and access to resources – the offer may be refused.

Sufficient conditions and programme theories

The above processes and issues illustrate Pawson *et al*'s (2004: 5) contention that 'intervention chains are long and thickly populated. Interventions carry not one, but several implicit mechanisms of action'. We have noted Coakley's (1998) contention that sports are *sites* for socialisation experiences, not *causes* of socialisation outcomes. Such perspectives shift analysis from families of programmes (sport) to *families of mechanisms* – the processes, relationships and experiences that *might* achieve the desired impacts and, perhaps, outcomes. In terms of investment decisions and programme development there is a need to clarify programme theories, or theories of behaviour change, which inform, or should inform, programme design and practice (Coalter, 2007, 2011, 2013). A programme theory is a sequence of *presumed* causes/actions/processes and effects (Weiss, 1997) and this approach describes mechanisms, examines the theoretical underpinnings of programmes, serves as a framework for evaluation and provides some basis for generalisation to inform programme design.

A framework for developing a programme theory

Given the diversity of participants, programmes, processes, relationships and desired impacts and outcomes it is not possible to develop a definitive or prescriptive programme theory – each programme may require its own programme theory to reflect its context, although progress requires a search for middle-range commonalities. Figure 49.1 illustrates that the variety of programmes can be placed on a continuum which includes a variety of components.

Inputs 1: methods of recruitment

There is a continuum, ranging from open access programmes that provide free or highly subsidised activities to *self-selecting* young people, to those aimed solely at those deemed to be at-risk and recruit either via referral or targeted street work.

Inputs 2: the nature of participants

The method of recruitment has substantial implications for the nature, extent and severity of the social and personal issues which programmes seek to address. Targeted programmes are most likely to recruit participants who are characterized by the issues with which the programmes are concerned. However, open access, self-selecting, programmes may be based on a vague mixture of a *deficit* view of participants and an *environmental determinism* that assumes that young people from deprived communities are uniformly deficient. Without evidence of the nature and distribution of the issues that the programme is seeking to address, it is not possible to establish meaningful performance indicators and assess effectiveness. Even more importantly, the lack of such information limits greatly the ability to design and deliver appropriate programmes, resulting in sports programmes that are simply assumed to be able to address poorly understood issues. This is why the box at the bottom of the Inputs 2 column has a question

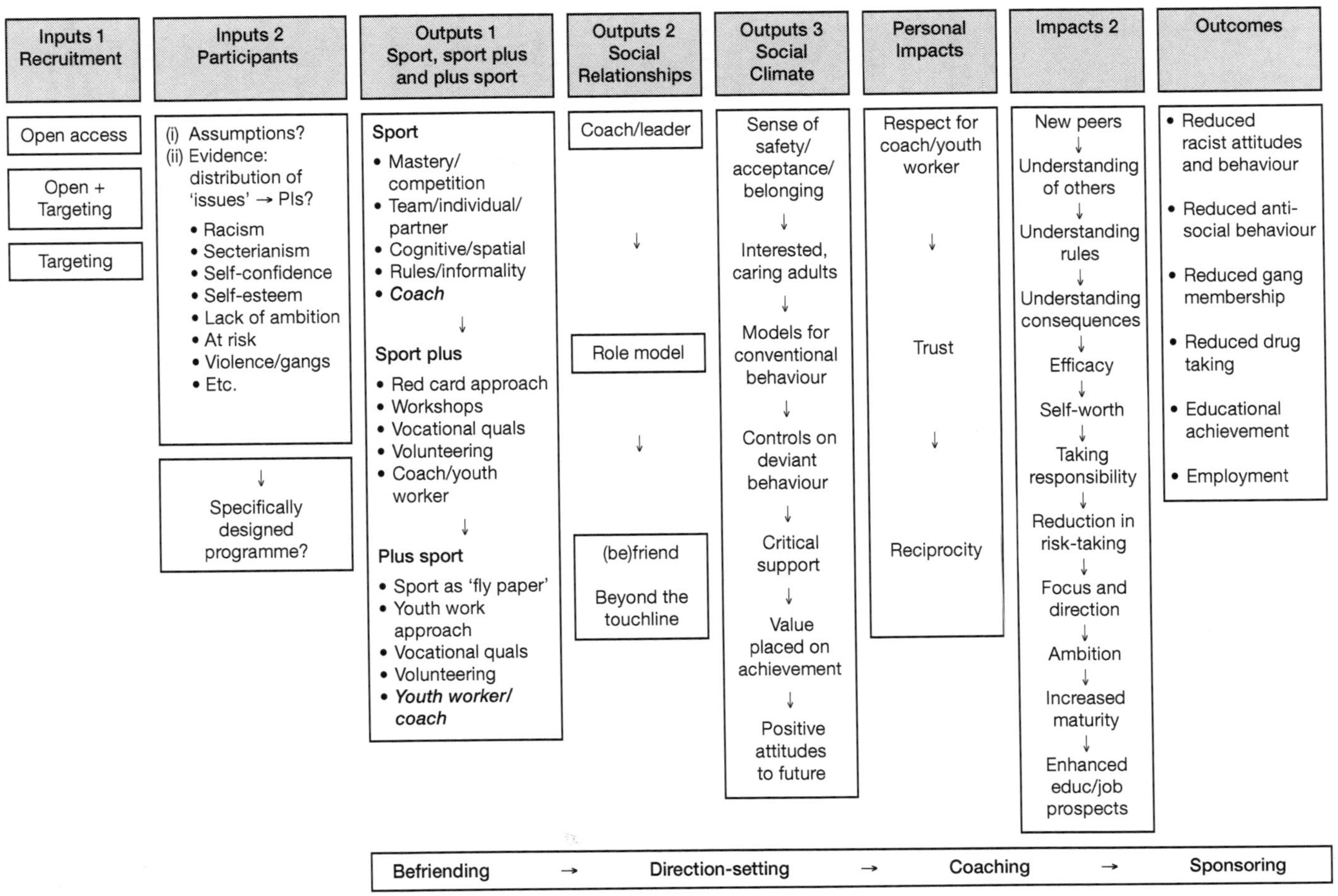

Figure 49.1 Programme Theory

mark – are programmes simply generic sports programmes, or are they based on an understanding of the causes, distribution and possible solution to assumed problems?

Outputs 1: the nature and type of programme: from sport to plus sport

There is a continuum of programmes based on the balance between sport and other components. Programmes range from:

- the provision of sporting opportunities, assuming that unexamined 'inherent properties' of sport will address certain issues; via
- *sport plus* programmes in which sports are supplemented by other activities (e.g. workshops on drug use; racism; sectarianism); to
- *plus sport*, where sport is a *fly paper* to attract young people to programmes in which the main developmental work is undertaken via a range of non-sporting and personally intense activities.

Within these contexts, the types of sport can also take various forms. For example, sports may:

- Be individual, partner or team-based. These involve different types of social relations and experiences, which may or may not be relevant to the issues being addressed.
- Emphasise individual task/mastery or competition. Research points to the effectiveness of a mastery orientation for vulnerable young people. In this approach, participants' skills are matched with the challenges they face and they are provided with positive encouragement and support and experiences of personal success.
- Be norm-based (i.e. subject to external judgements) or criterion-based (personal judgements of progress).
- Require spatial skills (e.g. football) or motor skills (e.g. gymnastics).
- Emphasise rules or informality. While it is often assumed that part of the positive impact of sport is the experience of rule-governed behaviour, research suggests that some adolescents reject organised, competitive sport because it contains components similar to those that they have previously failed to resolve and prefer games with fewer and less specified rules.

Finally, some programmes, mostly *sport plus*, offer the opportunity to undertake coaching qualifications and to volunteer within the programmes. Such experiences are highly valued and contribute to the achievement of some of the desired impacts and outcomes.

Outputs 2: social relationships

The combination of types of programmes and types of delivery personnel define the nature of social relationships within a programme – a key factor in effectiveness.

The *coach/leader role*, which is the predominant one in open access sports programmes, is relatively impersonal and tends to be confined to the organisation and delivery of the sessions, with limited ability to develop personal relationships with large numbers of participants. On the other hand, the various forms of the (be) friending role – *coach/youth worker, youth worker/coach* – in which a degree of trust and intimacy is developed and often goes 'beyond the touchline', are more characteristic of *sport plus* and *plus sport* approaches.

Outputs 3: social climate

The nature of the activity and the social relationships are fundamental to establishing the social climate. Some may simply rely on sport's presumed inherent properties – team work, rule-governed behaviour, the development of social skills, learning to respect and cooperate with others – although such experiences and impacts are not inevitable, as the sporting environment varies widely.

More generally, most programmes seek to provide an environment where young people feel a sense of safety and acceptance. Although they would be unlikely to continue to participate if this was not the case, it also provides the context for developmental work. Within this context, interested and caring adults are able to construct positive social relationships with young people, although the emotional depth of these will vary with the nature of the relationships implied in Outputs 1 and 2. Also, reflecting the variety of contexts and relationships, the coaches/leaders/youth workers can act with varying effectiveness as role models, mentors and (be) frienders. Within these contexts, varying types and degree of control on deviant behaviour are exercised – ranging from formal sanctions to self-control based on respect and reciprocity.

Contexts that place a high value on achievement and positive attitudes to the future are more likely to be those characterised by a *sport plus* and (be) friending and mentoring approach. This also relates to *direction-setting*, in which self-reflection is promoted via the discussion of alternatives to enable participants to consider their loyalties, values and ambitions.

Personal impacts: laying the basis for changed attitudes and behaviour

The social relationships, the social climate and the components of direction-setting may lead some participants to develop the basis for changing their values, attitudes and behaviours. In data presented above, the development of *respect* for the leader/role model/mentor was a key basis for the development of trust and reciprocity – the desire not to disappoint the leader/mentor and to conform to his/her expectations. This increases the influence of the leaders/mentors and the possibility that participants will change their values, attitudes and behaviour. Such changes are most likely to occur in the smaller scale and more intensive *sport plus* and *plus sport* programmes, where role modelling is central to the programme approach and are likely to be reinforced via Pawson's (2006) 'coaching stage', in which participants are encouraged and persuaded to acquire the skills and assets required to pursue education, training or employment.

Impacts 2

The precise nature of the desired positive impacts will vary between programmes. Further, the ability to achieve some of them will be dependent on the mixture of the inputs, outputs and personal impacts outlined above. Any changes in attitudes and behaviour might also reflect psychological changes in perceived self-efficacy and self-esteem, although such changes are more likely to be systematically promoted and supported in *sport plus* and *plus sport* organisations. It will be such organisations that are most likely directly to encourage and support an increased focus and sense of direction and to provide opportunities that enhance educational and employment prospects.

In some cases, the vital connection with education or the labour market is provided via *sponsorship* (Pawson, 2006) – that is, the organisation's personnel use their networks to assist the mentee to gain relevant contacts and opportunities. If the aim is to enable young people to enter the mainstream, programmes based on an overly individualised version of this process, ignoring the wider context in which they live, may not provide the full support that young people need. Programmes that aim simply to develop individuals' perceived self-efficacy or self-esteem, or encourage ambition, may underestimate the difficulties that many at-risk young people face in continuing in education or entering the labour market.

Outcomes

Given the variety of contexts and programmes, the desired outcomes will vary. Figure 49.1 cannot be read as implying a simple unilinear path from Recruitment to the achievement of the desired Outcomes. The key assumption underpinning a programme theory approach is that the various activities, processes, relationships and experiences are designed and delivered in such a way as to maximise the *possibility* of achieving desired outcomes. In a sense, programmes need to start with the desired outcomes and work backwards. What are the elements in the programme that will change sectarian attitudes? What are the experiences that will lead to an end to gang membership? In other words, such outcomes have to be formulated within an appraisal of what each programme can realistically seek to achieve.

For example, open access, self-selecting traditional sports programmes might seek to change individuals' attitudes to (say) race or act as crime diversion schemes. However, the more fundamental changes in values, attitudes and behaviours that underpin crime reduction, reduced drug taking or improved employment prospects are more realistically related to more intensive *sport plus* and *plus sport* approaches.

Reading Figure 49.1

In Figure 49.1 the vertical columns contain possible components and programmes will contain particular combinations. The various elements are listed in a broadly hierarchically way, from relatively superficial components (which one might expect in all programmes) to more fundamental aspects dealing with issues of vulnerability and risk. Research evidence indicates that the most effective interventions will contain most of the elements towards the bottom of the vertical columns and will not rely on a simple one-dimensional notion of the 'power' of sport.

The more fundamental changes in values and attitudes that underpin the outcomes of crime reduction and reduced drug taking are more realistically related to more intensive *sport plus* and *plus sport* approaches. Depending on the degree of social vulnerability, or at-risk status, such impacts tend to be achieved via particular social climates, longer term social relationships and forms of direction-setting and coaching. However, care needs to be taken in attributing simple cause-and-effect relationships between participation, measured impacts and strategic outcomes, as many young people will also be going through a process of emotional development and maturity, which may also lead to changes in attitude and behaviour.

Because of space restrictions, the use of the framework can be illustrated via only one example (working from left to right in Figure 49.1).

Targeted programmes

These will broadly:

* Adopt at least a *sport plus* approach, or may see sport as a 'fly paper' to attract participants to youth-work type programmes.

- Adopt a role model or even a be-friending or mentoring approach. This also contains the possibility of using peer leaders.
- Place a strong and systematic emphasis on values and attitude change, behavioural modification and achievement. This can be reflected in the hidden curriculum and/or via various workshops and discussions.
- Develop relationships of respect, trust and reciprocity as a basis for behaviour change.
- Assist in and systematically promote the development of self-worth, ambition and direction among participants. Again, such impacts will not be left to the 'power' of sport.

It is suggested that this tentative programme theory framework can be used as a template to enable providers to think about how they recruit, design and deliver their programmes and seek to define and achieve their impacts and (maybe) outcomes. It is presented as tentative and others are invited to interrogate, disagree and/or develop the proposed programme theory through practice and research. Finally it is important to remember Pawson *et al*'s (2004: 7) contention that:

> It is through the workings of entire systems of social relationships that any changes in behaviours, events and social conditions are effected . . . Rarely if ever is the same programme equally effective in all circumstances because of the influence of contextual factors.

References

Bandura, A. (1994). Self-efficacy. In V.S. Ramachaudran, ed. *Encyclopedia of Human Behavior* Vol 4. New York: Academic Press. pp. 71–81.

Coakley, J. (1998). *Sport in Society: Issues and Controversies* (6th edition). Boston, MA: McGraw Hill.

Coalter, F. (2007). *A Wider Social Role for Sport: Who's Keeping the Score?* London: Routledge.

Coalter, F. (2011). *Sport, Conflict and Youth Development*. London: Comic Relief.

Coalter, F. (2013) *Sport for Development*. London: Routledge.

Collins, M. and Kay, T. (2014) *Sport and Social Exclusion* (2nd edition). London: Routledge.

Crabbe, T. (2008). Avoiding the numbers game: Social theory, policy and sport's role in the art of relationship building. In: M. Nicholson R. M and Hoye (eds) *Sport and Social Capital*. London: Elsevier. pp. 21–37.

Fox, K. (2000). The influence of exercise on self-perceptions and self-esteem. In S.J.H. Biddle, K.R. Fox and S.H. Boucher (eds). *Physical Activity and Psychological Well-being*. London: Routledge. pp. 89–117.

Gambone, M. and Arbreton, A. (1997). *Safe Havens: The Contributions of Youth Organizations to Healthy Adolescent Development*. Philadelphia: Public/Private Ventures.

Hartmann, D. (2003). Theorising sport as social intervention: A view from the grassroots. *Quest*, 55(2), 118–140.

Lyle, J. (2006). *Sporting Success, Role Models and Participation: A Policy Related Review* Research Report No. 101. Edinburgh: sportscotland.

MacCallum, J. and Beltman, S. (2002) *Role Models for Young People: What Makes an Effective Role Model Program?* Hobart: National Youth Affairs Scheme.

Nichols, G. (2007). *Sport and Crime Reduction: The Role of Sports in Tackling Youth Crime*. London: Routledge.

Nichols, G. and Crow, I. (2004). Measuring the impact of crime reduction interventions involving sports activities for young people. *Howard Journal of Criminal Justice*, 43(3), 267–83.

Pajares, F. (2002). *Overview of Social Cognitive Theory and of Self-Efficacy*. Available online at: www.emory.edu/EDUCATION/mfp/eff.html [Accessed 12 November 2012].

Patriksson M (1995) Scientific Review Part 2 in *The Significance of Sport for Society – Health, Socialisation, Economy: A Scientific Review*. Prepared for the 8th Conference of European Ministers responsible for Sport, Lisbon, 17–18 May. Strasbourg: Council of Europe Press.

Pawson, R. (2006). *Evidence-Based Policy: A Realist Perspective*. London: Sage.

Pawson, R. and Tilley, I. (2004). *Realist Evaluation*. Paper prepared for the British Cabinet Office. Available online at: www.communitymatters.com.au/RE_chapter.pdf [Accessed 20 November 2011].

Pawson, R., Greenhalgh, T., Harvey, G. and Walshe, K. (2004). *Realist Synthesis: An Introduction*. ESRC Research Methods Programme: University of Manchester. RMP Methods Paper 2/2004.

President's Council on Physical Fitness and Sports (2006). *Sports and Character Development*. Research Digest Series, 7/1, Washington, DC: President's Council on Physical Fitness and Sports.

Putnam, R. (2000). *Bowling Alone*. London: Simon and Schuster.

Sandford, R., Armour, K. and Warmington, P. (2006). Re-engaging disaffected youth through physical activity programmes. *British Educational Research Journal*, 32(2), 251–71.

Spaaij, R. (2011). Sport as a vehicle for social mobility and regulation of disadvantaged urban youth. *International Review for the Sociology of Sport*, 44(2), 247–64.

Tacon, R. (2007). Football and social inclusion: Evaluating social policy. *Managing Leisure: An International Journal*, 12(1), 1–23.

Taylor, P. (1999). *External Benefits of Leisure: Measurement and Policy Implications*. Presentation to Tolern Seminar. London: Department of Culture, Media and Sport.

Taylor, P., Crow, I., Irvine, D. and Nichols, G. (1999). *Demanding Physical Activity Programmes for Young Offenders Under Probation Supervision*. London: Home Office.

Weiss, C. (1997). How can theory-based evaluation make greater headway? *Evaluation Review*, 21(4), 501–24.

West, S. and Crompton, J. (2001). A review of the impact of adventure programs on at-risk youth. *Journal of Park and Recreation Administration*, 19(2),113–40.

Witt, P and Crompton, J. (1997). The protective factors framework: a key to programming for benefits and evaluating results. *Journal of Parks and Recreation Administration*, 15(3), 1–18.

50

ENACTING YOUTH SPORT POLICY

Towards a micro-political and emotional understanding of community sports coaching work

Ben Ives, Laura Gale, Lee Nelson and Paul Potrac

Introduction

There has been a tendency for governments to become increasingly interventionist in setting the sport policy agenda and the sport development work that subsequently arises from it (Bloyce and Smith, 2010). Indeed, state agencies in many Western nations have utilised sport and physical activity as a vehicle for achieving a variety of sporting and, especially, non-sporting policy objectives (Houlihan and Green, 2008). These have included reducing crime, developing pro-social behaviour, overcoming social isolation and exclusion, rebuilding communities, developing healthy lifestyles and raising educational aspirations and attainment (Bergsgard *et al.*, 2007; Bloyce and Smith, 2010; Coalter, 2013). Examples of this provision include diversionary schemes for youth from remote Aboriginal communities in Australia (Senior *et al.*, 2012) and Midnight Basketball leagues in the United States (Hartmann and Depro, 2006). Similarly, Green (2008, p. 130) highlighted how the United Nations (UN) also subscribes to the view that sport is a positive and effective socialising agent. In this regard, the UN has emphasised the convening role that sport and physical activity has to play in enhancing 'economic and social development, improved health, and a culture of peace and tolerance'.

In the context of the United Kingdom (UK), the coalition government's Youth Sport Strategy has seen Sport England allocate a budget of in excess of £1 billion to reduce the number of young people dropping out of regular participation in sport and physical activity (Department for Culture, Media and Sport [DCMS]/Sport England, 2012). These funds have been invested in a variety of schemes, such as Sportivate, Active England, Street Games and Games4life. More recently, as part of its recent Youth Insights programme (2014), Sport England has also sponsored initiatives such as Wheelscape, Run Dem Crew and Morning Glory. As in many other nations, the use of sport for development in the UK is not only an 'important aspect overall welfare provision, but it is also an important element of the economy in terms of job creation' (Bergsgard *et al.*, 2007, p. 3–4).

From a conceptual standpoint, such provision can be broadly classified into three categories (Bloyce and Smith, 2010; Coalter, 2007, 2010, 2013). The first is where *sport* provision, either by external affirmation or implicit assumption, is considered to 'have inherent developmental properties for participants and communities' (Coalter, 2013, p. 24). The second refers to occasions where sport is used to develop young people through sport (e.g. health, social skills, educational attainment, and confidence). This broad category is considered to consist of two sub-sets that could be labelled as *sport plus* or *plus sport*. The former refers to occasions where 'sports are adapted and often augmented with parallel programmes in order to maximise their potential to achieve developmental objectives', while the latter is when 'sport's popularity is used as a type of "fly paper" to attract young people to programmes of education and training' (Coalter, 2013, p. 24). In terms of the latter, 'the systematic development of sport is rarely a strategic aim' (Coalter, 2013, p. 24). Of course, while these ideal types can be separated for analytical purposes, Coalter (2013) acknowledged that they are not always clearly distinguishable in practice. In both cases, outcomes are pursued 'via varying mixtures of organisational values, ethics and practices, symbolic games, and more formal didactic approaches' (Coalter, 2013, p. 24).

The use and value ascribed to sport and physical activity to achieve a variety of sporting and non-sporting goals has attracted considerable critical attention in recent years (e.g. Bloyce and Smith, 2010; Coalter, 2007, 2010, 2013; Collins and Kay, 2014; Crabbe, 2008; Kay, 2009; Skinner *et al.*, 2008; Smith and Waddington, 2004). In this respect, scholars have increasingly focused their investigative lenses on a variety of issues that include project workers' experiences of monitoring and evaluating programmes and the fundamental programme theories that underpin them (e.g. Coalter, 2011; Draper and Coalter, 2014). Such inquiry has played an important role in helping us to better appreciate how 'social interventions are always complex systems thrust amid complex systems' (Pawson, 2006, p. 35). Furthermore, it has also led to a situation where we need to better appreciate and engage with the pathos and ambiguity that surrounds the use of sport as a tool for development (Bloyce and Smith, 2010; Coalter, 2013).

While the advances outlined above are important, there remains a dearth of empirical research addressing the working lives of those community sports coaches who are charged with the responsibility of enacting policy initiatives at the micro (face-to-face) level of practice (Gale, 2014; Cronin and Armour, 2013). Unlike those employed in other forms of caring and pedagogical work (e.g. teachers, nurses, social workers), we know very little about the many aspects of community sports coaches' work and its interconnections with their wider lives. This not only includes *how* and *why* community sports coaches attempt to achieve desired policy goals in the ways that they do, but also their understandings of the everyday demands and dilemmas that they experience in their work. Similarly, researchers have also given little consideration to exploring how community sports coaches experience wider contemporary employment trends, such as reduced funding and organisational rationalisation, flexible working hours, vulnerability in the form of zero-hours or short-term employment contracts, increased scrutiny and measurement of work-place performance, and unclear career pathways. The acquisition of such knowledge would seem important, as it has been increasingly acknowledged that (youth sport) policies are not simply implemented but are, instead, actively translated, interpreted, reconstructed and enacted by a range of social actors and stakeholders that includes community sports coaches (c.f. Ball *et al.*, 2012).

In drawing upon the work of Ball *et al.* (2012), it is perhaps important to recognise that community sports coaches are not merely automatons or technicians engaged in the linear and straightforward delivery of particular policy goals, objectives and initiatives. Instead, like all the social actors involved in the enactment of policy, they have aspirations, hopes, fears and worries and are bound up in networks of relations that are influenced by economic and social forces, institutions, people and interests, and, sometimes, pure chance (Ball *et al.*, 2012; Taylor *et al.*, 1997). Unfortunately, the scholarly understanding of community sports coaching work has yet to adequately consider and explore these realities (Gale, 2014). In order to address the situation described above, this chapter seeks to present some initial findings from a wider research agenda addressing the micro-political and emotional challenges faced by community sports coaches working in youth sport settings. Specifically, the findings presented in this chapter focus on some of the everyday demands and dilemmas that two community sports coaches (Greg and James) experienced when implementing a government funded initiative aimed at increasing young people's participation in sport and physical activity.

At the time of the study, Greg was aged 18 years and had been employed as community sports coach at Coaching 'R' Us (a pseudonym), a charitable enterprise, for just over two years. James was 21 years of age and worked as a community sports coach for approximately four years at Get Active Coaching (a pseudonym), a private sector company. Both Coaching 'R' Us and Get Active Coaching worked in partnership with local authorities and contracted to deliver the aforementioned scheme in two socially deprived communities in the UK.

Data for the study were collected in two inter-related phases. Phase I entailed the use of participant observation to explore the behaviours and interactions of Greg and James as they sought to realize the programme outcomes in practice. Following the observations, Greg and James participated in a series of in-depth, one-to-one, informal interviews. These interviews sought to generate greater insight into the ideas, thoughts, opinions, feelings, and meanings that Greg and James ascribed to their experiences in the field (Purdy, 2014). The fieldnotes and interview transcripts for each coach were subjected to an iterative and recursive process of analysis that occurred alongside data collection and writing (Taylor, 2014; Tracey, 2013). That is, we worked 'back and forth between data and theory, the understanding and questioning of the data' (Taylor, 2014 p. 182) from the second we started our investigation until this chapter was accepted for publication. While we generated several interrelated themes across Greg's and James' stories, the focus of this chapter is delimited to two important facets. These are:

1 Greg's understanding of the 'target hitting' culture of community sports coaching work and those strategies that he used to safeguard his earnings and future job prospects.
2 James' thoughts and experiences regarding the emotionally demanding nature of community coaching work and the associated need to manage his emotions in particular ways to protect and advance his employment.

Greg's story: targets, vulnerability and self-interest

In his role with Coaching 'R' Us, Greg was required to improve the health and well-being of young people in a socially deprived community in northern England through fostering their engagement in rugby-focused activity. His coaching sessions took place on a Monday evening on a multi-purpose outdoor sports facility, lasted between 30 and 120 minutes, and typically attracted up to twenty participants. One of the key issues that we identified during the participant observation phase was the emphasis that Greg appeared to place upon ensuring that the participant contact details and attendance register were kept up-to-date. Indeed, Greg was reluctant to begin each of the observed coaching sessions until these administrative duties had been completed to his satisfaction. Collecting this information was not always a straightforward affair for Greg, as some of the participants were less than willing to provide the information or signatures that he requested. Accordingly, this task often took Greg between 10 and 50 minutes to complete. The following fieldnote extract is illustrative of the types of interactions that often occurred in this regard:

The Chase: Coaching 'R' Us Session 8 (15 April 2013)

Greg entered the astroturf, "Guys, please come and fill the register in. I need your details." The participants ignored Greg. "Guys, come on?" The participants didn't move. Greg marched over towards Ed, a participant, "Hey Ed, can you fill this form out?" "I don't want to give my details" Ed replied. "Come on Ed, it's simply so we know how many is here." Ed looked towards Greg, "Alright, I'll do it." Once Ed had filled out a participation information sheet, Greg walked over to Richard, another participant, "Hey Rich, can you fill this form out?" "Not a chance" Richard replied. "Well I'm afraid you're going to have to leave. You can't be here if you don't give me your details", Greg explained. Richard grabbed a participant information sheet from Greg's hands and started to fill it out. Once Richard had completed the form, Greg walked over to another participant, "Hey Billy, can you fill this in?" . . .

When asked why he placed so much emphasis on the administrative element of his work with the young people, Greg revealed how he believed that his employer principally judged his performance in relation to the number of participants that attended his sessions. Greg understood that Coaching 'R' Us largely judged his pedagogical effectiveness in relation to documents he compiled, namely the completed registers and participant details forms. Interestingly, Greg shared how his view on this matter was principally shaped through a 'meeting' he had with his line manager shortly before the start of the scheme. At the meeting, Greg was told that not only was the income awarded to the company determined by the achievement of pre-defined sessional participation targets, but that his wage would also be measured in this way. Simply put, the failure to demonstrate required levels of participation meant a reduction in the monies paid to Coaching 'R' Us and, resultantly, the wages that Greg would receive for his work. He explained:

> My boss said that if I didn't collect the register and hit the numbers then I won't be getting paid for delivering the session because they won't be getting the funding. We never spoke about the content or the quality of the session. He just said 'We need to hit these targets to help fund different parts of the company and pay salaries and if you're not meeting the targets we are not going to pay you.'

Perhaps unsurprisingly, Greg was aggrieved by this situation as he believed that his performance and salary 'should' be based on the content and quality of his coaching, not solely by the number of young people that attended these sessions. Greg's frustration regarding this matter was further exacerbated by his belief that he, ultimately, had little or no control over the number of people who turned up to his sessions each week. He noted:

> It made me angry because obviously I feel that the numbers are out of my control. I can't help it if something else is going on or they don't particularly want to come to the session. They have made it out like I am not doing my job properly if I am not getting the numbers on the session but it isn't, it's down to external factors [e.g. the

weather, time of the session, and location]. If I go down to the session and try to get them involved and they don't want to join in or they are not there that is not my fault.

Greg explained how he had initially wanted to voice his concerns to his line manager, but was dissuaded from doing so by his parents, who explained that such complaints might endanger his continued employment with the company. Heeding this 'sage' advice, Greg instead chose to engage in strategies that he believed would address the demands and expectations of his employer. These included offering each participant a reward (e.g. a key-ring or water bottle) in exchange for their attendance and prioritising the attainment of contact details and completed registers at the start of every session. Greg ultimately hoped that these actions would help to protect his earnings and increase the possibility of him moving from a zero-hours contract to the full-time position with the company that he desired. In his own words:

> When I realised we were getting judged by numbers, I had to change my approach and getting the participants details became the most important thing. I had to do that because if I didn't collect them I didn't get paid. I was also looking for a full-time position and I knew I would never have a chance of getting a full-time job unless I delivered against these targets.

When making sense of Greg's experiences, we found Kelchtermans' (2002a, 2002b, 2009, 2011) work addressing the micro-political nature of teachers' careers and everyday organisational life to be a particularly useful explanatory framework. Kelchtermans' analysis focused on how individuals develop their *micropolitical literacy* regarding the contested nature of organisational life. That is, 'the competence to understand the issues of power and interests' in a particular organisational setting (Kelchtermans 2005, p. 1004). From Kelchtermans' perspective, this literacy encompasses three interrelated features: a *knowledge aspect* (i.e. 'ability to acknowledge and understand ["read"] the micropolitical character of a particular situation'), an *operational aspect* (i.e. 'the repertoire of micropolitical strategies and tactics teachers manage to skilfully and effectively apply in order to influence the situation') and an *experiential aspect* (i.e. 'how one feels about one's micropolitical understanding and actions') (Kelchtermans, 2005, p. 1004). Kelchtermans' (2009) theorising also highlighted how teachers' work is characterised by *structural vulnerability*. This refers to a reality whereby teachers are never in total control of the situation in which they find themselves, are unable to fully prove or guarantee the effectiveness of their choices and actions, and, as such, occupy a position where their decisions can always be challenged or questioned by others (Kelchtermans, 2009). Such a reality, according to Kelchtermans (2009), can elicit a range of strong emotions in individual teachers (e.g. anxiety, anger and frustration).

When exploring Greg's story in relation to Kelchtermans' theorising, we would argue that Greg had simultaneously developed the necessary *knowledge aspect* to 'read' the micropolitical reality of his situation while also recognising his own vulnerability as an employee. In terms of his micro-political literacy, Greg appeared to be acutely aware of the need to successfully fulfil the participation targets set by his employers if he was to protect his immediate income and also impress his employers enough to be offered a full-time coaching position in the future. Moreover, his recognition of these realities of working life was not a straightforward or unproblematic affair. Indeed, Greg's understanding of the vulnerability of his position led him to experience strong degrees of anger, anxiety, and frustration. In an effort to reduce this vulnerability, Greg engaged in the *operational aspect* of micro-political literacy when he prioritised the recording of participant contact details and rewarding them (e.g. key-rings and water bottles) for their attendance. For us at least, the importance that Greg attached to this aspect of his work seemed to overshadow his attempts to facilitate the stated goals and objectives of the programme that he was helping to deliver and is an issue that warrants further examination more widely in the context of community sport coaching work.

We also believe that Greg's thoughts, feelings and actions could also be understood in relation to wider debates regarding neo-liberal working practices and the rise of precarious work in the UK more widely. With regard to the former, Houlihan and Green (2008) have outlined the radical changes to government spending. In particular, they identified a shift towards the competitive tendering of government contracts that required service providers to fulfil a variety of key performance indicators in order to obtain the full financial value of awarded contracts (DCMS/Sport England, 2012). This approach to funding has seen many public and private sector organisations and companies, such as Coaching 'R' Us, increasingly use part-time and zero-hour contracts as a means of managing their financial flexibility, reducing staffing costs and optimising profit margins. Given the employment practices to which Greg was subject, it could be argued that he was engaged in precarious work. That is, his employment was 'uncertain, unpredictable, and risky from the point of view of the worker' (Kalleberg, 2009 p. 2). It was unsurprising, then, that Greg opted to practice in a defensive manner and do what he felt he needed to do in order to survive, and hopefully thrive, in his working role (Gilbourne, 2013).

James' story: emotions? I bottle them up. I have to.

As an employee of Get Active Coaching, James was required to deliver a multi-sports initiative to children in a socially deprived urban neighbourhood in southern England. His weekly, two-hour long, coaching sessions took place at a local youth centre and attracted between 15 and 35 participants. A striking feature that we took from our engagement with James was his belief that he had to strategically control and manage the emotions that he displayed to the participants and other people present in the youth club setting (e.g. various youth centre staff), especially when dealing with anti-social behaviour. By way of an example, the fieldnote excerpt below is typical of how James attempted to address such incidents:

"STOP THAT NOW!": Get Active Coaching Session 3 (14 June 2013)

Sam, a participant, had just thrown a badminton racket towards the wall of the sports hall after losing a badminton match. James jumped up from his seat, clenched his fists and glowered towards Sam, "STOP THAT NOW! WHAT DO YOU THINK YOU'RE DOING? YOU CANNOT BEHAVE LIKE THAT HERE OR ANYWHERE ELSE." By the time James had finished berating Sam his face was red as lava and contorted with rage – his nostrils were flaring, his eyebrows were pulled down and together and his eyes were narrowed into slits, through which the barest glimpses of his dark contracted pupils could be seen. Sam raised his arms above his shoulders with his palms facing towards James, "I'm sorry James, I didn't mean it, it just happened." With his eyes still riddled with fury James silently marched towards Sam. "James, I am sorry, I am really sorry", Sam cried out again. James suddenly stopped two feet short of Sam where he lowered his head, unclenched fists and put his left hand in his left trouser pocket. After a moment's pause for a deep breath, James raised his head and made eye contact with Sam, "Look Sam, you can't do things like that. You can't just smash stuff up because you've lost a game of badminton." "I know James, I am really sorry." James raised his right arm and placed it about Sam's left shoulder, "I am serious mate, you've got to learn to control your anger otherwise you'll get in serious trouble." Sam looked up towards James, "I will, I promise." James smiled towards Sam, "Get back to your badminton match."

When asked about the emotions that he felt and displayed in such situations, James revealed how he initially sought to present an 'angry and disappointed' front (Goffman, 1959). James hoped that doing so would bring events to a halt and evidence to the young people attending his session that such behaviours would not be tolerated. While James used negative emotional displays to gain the attention of his participants, he was also aware that the sustained use of such observable behaviours could alienate him from the group. This was something that he wanted to avoid for fear of the damage this could do to his reputation in the eyes of the youth club staff and, importantly, his employers. In light of this, James explained that he would quickly transition back to a more calm and friendly persona. He believed that this shift from a negative to a positive emotional display helped him to maintain the participants respect and, in turn, reduced the likelihood of them reoffending in subsequent sessions. He explained:

> When the kid first misbehaves you have got to come down on them hard to make sure that they know that they can't behave like that and that means presenting angry and disappointed emotions but after that initial burst you have to calm it down a bit . . . If you don't do that the participant[s] will just think you're a w★★ker and won't take on board anything you say . . . But by being angry at the start and then calming down you let them know that you're disappointed in their behaviours and that they are in the wrong, and you also maintain their respect which means that they are less likely to kick off again.

Importantly from our perspective, James described how his outlook was based on his understanding that his employer, Get Active Coaching, held the behaviour management skills of their coaching staff in very high regard. Indeed, prior to the start of the scheme, his line manager told James that failure to effectively manage his participants' behaviours might result in reduced working hours or, worst still, him being sacked. Despite wanting to 'swear', 'shout and bawl', and generally go 'wild' at those misbehaving young people in his sessions, James decided to refrain from revealing his 'true' feelings, preferring instead to present the emotions discussed above. James thought that displaying his 'real' thoughts and accompanying emotions would not only be unproductive in terms of his desire to prevent further anti-social behaviour in the future, but would also likely have resulted in him being disciplined or released from his coaching position. He noted:

> By them being idiots they were putting my job on the line and that made me extremely angry but I tried to hide how I felt . . . I knew that I couldn't just go crazy at someone and press my head against theirs . . . That is not professional at all and I knew if I did I would have lost my job . . . Get Active Coaching would not employ a coach who physically and verbally abuses a participant . . . So it was imperative that I controlled my emotions . . . Yes, I initially had to be firm with the participants to stop them from misbehaving and let them know that they were in the wrong but I had to make sure that I didn't swear and just shout and ball.

We believe that Hochschild's (1983, 2000) theorising of emotions offers a particularly valuable sense-making framework for understanding James' thoughts, feelings, and actions. In her seminal work, Hochschild investigated how flight attendants and bill collectors managed their emotional experiences and displays in accordance with the rules and ideologies of their respective workplace environments. Central to Hochschild's (2000, p. 7) theorising is *emotional labour*, which she defined as:

> Labour that requires one to induce or suppress feeling in order to sustain the outward countenance that produces the proper state of mind in others [such as] the sense of being cared for in a convivial and safe place. This kind of labour calls for communication of mind and feeling, and it sometimes draws on a source of self that we honour as deep and integral to our individuality . . . Emotional labour is sold for a wage and, therefore, has exchange value.
>
> *(Hochschild, 2000, p. 7)*

According to Hochschild's analysis, emotional labour is operationalised through the application of *deep acting* or *surface acting*. Deep acting refers to those instances whereby a person induces and actually experiences an emotion that is subsequently displayed to others. Surface acting differs from deep acting in that in surface acting the individual deceives others about what he or she really feels, but does not deceive himself or herself. That is, the individual displays emotions that he or she is not necessarily experiencing (Hochschild, 1983, 2000).

When considered in light of Hochschild's theorising, it could be argued that James engaged in *emotional labour* through the application of *surface acting*. That is, for a wage, James managed his emotional displays in accordance with the perceived expectations of his employer, Get Active Coaching. In this respect, James had learned through experience that there were certain *display rules* (i.e. those emotions that should and should not be displayed within this social setting) that he felt obliged to comply with if he were to achieve his career goals (Hochschild, 1983). Such instrumental thinking (and action) was also evident in terms of the emotional personas that he presented to the young people attending his coaching sessions. Specifically, he suppressed and refrained his 'true' thoughts and feelings in a concerted effort to influence the behaviours of the community sports participants towards desired ends.

Summary

This chapter sought to provide some initial insights into the tensions and dilemmas that Greg and James experienced when enacting a government funded initiative to increase young people's participation in sport and physical activity. In particular, we hope that the accounts offered in this chapter have illustrated at least some aspects of the inherently micro-political and emotional nature of community sports coaching work and, relatedly, the messy nature of policy enactment within the context of youth sport. While we emphasised the micropolitical analysis in Greg's story and the emotional features of James' story, it is important to point out that we did this purely for analytical clarity. We are not, of course, suggesting that Greg found his coaching work to be devoid of emotion or that micropolitics were absent from James' experience in the field. Indeed, given the findings of our on-going and completed work to date (e.g. Gale, 2014; Ives, 2014; Potrac *et al.*, 2013; Thompson *et al.*, 2014), we believe that emotions and micro-politics are inextricably interlinked features of coaching, be it in performance or participation settings (Kelchtermans, 2005; Potrac *et al.*, 2013).

We would also argue that ethnographic studies of community sports coaches' work, lives, and careers have much to offer in terms of complementing related research in youth sport, which addresses important issues such as the design, delivery, monitoring and evaluation of various programmes and interventions (Coalter, 2013; Smith and Waddington, 2004). From our standpoint, it has the potential to probe beneath the glossy surface veneer of sport as a tool for development by challenging the predictive certainty that, some (e.g. Coalter, 2013) would argue, have typified the academic literature in this area. Indeed, it is perhaps only by recognising the ambiguity, pathos and dynamic complexity of community sports coaching work and policy enactment that we can develop a less naïve and more reality-grounded understanding of this topic area. In echoing the eloquent thoughts of Coalter (2013), such knowledge would appear to be essential if researchers, policy makers, educators and practitioners are to contribute to the provision of positive and purposeful experiences for the young people in their charge.

Future research

In reflecting the call of Potrac *et al.* (2013) in sports coaching, we believe that it is important for scholars of youth sport to better consider how 'emotion and cognition, self and context, ethical judgement and purposeful action' (Kelchtermans, 2005, p. 996) are all inter-twined in community sports coaches' enactment of health and social policy. In order to generate such reality-grounded insights, future research addressing the working lives and practices of community sports coaches might seek to examine the following issues and topics:

1   How community sports coaches enact health and social policy directives with youth populations at the micro-level of community sport.
2   Why they act as they do to achieve these outcomes.
3   What they consider to be the everyday challenges, tensions and dilemmas that they experience in their work.
4   How and why they attempt to navigate these issues in the ways that they do.
5   How they understand various coach education and development courses to have prepared (or not prepared) them for the everyday demands of working with young people.
6   What assistance they would like to receive in terms of enhancing their abilities to facilitate the achievement of various health and social policy goals.
7   How they understand the employment demands of community sports work to impact upon their health and well-being, as well as their inter-personal relationships with others both inside and outside of the workplace.

In exploring topics such as these, we encourage researchers to generate rich and detailed accounts of the experiences of both neophyte and experienced community sports coaches through various forms of representation (Huggan *et al.*, 2014), which could include (auto)ethnographic accounts, poetry, film, ethnodrama, (modified) realist tales, photography and confessional tales, among others (Groom *et al.*, 2013). Such knowledge has, we believe, much to offer in both theoretical and practical terms and could be used to benefit those involved in the management and delivery of youth sport.

References

Ball, S. J., Maguire, M. and Braun, A. (2012). *How schools do policy: Policy enactments in secondary schools.* London: Routledge.

Bergsgard, N.A., Houlihan, B., Mangset, P., Nodland, S.I. and Rommetvedt, H. (2007). *Sport policy: A comparative analysis of stability and change.* Oxford: Elsevier.

Bloyce, D. and Smith, A. (2010). *Sport policy and development: An introduction.* London: Routledge.

Coalter, F. (2007). *Sport a wider social role: Who's keeping score?* London: Routledge.

Coalter, F. (2010). The politics of sport-for-development: Limited focus programmes and broad gauge problems? *International Review for the Sociology of Sport, 45*(3), 295–314.

Coalter, F. (2011). *Sport, conflict and youth development*. London: Comic Relief.

Coalter, F. (2013). *Sport for development: What game are we playing?* London: Routledge.

Collins, M. and Kay, T. (2014) *Sport and social exclusion* (2nd edition). London: Routledge.

Crabbe, T. (2008). Avoiding the numbers game: social theory, policy and sport's role in the art of relationship building, in M. Nicholson and R. Hoye (eds) *Sport and Social Capital*, Oxford: Butterworth-Heinemann.

Cronin, C. and Armour, K.M. (2013). Lived experience and community sport coaching: A phenomenological investigation. *Sport, Education and Society*. DOI: 10.1080/13573322.2013.858625.

Department for Culture, Media and Sport/Sport England (DCMS/SE). (2012). *Creating a sporting habit for life: A new youth sport strategy*. London: DCMS.

Draper, C. and Coalter, F. (2013) "There's just something about this club. It's been my family." An analysis of the experiences of youth in a South African sport-for-development programme, *International Review for the Sociology of Sport*. DOI: 10.1177/1012690213513783

Gale, L. (2014). Understanding community coaches' experiences of everyday coaching practice: A narrative-biographical study. University of Hull: Unpublished PhD thesis.

Gilbourne, D. (2013). Heros, toxic ferrets and a large man from Leeds. *Sports Coaching Review*, 2(2), 86–97.

Goffman, E. (1959). *The presentation of the self in everyday life*. London: Penguin Books.

Green, M. (2008). Non-governmental organisations in sports development, in V. Girginov (ed.) *Management of Sports Development*, Oxford: Butterworth-Heinemann.

Groom, R., Nelson, L., Potrac, P. and Smith, B. (2014). Writing and representing research. In L. Nelson, R. Groom and P. Potrac (eds), *Research methods in sports coaching* (pp. 87–97). London: Routledge.

Hartmann, D. and Depro, B. (2006). Rethinking sports-based community crime prevention: A preliminary analysis of the relationship between midnight basketball and urban crime rates. *Journal of Sport and Social Issues*, 30, 180–196.

Hochschild, A. (1983/2000). *The managed heart*. Berkley, CA: University of California Press.

Houlihan, B. and Green, M. (2008). Modernization and sport: The reform of Sport England and UK Sport. *Public Administration, 87(3)*, 678–698.

Huggan, R., Nelson, L. and Potrac, P. (2014). Developing micropolitical literacy in professional soccer: a performance analyst's tale. *Qualitative Research in Sport, Exercise and Health*. DOI 10.1080/2159676X.2014.949832

Ives, B. (2014). *Exploration into the day-to-day realities of community sports coaching.* University of Hull: Unpublished PhD thesis.

Kalleberg, A.L. (2009). Precarious work, insecure workers: Employment relations in transition. *American Sociological Review*, 74, 1–22.

Kay, T. (2009). Developing through sport: Evidencing sport impacts on young people. *Sport in Society*, 12(9), 1177–1191.

Kelchtermans, G. (2005). Teachers' emotions in educational reforms: Self-understanding, vulnerable commitment and micropolitical literacy. *Teaching and Teacher Education, 21*, 995–1006.

Kelchtermans, G. (2009). Who I am in how I teach is the message: Self-understanding, vulnerability and reflection. *Teachers and Teaching; Theory and Practice, 15(2)*, 257–272.

Kelchtermans, G. and Ballet, K. (2002a). Micropolitical literacy: Reconstructing a neglected dimension in teacher development. *International Journal of Educational Research, 37*, 755–767.

Kelchtermans, G. and Ballet, K. (2002b). The micro-politics of teacher induction. A narrative -biographical study on teacher socialisation. *Teaching and Teacher Education, 18*, 105–120.

Pawson, R. (2006). *Evidence-based policy: A realist perspective*. London Routledge.

Potrac, P., Jones, R.L., Purdy, L., Nelson, L. and Marshall, P. (2013). Towards an emotional understanding of coaching practice: A suggested research agenda. In P. Potrac, W. Gilbert and J. Denison (eds), *Routledge handbook of sports coaching* (pp. 235–246). London: Routledge.

Purdy, L. (2014). Interviews. In L. Nelson, R. Groom and P. Potrac (eds), *Research methods in sports coaching* (pp. 161–170). London: Routledge.

Senior, K., Ivory, W., Chenhall, R., Cunningham, T., Nagel, T., Lloyd, R. and McMahon, R. (2012). *Developing successful diversionary schemes for youth from remote Aboriginal communities*. Darwin, Australia: Criminology Research Advisory Council.

Skinner, J., Zakus, D. H. and Cowell, J. (2008). Development through sport: Building social capital in disadvantaged communities. *Sport Management Review*, 11(3), 253–275.

Smith, A. and Waddington, I. (2004). Using "sport in the community schemes" to tackle crime and drug use among young people: Some policy issues and problems. *European Physical Education Review*, 10, 279–297.

Sport England (2014). *The challenge of growing youth participation in sport: Youth Insights Pack*. London: Sport England. Taylor, S., Rizvi, R., Lingard, B. and Henry, M. (1997). *Education policy and the politics of change*. London: Routledge.

Taylor, W. (2014). Analysis of qualitative data. In L. Nelson, R. Groom and P. Potrac (eds), *Research methods in sports coaching* (pp. 181–191). London: Routledge.

Thompson, T., Potrac, P. and Jones, R.L. (2014). 'I found out the hard way': Micro-political workings in professional football. *Sport, Education and Society*. DOI 10.1080/13573322.2013.862786

Tracy, S.J. (2013). *Qualitative research methods: Collecting evidence, crafting analysis, communicating impact*. Chichester: John Wiley.

INDEX

Made in the USA
San Bernardino, CA
20 September 2018